Clinical PET-CT in Radiology

Paul Shreve · David W. Townsend
Editors

Clinical PET-CT in Radiology

Integrated Imaging in Oncology

Springer

Editors
Paul Shreve
Advanced Radiology Services
Grand Rapids, MI
USA
pshreve@earthlink.net

David W. Townsend
Head, PET and SPECT Development
Singapore Bioimaging Consortium
Singapore
david_townsend@sbic.a-star.edu.sg

ISBN 978-0-387-48900-1 e-ISBN 978-0-387-48902-5
DOI 10.1007/978-0-387-48902-5
Springer New York Dordrecht Heidelberg London

Printed on acid-free paper

Springer is part of Springer Science+Business Media (www.springer.com)

Preface

It has been nearly a decade since the first PET-CT scanners became commercially available. At the time of the initial launch of clinical PET-CT scanners it was thought at most 30% of the PET scanner market would be in the form of PET-CT scanners. Within only a few years (by 2006), however, PET-CT scanners replaced stand-alone PET scanners completely in commercial offerings, and today over 5,000 PET-CT scanners have been delivered worldwide. The remarkably rapid adoption of PET-CT is not entirely surprising, as the overwhelming clinical application of PET-CT has been body oncology imaging, and the merging of the anatomic and metabolic information provided by CT and FDG PET scans was a natural and already ongoing practice for body oncology imaging.

The original intent of PET-CT was to provide clinical CT and clinical PET in one scan procedure with the images sets inherently registered and aligned to facilitate interpretation of both modalities. The notion of merging the anatomic information of CT with the metabolic information of PET was suggested by a cancer surgeon in the early 1990s, but in fact the practice of integrating the interpretation of complimentary imaging modalities for clinical diagnosis has been ongoing in disease-based or organ system-based medical imaging subspecialties. This trend has accelerated recently with the widespread application of PACs and teleradiology as well as continued refinements in image registration and image fusion software. The acceptance of PET-CT hybrid scanners has more recently led to commercial SPECT-CT hybrid scanners and to the tentative development of PET-MRI scanners; the concept of hybrid imaging and multimodality imaging diagnosis is a broad and pervasive process occurring in medical imaging.

Since the introduction of commercial PET-CT scanners, published textbooks have approached the subject mainly from a nuclear medicine perspective, including applications to neurologic and cardiac imaging, and discussion of PET radiotracers other than FDG. The true necessity of the hybrid scanner applies to body imaging and in particular the vast majority of applications of clinical PET-CT today remain in body oncology imaging. In this textbook we bring together all aspects of PET-CT relevant to clinical body oncology imaging using clinical CT and clinical FDG PET. The intent is to provide practicing imaging physicians with both a comprehensive and practical text, which treats PET-CT as an integrated anatomic-metabolic medical imaging procedure applied to cancer imaging that it currently is, and was always intended to be. Ample coverage of the relevant physics and clinical oncology is included for reference. The physics and instrumentation chapters are oriented to provide an overview of the available technology and some of the physical concepts without entering into excessive detail. The clinical chapters are structured to provide concise and structured background regarding the clinical management of each cancer and the role of PET-CT imaging in all phases of patient management. It is assumed the reader has some background in both PET and CT interpretation. The intent of each clinical chapter is to help the imaging physician more completely understand the relationship and role of the integrated modality imaging with respect to the overall treatment of the cancer patient. We hope that this text will be a valuable companion for the imaging physician and further establish PET-CT in the mainstream of cancer imaging.

David Townsend, Ph.D.
Singapore

Paul Shreve, M.D.
Grand Rapids, Michigan

Contents

Contributors

Harry Agress Jr. M.D.
Chairman, Department of Radiology, Hackensack University Medical Center, Hackensack NJ, USA

Gerald Antoch, M.D.
Professor, Department of Diagnostic and Interventional Radiology, University Hospital Essen, Essen, Germany

Suzanne L. Aquino, M.D.
Consultant, NightHawk Radiology Services, Scottsdale AZ, USA

Thomas Beyer, Ph.D.
Professor, Department of Nuclear Medicine, University Hospital Essen, Essen, Germany and cmi-experts GmbH Zurich, Switzerland

Michael Blake, M.D., B.Sc., MRCPI, FFR (RCSI), FRCR
Director of Abdominal PET-CT, Department of Abdominal Imaging and Intervention, Massachusetts General Hospital, Boston MA, USA

Todd M. Blodgett, M.D.
Assistant Professor, President, FRG Molecular Imaging, Department of Radiology, University of Pittsburgh Medical Center, Foundation Radiology Group, Pittsburgh PA, USA

Andreas Bockisch, M.D., Ph.D.
Director, Clinic and Policlinic for Nuclear Medicine, Department of Nuclear Medicine, University Hospital Essen, Essen, Germany

Trond Velde Bogsrud, M.D.
Researcher, Department of Diagnostic Imaging, Division of Nuclear Medicine, University Clinic, The Norwegian Radium Hospital/Rikshospitalet University Hospital, Montebello Oslo, Norway

Barton F. Branstetter, IV M.D.
Associate Professor, Director, Head and Neck Imaging, Clinical Director of Neuroradiology, Departments of Radiology, Otolaryngology and Biomedical Informatics, University of Pittsburgh Medical Center, Pittsburgh PA, USA

Jacqueline Brunetti, M.D.
Associate Clinical Professor, Medical Director, Department of Radiology, Columbia University College of Physicians and Surgeons, Holy Name Hospital, Teaneck NJ, USA

Carlos A. Buchpiguel, M.D., Ph.D.
Associate Professor, Director PET-CT Laboratory, Department of Radiology, São Paulo University School of Medicine, Hospital do Coração, São Paulo, Brazil

Chuong Bui, MBBS, FRACP
Clinical Lecturer, Medicine, Staff specialist, Nepean Clinical School, Nuclear Medicine Department, Nepean Hospital, The University of Sydney, NSW, Australia

Jonathan P.J. Carney, Ph.D.
Assistant Professor, Department of Radiology, University of Pittsburgh Medical Center, Pittsburgh PA, USA

Natalie Charnley, MBChB, MRCP, FRCR
Researcher, University of Manchester Wolfson Molecular Imaging Centre, Preston, Lanchester, United Kingdom

Gary J.R. Cook, MBBS, M.Sc., M.D., FRCR, FRCP
Consultant Nuclear Medicine Physician, Department of Nuclear Medicine and PET, Royal Marsden Hospital, Surrey, United Kingdom

Thomas F. DeLaney, M.D.
Associate Professor, Medical Director, Department of Radiation Oncology, Harvard Medical School, Northeast Proton Therapy Center, Massachusetts General Hospital, Boston MA, USA

Sukru Mehmet Erturk, M.D.
Associate Professor, Department of Radiology, Sisli Etfal Training and Research Hospital, Istanbul, Turkey

James W. Fletcher, M.D.
Professor, Director, Division of Nuclear Medicine/PET, Director, PET Imaging Center, Division of Nuclear Medicine/PET, Department of Radiology, Indiana/Purdue University, Indiana University School of Medicine, Indianapolis IN, USA

Michael M. Graham, M.D., Ph.D.
Professor, Department of Radiology-Nuclear Medicine, University of Iowa, Iowa City IA, USA

Ian D. Hay, M.D., Ph.D.
Professor, Section of Endocrinology, Department of Internal Medicine, Mayo Clinic, Rochester MN, USA

Terry Jones, D.Sc., F Med Sci
Professor, The PET Research Advisory Company, Cheshire, United Kingdom

Laurie B. Jones-Jackson, M.D.
Assistant Professor of Clinical Radiology & Radiological Sciences, Vanderbilt University Medical Center, Nashville TN, USA

Joseph J. Junewick, M.D.
Chairman, Department of Radiology, Spectrum Health Hospitals, Grand Rapids, Advanced Radiology Services, PC, Grand Rapids Division, Grand Rapids MI, USA

Marc Kachelrieß, Dipl.-Phys
Professor, Department of Medical Imaging, Institute of Medical Physics (IMP), University of Erlangen Nuremberg, Erlangen, Germany

Mannudeep Kalra, MBBS, M.D., DNB
Director of MGH, Department of Radiology, Center for Evaluation of Radiologic Technologies, Massachusetts General Hospital, Boston MA, USA

Lale Kostakoglu, M.D.
Professor, Section of Nuclear Medicine, Department of Radiology, Mt. Sinai Medical Center, New York, NY, USA

Vikram Krishnasetty, M.D.
Private Practice, Columbus Radiology Corporation, Columbus OH, USA

Hilmar Kuehl, M.D.
Senior Physician, Department of Diagnostic and Interventional Radiology, University Hospital Essen, Essen, Germany

Steven Kymes, Ph.D., MHA
Research Assistant Professor, Department of Ophthalmology and Visual Sciences, Washington University School of Medicine, St. Louis MO, USA

Val J. Lowe, M.D.
Professor, Department of Radiology, Division of Nuclear Medicine, Mayo Clinic, Rochester MN, USA

Carolyn Cidis Meltzer, M.D.
Associate Dean for Research, Professor and Chair, Department of Radiology, School of Medicine, Emory University Hospital, Emory University School of Medicine, Atlanta GA, USA

Marisa H. Miceli, M.D.
Resident, Department of Internal Medicine, Oakwood Hospital and Medical Center, Dearborn MI, USA

Sanjay Paidisetty, BS
Intern, Department of Radiology, University of Pittsburgh Medical Center, Pittsburgh PA, USA

Edwin L. Palmer, M.D.
Associate Radiologist, Nuclear Imaging – Division of Molecular Imaging & PET-CT, Massachusetts General Hospital, Boston MA, USA

Pat Price, M.D., FRCP, FRCR
Professor, Imaging Department, Imperial College, London, United Kingdom

Robert E. Reiman, MSPH, M.D.
Assistant Clinical Professor, Radiation Safety Division, Duke University Medical Center, Durham NC, USA

Dushyant Sahani, M.D.
Medical Director of CT Services, Department of Abdominal Imaging and Intervention, Massachusetts General Hospital, Boston MA, USA

James A. Scott, M.D.
Associate Professor, Department of Radiology, Massachusetts General Hospital, Boston MA, USA

Anthony F. Shields, M.D., Ph.D.
Professor of Medicine and Oncology, Department of Internal Medicine, Karmanos Cancer Institute, Wayne State University, Detroit MI, USA

Paul Shreve, M.D.
Advanced Radiology Services, P.C., Michigan State University College of Human Medicine, Spectrum Health Lemmen-Holten Cancer Center, Grand Rapids MI, USA

James Slattery, MRCPI, FFR (RCSI), FRCR
Fellow, Division of Abdominal Imaging and Interventional Radiology,
Massachusetts General Hospital, Boston MA, USA

Nancy M. Swanston, CNMT, PET, RT(N)
Manager, Diagnostic Imaging, Division of Diagnostic Imaging, The University
of Texas M.D., Anderson Cancer Center, Houston TX, USA

Mark Tann, M.D.
Associate Professor of Clinical Radiology, Department of Radiology and Imaging Sciences,
Indiana University School of Medicine, Indianapolis IN, USA

Rick Tetrault, CNMT, RT(N), PET
Administrative Director of Imaging Services, Department of Radiology, Dana-Farber Cancer
Institute, Boston MA, USA

David W. Townsend, Ph.D.
Head, PET and SPECT Development, Singapore Bioimaging Consortium, Singapore

Timothy G. Turkington, Ph.D.
Associate Professor, Department of Radiology and Department of Biomedical Engineering,
Duke University and Duke University Medical Center, Durham NC, USA

Annick D. Van den Abbeele, M.D.
Chief, Founding Director, Department of Imaging, Center for Biomedical Imaging
and Oncology, Dana-Farber Cancer Institute, Boston MA, USA

Patrick Veit, M.D.
Radiologist, Department of Diagnostic and Interventional Radiology,
University Hospital Essen, Germany

Ronald C. Walker, M.D., FACNM
Professor, Clinical Radiology & Radiological Sciences, Vanderbilt University Medical
Center, Nashville TN, USA

Yat Yin Yau, MBBS (OLD), FHKCR, FHKAM
Associate Professor, Director, Diagnostic Imaging, Nuclear Medicine and PET-CT,
Department of Radiology, University of Hong Kong, Hong Kong Adventist Hospital,
Hong Kong, China

Chapter 1
Principles, Design, and Operation of Multi-slice CT

Marc Kachelriess

Major technical improvements in CT have been taken place since its introduction in 1972 by Godfrey N. Hounsfield (Fig. 1.1). Even in daily clinical routine whole-body CT scans with isotropic submillimeter resolution within a single breath-hold are available. The high spatial resolution combined with volumetric imaging enables CT angiography (CTA) and virtual endoscopy to be performed. In addition CT's high temporal resolution in combination with dedicated image reconstruction algorithms provides superb images of the heart with few motion artifacts.

True 3D data acquisition became available with the introduction of spiral CT in 1989 by W.A. Kalender [1–3]. Spiral CT requires the scanner to rotate continuously and acquire data continuously. During the spiral scan the patient is translated through the CT gantry. Relative to the patient the focal spot and the detector move along a spiral or helical trajectory (Fig. 1.2). The symmetry of the scan trajectory allows for an arbitrary and retrospective selection of the longitudinal image position (z-position). The continuous axial sampling is required for high-quality 3D displays and led to a renaissance of CT [3].

As an enhancement to single-slice spiral CT (SSCT) multi-slice spiral CT (MSCT) scanners became available in 1998. They further improve the scanner's volume coverage, z-resolution, and scan speed. For example, typical chest exams are carried out with collimations of 1×5 mm in 36 s with single-slice, 4×1 mm in 30 s with 4-slice, and 16×0.75 mm in 10 s with 16-slice scanners. Today, even 64×0.5 mm scans rotating with up to three rotations per second can be used (see Fig. 1.2).

This chapter is an introduction to the basics of clinical CT. It covers technological issues such as tube and detector design, image reconstruction algorithms, as well as special techniques such as cardiac CT or dynamic CT. The reader will further get an overview of the relations between image quality and dose and will become familiar with dose reduction methods that are provided by the manufacturers as well as dose reduction techniques that can be readily applied to optimize scan protocols.

M. Kachelriess (✉)
Department of Medical Imaging, Institute of Medical Physics, University of Erlangen Nuremberg, Henkestr. 91, Erlangen 91052, Germany
e-mail: marc.kachelriess@imp.uni-erlangen.de

Basic CT Principles

From radiography we know that the information available from a single projection is limited. The information can be increased by taking two projections, typically anteroposterior and lateral. However, the radiographic images still show a superposition of all the objects that have been irradiated. Further increasing the number of projection directions (views) is of little help since the observer is not able to mentally solve the superposition problem and to "reconstruct" the internal information of the object (Fig. 1.3).

Fortunately it can be shown that a complete reconstruction of the object's interior is mathematically possible as long as a large number of views have been acquired over an angular range of 180° or more. This acquisition scheme is implemented in computed tomography scanners by using an x-ray tube that rotates around the patient. On the opposing side of the x-ray tube a cylindrical detector consisting of about 10^3 channels per slice is mounted (Figs. 1.2 and 1.4). The shape of the x-ray ensemble is called a fan-beam when the detector consists of only few slices and is called cone-beam when the detector approaches an area detector. During a full rotation 10^3 readouts of the detector are performed per detector slice. Altogether about 10^6 intensity measurements are taken per slice and rotation.

Physically, x-ray CT is the measurement of the object's x-ray absorption along straight lines. For I_0 incident quanta and an object layer of thickness d and attenuation coefficient μ the number I of quanta reaching the detector is given by the exponential attenuation law as

$$I = I_0 e^{-\mu d}.$$

The negative logarithm p of each intensity measurement I gives us information about the product of the object attenuation and

P. Shreve and D.W. Townsend (eds.), *Clinical PET-CT in Radiology: Integrated Imaging in Oncology*,
DOI 10.1007/978-0-387-48902-5_1, © Springer Science+Business Media, LLC 2011

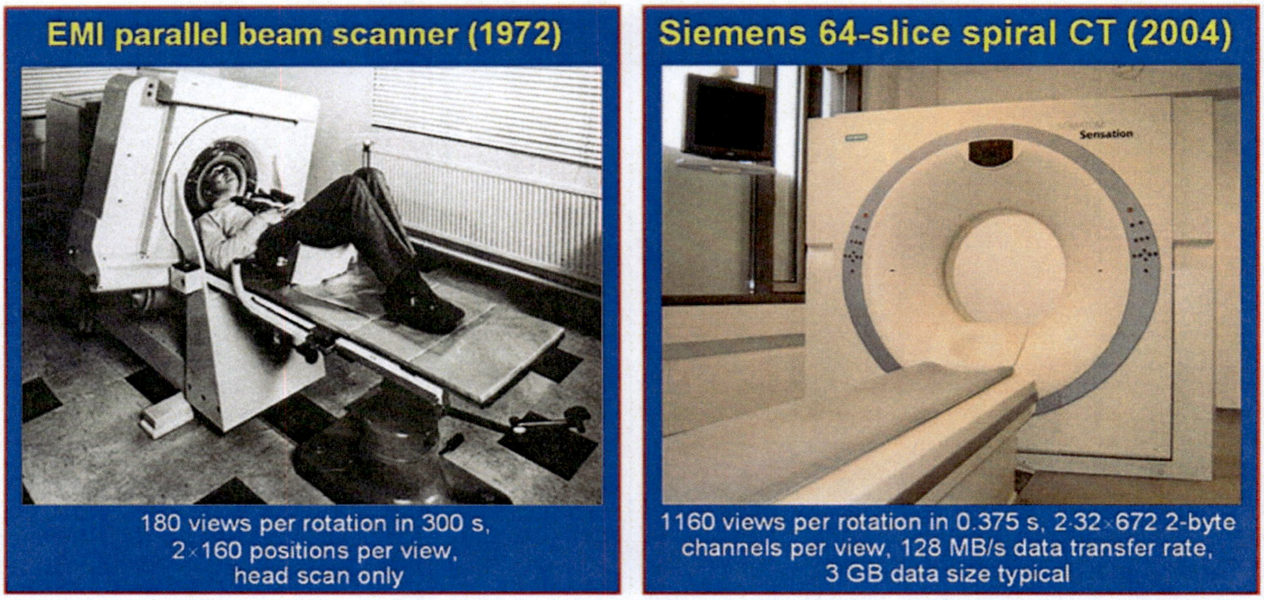

Fig. 1.1 Today, subsecond true 3D cone-beam scans with submillimeter spatial resolution and 50–100 ms temporal resolution are routinely available

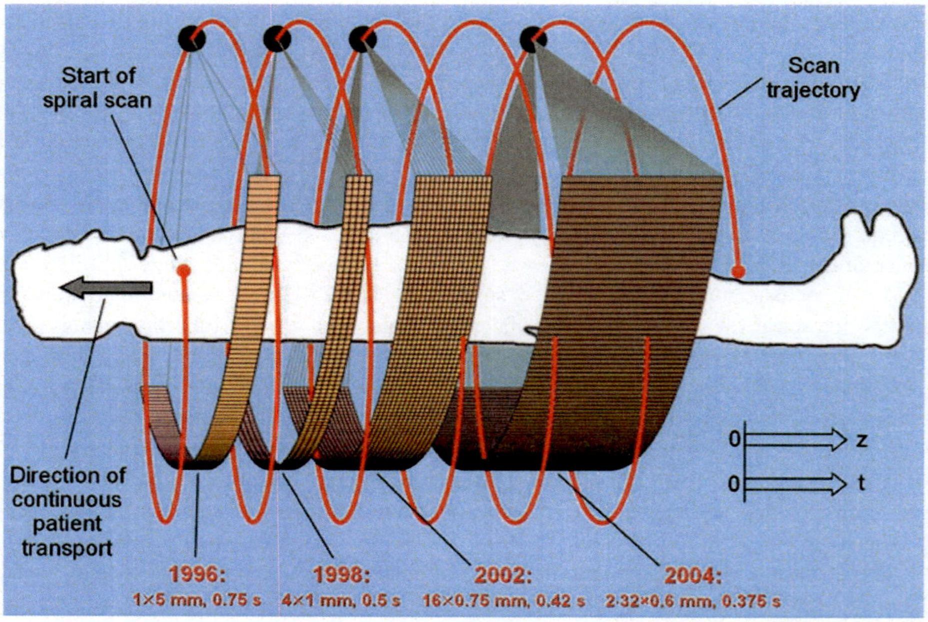

Fig. 1.2 Spiral CT scan principle and four generations of CT scanners. The collimation is given in the form $M \times S$, with M being the number of simultaneously acquired slices and S being the collimated slice thickness

thickness. For nonhomogeneous objects the attenuation coefficient is a function of x, y, and z. Then, the projection value p corresponds to the line integral along line L of the object's linear attenuation coefficient distribution $\mu(x, y, z)$:

$$P(L) = -In\frac{I(L)}{I_0} = \int_L dL\,\mu(x, y, z)$$

I_0 is the primary x-ray intensity and is needed for proper normalization. It is proportional to the tube current.

We are interested in obtaining knowledge of $\mu(x, y, z)$ by reconstructing the acquired data $p(L)$. The process of computing the CT image $f(x, y, z)$ – the CT image is an accurate approximation to $\mu(x, y, z)$ – from the set of measured projection

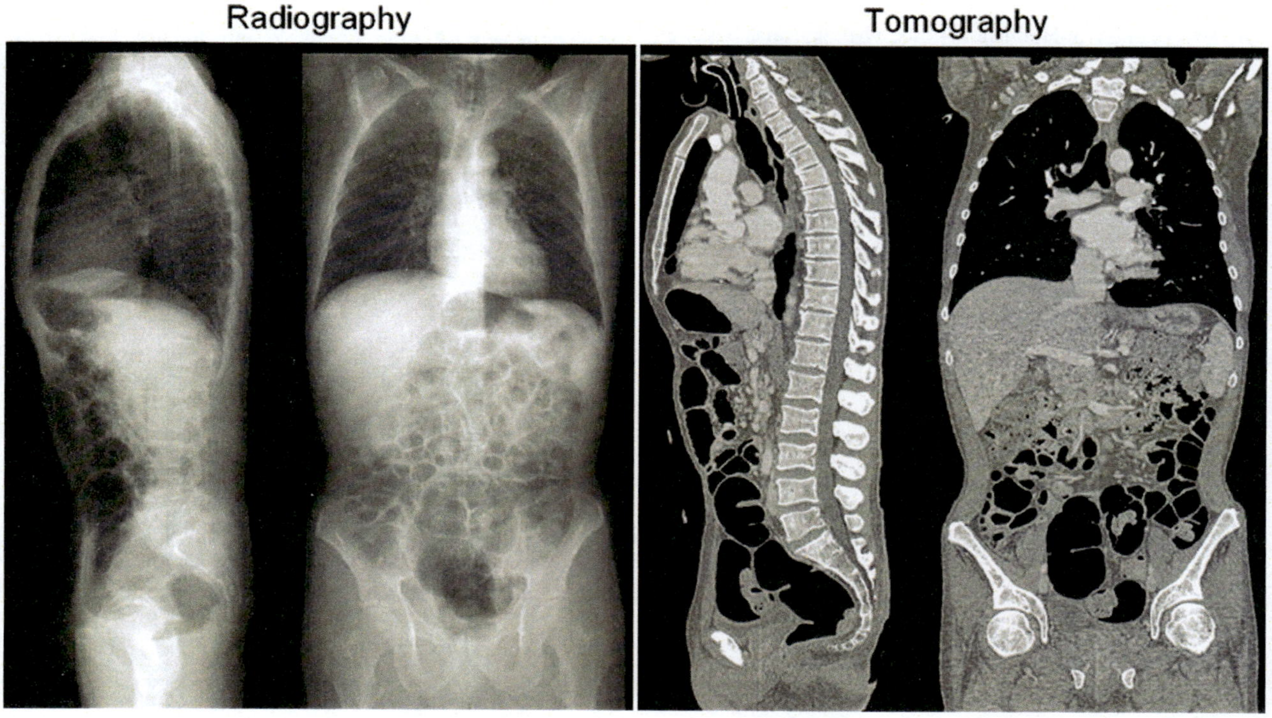

Fig. 1.3 Radiography provides only limited information due to the superpositioned information of several objects. Typically, only one or two projections are acquired. CT, in contrast, allows one to derive the complete volumetric information from a very large number of projections

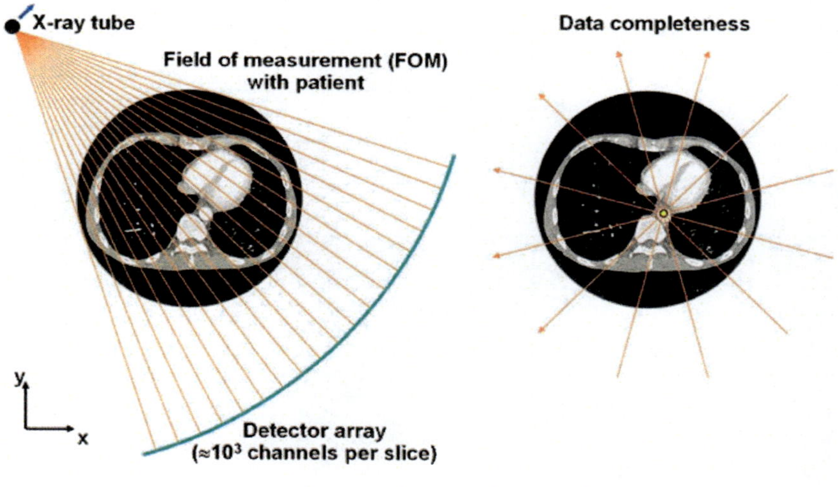

Fig. 1.4 X-ray CT is the measurement of x-ray photon attenuation along straight lines. An object point can be reconstructed as long as it has been viewed by the x-rays under an angular interval of 180° or more. If this applies to all object points within the field of measurement the data are said to be complete

values *p(L)* is called *image reconstruction* and is one of the key components of a CT scanner. For single-slice CT scanners images can be reconstructed slice-by-slice and image reconstruction is rather simple. It consists of a filtering of the projection data with the reconstruction kernel followed by a backprojection into image domain and can be formulated as

$$f(x,y) = \int_0^{\pi} d\vartheta p(\vartheta,\xi) * k(\xi)\big|_{\xi = x\cos\vartheta + y\sin\vartheta}.$$

This so-called filtered backprojection (FBP) is implemented in all clinical CT scanners. Several reconstruction kernels $k(\xi)$ are available to allow image sharpness (spatial resolution) and image noise characteristics to be modified.

The image values $f(x,y,z)$ are converted into CT values prior to storage by applying the linear function

$$CT = \frac{f - \mu_{\text{water}}}{\mu_{\text{water}}} 1{,}000\,HU.$$

where HU stands for Hounsfield units. The relation is based on the requirement that air (zero attenuation) has a CT value of –1,000 HU and water has a value of 0 HU. The CT values have been introduced by Hounsfield to replace the μ values by an integer quantity. We can interpret the CT value of a pixel or voxel as being the density of the object relative to the density of water at the respective location. For example, 200 HU means that the object density at that location is 1.2 times the density of water. An illustration of the CT scale is shown in Fig. 1.5. CT values range from –1,000 to 3,000 HU except for very dense materials such as dental fillings or metal implants.

CT images are usually displayed as grayscale images. The mapping from CT values to gray values can be controlled by the user to optimize contrast. In CT the display window is usually parameterized by the center C and width W. Values between $C - W/2$ and $C + W/2$ are linearly mapped to the gray values ranging from black to white, whereas values below and above that "window" are displayed black and white, respectively (Fig. 1.6). For example, the window (0, 600) means that it is centered at 0 HU and has a width of 600 HU. Thus, values in the range from –300 HU to 300 HU are mapped to the gray values; values below –300 HU are displayed black and values above 300 HU are displayed white.

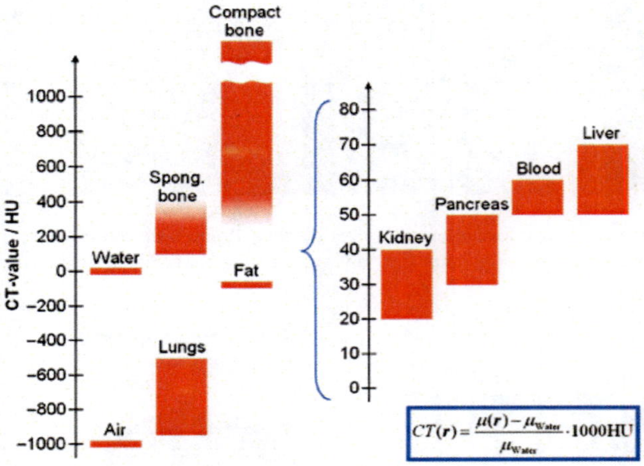

Fig. 1.5 Ranges of CT values of the most important organs

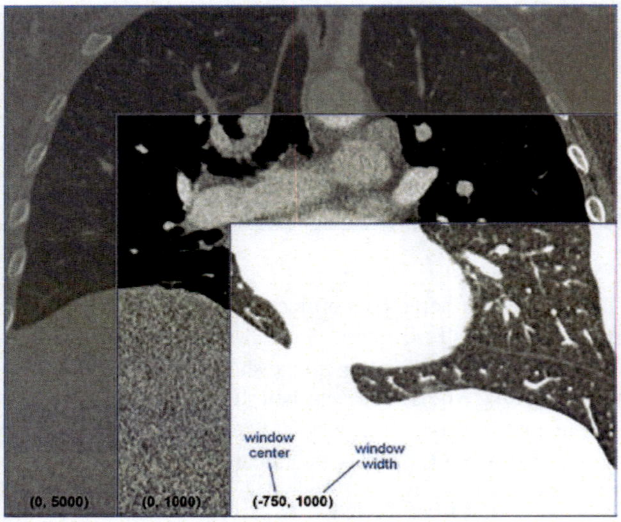

Fig. 1.6 CT image of the thorax displayed with three different window settings

CT Design

A clinical CT scanner consists of the patient table, the gantry, the reconstruction, and viewing PCs and a cooling system. The main purpose of the patient table is to move the patient through the gantry during the scan. Only then can complete anatomic regions be acquired. Further, the table's vertical degree of freedom allows it to be lowered until the patient can comfortably lie down. The gantry comprises a stationary part and a rotational part. Power and data are transferred via slip rings. Continuous rotation and continuous data acquisition are supported. The components carried by the gantry are the x-ray tube and the x-ray detector.

Two kind of tubes are in use today. A typical x-ray tube consists of a vacuum-filled tube envelope. Inside the vacuum is the cathode and a rotating anode with one bearing Fig. 1.7 (*left*). This conventional concept has the disadvantage that tube cooling is inefficient and that the one-sided bearing cannot tolerate high forces. It is also difficult to lubricate bearings in a vacuum. To improve these conventional tubes, vendors try to maximize the heat capacity (expressed in mega heat-units, or MHU) to minimize cooling delays. Recently, a new CT tube has become available where the cathode, the anode, and the envelope together rotate in the cooling medium Fig. 1.7 (*right*). Due to the direct contact to the cooling oil, there is no need to store the heat and thus there will be no cooling delays [4].

Data transfer rate limitations imply a restriction on the number of slices that can be read out simultaneously. Often, scans with fast rotation time acquire fewer slices than scans with slower rotation times. One therefore distinguishes between the number of detector rows that are built into a detector and the number of slices M that can be read out simultaneously. Obviously, the number of slices M is the critical parameter for the user, and not the number of detector rows. Electronic combination (binning) of neighboring rows is used to generate thicker collimated slices and to make use of all detector rows available. An example of modern detector technology is shown in Fig. 1.8. The adaptive array technology has a higher x-ray sensitivity and requires less patient dose than the matrix array detectors since binning to lower spatial resolution includes less detector gaps (septa) with adaptive detectors than

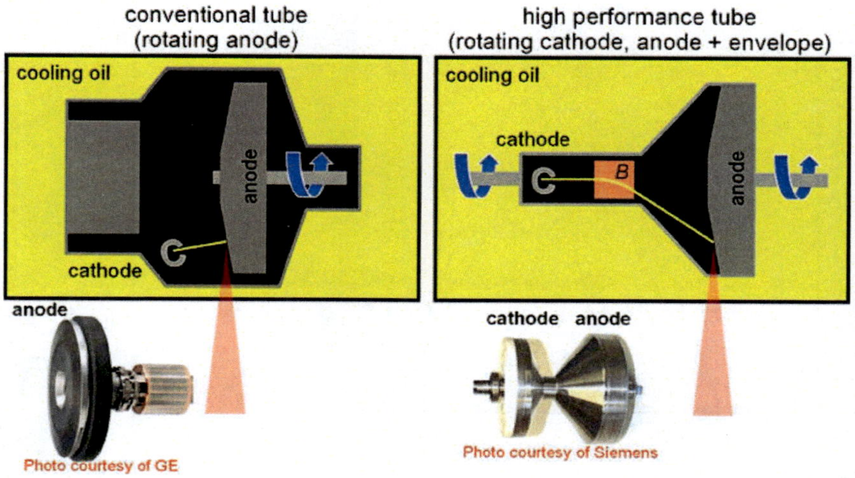

Fig. 1.7 Conventional x-ray tube versus rotating envelope technology (courtesy General Electric, Piscataway, NJ; and Siemens, Munich, Germany)

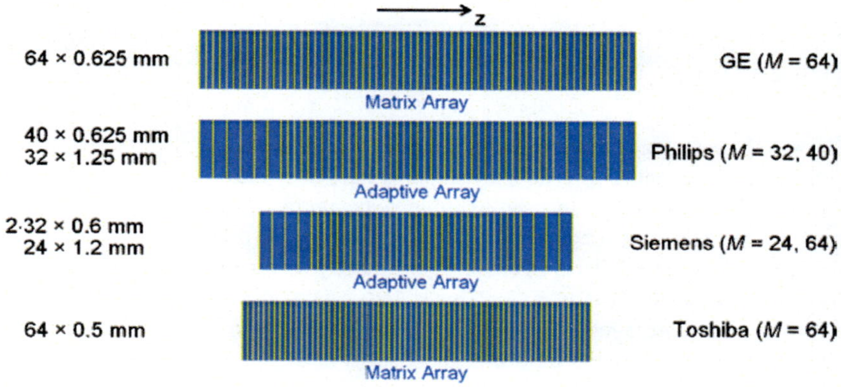

Fig. 1.8 Detector concepts available in 2004. Due to a flying focal spot that jumps back and forth in the longitudinal direction the Siemens detector allows to acquire 64 slices while it provides only 32 high resolution detector rows. It is the only scanner that fulfills the Nyquist sampling criterion in the z-direction

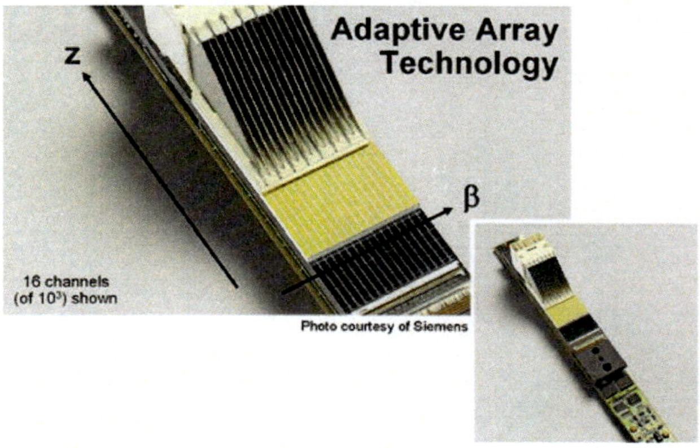

Fig. 1.9 Photo of a 40-row 64-slice adaptive array detector (courtesy Siemens, Munich, Germany)

with matrix detectors. A photo of a typical 64-slice detector is shown in Fig. 1.9; data transfer rates of up to 300 MB per second are achieved with such a system.

The Siemens Sensation 64 scanner has a distinctive feature that allows 64 slices to be acquired from only 32 rows: the *z*-flying focal spot (zFFS). Between two adjacent readings the focal spot jumps back and forth on the tube anode (a few thousand times per second) to double the sampling distance. Slices of 0.6 mm thickness are acquired at a sampling distance of 0.3 mm (Fig. 1.10). This so-called double sampling, that fulfills the Nyquist sampling condition, improves spatial resolution and reduces spiral windmill artifacts [5].

Advanced CT Principles

Before a CT scan can be started the acquisition software must register the patient. Basic information that is required are the patient name, patient age (birth date), and patient sex. Then, the patient is placed on the table. If required, contrast injection is prepared, ECG leads are applied, spirometric devices are attached, or other preparations are done. Often, the patient is instructed how to behave during the scan to be prepared for the breath-hold commands. In parallel, scan protocols can be selected and scan parameters can be modified.

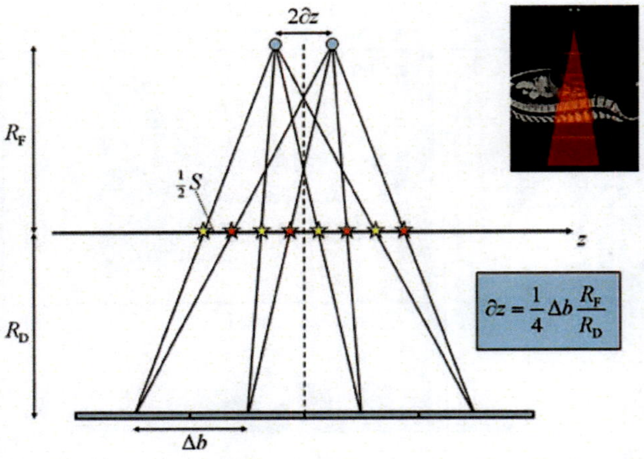

Fig. 1.10 Illustration of the zFFS. Double sampling is indicated by the yellow and red stars

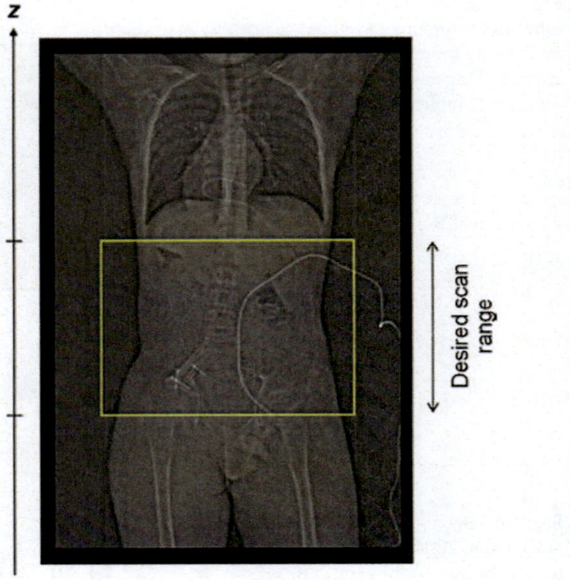

Fig. 1.11 The topogram is a digitally enhanced version of a radiographic projection used to graphically select the desired scan range

Topogram

Most CT scans start by acquiring an overview radiographic image of the patient. This is done by stopping the gantry rotation and by moving the table through the gantry during data acquisition. The image obtained is known as the topogram, the scanogram, or the scout view (Fig. 1.11). It mainly serves to determine the final CT scan range. This is done by the placement of one or more rectangular ROIs that define the z-positions of scan start and end for one or more scans of the same patient. Internally, the scanner may further utilize the topogram information to compute a patient specific tube current control curve that will be used during the scan (see below).

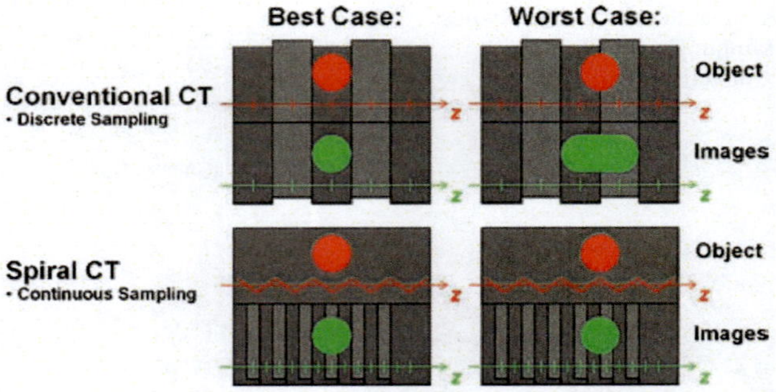

Fig. 1.12 Sampling in conventional CT is sparse, and objects may be imaged differently when their position relative to the slice center varies. This may not happen with spiral CT scans where sampling in z is (almost) continuous

Conventional CT

Before the introduction of spiral CT a CT scan consisted of a rotation about the stationary object followed by a translation of the patient by one slice thickness (for today's multi-slice scanners the scan increment is M times the slice thickness). This scan mode is called conventional CT or step-and-shoot CT, and we may also refer to the combination of several circle scans as a sequence scan or a sequential scan.

Image reconstruction for sequence scans is fairly easy since each slice can be reconstructed separately using filtered backprojection. There are two major drawbacks in conventional CT. First, step-and-shoot scans are rather slow due to the interscan delay when shifting the patient. Second, z-sampling is rather inadequate and there is no true longitudinal translation invariance. This means that scan results may randomly depend on the absolute location of objects, especially for thick slices (Fig. 1.12).

Spiral CT

Today, most scans are carried out in spiral mode. In the late 1980s, just after continuously rotating scanners became available, this scan mode was introduced by Willi A. Kalender [1–3]. It performs continuous data acquisition while the patient moves at constant speed through the gantry (cf. Fig. 1.2). To obtain high-quality images the z-interpolation is required as an additional image reconstruction step. Given a desired reconstruction position z_R the z-interpolation uses projection data acquired at positions adjacent to that plane to synthesize virtual scan data corresponding to a circular scan at $z = z_R$ (Fig. 1.13). Typically, but not necessarily, linear

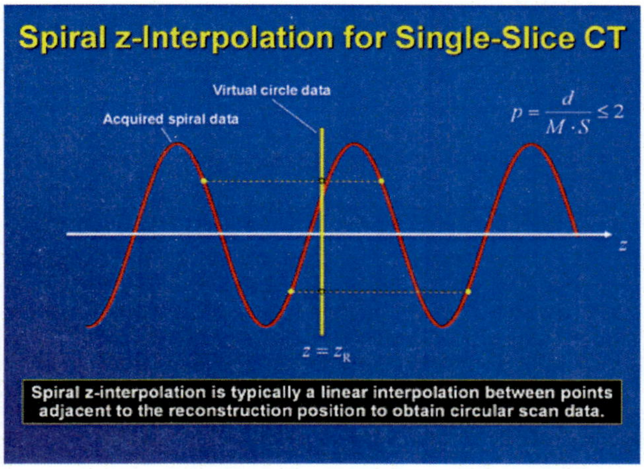

Fig. 1.13 Illustration of the spiral z-interpolation principle. A similar technique, the so-called z-filtering, is applied for multi-slice CT scanners with up to four slices

interpolation is used and a similar principle holds for multi-slice scanners with $M \leq 4$ slices. The virtual circle scan, obtained by z-interpolation or z-filtering, is then reconstructed using FBP.

There are two major advantages in spiral CT. First, the continuous data acquisition yields continuous data even in the case of patient movement or breathing because there is no interscan delay as in the step-and-shoot case. Consequently, with spiral CT no anatomic details can be lost or imaged twice, as could be the case with conventional CT. Second, the possibility of retrospectively selecting the reconstruction positions z_R allows images to be reconstructed at finer intervals than dictated by the collimated slice thickness S (see Fig. 1.12). It is recommended that images are reconstructed at an interval that is equal to or less than half the collimated slice thickness (Nyquist theorem). Only then will 3D displays be of high quality and show no step artifacts and multiplanar reformations (MPRs) will yield image quality equivalent to the primary, transaxial images.

The table increment d per rotation is a new degree of freedom in spiral CT. In contrast to conventional CT it typically differs from the slice collimation $W_{tot} = M\ S$. One uses the so-called pitch value to make the definition of the table increment relative [6]:

$$p = \frac{d}{W_{tot}}.$$

Small pitch values yield overlapping data and the redundancy can be used to decrease image noise (more quanta contribute to one z-position) or to reduce artifacts. For example, with a pitch of 0.5 each z-position will be imaged by two full rotations and the data are highly redundant. These redundant data can be used to reduce image noise by accumulating the dose in the final image. Alternatively one uses the redundancy of data obtained from low pitch values to perform cardiac imaging, as we will see below. Large pitch values increase the scan speed and complete anatomical ranges can be covered very fast. Typical pitch values lie between 0.2 and 1.5, for single-slice scanners pitch values up to 2 are reasonable.

Cone-Beam CT

In 1998, the race to introduce more slices began with the introduction of 4-slice scanners. The advantages of multi-slice scanning are more than obvious: Scan time can be reduced or spatial resolution can be increased by a factor of M. In fact, the typical scan modes were a combination of both options and are illustrated in Fig. 1.2.

With single-slice or 4-slice scanners, each acquired slice can be regarded as being (approximately) perpendicular to the axis of rotation. This simplifies image reconstruction considerably. However, with scanners that acquire more than four slices simultaneously one must not neglect the cone-beam nature (Fig. 1.14). Image reconstruction becomes a challenging problem because it must now take the cone angle explicitly into account.

Today, two classes of cone-beam algorithms are implemented in the commercial software of clinical 16- to 64-slice

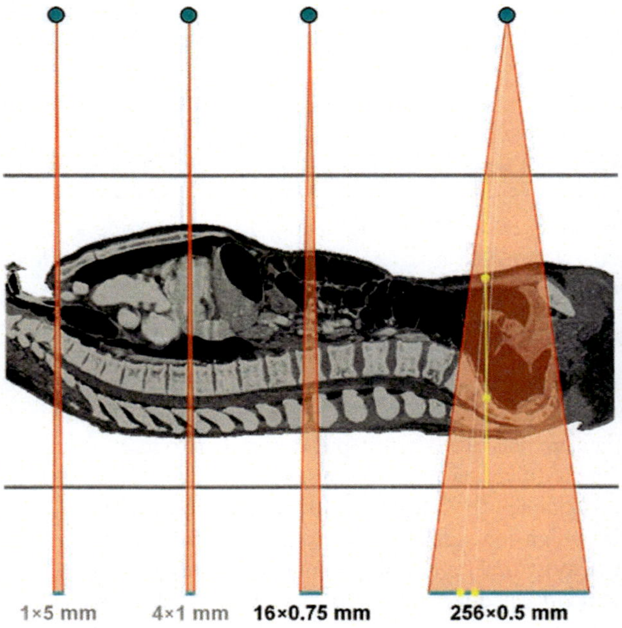

Fig. 1.14 For larger cone angles (more than $M = 4$ slices) one may not neglect the obliqueness of the rays anymore. A slice-by-slice reconstruction as done for single and 4-slice scanners would yield significant cone-beam artifacts. Thus, dedicated cone-beam reconstruction is required

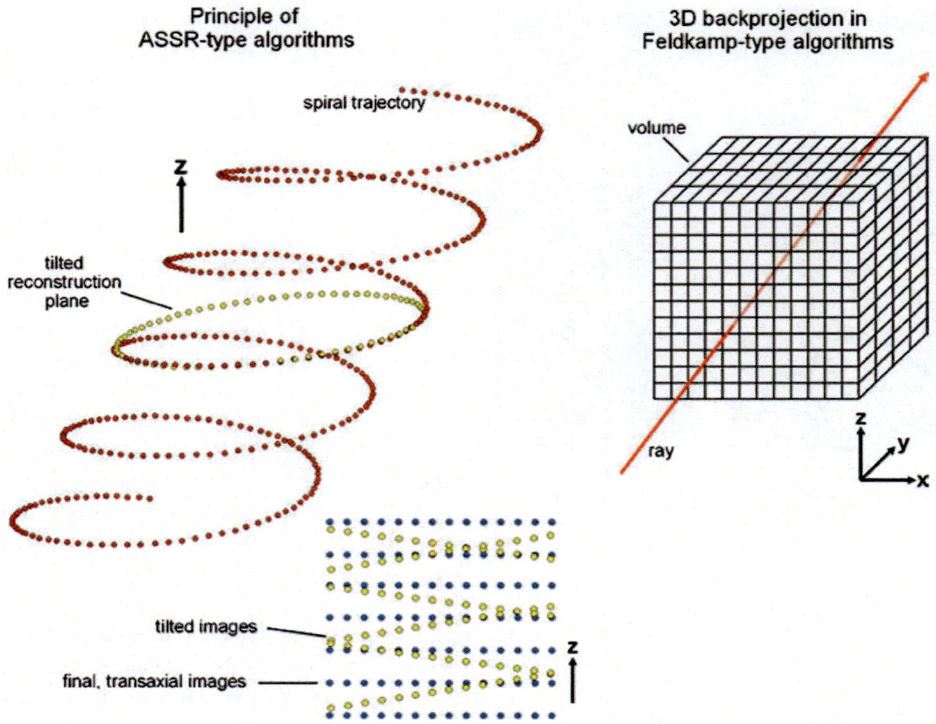

Fig. 1.15 Basic principles of ASSR-type and Feldkamp-type reconstruction. The ASSR illustration shows how a reconstruction plane fits nicely into the spiral trajectory, and it further depicts the volume interpolation procedure to convert from tilted images to Cartesian images. The Feldkamp illustration shows the principle of 3D backprojection

CT scanners: modifications of the advanced single-slice rebinning (ASSR) algorithm [7] and adapted versions of the Feldkamp algorithm [8].

The advanced single-slice rebinning ASSR fits 180° segments of circles to the spiral trajectory. This can be done with high accuracy as long as one allows these circles to tilt with respect to the x-y plane [7]. The tilted planes are called *reconstruction planes*. A rebinning (resorting) of the acquired cone-beam data is performed to obtain virtual 2D scans along these reconstruction planes. Then, a standard 2D image reconstruction of these tilted virtual circle data follows and yields tilted images. ASSR uses many adjacent and overlapping reconstruction planes to sufficiently cover the whole volume. As soon as enough tilted images are available the data are resampled in the spatial domain to obtain a standard Cartesian volume that can be stored and viewed (Fig. 1.15).

Compared to Feldkamp-type image reconstruction, ASSR is of high computational efficiency. Backprojection, which is the most time-consuming component during image reconstruction, is done in two dimensions with ASSR-type algorithms, whereas a 3D backprojection is required for Feldkamp-type algorithms. Further, ASSR allows the available 2D reconstruction hardware to be used, thereby minimizing development costs. However, the ASSR approach is limited to approximately $M = 64$ slices [7] and data for scanners with many more slices should be reconstructed using a modified Feldkamp algorithm.

Feldkamp-type reconstruction is an extension of 2D filtered backprojection reconstruction to three dimensions [8]: The data are convolved and then backprojected. Here, the backprojection is done in 3D cone-beam geometry (Fig. 1.15). A highly versatile modified Feldkamp algorithm is the extended parallel backprojection (EPBP) (Fig. 1.16) [9]. The algorithm is dedicated to clinical CT, reconstructs circular, sequential, and spiral scans and allows 100% dose usage and arbitrary pitch values. These benefits are not automatically available with other Feldkamp-type reconstruction algorithms. Further, EPBP is able to perform phase-correlated reconstruction of cone-beam data and is therefore the first real cone-beam cardiac CT algorithm.

Cardiac CT

The driving force of CT development is retrospectively gated CT of the heart. High-quality imaging of the human heart is possible only with high-end technology. Spiral CT, subsecond rotation times, and multi-slice data acquisition, that have become available within the past few years, are a

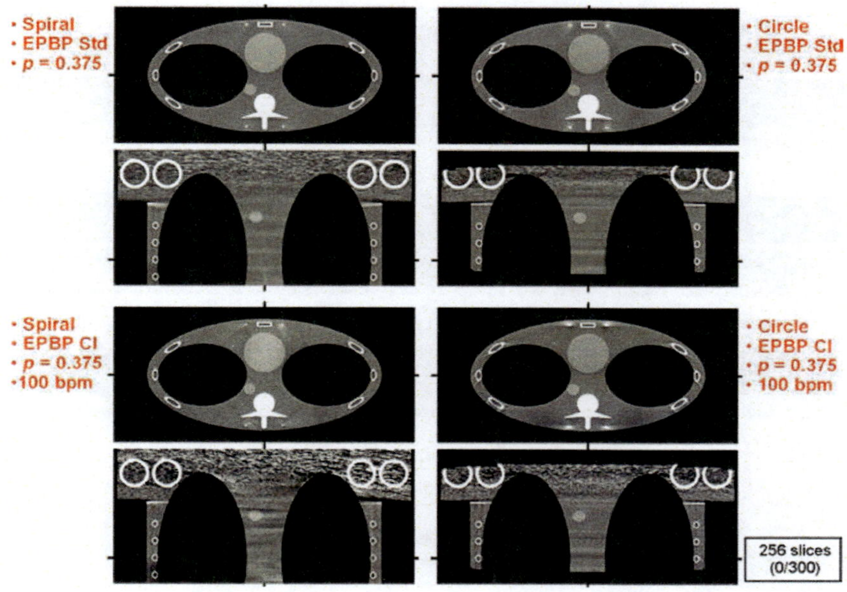

Fig. 1.16 EPBP reconstruction of 256-slice data. Each quadrant shows an axial slice and a coronal MPR. The upper images show standard reconstructions, the lower images show phase-correlated cardiac CT reconstructions. For the left column spiral data and for the right column circle data have been simulated (From [9], with permission)

prerequisite for cardiac CT. Cardiac spiral CT started with the introduction of dedicated phase-correlated reconstruction algorithms for single-slice spiral CT in 1997 [10–12]. These were generalized to the case of multi-slice spiral CT (MSCT) data acquisition [13–15], and recently, to cone-beam acquisition for scanners with up to 256 slices or more [11, 16].

The difficulty with imaging the human heart is the inherent motion artifacts that, for adequate image quality, require dedicated scan protocols and reconstruction algorithm. To reduce motion artifacts cardiac CT synchronizes either the scan or the image reconstruction with a synchronization signal that reflects cardiac motion. Typically, one uses the ECG signal that is acquired simultaneously with the CT data, for synchronization [12]. Alternatively, there is the possibility to derive a motion function, the kymogram, directly from the acquired raw data [17].

The possibility to carry out a sequence scan that is triggered by the patient ECG is known as prospective gating. To minimize motion artifacts, an angular range of slightly more than 180° plus fan-angle is acquired in contrast to the usual 360° that are used for standard sequence scans. Image reconstruction for prospectively gated cardiac scans is equivalent to standard sequence image reconstruction and consists of filtered backprojection. Drawbacks of prospective gating are that: (1) one cannot retrospectively correct for the timing window; (2) the scan time is rather long due to the interscan delays; and (3) image quality is inferior since it is a sequence and not a spiral acquisition protocol.

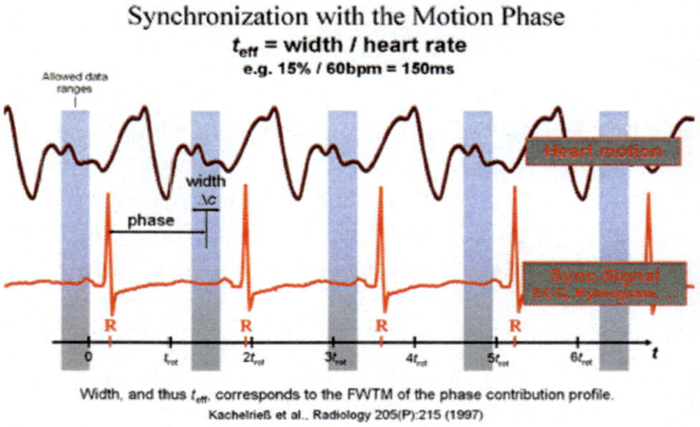

Fig. 1.17 Synchronization of the sinogram data with the motion phase (From [10], with permission)

In contrast to prospective gating, phase-correlated spiral CT consists of a continuous spiral CT scan covering the heart combined with the simultaneous acquisition of a motion function (ECG, kymogram). Image reconstruction, which is a key issue for phase-correlated CT, eliminates the data acquired in undesired motion phases and utilizes only allowed data ranges (Fig. 1.17). It is important to note that the definition of allowed and forbidden data ranges is applied retrospectively and specified by the user. If the reconstructed images do not meet expectations, another reconstruction may be performed with a different timing window. Typically, the location of the timing window is specified relative to the

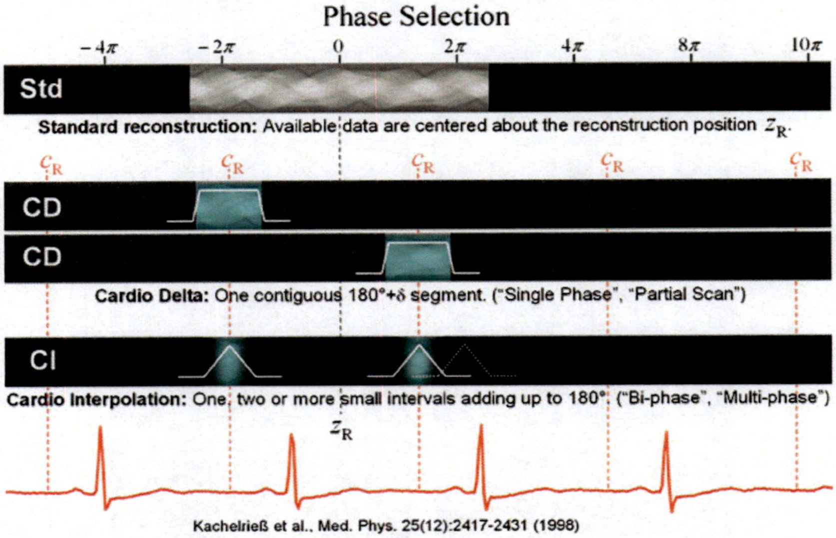

Fig. 1.18 Principle of retrospectively gated cardiac CT. One or more data segments are combined to yield a complete 180 degree data range with maximum temporal resolution (From [12], with permission)

R-peaks of the ECG and Fig. 1.17 shows allowed data ranges located at about 75% of R-R.

To be able to carry out phase-correlated image reconstruction enough data must be acquired. The data completeness condition (see Fig. 1.4) requires each z-position to be covered by at least 180° plus fan-angle. Since we also need to be able to select the timing window at that z-position coverage must be increased by the duration of at least one heartbeat. Summarizing, a given z-position must be covered by 180° plus fan-angle plus one heart cycle. This is achieved by using very small spiral pitch values. Typical values range from 0.2 to 0.4. Obviously, patients with a low heart rate require a lower pitch than patients with a high heart rate. Similarly for scanners with very fast rotation, the pitch value is generally less than with slower rotation scanners.

As soon as the data are acquired, the image reconstruction algorithm determines the optimal allowed data ranges. It is possible to combine data segments from more than one heart cycle. Under certain circumstances up to three heart beats can contribute to one image. The advantage of these multiphase reconstructions is the improved temporal resolution since the sum of the sizes of all segments make up the 180° completeness range (Fig. 1.18). For example, with three segments (depending on the patient heart rate and scanner rotation time) only slightly more than 60° of scan data may be required from each heart cycle.

Retrospectively phase-correlated image reconstruction achieves high quality images of the heart-especially in combination with multi-slice CT scanners and thin slice thicknesses. The cardiac images are used to perform either an automated quantification of coronary calcium or a CT angiography of the coronary arteries (Fig. 1.19) [3, 18].

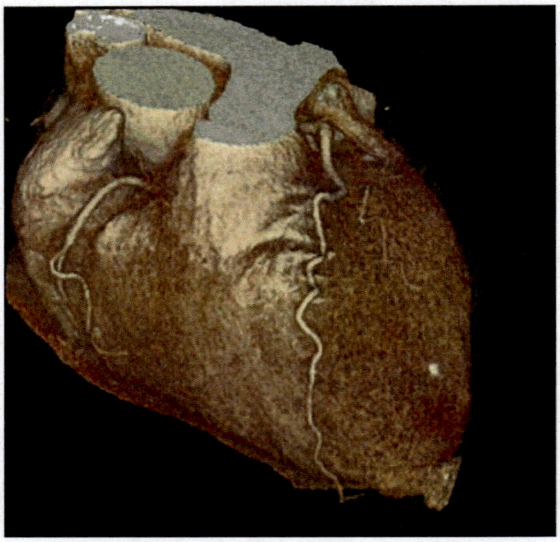

Fig. 1.19 Routine examinations achieve extremely high image quality today. This image is a scan of the human heart with a high-speed multislice CT scanner and a rotating envelope tube (data courtesy Dieter Ropers, Erlangen, Germany)

Since cardiac CT makes use of only a fraction of the data available there are some image noise issues or, alternatively, dose issues. To obtain high-quality images the tube current must be increased and thereby so will the patient dose. One possibility to reduce patient dose in phase-correlated cardiac CT is to modulate the tube current as a function of the patient ECG. For those projections that are in a slow motion phase and therefore are likely to be used in subsequent image reconstruction the tube current is increased, whereas it is decreased (but not switched off) for projections that are unlikely to contribute to the image. This ECG-pulsing is related to the dose modulation techniques that will be discussed later in the dose and image quality section.

Additionally, novel display techniques help to improve the signal-to-noise ratio. Fig. 1.20 shows the possibility to perform slabs in the z-direction, and in the temporal direction (t-direction), and to combine both effects. Whereas the standard image (0.5-mm voxel size, isotropic resolution) suffers from image noise we find a significant reduction of noise in the other three images where voxels perpendicular to the slice shown have been used for averaging [19].

Dynamic CT

Another mode of CT operation is dynamic CT. Dynamic CT covers an organ of interest multiple times to monitor the concentration of contrast agents over time [20]. Thus information about blood flow or perfusion can be obtained. It can be achieved by repeatedly scanning some organ of interest or by performing a spiral scan with very low pitch and applying similar principles as for cardiac CT. Often, dynamic CT consists of multiple circle scans and therefore the coverage of complete organs is not guaranteed with the axial coverage of current detectors.

With the advent of cone-beam CT dynamic studies of the heart will become possible by performing a multiple-circle scan (no table motion) of the heart and combining the principles of phase-correlation and dynamic CT. In fact we can see from Fig. 1.21 that such five-dimensional data have been acquired and the feasibility of phase-correlated dynamic CT has been demonstrated [21, 22].

The most frequent application of dynamic CT is the automatic triggering of a standard or phase-correlated CT scan. These are often carried out with intravenous contrast agent (iodine-based) and the dynamic scan is useful for tracking the contrast bolus before the final scan is started. This so-called bolus tracking is a dynamic scan where one slice of interest is scanned repeatedly (e.g., in intervals of 5 or 10 s) until the density within some predefined ROI exceeds a threshold. Exceeding the threshold indicates that the contrast bolus has arrived and the full CT scan is automatically triggered.

Dose and Image Quality

The annual effective dose due to natural radiation is of the order of 2 to 3 mSv. A typical CT scan adds between 1 and 20 mSv, or even more, to that dose. Consequently, dose in CT must be regarded critically. Often press commentaries refer to CT as a "high-dose modality", which is perceived by the public as something dangerous. It is rarely explained that the CT acquisition provides an enormous amount of information. The amount of data made available by a CT scan is orders of magnitude larger than that of any other medical imaging modality.

Since CT dose is inherently related to CT image quality, we discuss parameters and methods that have direct impact on dose and image quality issues. Probably the most basic parameter in CT imaging is the effective mAs-product $(I \cdot t)_{\text{eff}}$ or mAs_{eff}. It is a measure of the number of x-ray photons that enter a given z-position (transaxial slice) of the patient. The effective tube current and time product is defined as the mAs-product per rotation divided by the pitch value:

$$(I \cdot t)_{\text{eff}} = (I \cdot t)_{360} / \, p$$

For sequence scans it is equal to the product of tube current and rotation time: in this case the table increment d equals the total collimation $M\ S$ and therefore $p = 1$. Typical effective mAs values range from 10 to 500 mAs. Low values yield high image noise and vice versa. The standard deviation of the image noise is inversely proportional to the square of the effective mAs: reducing noise by 50% requires a fourfold increase of mAs_{eff}.

It is important to emphasize that the selection of the effective mAs value (as is possible with most MSCT scanners) yields an image quality independent of the pitch value, i.e., independent of the degree of scan overlap. Fig. 1.22 shows an experiment where scans were performed with 165 mAs_{eff}, a rotation time of 0.5 s and three different pitch values. The actual tube current computed by the scanner ranges from 198 to 461 mA such that image noise σ and thus dose and image quality remain constant. Thus, for scanners that adapt the tube current, the same noise, image quality, and dose are achieved with MSCT regardless of the pitch value.

Another important parameter is spatial resolution, where particularly in the longitudinal direction, resolution is determined by the slice thickness, and there is a large range of possible values. The collimated slice thickness S determines the thickness of one cross-section as it is measured during the scan. During image reconstruction the so-called effective slice thickness S_{eff} can be used to reconstruct images thicker than S. Thicker slice images show reduced image noise. Typical values for the collimated slice thickness range from 0.5 to 2.5 mm with modern 16-slice CT scanners. The effective slice thickness typically ranges from 0.5 to 10 mm. Compared to the z-resolution there is less freedom in choosing the in-plane resolution Δr. It can be modified to some

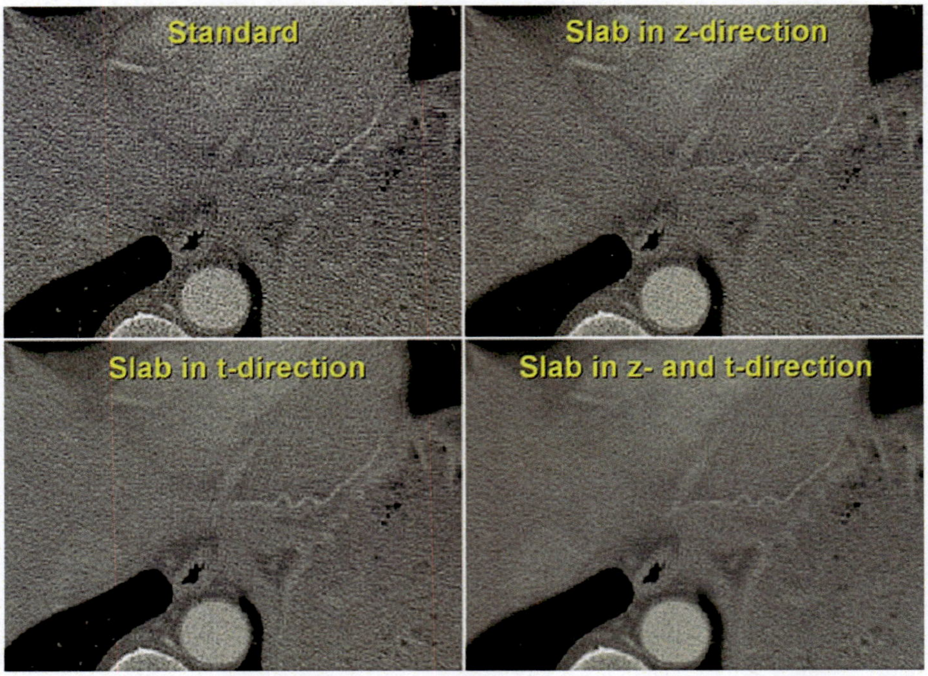

Fig. 1.20 Image noise in cardiac CT can not only be reduced by performing slabs orthogonal to the image plane, but also in the temporal direction. Combined spatial and temporal slab techniques yield a minimum of image noise or, alternatively, a minimum of patient dose

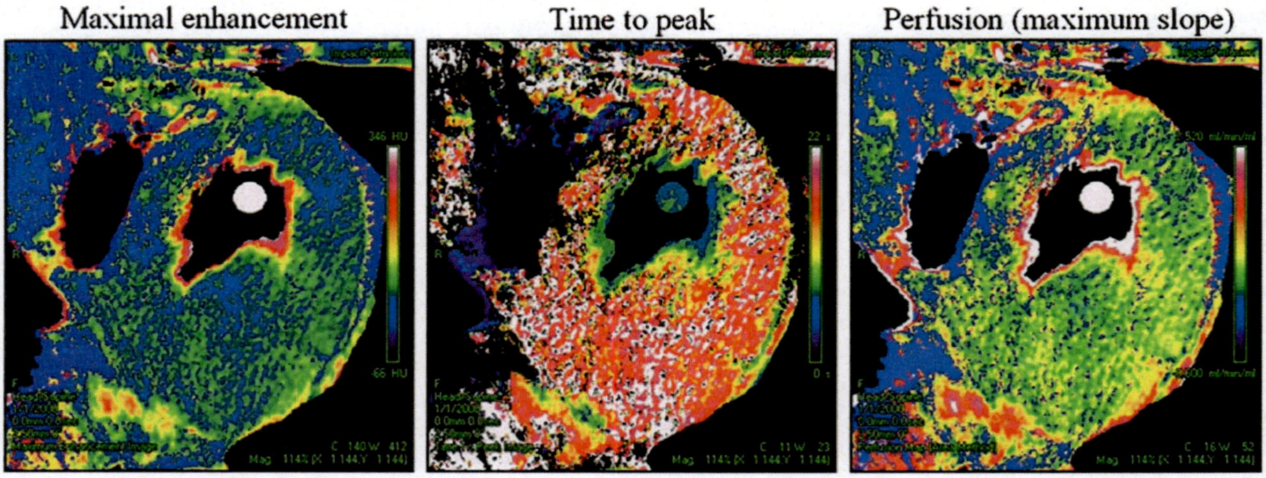

Fig. 1.21 Dynamic study of the heart using a four-slice spiral CT scanner. The acquisition of phase-correlated dynamic data was done with a 4 × 5 mm collimation and a multiple circle ECG-correlated scan with a total duration of 30 s (from [22]). The color coded images show the maximal enhancement, the time to peak enhancement and the cardiac perfusion of the z = 5 mm slice at 70% of R-R

extent by choosing the reconstruction kernel but one cannot directly enter a desired value of, for example, 1.5 mm.

Quantitatively,

$$\sigma^2 \propto \frac{1}{(I\,t)_{\mathrm{eff}}\; S_{\mathrm{eff}}\; \Delta r^3} \tag{1.1}$$

relates spatial resolution, effective tube-current, and image noise σ. The constant of proportionality depends in a complicated way on the patient size and density, tube voltage, and prefiltration. This equation shows that a 16-fold increase of dose (or $\mathrm{mAs}_{\mathrm{eff}}$) is required to improve spatial resolution by a factor of 2 in all three dimensions with pixel noise

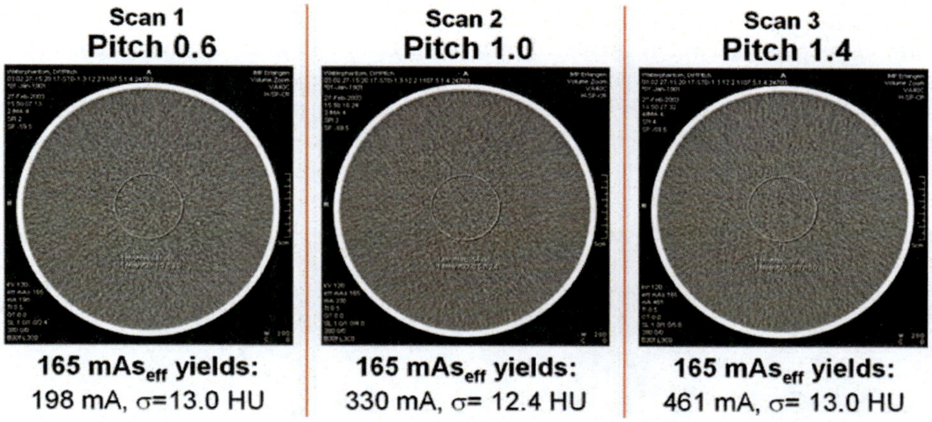

Fig. 1.22 Multi-slice scanners compensate for the effect of scan overlap by adjusting the actual (physical) tube current

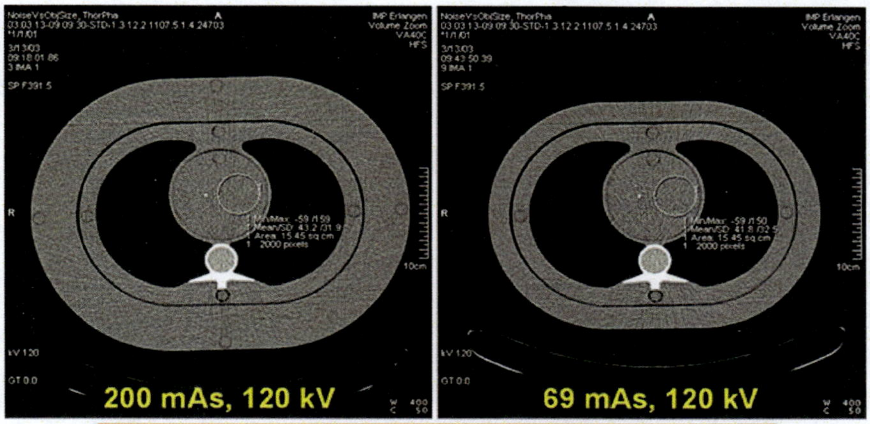

	40 cm × 30 cm	35 cm × 25 cm	HVL$_{eff}$
80 kV	957 mAs	287 mAs	2.9 cm
120 kV	200 mAs	69 mAs	3.3 cm
140 kV	142 mAs	51 mAs	3.4 cm

Fig. 1.23 The optimal mAs and thus the minimal patient dose can be achieved only if the patient shape is taken into account. To do so it is important to have an idea of the half-value layer of typical cross-sections

σ constant. Since the above equation is strongly object dependent, a simple experiment was conducted to demonstrate this dependence. A thorax phantom [23] equipped with extension rings of different thicknesses was used to mimic a standard and an obese patient. The diameter of the obese patient is 5 cm larger than a standard patient diameter. The obese patient was scanned with 200 mAs$_{eff}$ at 80, 120, and 140 kV, respectively. The mAs value for a standard patient was adjusted to yield the same image quality (image noise) as for the obese patient. The results are shown in Fig. 1.23. The critical parameter that determines the change in object size requires a twofold change in mAs$_{eff}$ is the half value layer (HVL); in the thorax region the HVL is in the order of 3–5 cm.

Another parameter that plays a significant role in protocol optimization is the total scan length or scan range. Although this issue is somewhat obvious, it is worth mentioning that a scan range that exceeds the organ of interest is a waste of dose. For example, consider a cardiac CT scan where, typically, the organ of interest has a longitudinal extent of not more than 15 cm. If the operator adds a 5-cm "safety-region" on either side, dose is increased by more than 60% compared to scanning only the required range.

To experience the effect of scan range, object shape or tube voltage and thereby to optimize scan protocols phantom experiments can be carried out easily. Adequately sized water phantoms are available with each CT scanner and comparisons should be performed at equal image quality (i.e., same noise and same resolution). Further, dose tutoring software is available to perform mAs-optimization [24]. Acquired raw data are used to add virtual noise, which converts the data to a lower mAs value. This tool helps to iteratively seek for the optimal scan parameters and learn more about the relationship between patient shape and image noise (Fig. 1.24).

Although not a scan parameter, individual dose assessment can be a useful educational tool that might not only be used for patient information but also help to optimize scan protocols. To directly assess scanner-, scan protocol-, and organ-specific dose values, dose calculators have become available. Based on Monte Carlo dose calculations [25],

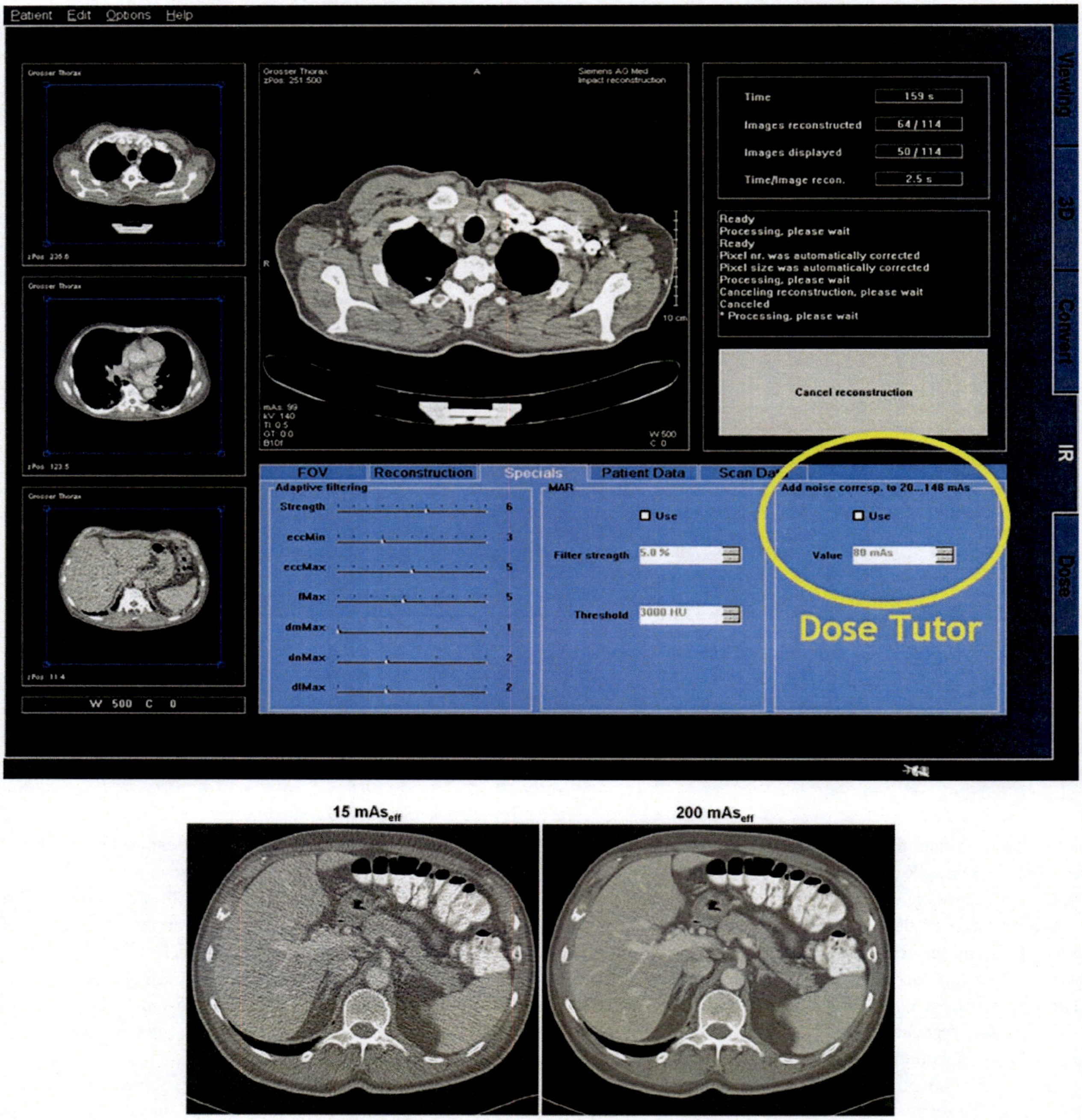

Fig. 1.24 Dose tutors (e.g., refer to [24]) allow one to retrospectively adjust the tube current and thereby iteratively seek for the optimal scan protocol.

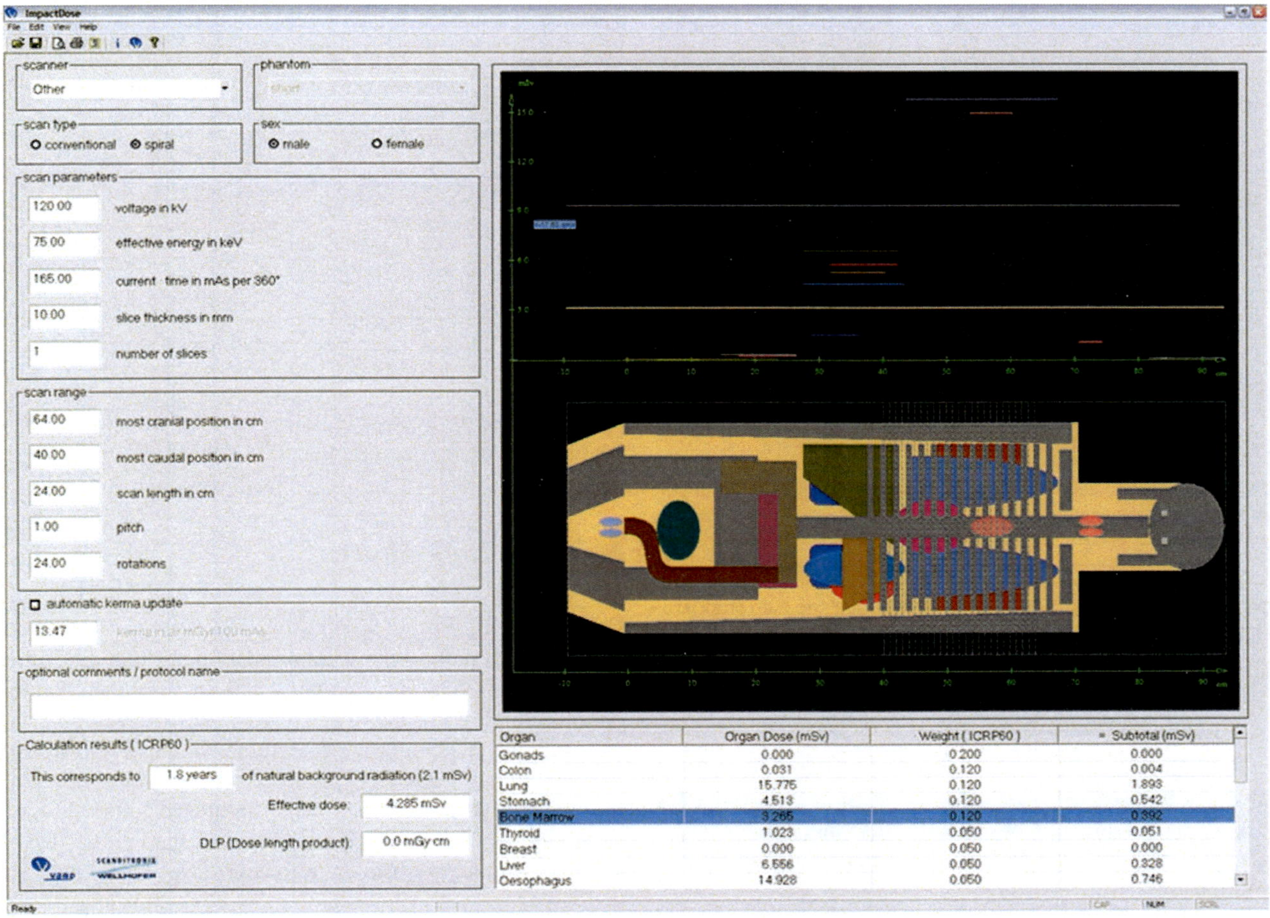

Fig. 1.25 Organ dose values and the weighted effective dose are provided by dose calculation software as a function of the scanner, the anatomic region scanned, and the scan parameters used (refer to [24, 26])

organ dose and effective dose values are computed in real time (Fig. 1.25).

Penumbra Effects

A fundamental difference between single-slice and multi-slice scanners is the longitudinal x-ray or dose profile. Theoretically, there should be no difference in dose usage if comparisons are performed at equal spatial resolution and equal image noise. Practically, however, penumbra effects in the axial dose-profile play an important role.

Due to the finite size of the x-ray tube focal spot, the desired rectangular distribution of primary x-rays in the *z*-direction cannot be achieved. In reality, the dose profile is approximated by a trapezoidal function. The shape of this function is a function of scanner-dependent geometric parameters: the size *F* of the focal spot, the distance *D* of the prepatient collimation to the focal spot, and the distance R_F of the focal spot to the center of rotation (isocenter). The relations are illustrated in Fig. 1.26. The triangular tails of the profile are called the penumbra, while the rectangular uniform region is called the umbra. The figure also takes into account the effect of a flying focal spot in the z-direction, as at least one manufacturer offers in the 64-slice scanner. The distance of the two focal spot positions is denoted as Δ. It is approximately equal to the collimated slice thickness S.

In contrast to SSCT, it is not possible with MSCT to use the penumbra regions for imaging. This implies some dose increase with multi-slice CT. With the zFFS we even expect

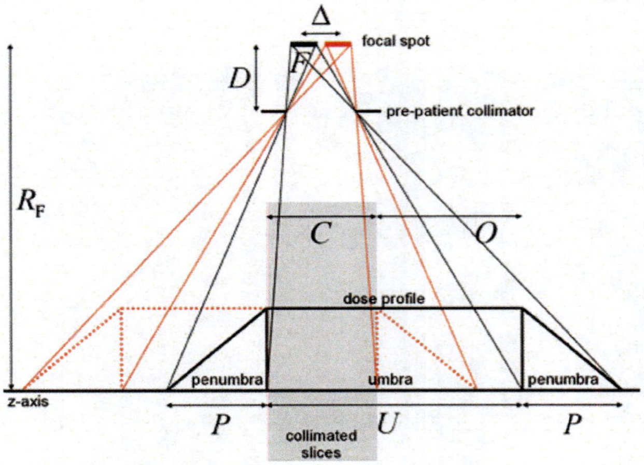

Fig. 1.26 Finite-sized focal spots yield trapezoidal primary dose profiles, whereas rectangular profiles are desired. The penumbra size P is constant, while the size of the umbra varies with the collimation

some further increase in patient dose since the two trapezoidal profiles are shifted by the offset

$$O = \frac{R_F - D}{D}\Delta$$

with respect to each other. Only the overlapping uniform area can be used for imaging and it must at least cover the desired collimation C. Consequently, the umbra size in multi-slice CT must be $U = C + O$ or larger. For the penumbra size we find

$$P = \frac{R_F - D}{D}F$$

accordingly. The total dose is proportional to $P + U$, whereas the dose used for imaging is proportional to C. Hence, the ratio of applied dose to the dose used for imaging is given by

$$1 + \frac{P+O}{C}.$$

The geometric dose increase, compared to SSCT, is given by the second term which evaluates to

$$\frac{R_F - D}{D}\frac{F+\Delta}{C}.$$

Inserting typical values for modern MSCT scanners (R_F = 600 mm, D = 200 mm, F = 0.5 mm) yields a penumbra size of P = 1 mm. Table 1.1 gives examples for MSCT scanners with typical collimations using $\Delta = 0$ without double z-sampling and $\Delta = S$ with zFFS:

Apparently, the dose increase compared to single-slice CT becomes smaller for larger collimations and becomes negligible with the acquisition of 32 slices or more. However, the zFFS yields a slightly lower dose efficiency, which becomes worse for decreasing collimated width.

Table 1.1 Examples for MSCT scanners with typical collimations using $\Delta = 0$ without double z-sampling and $\Delta = S$ with zFFS

Collimation	C	Geometric dose increase (%)
4 × 1 mm	4 mm	25
4 × 2.5 mm	10 mm	10
4 × 5 mm	20 mm	5
16 × 0.75 mm	12 mm	8
16 × 1.5 mm	24 mm	4
32 × 0.6 mm	19.2 mm	5
2·32 × 0.6 mm	19.5 mm (zFFS)	11
64 × 0.5 mm	32 mm	3

Manufacturers' Efforts

Besides issues of protocol optimization, there are a number of technical methods and implementations that are provided by the scientific community and the manufacturers to optimize dose usage and image quality. Basic developments are concerned with tube and detector technology. Improving the tube output, decreasing the focal spot size, and reducing the off-focal radiation directly influence dose usage. Anatomy-dependent prefiltration and shaped filters have significant potential to reduce patient dose, especially for pediatric applications. Detector technology aims at producing faster detectors with higher spatial resolution and higher absorption efficiency. In the future, energy resolving detectors for CT may become available, which would have a positive impact on image quality and thereby on patient dose reduction.

A method directly related to dose optimization is the automatic exposure control (AEC). AEC controls the tube current according to the patient cross-section. This automatic adaptation decreases the tube current for rays of low attenuation (typically the anterior-posterior direction) and increases the tube current for rays of high attenuation (lateral projections) [26–28]. It further compensates for the global changes in the patient cross-section. For example, a lower mean tube current value is used in the head and neck regions than in the shoulder and thorax regions (Fig. 1.27) [29, 30]. Significant dose reduction values are achievable with AEC. Today, implementations based on topogram (or scout view) data that are used to extract the required attenuation information as a function of the rotation angle and the z-position are available from most manufacturers.

A purely software-based dose reduction approach is raw data-based adaptive filtering. Noise is removed from the acquired sinogram by performing dedicated raw data

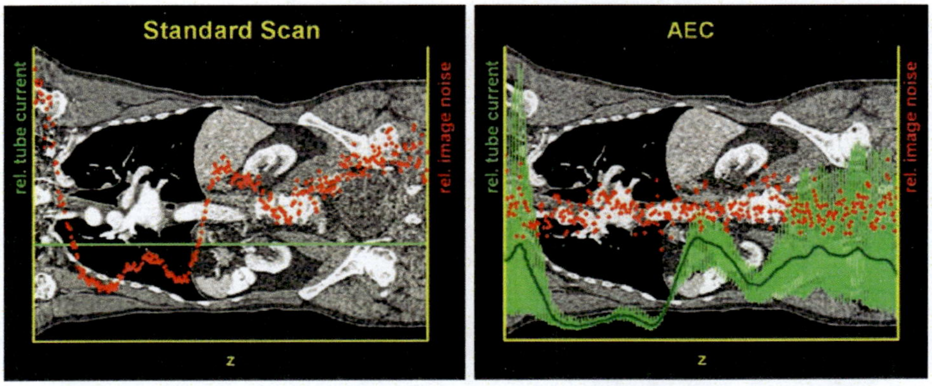

Fig. 1.27 A constant tube current (*green curve*) yields varying image noise (*red dots*). AEC can achieve a desired image noise profile with reduced radiation and improved image quality

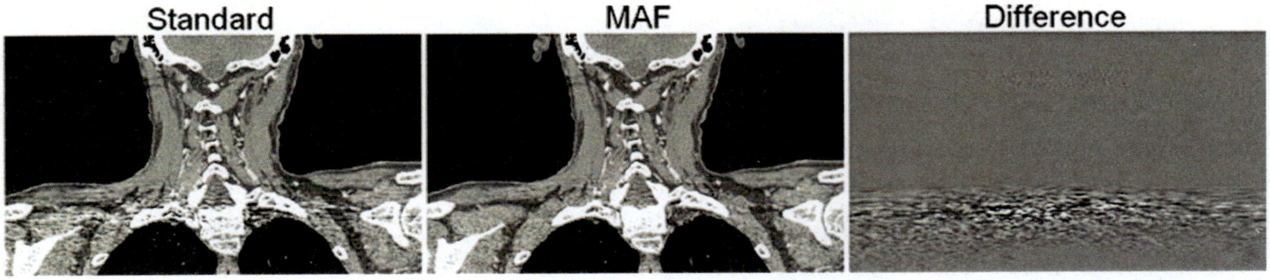

Fig. 1.28 Multi-dimensional adaptive filtering significantly reduces image noise and correlated noise structure (*streaks*). The subtraction image shows that there is no loss in resolution

preprocessing prior to image reconstruction [31–35]. A highly effective method is multidimensional adaptive filtering (MAF) that is especially suited for multi-slice and cone-beam CT scanners (Fig. 1.28). It allows image noise in cross-sections of high eccentricity to be reduced such as the pelvis, thorax, or shoulder without affecting spatial resolution [36, 37]. Thereby, the visibility of low-contrast objects can thus be greatly improved [38].

Summary

Recently, CT imaging has become a true 3D modality that allows complete anatomic regions to be imaged within a few seconds at an isotropic spatial resolution of 0.5–0.7 mm (Fig. 1.29). Modern scanners are cone-beam spiral CT scanners rotating at two to three revolutions per second. The measurement of x-ray attenuation corresponds to the measurement of line integrals through the object. Image reconstruction, which is usually based on filtered backprojection, yields quantitative images that represent the distribution of the attenuation coefficient $\mu(x, y, z)$ converted to Hounsfield units for display. Image noise is in the range of 10–50 HU for typical scans and therefore corresponds to a low relative error of 1–5%.

The improved performance of modern scanners has led to an increased use of CT scanning and, unfortunately, also to an increase in dose. For example, phase-correlated cardiac CT has become an important application, but due to the phase-correlation and the collection of redundant data each exam corresponds to a dose equivalent to 5–10 years of natural background radiation. Several issues of dose reduction (at given image quality) have been discussed in this chapter. Among the most important are user education and protocol optimization. Manufacturers further provide advanced x-ray filtration, tube modulation, automatic exposure control and adaptive filtering techniques to keep dose values at an acceptable level. Exploiting all possibilities will certainly help to significantly reduce dose (Fig. 1.30), and therefore pave the way for scanners with even higher resolution and improved image quality in the future.

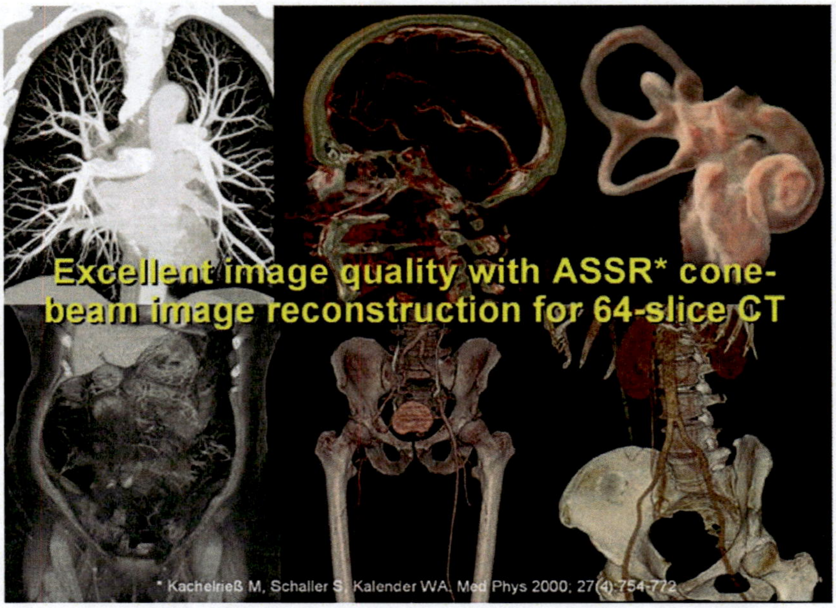

Fig. 1.29 Routine data acquired on a 16-slice CT scanner. Not only the quality of the CT images themselves, but also the display techniques have improved. Here, so-called volume renderings are shown. (Data courtesy of the Department of Diagnostic Radiology, Erlangen, Germany.) (From [7], with permission)

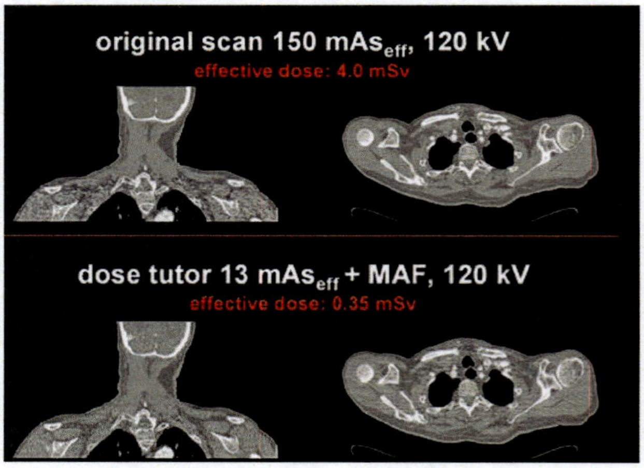

Fig. 1.30 Combining the possibility of retrospective dose reduction using the dose tutor with the capability to perform multidimensional adaptive filtering nicely illustrates the potential of dose reduction

References

1. Kalender WA, Seissler W, Vock P. Single-breath-hold spiral volumetric CT by continuous patient translation and scanner rotation. Radiology 1989;173(P):414.
2. Kalender WA, Seissler W, Klotz E, Vock P. Spiral volumetric CT with single-breathhold technique, continuous transport, and continuous scanner rotation. Radiology 1990;176(1):181–183.
3. Kalender WA. Computed tomography. Fundamentals, system technology, image quality, applications, 2nd edn. Erlangen: Publicis MCD, 2005.
4. Schardt P, Deuringer J, Freudenberger J, Hell E, Knüpfer W, Mattern D, et al. New x-ray tube performance in computed tomography by introducing the rotating envelope tube technology. Med Phys 2004; 31(9):2699–2706.
5. Kachelriess M, Knaup M, Penssel C, Kalender WA. Flying focal spot (FFS) in cone-beam CT. IEEE Medical Imaging Conference Program, San Diego, 2005.
6. Medical electrical equipment. Part 2–44: Particular requirements for the safety of X-ray equipment for computed tomography. Geneva: International Electrotechnical Commission, 1999.
7. Kachelriess M, Schaller S, Kalender WA. Advanced single-slice rebinning in cone-beam spiral CT. Med Phys 2000;27(4):754–772.
8. Feldkamp LA, Davis LC, Kress JW. Practical cone-beam algorithm. J Opt Soc Am 1984;1(6):612–619.
9. Kachelriess M, Knaup M, Kalender WA. Extended parallel backprojection for standard 3D and phase-correlated 4D axial and spiral cone-beam CT with arbitrary pitch and 100% dose usage. Med Phys 2004;31(6):1623–1641.
10. Kachelriess M, Kalender WA. ECG-based phase-oriented reconstruction from sub-second spiral CT scans of the heart. Radiology 1997;205(P):215.
11. Kachelriess M, Kalender WA, Karakaya S, Achenbach S, Nossen J, Moshage W, et al. Imaging of the heart by ECG-oriented reconstruction from subsecond spiral CT scans. In: Glazer G, Krestin G (eds.). Advances in CT IV. Heidelberg: Springer-Verlag, 1998: 137–143.
12. Kachelriess M, Kalender WA. Electrocardiogram-correlated image reconstruction from subsecond spiral CT scans of the heart. Med Phys 1998;25(12):2417–2431.
13. Kachelriess M, Ulzheimer S, Kalender WA. ECG-correlated imaging of the heart with subsecond multi-slice spiral CT. IEEE Trans Med Imaging (Special issue) 2000;19(9):888–901.

14. Taguchi K, Anno H. High temporal resolution for multislice helical computed tomography. Med Phys 2000;27(5):861–872.
15. Flohr T, Ohnesorge B, Kopp AF, Becker C, Halliburton SS, Knez A. A reconstruction concept for ECG-gated multi-slice spiral CT of the heart with pulse-rate adaptive optimization of spatial and temporal resolution. Radiology 2000;217(P):438.
16. Kachelriess M, Fuchs T, Lapp R, Sennst D-A, Schaller S, Kalender WA. Image to volume weighting generalized ASSR for arbitrary pitch 3D and phase-correlated 4D spiral cone-beam CT reconstruction. Proceedings of the 2001 International Meeting on Fully 3D Image Reconstruction, CA, Monterey, 2001.
17. Kachelriess M, Sennst D-A, Maxlmoser W, Kalender WA. Kymogram detection and kymogram-correlated image reconstruction from sub-second spiral computed tomography scans of the heart. Med Phys 2002;29(7):1489–1503.
18. Ulzheimer S, Kalender WA. Assessment of calcium scoring performance in cardiac computed tomography. Eur Radiol 2003;13: 484–497.
19. Lapp RM, Kachelriess M, Fuchs TO, Kalender WA. Variable isotropic resolution in computed tomography using spatial domain filtering. Radiology 2003;225(P):254.
20. Kalender WA, Suess C. Functional imaging with x-ray. In: von Schulthess GK, Henig J (eds.). Functional Imaging. Philadelphia: Lippincott-Raven, 1998:217–240.
21. Kachelriess M. Phase-correlated dynamic CT. IEEE International Symposium on Biomedical Imaging, Arlington, VA, 2004.
22. Ulzheimer S, Muresan L, Kachelriess M, Roemer W, Achenbach S, Kalender WA. Considerations on the assessment of myocardial perfusion with multislice spiral CT (MSCT) scanners. Radiology 2001;22(P):458.
23. http://www.qrm.de.
24. http://www.ct-imaging.de/en/.
25. Schmidt B, Kalender WA. A fast voxel-based Monte Carlo method for scanner- and patient-specific dose calculations in computed tomography. Phys Med 2002;18(2):43–53.
26. Kalender WA, Schmidt B, Zankl M, Schmidt M. A PC program for estimating organ dose and effective dose values in computed tomography. Eur Radiol 1999;9:555–562.
27. Gies M, Kalender WA, Wolf H, Suess C, Madsen MT. Dose reduction in CT by anatomically adapted tube current modulation. I. Simulation studies. Med Phys 1999;26(11):2235–2247.
28. Kalender WA, Wolf H, Suess C. Dose reduction in CT by anatomically adapted tube current modulation. II. Phantom measurements. Med Phys 1999;26(11):2248–2253.
29. Kachelriess M, Leidecker C, Kalender WA. Image quality-oriented automatic expo-sure control (iqAEC) for spiral CT. Radiology 2001;221(P):366.
30. Leidecker C, Kachelriess M, Kalender WA. Comparison of an attenuation-based automatic exposure control (AEC) to alternative methods utilizing localizer radiographs. Eur Radiol 2004;14(Suppl 2):247.
31. Eklundh JO, Rosenfeld A. Imaging smoothing based on neighbor linking. IEEE Trans Pattern Analy Machine Intel 1981;3(6):679–683.
32. Keselbrener L, Shimoni Y, Akselrod S. Nonlinear filters applied on computerized axial tomography. Theory and phantom images. Med Phys 1992;19(4):1057–1064.
33. Lauro KL, Heuscher DJ, Kesavan H. Bandwidth filtering of CT scans of the spine. Radiology 1990;177:307.
34. Hsieh J. Generalized adaptive median filter and their application in computed tomography. SPIE Proc 1994;2298:662–672.
35. Hsieh J. Adaptive streak artifact reduction in computed tomography resulting from excessive x-ray photon noise. Med Phys 1998;25(11): 2139–2147.
36. Kachelriess M, Watzke O, Kalender WA. Generalized multi-dimensional adaptive filtering for conventional and spiral single-slice, multi-slice, and cone-beam CT. Med Phys 2001;28(4):475–490.
37. Kachelriess M, Kalender WA. Inventors. Patent Specification DE 198 53 143, assignee. Germany. 2000.
38. Baum U, Lell M, Kachelriess M, Greess H, Kalender WA, Bautz WA. Raw data-based 3D adaptive filtering for CT scans of the cervicothoracic region: clinical evaluation. Radiology 2000;217(P):413.

Chapter 2
PET Imaging Basics

Timothy G. Turkington

PET Radiotracers

Positron emission tomography (PET) imaging is the injection (or inhalation) of a substance containing a positron emitter, the subsequent detection of the emitted radiation by a scanner, and the computation of a digital image that represents the distribution of the radiotracer in the body.

Nuclide is the name for a specific combination of protons and neutrons that make up a nucleus, and a *radionuclide* is a nonstable nuclide, which will eventually decay. The most common nomenclature for nuclides is to specify the element name or symbol (which in turn specifies the number of protons) and the mass number, which is the sum of protons and neutrons. Typical ways to designate the nuclide with eight protons and eight neutrons are fluorine-18, ^{18}F, and [F-18]. Many radionuclides emit a positron upon decaying. The positron is a subatomic particle identical to the electron in some ways, but opposite in all the ways that particles can be opposite. It therefore has the same mass as an electron, but opposite charge. The symbol e^+ is used to represent the positron.

The time-dependence of the radioactive decay of a radionuclide is typically expressed as its half-life. The half-life is the time during which half of the substance decays. Such a parameterization is appropriate for an exponentially decaying process.

While many radionuclides decay via positron emission, only a few have been used much for PET imaging. The most commonly used are:

Nuclide	Half-life
C-11	20.3 min
N-13	10 min
O-15	124 s
F-18	110 min
Rb-82	75 s

T.G. Turkington (✉)
PET Facility, DUMC 3949, Durham, NC, 27710, USA
e-mail: timothy.turkington@duke.edu

The first four are produced by a particle accelerator (usually a cyclotron). For example, to produce fluorine-18, a beam of accelerated protons hits a target containing water with oxygen-18. From the interaction of a proton and oxygen-18 nucleus, a fluorine-18 nucleus and neutron are emitted.

Rubium-82 comes from the decay of strontium-82, which has a 25-day half-life. A generator containing strontium-82 can be used for approximately 1 month to provide rubidium-82 doses.

Coincidence Detection Physics

Positron Annihilation

After a positron is emitted, it travels a short distance (~1 mm) in tissue, losing energy by exciting and ionizing nearby atoms. Once it has lost almost all kinetic energy, it annihilates with a nearby electron. The product of this annihilation is a pair of photons. Conservation of energy and momentum dictate that the two photons depart in opposite directions, each with energy 511 keV.

Coincidence Detection

The emission of two photons from positron decay is shown in Fig. 2.1. Three possible trajectories are shown. Of all the possible trajectories, only a few, such as the ones shown, would be directed toward the depicted ring of detectors. One pair is shown making a signal in the corresponding detectors. The detectors consist of a scintillator, which converts energy from the 511-keV photon into many lower-energy light photons, and a photomultiplier, which converts the light into an electronic pulse. The creation of two electronic pulses at the same time ("in coincidence") is a signal that there was an annihilation somewhere in the column or line of response (LOR) connecting the associated detectors. During the scan, coincidence counts are recorded for each LOR. The number of coincidence counts obtained on a particular LOR indicates

P. Shreve and D.W. Townsend (eds.), *Clinical PET-CT in Radiology: Integrated Imaging in Oncology*,
DOI 10.1007/978-0-387-48902-5_2, © Springer Science+Business Media, LLC 2011

the amount of radioactivity present along that line during the scan. A parallel set of LORs then measures a projection of the radioactivity distribution, as illustrated in Fig. 2.2. This information is similar to what would be obtained with a collimated gamma camera at a particular angle. An important difference between PET and single photon imaging is that a gamma camera is measuring one projection at a time, whereas a PET camera is measuring all angles simultaneously.

Image Reconstruction

It is typical to store and display the raw data from a PET detector ring in a sinogram. In this format, the lines of response are sorted into parallel subsets, each of which represents a projection angle. Each subset (or angle) is represented by a row in an image. The image reconstruction process starts with raw data (sinograms) and produces cross-sectional images that represent that radioactivity distribution. Many algorithms have been proposed and used for this task. The images of Fig. 2.3 show the results of two popular algorithms for reconstructing PET images, filtered backprojection (FBP), and ordered subsets expectation maximization (OSEM), an iterative algorithm.

The images that result from PET provide quantitative information. After corrections (to be described) and image reconstruction, each image is a pixel-by-pixel representation of the radiotracer concentration at scan time. In some cases, scan protocols are performed to provide more physiologically

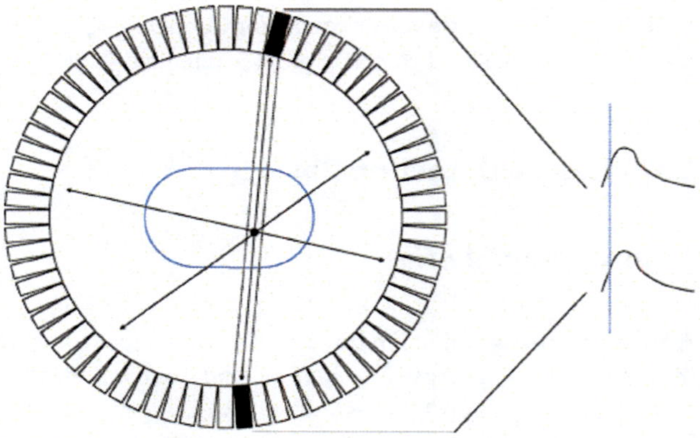

Fig. 2.1 Emission and detection of photons from annihilation point. Three possible trajectories are shown for a specific annihilation site. Many other trajectories are possible, the vast majority of which will not be in the plane of the detector ring. Two detectors indicate hits, and the system records a count for that line of response. The shaded area shows all possible locations from which the two photons could have originated and be detected in these two detectors

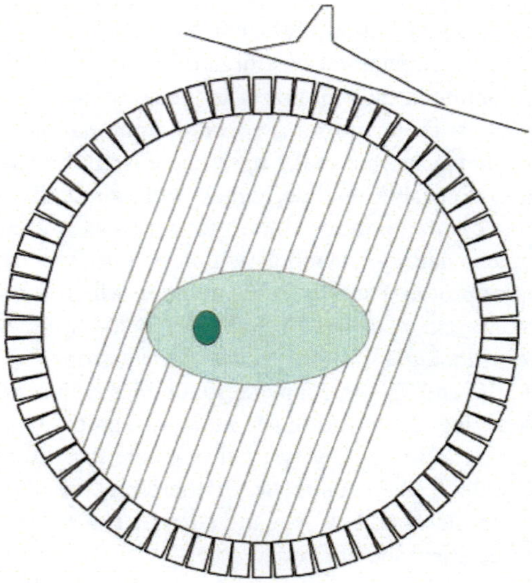

Fig. 2.2 Radioactivity measurement shown for a parallel set of lines of response, equivalent to a projection of the radioactivity distribution. There is a uniform background in the body with a single hot lesion

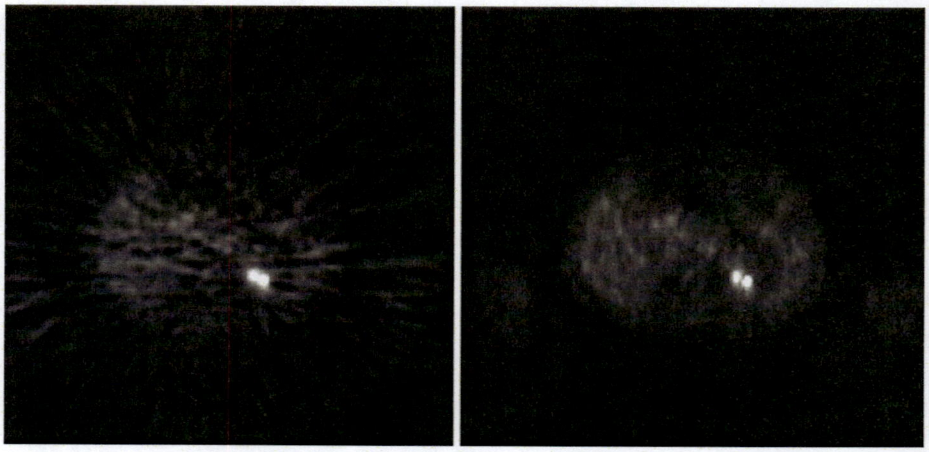

Fig. 2.3 Images reconstructed from the same raw data reconstructed with filtered backprojection (FBP) at left and ordered subsets expectation maximization (OSEM) at right. The most noticeable difference is the noise structure and the prevalence of noise at different activity levels. With FBP, the noise level is similar throughout the image. With OSEM, and other iterative algorithms, the noise levels are highest where the radioactivity levels are highest

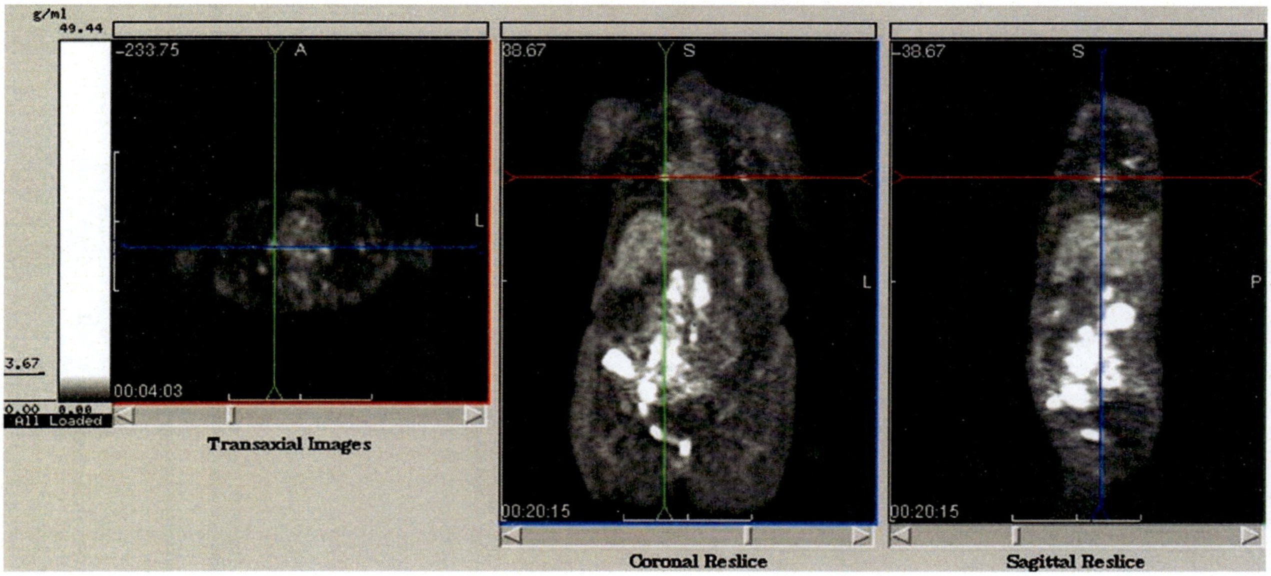

Fig. 2.4 Orthogonally reformatted images from a multi-slice PET acquisition

meaningful quantitation, such as glucose metabolic rate, or blood flow. In general, these require knowledge of the radiotracer concentration in the arterial blood, finely sampled, starting at injection time. Often, they also require the acquisition of dynamic data, that is, repeated scans starting at injection time that show the time course of radiotracer in the tissue of interest.

When multi-slice data are acquired and reconstructed (which is typical for all modern PET systems), it is possible to reformat the data into orthogonal planes, as shown in Fig. 2.4. Additional, oblique planes can be produced, as is typically done with cardiac PET and some brain protocols.

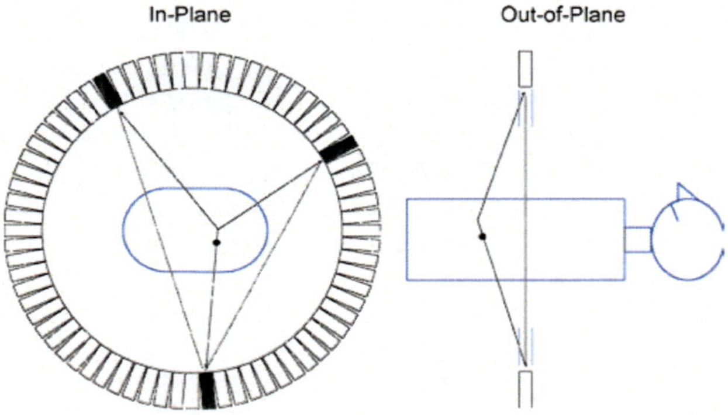

Fig. 2.5 At left two scatter possibilities for an emission photon pair. One leads to a coincidence appearing to come from within the body, and the other leads to a coincidence appearing to come from outside the body. At right is a side view depicting a different scattered event. This event appears to come from within the imaging plane, even though it does not. Shields places in front and behind the detector ring (*dashed line*) would preclude such an event from being detected. On a multi-ring PET system, thin shields can be placed at each of the seams between rings to provide the same effect. In this case they are called septa

Background Events

Background events in PET imaging include the scattered event and the random event. The presence of these background events is detrimental to the quality of the resulting images.

Scattered Events

In a scattered event, one or both of the photons scatters in body tissue, changing direction and losing energy, but it is still detected. In Fig. 2.5 (*left*), two different possible trajectories for a scattered photon are shown. In each case, the resulting line of response does not contain the annihilation location. In one case, the line of response is entirely outside the body, which is a phenomenon unique to PET. (In single-photon emission or transmission modalities, scattered radiation always appears to come from the scattering medium.) In Fig. 2.5 (*right*), a side view of the detector ring is shown, along with a scattered event originating outside the detector ring. Such events add background due to radioactivity outside the field of view. In general, scattered events will have in-plane and out-of-plane components. To limit the number of events with substantial out-of-plane components, shielding can be used in front of and behind the detector ring. Such shields are called septa. In addition to reducing the number of detected scattered events, the septa also reduce the number of events lost to detector dead time and the number of random events.

Random Events

A random event is depicted in Fig. 2.6. The two photons measured are from different annihilations. While it is possible to measure four photons simultaneously from simultaneous annihilations, the probability of all four photons leaving the body unscattered is quite small, and measuring only two photons as depicted in Fig. 2.6 is much more likely than measuring three or four.

The rate at which random coincidences will be measured between detectors A and B is given by

$$R_R = 2\tau R_A R_B, \tag{2.1}$$

were R_A and R_B are the rates at which detectors A and B are detecting photons, respectively, and 2τ is the size of the timing window. This timing window, analogous to the energy window used to discriminate between scattered and nonscattered photons, is set large enough to allow true events to be accepted, but small enough to exclude as many random events as possible. Imprecision in the timing of individual photons is a limit of the detection process, but varies for different detector materials.

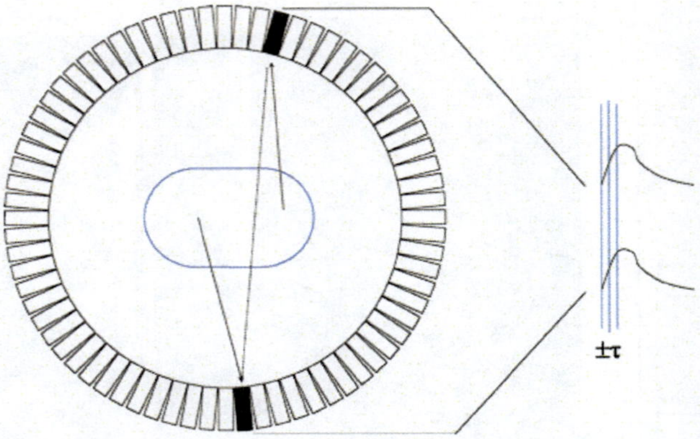

Fig. 2.6 A random event. Annihilation photons from two independent decays are emitted and detected at approximately the same time

Background Events and Count Statistics

Counts measured during a PET scan include true, scattered, and random events:

$$P = T + S + R, \tag{2.2}$$

where *P*, *T*, *S*, and *R*, are the prompt, true, scattered, and random events, respectively, "prompt" being the term for any in-time coincidence. Since it is desired to reconstruct images with *T* events only, an estimate of true events, *T'*, is obtained as follows:

$$T' = P - S' - R', \tag{2.3}$$

where S′ and R′ are estimates of the number of scattered events and random events. These estimates come from the scatter correction and random correction algorithms.

Even with accurate corrections for scattered and random events, there is an inherent detrimental effect of this background. The statistical quality of data with background present is inherently worse than that with no background present. For the *T′* calculated as above, the variance of *T′* is

$$\langle T' \rangle = \langle P \rangle + \langle S' \rangle + \langle R' \rangle, \tag{2.4}$$

where ⟨⟩ represents the variance on the enclosed quantity. That is, the variance of *T* is at least as large as the variance in the prompts measurement, which is dictated by Poisson statistics, and this is worse than the variance on T if there were no background at all.

The noise equivalent count (NEC) parameter has been developed to provide an estimate of image signal to noise ratio as a function of *T*, *S*, and *R*. A simplified version is

$$NEC = \frac{T}{\left(1 + S/T + R/T\right)}. \tag{2.5}$$

This could refer to the statistical quality of data on a specific line of response, or the image quality resulting from all lines of response. In the latter case, background is only considered for lines of response that are within the imaged object. This particular formulation assumes noiseless scatter and random corrections. If the corrections are themselves noisy (such as the delayed event correction for random events), then the terms in the denominator are even larger. With no background, NEC = *T*. As background increases, NEC decreases for a fixed number of trued events.

Extended Axial Field of View and 3D PET

To obtain as many true counts as possible, PET systems incorporate multiple rings of detectors. While this would be of little or no benefit for imaging a single slice of the body, the typical task of whole body imaging can be done with more time spent on each body section if the scanner's axial field of view is greater (assuming a fixed total time is allowed for the whole body scan). Available systems have 18–52 rings of detectors, providing a total axial field of view of at least 15 cm and up to almost 22 cm.

In multi-ring 2D PET, the septa are positioned at the seam between each crystal ring. Coincidences are recorded for photons detected within the same ring (direct planes), and for photons detected in adjacent rings (cross-planes).

In 3D PET, events are recorded regardless of which rings the two photons hit. Since the septa themselves limit the axial acceptance angle, they must be removed for all possible photon trajectories to actually be detected. Compared to the 2D mode of acquisition, 3D PET increases the system sensitivity for true events (approximately fivefold, but varying depending on the specifics of the septa and other factors). The fraction of events that are background rises dramatically, though as well, since septa are not present to limit scattered and random events. In addition, for a specific amount of radiation leaving the body, the individual detectors are much more likely to be hit without septa, and therefore dead-time issues are greater in 3D PET if the injected dose is kept constant.

The clearest benefit of 3D PET is in imaging the brain, where the scatter and random fractions are relatively low. In some applications, a lower injected dose must be used than could have been used in 2D, because of excessive losses due to dead time and the statistical effects of the random events.

The desire to benefit from the increased sensitivity of 3D PET has driven the development of improved radiation detectors. Good energy resolution is one desired trait, since photons lose energy when Compton scattering. The better a detector's energy resolution, the better it can reject scattered photons. Better timing resolution is another desired characteristic. The more precisely the photons' arrival time can be measured, the smaller the timing window can be used, rejecting more random events while retaining true events. Faster scintillators also decrease the number of events lost to dead time.

Revisiting the NEC formula (2.5), 3D imaging has the following direct effects

Increase in T (demonstrated by increased system sensitivity):	+NEC
Increase in S/T (depending on body size and radioactivity distribution):	–NEC
Increase in R/T:	–NEC

In addition, there are indirect effects. For example, the injected dose may need to be lower for 3D, due to count-rate and random event considerations, directly detracting from the increase in T. The degree to which 3D scanning improves final image quality (if at all) depends on a variety of factors.

The currently available PET systems all achieve good image quality through different designs that capitalize on the properties of the detectors being used.

Spatial Resolution and Block Detectors

The spatial resolution of PET images is determined by several factors. Fundamental limits include the positron range (the scanner sees the annihilation location, not the emission location, which is of interest) and photon noncolinearity (the annihilation photon departure trajectories are not exactly 180° apart). Fortunately, these effects are relatively small.

An effect that can be controlled is the size of the detector. If events are always assigned to the correct detector (which is not always the case), smaller detectors yield improved spatial resolution. Several factors have limited the miniaturization of PET detector crystals. An important factor is that it is not feasible to couple each crystal to its own photomultiplier tube, if the crystals are small and numerous. A popular solution is to couple a matrix of crystals (6 × 6, 8 × 8, and up to 13 × 13) to a small number of photomultiplier tubes (four conventional tubes, or two tubes, each with two separate photosensitive regions, or a single tube with four independent quadrants). The relative pulse heights from the four photomultiplier signals are used to determine which crystal in the matrix was actually hit. This scheme leads to a large reduction in the required number of photomultipliers. For example, four photomultipliers on an 8 × 8 crystal matrix is one photomultiplier per 16 crystals. Using such a scheme, a PET system can have 10,000–20,000 crystals, each 4–6 mm in size, with only 1,000 photomultipliers. The reduction is even greater if a single, four-quadrant photomultiplier is used per block.

Attenuation

Attenuation is the loss of coincidence events through scatter or absorption of one or both of the annihilation photons in the body. While the photon energy is higher in PET than that of any single-photon emission radionuclide and the linear attenuation coefficient is relatively low, the requirement of detecting both photons yields a higher overall event-per-event attenuation probability. Fig. 2.7 depicts the quantitative attenuation considerations for coincidence imaging. Fig. 2.8 shows the probability of events surviving attenuation from a uniform distribution in a range of circular cylinder radii for both PET and 140 keV single photons. For objects the size of a head,

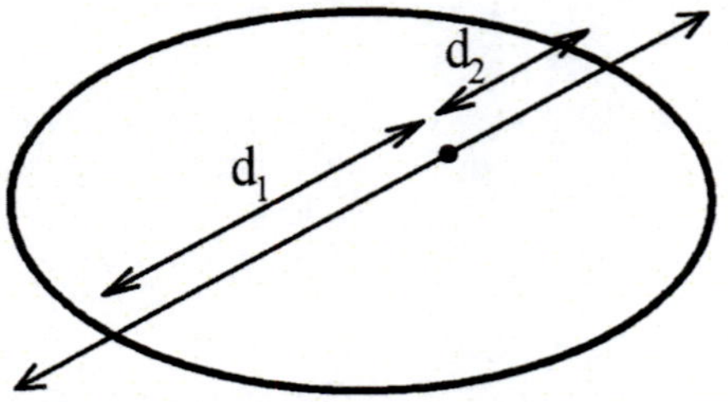

Fig. 2.7 Attenuation effects in PET. Each photon has an attenuation probability (shown for the uniform attenuation case), and the overall probability of both photons surviving is the product of the two. The result is that the overall probability for a specific line of response depends only on the summed trajectories of the two photons, independent of specific location on that line. (From Turkington TG, Attenuation correction in hybrid positron emission tomography. Semin Nucl Med 2000;30:255–267, with permission from Elsevier)

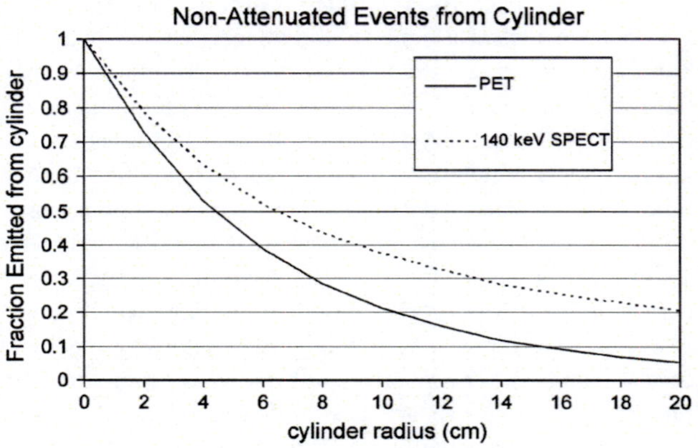

Fig. 2.8 Attenuation effects with increasing object size. For a uniform distribution of radioactivity in a circular cylinder of increasing radii, the probability of the event not being attenuated is shown for PET and for SPECT at 511 keV. (From Turkington TG, Attenuation correction in hybrid positron emission tomography. Semin Nucl Med 2000;30:255–267, with permission from Elsevier)

approximately 25% of photon pairs survive. For a small abdomen, approximately 10% survive. For a very large abdomen, the number surviving is not shown, but can be 1% or smaller.

This loss of events has several implications. First, image quality is degraded because of the decreased counts obtained from large body regions. This effect cannot be corrected. It can only be offset by using a higher injected dose (this is only possible if the scanner can accommodate the increased event rate; the individual detector rates do not decrease with size as quickly as coincidence rates), or a longer scan time. Given the wide range in attenuation differences between very large and very small patients (~10×) it would be very difficult to implement scan time variations of this magnitude in a busy setting. It is important to note that attenuation levels are independent of scanner design or operating parameters. However, attenuation affects are compounded by the effect of increased scatter fraction that occurs with larger bodies, as

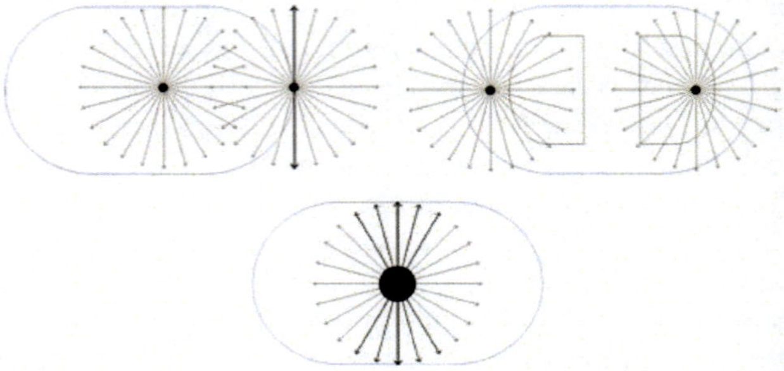

Fig. 2.9 Explanation of attenuation artifacts. *Upper left* depicts the tendency for radiation originating deeper in the body to suffer more attenuation, thereby appearing to have less uptake. The outer contour of the body is an extreme case, in which a narrow band of trajectories has no attenuation at all for either photon. The *upper right* depicts the effect of the lungs. Radiation originating in the lungs, or any other low-density area, will suffer less attenuation, even less than radiation from less-deep structures. At *bottom* is the effect typically seen with the bladder. Radiation emitted in the anterior-posterior direction is much more likely to be detected than radiation emitted in the lateral direction. The resulting reconstructed images show an elongation of the bladder in the direction of low attenuation, and depleted areas on the sides. This phenomenon would be true of any hot object with highly nonisotropic attenuation

well, and its additional effect on count statistics, as reflected in NEC.

Another implication of attenuation is the loss of quantitation in measurement of radioactivity concentration and other quantities derived from it. Tenfold or greater errors not only need to be corrected, but the correction must also be very accurate if any quantitative use is to be made.

An additional factor with attenuation is the introduction of image artifacts; that is, features that make the image qualitatively unrepresentative of the actual radioactivity distribution. Three general types of PET attenuation artifacts are explained in Fig. 2.9 and depicted in Fig. 2.10.

Attenuation Correction

While the statistical effect of lost counts and the resulting image noise cannot be compensated, quantitative accuracy can be restored and attenuation-related artifacts can be removed with attenuation correction. Attenuation correction generally means taking into account the attenuation factor for each line of response; that is, the probability that photons emitted along each line of response will survive. The reciprocal of this factor, the attenuation correction factor, can be applied for each line of response, resulting in an estimate of the number of counts that would have been attained on each LOR.

If the outer contour of the body is known, and if all of the tissue within that boundary is of uniform density, then the

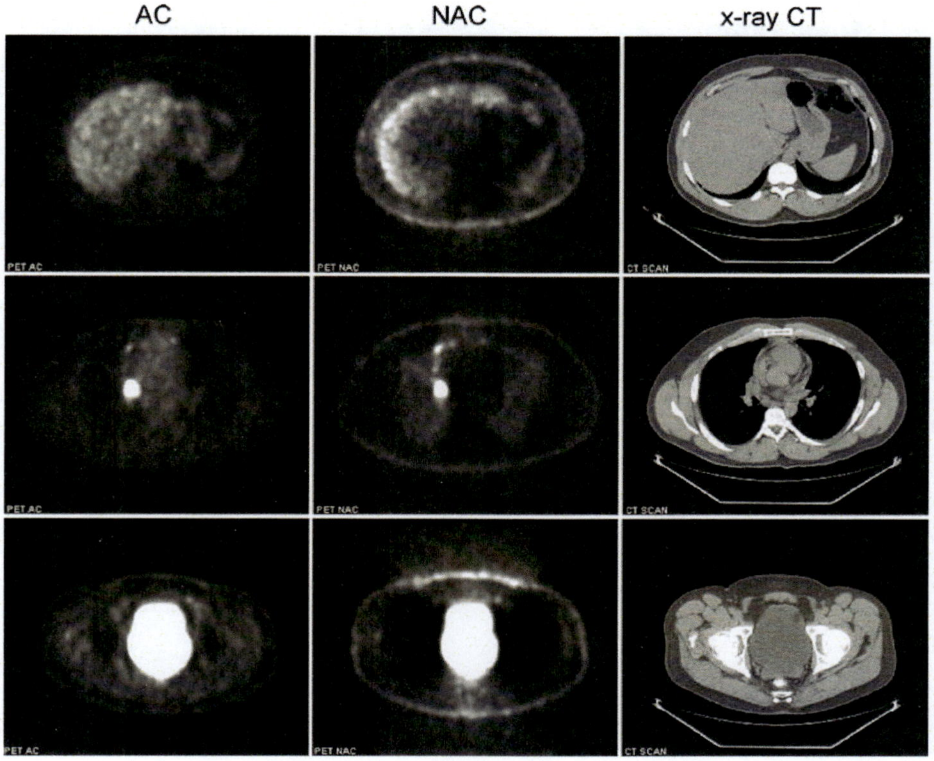

Fig. 2.10 Attenuation artifacts in PET. The three columns are attenuation-corrected PET (*left*), non-attenuation-corrected PET (*middle*), and x-ray CT (*right*) for anatomical reference. Notable artifacts in the non-corrected PET are the non-uniformity of the liver (*upper image*), the bright outer contour (all images), the apparent high activity in the lungs (*middle image*), the false high and low activity areas around the bladder (*lower image*). An additional effect is that concave areas in the body surface are not concave in the noncorrected image. That is, radioactivity shows up falsely in regions that were actually air. This phenomenon occurs internally, as well, for example in the top image a gaseous region adjacent to the liver shows activity falsely in the noncorrected image that is fixed by the attenuation correction

attenuation factor for each LOR can be calculated using the simple attenuation formula $e^{-\mu d}$, and the corresponding correction factor calculated and applied. These criteria are never strictly met in any section of the body, because of bone and lung, but it is common to use calculated attenuation correction for brain imaging if quantitation is not being used.

More accurate attenuation correction can be obtained with a transmission scan. A conventional scheme for PET transmission scanning uses one or more Ge-68 rods that orbit around the body, inside the detector ring for 1–5 min per bed position (Fig. 2.11). Ge-68 is a positron emitter, and therefore produces 511 keV photon pairs. The rod is as long as the axial field of view of the system. A transmission coincidence is measured similarly to an emission coincidence. Attenuation factors for each line of response are determined by dividing the counts obtained during a transmission scan by the counts obtained during a blank scan, which is a transmission scan performed with an empty gantry. Such radionuclide-based transmission scans have the benefits of using the same detectors as are used for emission events, and of having high accuracy, since the attenuation factors are determined with the same photon energy as is being corrected. The fundamental limit is that of statistics. There is a limit in the measurable transmission count rate, because of the PET detectors' limits (and exacerbated by the proximity of the source to the nearby detector ring). For a reasonable scan time (preferably shorter than the emission scan, since that provides the fundamental information), the limited number of counts translates into additional noise in the corrected emission image.

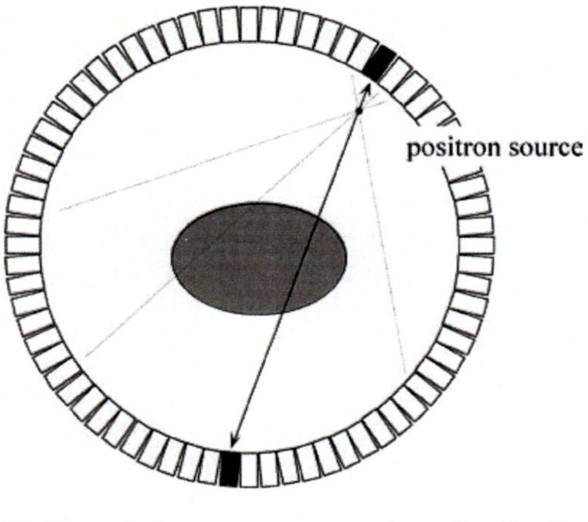

Fig. 2.11 Transmission scan geometry using a Ge-68 radionuclide source. The source orbits around the body, illuminating all possible lines of response, and by comparison with a blank scan, yielding the attenuation factors for each line

A third option for attenuation correction is to use x-ray CT as the transmission data. Much short scans provide much lower-noise corrections. The use of x-ray CT for PET attenuation correction and the other considerations for combined PET-CT scanners are discussed in a later chapter.

PET Quantitation

Quantitative use of PET data requires accurate corrections for attenuation, scatter, random events, and dead time. The first step in quantitation is producing images whose pixel values represent the radioactivity concentration of the imaged object. In addition to the various corrections, calibration factors must be determined to translate the corrected counts to radioactivity values.

PET can be used to measure physiologic parameters, such as blood flow, or glucose metabolic rate, quantitatively. Quantitative measurements such as these require knowledge of the arterial blood radioactivity concentration as a function of time, starting at the injection, and can require multiple time points to be imaged (dynamic scanning).

Short of quantitating physiological parameters, the SUV (standardized uptake value) is an index that normalizes for the injected dose and body size in a simple way. The SUV is calculated as

$$SUV = \frac{\mathit{Radioactivity\ concentration}}{(\mathit{Injected\ dose})/(\mathit{Body\ mass})}. \tag{2.6}$$

Dividing by the injected dose normalizes the measured concentration to yield a dose-independent index. Multiplying by body mass (or dividing by it in the denominator) normalizes for the effect that a larger body has more competing tissue than a small body, compared to a given size tissue of interest. An alternate perspective is that the SUV is the concentration of tracer measured in a region, divided by the average concentration throughout the body. Since some of the tracer will typically have been voided by the time of the scan, this is not exactly correct, and an SUV of 1 will therefore be higher than the body average. Individual pixels can be calculated as SUV values, and regions-of-interest statistics (typically maximum and mean) can be reported in SUV.

References

1. Cherry SR, Sorenson JA, Phelps ME. Physics in Nuclear Medicine, 3rd edn. Philadephia: Saunders, 2003.
2. Townsend DR, Bendriem B. The Theory and Practice of 3D PET. Dordrecht: Kluwer, 1998.
3. Turkington TG. Introduction to PET instrumentation. J Nucl Med Technol 2001;29:4-11.
4. Wernick MW, Aarsvold JN. Emission Tomography: the Fundamentals of PET and SPECT. San Diego: Elsevier, 2004.

Chapter 3
Design and Operation of Combined PET-CT Scanners

David W. Townsend

Introduction

The recent development of combined PET-CT instrumentation is an important evolution in imaging technology. Since the introduction of the first prototype computed tomography (CT) scanner in the early 1970s, tomographic imaging has made significant contributions to the diagnosis and staging of disease. Rapid commercial development followed the introduction of the first CT scanner in 1972 and within 3 years of its appearance more than 12 companies were marketing, or intending to market, CT scanners; about half that number actually market CT scanners today. With the introduction of magnetic resonance imaging (MRI) in the early 1980s, CT was, at that time, predicted to last another 5 years at most before being replaced by MRI for anatomic imaging. Obviously this did not happen, and today, with multi-slice detectors, spiral acquisition, and subsecond rotation times, CT continues to develop and play a major role in clinical imaging, especially for anatomic regions outside the brain.

Functional imaging, as a complement to anatomic imaging, has been the domain of nuclear medicine ever since the early 1950s. Initially, planar imaging with the scintillation (gamma) camera invented by Anger in 1958 was the mainstay of nuclear medicine. Even today, the widely used scintillation camera still follows Anger's original design, comprising a large sodium iodide crystal and collimator, with photomultiplier tubes as the photo detectors. In modern nuclear medicine, planar scintigraphy has been extended to tomography by the development of single photon emission tomography (SPECT), which can be helpful for certain clinical applications. Although early SPECT systems actually predated CT, the real growth in SPECT did not occur until after the appearance of CT when similar reconstruction algorithms to those used in CT were applied to the reconstruction of parallel projections from SPECT data acquired by a rotating gamma camera.

Functional imaging with positron-emitting isotopes was first proposed in the early 1950s as an imaging technique that could offer greater sensitivity than conventional nuclear medicine techniques with single photon-emitting isotopes. The SPECT collimator is eliminated and replaced by electronic collimation – the coincident detection of two photons from positron annihilation – greatly increasing the sensitivity of the imaging system. However, other than some early prototypes in the 1960s, instrumentation to image positron emitters did not emerge seriously until the 1970s, and the first commercial PET scanners date from around 1980, about the time MRI also became commercially available. PET was initially perceived as a complex and expensive technology requiring both a cyclotron to produce the short-lived PET radioisotopes and a PET scanner to image the tracer distribution in the patient. Consequently, during the 1970s, PET did not experience the explosive growth of CT, nor during the 1980s, the comparable growth of MRI. In fact, it was not until the 1990s that PET became recognized as an important technique for imaging cancer by mapping glucose utilization throughout the body with FDG. The elevated utilization of glucose by malignant cells allows cancerous tissue to be identified anywhere in the body, even though it may have no anatomic correlate that would allow identification on a CT scan. The effectiveness of FDG-PET imaging for diagnosing and staging malignant disease was officially recognized when the Centers for Medicare and Medicaid Services (CMS) approved reimbursement for a number of cancers in 1998. Following that decision, the application of FDG-PET for imaging cancer expanded rapidly, although still not at a rate that has ever fully rivaled the growth of the dominant anatomic imaging modalities CT and MRI during the 1970s and 1980s, respectively.

The corporate environments that developed these different imaging technologies, the medical specialties of radiology and nuclear medicine that were responsible for acquiring and operating them and the differing chronology of clinical

D.W. Townsend (✉)
Singapore Bioimaging Consortium,
11, Biopolis Way, #02-02 Helios,
Singapore 138667
e-mail: david_townsend@sbic.a-star.edu.sg

P. Shreve and D.W. Townsend (eds.), *Clinical PET-CT in Radiology: Integrated Imaging in Oncology*,
DOI 10.1007/978-0-387-48902-5_3,

acceptance described above each contributed to ensuring CT and PET followed separate and distinct developmental paths. Both modalities have their strengths; CT scanners image anatomy with high spatial resolution, although malignant disease can generally only be identified from the presence of abnormal masses or from size changes in lymph nodes. PET, on the other hand can identify a functional abnormality in, for example, a normal sized lymph node – although accurate localization of the node may be difficult, or even impossible, from the PET scan alone. To initiate the evolution in imaging technology that was required to physically integrate CT and PET [1] in a single device, initial skepticism from both the corporate environment and the medical profession had to be overcome. The key was to design and develop a research prototype PET-CT scanner within the context of NIH grant-funded collaboration between academia and industry. The first combined PET-CT prototype scanner was completed in 1998 [2] and clinical evaluation began in June of that year. The initial studies with the prototype [3–6] demonstrated a number of significant advantages of PET-CT: that functional abnormalities could now be accurately localized, that normal benign uptake of a nonspecific tracer such as FDG could be distinguished from uptake due to disease, and that confidence in reading both the PET and the CT increases significantly by having the anatomic and functional images routinely available and accurately aligned for every patient.

While it may seem that, in many cases, it would be equally effective to view separately acquired CT and PET images for a given patient on adjacent computer displays, with [7] or without software registration, experience in the past 4 years with commercial PET-CT scanners has highlighted numerous unique advantages of the new technology. While a number of these advantages were anticipated in the original PET-CT proposal, others were unexpected and have only emerged since the technology became more widely available for clinical imaging.

The purpose of this chapter is to review the design objectives of this emerging technology and present the status of current instrumentation, including that of CT-based attenuation correction. Operation of the technology within the clinical setting opens up new possibilities for disease diagnosis, staging and monitoring response to therapy. Such applications are discussed in depth in other chapters in this book, and thus only general protocol definitions and some specific refinements are presented here.

Design Objectives

The development of the first PET-CT prototype was initiated in 1992 with the objectives to integrate CT and PET within the same device, to use the CT images for the attenuation and scatter correction of the PET emission data, and to explore the use of anatomic images to define tissue boundaries for PET reconstruction. Thus, the goal was to construct a device with both clinical CT and clinical PET capability so that a full anatomic and functional scan could be acquired in a single session, obviating the need for the patient to undergo an additional clinical CT scan. The original prototype [2] combined a single-slice spiral CT (Somatom AR.SP, Siemens Medical Solutions, Forchheim, Germany) with a rotating ECAT ART scanner (CPS Innovations, Knoxville, TN), as shown in Fig. 3.1. The components for both imaging modalities were mounted on the same mechanical support and rotated together at 30 rpm. However, by the time the prototype became operational in 1998, neither the CT nor the PET components were state of the art. Nevertheless, the work convincingly demonstrated the feasibility of combining the

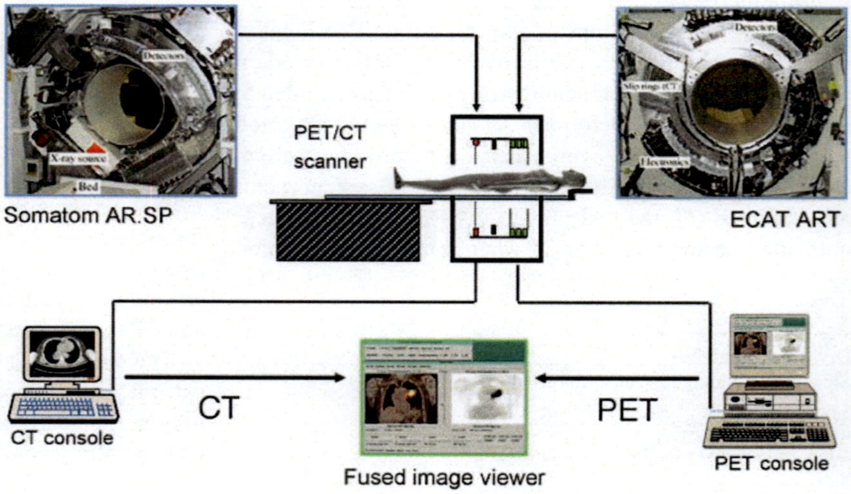

Fig. 3.1 The design of the original PET-CT prototype developed by Beyer et al. [2] showing schematically the combination of the CT and PET components on a single rotating support

two technologies into a single device that could acquire coregistered anatomic and functional images without the need for software realignment.

As mentioned, a number of important lessons emerged during the clinical evaluation program that followed the installation of the prototype and covered the years from 1998 until 2001 [3–6]. Over 300 cancer patients were scanned and the studies highlighted the advantages of being able to accurately localize functional abnormalities, to distinguish normal uptake from pathology, minimize the effects of both external and internal patient movement, and reduce scan time and increase patient throughput by using the CT images for attenuation correction of the PET data. Even during the initial evaluation it was evident that coregistered anatomy increases the confidence of physicians reading the study. Radiologists rapidly came to appreciate that coregistered functional images help to focus attention on regions of abnormal uptake, especially regions with no evident pathology on CT.

Despite concerns over the likely cost and operational complexity of combined PET-CT technology, the major vendors of medical imaging equipment nevertheless recognized a market for PET-CT. The first commercial design comprised a CT scanner and a PET scanner enclosed within a single gantry cover and operated from separate consoles. The design involved little integration at any level and was intended primarily to be the first commercial PET-CT scanner on the market, as indeed it was. The PET scanner included retractable septa and standard PET transmission sources were offered as an alternative to CT-based attenuation correction. Retractable septa allowed the device to acquire PET data in either 2D or 3D mode. Within a few months, another PET-CT design (Fig. 3.2) from a different vendor appeared that had no septa and acquired data fully in 3D [8]. Since no mechanical storage was required for retractable septa and standard PET transmission sources were not offered, the design was compact; the patient port was a full 70 cm diameter throughout and the overall tunnel length was only 110 cm. Integration of the control and display software allowed the scanner to be operated from a single console. As with these and most subsequent commercial designs, both the CT and the PET were clinical state-of-the-art systems, following the objectives of the original prototype. A more open concept PET-CT with spacing between the CT and PET scanners has since been offered by two other vendors, allowing greater access to the patient and reducing possible claustrophobic effects of the other designs.

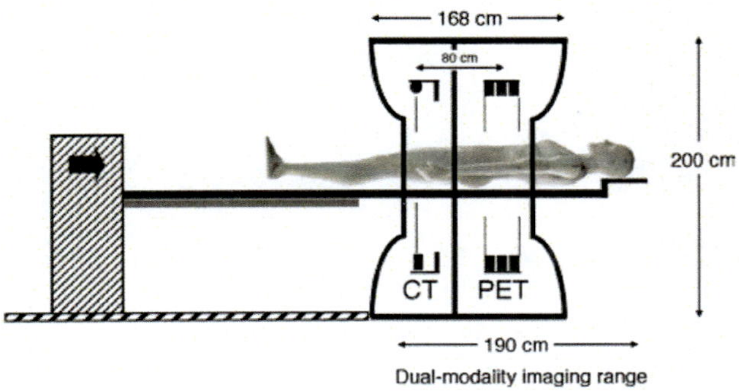

Fig. 3.2 A schematic of a current PET-CT scanner design marketed by Siemens as the *biograph* (Siemens Medical Solutions, Chicago). The design incorporates a multi-detector spiral CT scanner and an LSO PET scanner. The dimensions of the gantry are 228 cm wide, 200 cm high, and 168 cm deep. The separation of the CT and PET imaging fields is about 80 cm. The co-scan range for acquiring both CT and PET is up to 190 cm. The patient port diameter is 70 cm

The hardware integration of recent PET-CT designs, therefore, has remained rather minimal. The advantage is that vendors can then benefit more easily from separate advances in both CT and PET instrumentation. In the past few years, spiral CT technology has progressed from single to dual-slice, to 4, 8, 16, and, most recently, 64 and 128 slices; in parallel, CT rotation times have deceased to less than 0.4 s, resulting in very rapid scanning protocols. Advances in PET technology have been equally dramatic with the introduction of new faster scintillators such as gadolinium oxyorthosilicate (GSO) and lutetium oxyorthosilicate (LSO), faster acquisition electronics and higher resolution detectors (smaller pixels). Currently, a top-of-the-line PET-CT configuration might comprise a 128-slice CT scanner and an LSO-based PET scanner with 4-mm pixels. However, while the 128-slice CT configuration is targeted primarily for cardiac applications, the greatest impact of PET-CT to date has been in the oncology field for which a 16-slice CT scanner is generally considered adequate.

Current Technology for PET-CT

Currently six vendors offer PET-CT designs: GE Healthcare, Hitachi Medical, Philips Medical Systems, Toshiba Medical Corporation, Mediso Medical Imaging Systems and Siemens Healthcare. With respect to the offerings from the various vendors, GE Healthcare still offers BGO-based scanners with retractable septa that can acquire PET data in both 2D and 3D mode. The *Discovery* series incorporates PET detectors that are 4.7 mm × 6.3 mm × 30 mm in size and are configured with a 15.7 cm axial FOV and a 70 cm patient port. The PET components are combined with an 8-, 16- or 64-slice CT scanner. The most widely-installed models are the *Discovery* ST and the STE; the version with the 64-slice CT is the VCT. In 2008, GE announced the Discovery 600 (Fig. 3.3a), an oncology-oriented BGO-based PET/CT with a 70 cm patient port and a patient bed certified up to 500 lbs. More recently, GE announced the Discovery 690 (Fig. 3.3b),

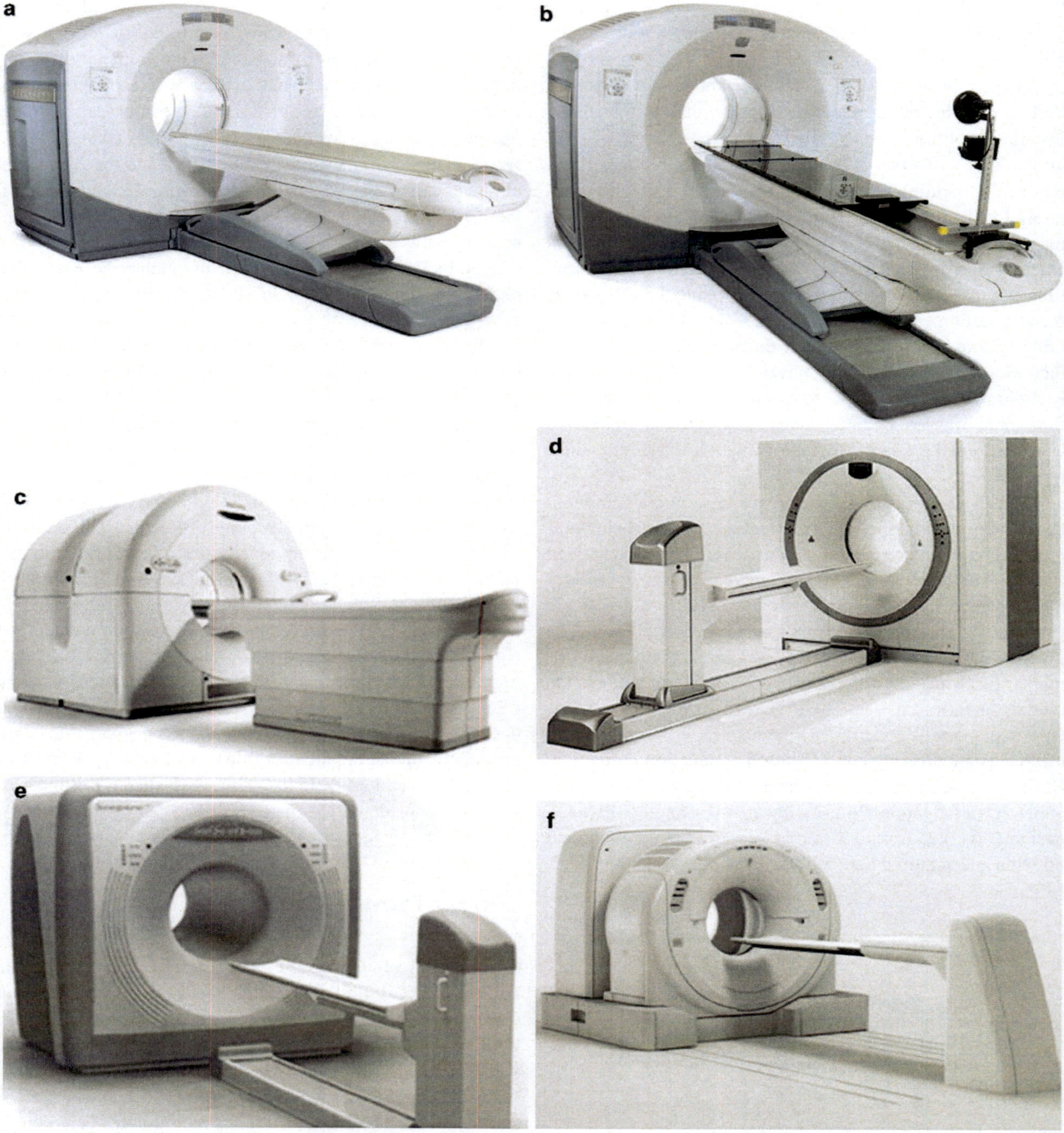

Fig. 3.3 Current commercial PET-CT scanners from five major vendors of medical imaging equipment: (**a**) GE Discovery PET/CT 600 for the BGO version (GE Healthcare); (**b**) GE Discovery PET/CT 690 for the Lutetium version (GE Healthcare); (**c**) *Gemini* (Philips Medical Systems); (**d**) *biograph* (Siemens Medical Solutions); (**e**) *SeptreP3* (Hitachi Medical Systems); (**f**) *Aquiduo* (Toshiba Medical Corporation)

an LYSO-based PET/CT scanner with 4.2 × 6.3 × 25 mm^3 detectors; this design also features time-of-flight (TOF) acquisition. The Discovery series features motion-free gating developed especially for tumors of the lung.

Philips Medical Systems has taken a different approach in their open design *Gemini* PET/CT (Fig. 3.3c). The design features a space between the CT and PET scanners that allows access to the patient while in the scanner. The original

Gemini GXL incorporated gadolinium oxyorthosilicate (GSO) detectors that were 4 mm × 4 mm × 30 mm. The detectors are somewhat different to the block-based systems employing instead a curved pixilated design with a continuous light guide (PIXELAR). The GXL incorporates a 6-, 10-, 16- or 64-slice CT scanner. The most recent model ranks as the first commercial TOF PET/CT scanner, the *Gemini* TF. This system is the same open design but with LYSO detectors, 4 mm × 4 mm × 22 mm in size. The scanner is operated with a short, 3.8 ns coincidence window and a TOF timing resolution of around 585 ps. Data acquisition is fully in 3D (no septa) and the axial FOV is 18 cm. The original patient port diameter was 70 cm, but recently Philips announced their Big Bore version that targets radiation oncology applications with an 85 cm diameter patient port and an integrated flat-table also certified up to a patient weight of 500 lbs.

The third of the major PET/CT vendors, Siemens Healthcare, offers the *Biograph* TruePoint PET/CT series of scanners (Fig. 3.3d). This design is also fully 3D acquisition and the block detectors are LSO with 4 mm × 4 mm × 20 mm pixels. The axial FOV can be either 16.2 cm or, with the extended FOV option (TrueV), 21.6 cm; the patient port is 70 cm and the detectors are operated with a 4.5 ns coincidence window. The *Biograph* TruePoint incorporates a 6-, 40-, or 64-slice Definition CT scanner. Recently, Siemens announced their first molecular CT (mCT), a new highly integrated design that features similar PET components to those of the *Biograph* TruePoint, together with a 64- or 128-slice CT scanner, a 78 cm patient port and a re-designed patient bed certified up to 500 lbs. The detectors are operated with a 4.1 ns coincidence window. The gantry depth is a full 20 cm less than that of the TruePoint and is therefore highly compact. PET image reconstruction is based on a system model that includes the point spread function of the scanner. The detectors from the Siemens Biograph are incorporated into the Aquiduo (Toshiba Medical; Fig. 3.3f) in combination with the 16-slice Aquillion CT scanner (Toshiba Medical); a unique feature of this device is that the bed is fixed and the CT and PET gantries move on floor mounted rails to image the patient.

While to date, with the exception of the Siemens mCT scanner, there has been little actual effort to increase the level of hardware integration, there has been significant effort to reduce the complexity and increase the reliability of system operation by adopting a more integrated software approach. In early designs, CT and PET data acquisition and image reconstruction were performed on separate systems accessing a common data base. Increasingly, functionality has been combined so as to reduce cost and complexity and increase reliability. Similar considerations of cost and complexity for the hardware may lead, in the future, to greater levels of integration. The likelihood is that these designs will be application-specific, incorporating a 16-slice CT for oncology and a 64-slice CT for cardiology. There will undoubtedly be a demand for more cost-effective, entry-level PET-CT designs for oncology such as the Hitachi *SceptreP3*. A scan of a 206 lb lymphoma patient acquired on a *Biograph* 16 HI-REZ PET-CT scanner is shown in Fig. 3.5 to illustrate state-of-the-art image quality; despite the large size of the patient, the coronal PET image (Fig. 3.5a) is of good quality, with the corresponding PET-CT image shown in Fig. 3.5b. Many more such examples will be found throughout this book.

Even though all PET-CT designs offer clinical quality CT and PET, many centers elect to operate with low-dose, non-diagnostic CT for attenuation correction and localization only. This approach does not therefore use the PET-CT to its

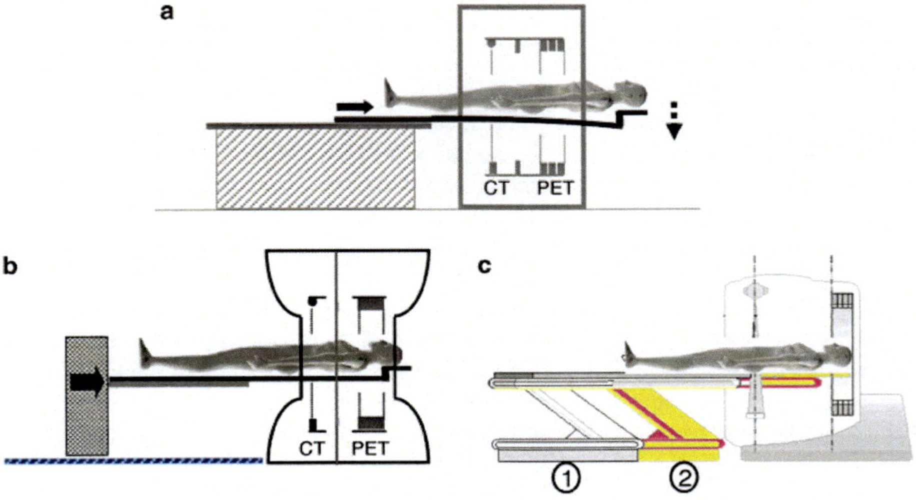

Fig. 3.4 (**a**) An illustration of the problem of the increasing bed deflection as the patient pallet moves through the scanner; this is caused by the changing cantilever point. Solutions include supporting the pallet throughout the tunnel, or (**b**) fixing the cantilever point such that the entire bed assembly moves on floor-mounted rails, and (**c**) a dual-position bed where position 1 is for the CT scan and position 2 is for the PET scan

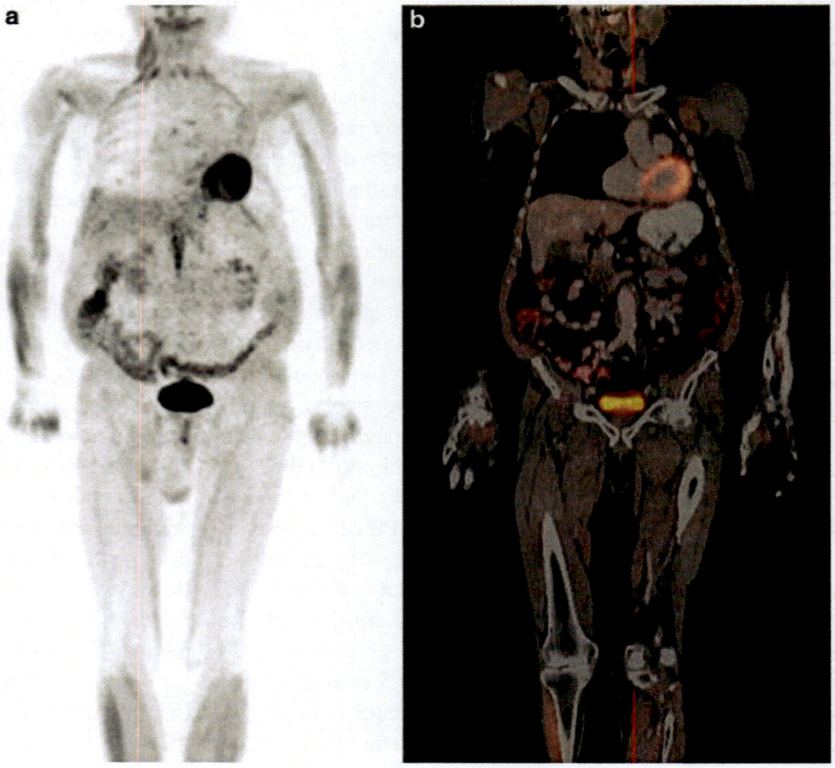

Fig. 3.5 A 206 lb lymphoma patient scanned on the PET-CT; the patient was injected with 10.1 mCi of ^{18}FDG and scanned 89 min post-injection. The PET scan was acquired with 4-min per bed position. The images show a coronal section of (**a**) the PET scan, and (**b**) the corresponding PET-CT scan

full, clinical potential and hopefully, as PET-CT is introduced more widely into clinical routine, direct referrals for PET-CT will increase. With over 5,000 PET-CT scanners installed worldwide, PET-CT now represents 100% of all PET sales. In the 9 years since the first commercial PET-CT was introduced, the modality has had a far-reaching impact on medical imaging, particularly for staging malignant disease and monitoring response to therapy.

CT-Based Attenuation Correction

The acquisition of accurately coregistered anatomic and functional images is obviously a major strength of the combined PET-CT scanner. However, as mentioned, an additional advantage of this approach is the possibility to use the CT images for attenuation correction of the PET emission data, eliminating the need for a separate, lengthy PET transmission scan. The use of the CT scan for attenuation correction not only reduces whole-body scan times by at least 40%, but also provides essentially noiseless ACFs compared to those from standard PET transmission measurements. Since the attenuation values are energy-dependent, the correction factors derived from a CT scan at mean photon energy of 70 keV must be scaled to the PET energy of 511 keV. The CT photon energy represents the mean energy of the polychromatic x-ray beam.

Scaling algorithms typically use a bilinear function to transform the attenuation values above and below a given threshold with different factors [11, 12]. The composition of biologic tissues other than bone exhibit little variation in their effective atomic number and can be well represented by a mixture of air and water. Bone tissue does not follow the same trend as soft tissue because of the calcium and phosphorus content and thus a different scaling factor is required that reflects instead a mixture of water and cortical bone. The break-point between the two mixture types has been variously set at 300 HU [11] and at 0 HU [12]. However, some tissue types, such as muscle (~60 HU) and blood (~40 HU), have Hounsfield units greater than zero and yet are clearly not a water-bone mix. A break-point around 100 HU would therefore appear to be optimal, as shown in Fig. 3.6. Hounsfield units define the linear attenuation coefficients normalized to water, and thus independent of the kVp of the x-ray tube. The scale factor for the air-water mix below approximately 100 HU will be independent of the kVp of the tube. This does not apply to the water-bone mixing and therefore the scale factor for bone will be kVp dependent [13]. The scaled CT images are first interpolated from CT to PET spatial resolution, scaled on a pixel-by-pixel basis using the function in Fig. 3.6, and

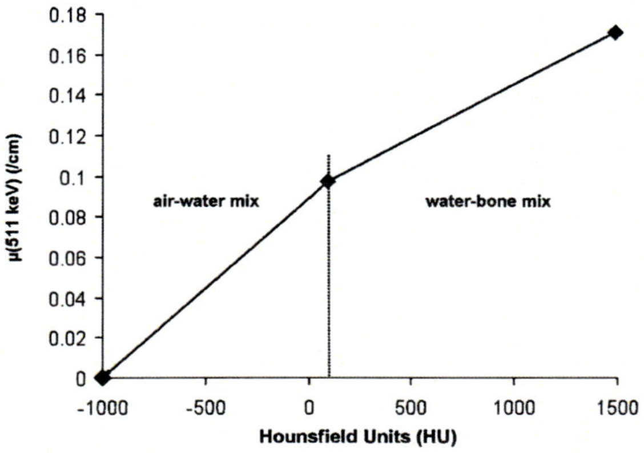

Fig. 3.6 The bi-linear scaling function used to convert CT numbers to linear attenuation values at 511 keV. The graph shows the linear attenuation coefficient at 511 keV as a function of the corresponding CT value (HU), based on measurements made with the Gammex 467 electron density CT phantom using tissue-equivalent materials. The separation between soft tissue (air-water mixing model) and bone-like tissue (water-bone mix) is around 100 HU

then the ACFs are generated by reprojection of the scaled images.

Intravenously injected iodinated contrast is used in CT to enhance attenuation values in the vasculature by increasing the photoelectric absorption compared with blood and resulting in a 40% change in attenuation. At the PET energy, where the photoelectric effect is negligible, the presence of contrast has only a 2% effect on attenuation. However, if contrast-enhanced pixels are misidentified as a water-bone mix, the scaling factor will be incorrect and the erroneously scaled pixels may generate artifacts in the PET image. Many thousands of PET-CT scans have now been performed in the presence of intravenous contrast and experience has shown that contrast administration does not generally cause a problem that could potentially interfere with the diagnostic value of PET-CT [14]. Oral contrast is administered to visualize the gastrointestinal tract and the distribution of the contrast material is rather variable, both in spatial distribution and level of enhancement. Modifications to the basic scaling algorithm have been introduced to distinguish oral contrast enhancement from bone [15], and strategies discussed elsewhere in this book have been developed that minimize or eliminate problems due to both intravenous and oral contrast. The modified algorithm can, to some extent, also reduce artifacts due to catheters and metallic objects in the patient. A more detailed discussion of artifacts arising from metallic objects can be found elsewhere in this book.

Avoiding the administration of contrast would, of course, eliminate all such problems. However, standard-of-care in CT dictates the use of either intravenous or oral contrast, or both, as in the case of the abdomen and pelvis. An obvious way to avoid such problems is to perform two CT scans: a clinical CT with appropriate contrast administration, and a low-dose, noncontrast CT for attenuation correction and coregistration. This two-scan approach, however, would further increase the radiation exposure to the patient.

One of the aspects of CT-based attenuation correction that has received the most attention over the past few years is the mismatch between CT and PET due to respiration. While the CT scan can be acquired with breathhold, especially with the new, fast CT scanners, such a procedure is obviously not possible with the lengthier PET scan. There are, therefore, a number of different respiration strategies that aim at minimizing the effects of this mismatch and reducing the incidence of artifacts, and they will be discussed in the next two chapters. A more detailed review of possible respiration protocols can be found in [16].

PET-CT Protocols

Data acquisition protocols for PET-CT, depending on the study, can be relatively complex, particularly when they involve a clinical CT and a clinical PET scan. Over the past 9 years since PET-CT technology first became commercially available, the initial rather simple and basic protocols have progressively become refined to correspond to accepted standards of care. Imaging protocols for oncology and cardiology are continuing to be refined and validated and it will be a while before they become as well established as the corresponding protocols for CT only. Issues of respiration, contrast media, operating parameters, scan time, optimal injected dose of FDG, and others must be carefully addressed before definitive PET-CT protocols for specific clinical applications emerge. Nevertheless, there are certain common features to the protocols, as shown schematically in Fig. 3.7, that illustrates a typical PET-CT scan.

As for any FDG-PET scan, following an injection of 10 to 15 mCi of FDG and a 90-min uptake period, the patient is positioned in the scanner. A 90-min uptake period is preferred over a 60-min period because increased washout of background activity and improved tumor-to-background ratios are obtained, even though a longer time is allowed for decay of the radionuclide. For all studies other than head and neck cancer, the patient is positioned in the scanner with the arms up in order to reduce attenuation that results from having the arms in the field-of-view; for head and neck cancer, the scan is acquired with arms down. The first step in the study (Fig. 3.7a) is the acquisition of a topogram, or scout scan that takes 10–15 s and covers a range of up to 200 cm. The total range to be scanned by both PET and CT is then defined on the topogram, based on the specific indication for the study (that is, skull base to abdomen for head and neck malignancies, and neck through upper thigh for most other

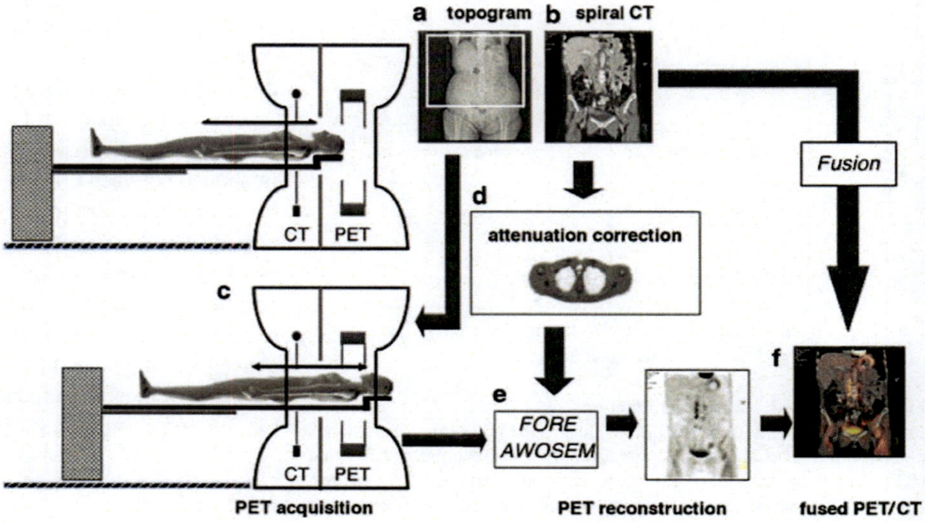

Fig. 3.7 A typical imaging protocol for a combined PET-CT study that includes: (**a**) a topogram, or scout, scan for positioning, (**b**) a spiral CT scan, (**c**) a PET scan over the same axial range as the CT scan, (**d**) the generation of CT-based ACFs, (**e**) reconstruction of the attenuation-corrected PET emission data, and (**f**) display of the final fused images

malignancies; for melanoma, the scan range covers head to toe, whenever possible). As mentioned above, an appropriate respiration protocol must be defined and implemented to minimize the mismatch between CT and PET. In the absence of respiratory gating, a good match is found if the CT is acquired with partial or full expiration, and the PET with shallow breathing. This is feasible with the 64-slice CT scanner where a scan of the thorax and abdomen can be as short as 6 s [17]. Problems posed by respiration mismatch are discussed elsewhere in this book. The whole-body CT scan is usually acquired with a slice width of about 5 mm that may not always correspond to standard clinical protocols. In some studies such as head and neck, a slice width of 3 mm or less may be preferred.

Upon completion of the spiral CT scan (Fig. 3.7b), the patient couch is advanced into the PET field-of-view and a multibed PET scan acquired over the same range as the CT (Fig. 3.7c). When the emission data are acquired in 3D, consecutive imaging fields typically overlap by 25% to average out the variations in signal-to-noise that would otherwise result. The reconstruction of the CT images occurs in parallel with the acquisition of the PET data, allowing the calculation of scatter and attenuation correction factors to be performed during the PET acquisition. The CT-based ACFs are calculated as described in the previous section (Fig. 3.7d), and once the acquisition for the first bed position is completed, PET reconstruction can begin (Fig. 3.7e). The 3D reconstruction is performed using Fourier rebinning (FORE) [18] and the attenuation-weighted ordered-subset algorithm (AWOSEM) [19]. Thus, within a few minutes of the acquisition of the final PET bed position, attenuation-corrected PET images are reconstructed and available for viewing, automatically coregistered with the CT scan by simply accounting for the axial displacement between the CT and PET imaging fields-of-view (Fig. 3.7f). The fused image is displayed as a combination of the individual CT and PET image pixel values v_{CT} and v_{PET}, respectively. Using an alpha blending approach, the fused image pixel value (v) is given by $\alpha v_{CT} + (1 - \alpha)v_{PET}$; for $\alpha = 0$, the fused image is PET only, while for $\alpha = 1$ the fused image is CT only. Then, for $0 < \alpha < 1$, the fused image represents the weighted combined pixel values of CT and PET.

While it is not feasible with current designs to acquire the CT and PET data simultaneously, scan times have been reduced significantly by the replacement of the lengthy PET transmission scan with the CT scan. In addition, as mentioned previously, the introduction of new PET technology such as faster scintillators (LSO, LYSO, and GSO) has reduced the emission acquisition time so that whole-body PET-CT acquisition times of 5–10 min are feasible with state-of-the-art systems [20]. Shorter imaging times lead to higher patient throughput, potentially creating logistical problems for imaging centers. To maintain high throughput, injection times must be carefully coordinated to ensure the constant availability of patients after a 90-min (±5 min) uptake period. It is essential to provide an adequate number of injection and uptake rooms.

In addition to the issues related to respiration and contrast, a topic of ongoing debate is the clinical role of the CT scan. Obviously a low-dose (≤40 mAs) CT scan would be adequate for attenuation correction and localization, whereas a full-dose CT scan (≥130 mAs) is required for clinical purposes. The decision to acquire a clinical CT scan depends on many factors, including whether or not such a scan was ordered by the referring physician, whether the patient has recently had a clinical CT, and whether the scan will be reviewed by a radiologist when the PET-CT study is read. Obviously the decision, which may be application-specific, will dictate the protocol and the parameters of the CT scan. Increasingly, as PET-CT becomes established in clinical routine, the acquisition of both a clinical CT and a clinical PET scan should become standard practice. Referring physicians will be advised to consider a PET-CT immediately rather than ordering first a CT, which might be equivocal, and then requiring a PET scan. Such an approach will ensure the best use is made of costly imaging equipment. More details on these and other practical issues can be found elsewhere in this book.

Finally, while there are many technical reasons to prefer the combined PET-CT approach over software image fusion, the convenience to both patient and physician should not be underestimated. For the patient, one appointment and a single scan session is required to obtain complete anatomic and functional information related to his or her disease. For the physician, the potential to have accurately registered CT and PET images available at the same time and on the same viewing screen offers unique possibilities. The added confidence in reading and interpreting the study comes from the accurate localization of tracer accumulation, the distinction of normal uptake from pathology, and the verification that a suspicious finding can be confirmed by the other modality. In some cases, such a suspicious finding on one modality invites a closer examination of the other modality, a retrospective image review that can take place immediately after the PET-CT scan has concluded.

Conclusions

Combined PET-CT scanners have been in production for over 9 years, and the technology has undergone rapid evolution. For PET, the introduction of new scintillator materials, detector concepts, and electronics is resulting in performance improvements in count rate, spatial resolution, and signal-to-noise. At the same time, the increasing number of detector rows and reduction in rotation time are transforming whole-body CT performance. The combination of high performance CT with high performance PET is a powerful imaging platform for the diagnosis, staging, and therapy monitoring of malignant disease. It is likely that there will then be a demand for a design that offers less performance at less cost. To meet this demand, an entry level or mid-range PET-CT is required, possibly in a form similar to the original prototype of PET detectors mounted on the same rotating assembly as the CT. Since the performance of the PET components is the limitation on the overall imaging time, institutions requiring high throughput and large patient volumes will always demand the highest PET performance. Nevertheless, a 16-slice CT scanner should be adequate for most oncology applications, with a 64- or 128-slice CT more appropriate for PET-CT applications in cardiology. As the current PET-CT technology becomes more widespread, appropriate future designs of this concept will doubtless emerge.

References

1. Townsend DW, Cherry SR. Combining anatomy with function: the path to true image fusion. Eur Radiol 2001;11:1968–1974.
2. Beyer T, Townsend DW, Brun T, et al. A combined PET/CT scanner for clinical oncology. J Nucl Med 2000;41:1369–1379.
3. Charron M, Beyer T, Bohnen NN, et al. Image analysis in patients with cancer studied with a combined PET and CT scanner. Clin Nucl Med 2000;25:905–910.
4. Meltzer CC, Martinelli MA, Beyer T, et al. Whole-body FDG PET imaging in the abdomen: value of combined PET/CT. J Nucl Med 2001;42:35P.
5. Meltzer CC, Snyderman CH, Fukui MB, et al. Combined FDG PET/CT imaging in head and neck cancer: impact on patient management. J Nucl Med 2001;42:36P.
6. Kluetz PG, Meltzer CC, Villemagne VL, et al. Combined PET/CT imaging in oncology: impact on patient management. Clin Positron Imaging 2000;3:223–230.
7. Hawkes DJ, Hill DL, Hallpike L, Bailey DL. Coregistration of structural and functional images. In: Valk P, Bailey DL, Townsend DW, Maisey MN (eds.). Positron Emission Tomography: Basic Science and Clinical Practice. New York: Springer, 2003;181–197.
8. Townsend DW, Beyer T, Blodgett TM. PET/CT scanners: a hardware approach to image fusion. Semin Nucl Med 2003;33(3): 193–204.
9. Brambilla M, Secco C, Dominietto M, Matheoud R, Sacchetti G, Inglese E. Performance characteristics obtained for a new 3-dimensional lutetium oxyorthosilicate-based whole-body PET/CT scanner with the national electrical manufacturers association NU 2-2001 standard. J Nucl Med 2005;46:2083–2091.
10. Surti S, Kuhn A, Werner ME, Perkins AE, Kolthammer J, Karp JS. Performance of Philips Gemini TF PET/CT scanner with special consideration for its time-of-flight imaging capabilities. J Nucl Med 2007;48:471–480.
11. Kinahan PE, Townsend DW, Beyer T, Sashin D. Attenuation correction for a combined 3D PET/CT scanner. Med Phys 1998;25: 2046–2053.
12. Burger C, Goerres G, Schoenes S, et al. PET attenuation coefficients from CT images: experimental evaluation of the transformation of CT into PET 511-keV attenuation coefficients. Eur J Nucl Med Mol Imaging 2002;29:922–927.
13. Rappoport V, Carney J, Townsend DW. X-ray tube voltage dependent attenuation correction scheme for PET/CT scanners. IEEE MIC Abstract Book 2004;M10-76:213.
14. Yau YY, Chan WS, Tam YM, et al. Application of intravenous contrast in PET-CT: does it really introduce significant attenuation correction error. J Nucl Med 2005;46:283–291.
15. Carney JP, Townsend DW. CT-based attenuation correction for PET/CT scanners. In: von Schultess G (ed.). CLINICAL PET, PET/CT and SPECT/CT: Combined Anatomic-Molecular Imaging. Philadelphia: Lippincott Williams & Wilkins, 2003:46–58.
16. Townsend DW. Dual modality imaging: combining anatomy and function. J Nucl Med 2008;49(6):938–955.

17. Townsend DW, Yap JT, Carney JPJ, et al. Respiratory gating with a 16-slice LSO PET/CT scanner. J Nucl Med 2004;45(5): 165P.
18. Defrise M, Kinahan PE, Townsend DW, Michel C, Sibomana M, Newport DF. Exact and approximate rebinning algorithms for 3D PET data. IEEE Trans Med Imag 1997;16: 145–158.
19. Comtat C, Kinahan PE, Defrise M, et al. Fast reconstruction of 3D PET data with accurate statistical modeling. IEEE Trans Nucl Sci 1998;45:1083–1089.
20. Halpern B, Dahlbom M, Quon A, et al. Impact of patient weight and emission scan duration on PET-CT image quality and lesion detectability. J Nucl Med 2004;45:797–801.

Chapter 4
CT-Based Attenuation Correction for PET

Jonathan P.J. Carney

In positron emission tomography (PET) imaging the fundamental measurement is the detection in coincidence of co-linear 511-keV photons originating from the annihilation of a positron, which itself is the product of a radioactive isotope (Fig. 4.1, *left*). The goal is the reconstruction of the spatial distribution of the positron-emitting isotope in the body, though what is in fact being reconstructed is the distribution of the annihilation event locations, which gives an estimate of the isotope distribution that is blurred according to the mean free path of the positron in the body [1]. Furthermore, since the positron is not generally at rest at the time of annihilation, the coincident photons will be approximately but not strictly colinear. The actual spatial resolution of PET cameras, ranging from approximately 4.5 to 6 mm for current clinical PET-CT designs, depends on these effects, together with effects of crystal size and event localization in the case of block detector designs [2]. When we speak of measuring the radioactive tracer distribution in the body we understand that what is really being measured is the annihilation event distribution, though the difference is not significant at these resolutions for low-energy emitters such as ^{18}F.

The measured number of true colinear coincidence events between two detectors is related to the integral of the isotope concentration (strictly, the annihilation event rate) along the line of response (LOR) connecting the detectors. However, for any annihilation event there is a finite probability that one or both photons interact with the body before reaching the detectors, such that the colinear coincidence is not detected (Fig. 4.1, *right*). Either no coincidence is detected due to the photon being scattered out of the gantry or rejected through energy discrimination, or a scatter coincidence may be detected as shown. The purpose of performing attenuation correction in the PET data reconstruction is to account for this loss of signal, so as to recover the true tracer distribution. The problem of attenuation correction in coincidence imaging is much simpler than the corresponding problem in single-photon emission computed tomography (SPECT) imaging. This is because the probability of attenuation does not depend on the position of the event along the line of response. In SPECT the probability of the emitted photon being attenuated, and the event not being available for measurement, depends on the location of the emission event. If the event occurs at a distance D from the detector, the probability p_D of the photon being attenuated (i.e., interacting) before reaching the detector is

$$P_D = e^{-\int_D \mu(x)dx}, \tag{4.1}$$

where $\mu(x)$ is the photon linear attenuation distribution, and the integral is along the direct path from the event location to the detector. The photon linear attenuation $\mu(x)$ expresses the local probability per unit length of a photon being attenuated by a medium through which it is traversing [3]. It is dependent on the energy of the photon, as the underlying atomic processes are energy dependent.

However, in coincidence imaging the net probability of attenuation affecting a particular coincidence event does not depend on the position of the annihilation event along the line of response. For each of the annihilation photons, the probability of attenuation does, of course, depend on the individual distances from event to detector. The probability p of a coincidence event not being detected depends on the product of the probabilities of each 511-keV photon being attenuated, i.e.,

$$\begin{aligned} p = p_{D_1} \cdot p_{D_2} &= e^{-\int_{D_1} \mu(x)_{511\,\text{keV}} dx} \cdot e^{-\int_{D_2} \mu(x)_{511\,\text{keV}} dx} \\ &= e^{-\int_{D_1+D_2} \mu(x)_{511\,\text{keV}} dx}, \end{aligned} \tag{4.2}$$

and the integration ranges can be combined into a single integral along the whole line of response connecting the two detectors. Referring again to Fig. 4.1, the probability of attenuation affecting the coincidence event shown depends only on the integral along the total distance $D_1 + D_2$ which is fixed, even though the distances D_1 and D_2 vary according to the position of the annihilation event along the line of response.

J.P.J. Carney (✉)
Department of Radiology,
University of Pittsburgh Medical Center,
200 Lothrop St, Pittsburgh, PA, 15213, USA
e-mail: carneyjp@upmc.edu

P. Shreve and D.W. Townsend (eds.), *Clinical PET-CT in Radiology: Integrated Imaging in Oncology*,
DOI 10.1007/978-0-387-48902-5_4, © Springer Science+Business Media, LLC 2011

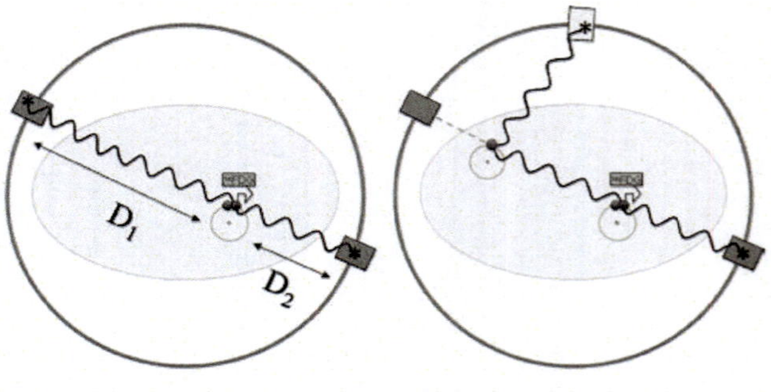

Fig. 4.1 *Left.* A useful event occurs when a positron annihilates to produce two back-to-back 511 keV photons that are detected. *Right.* There is a finite probability that one or both photons subsequently interact with the body, thereby reducing (attenuating) the number of detected useful events. The scattered photon may not be detected or may be detected as a scatter event as shown. The attenuation correction factor gives the ratio of useful events that would be measured in the absence of attenuation to the actual number of useful events detected

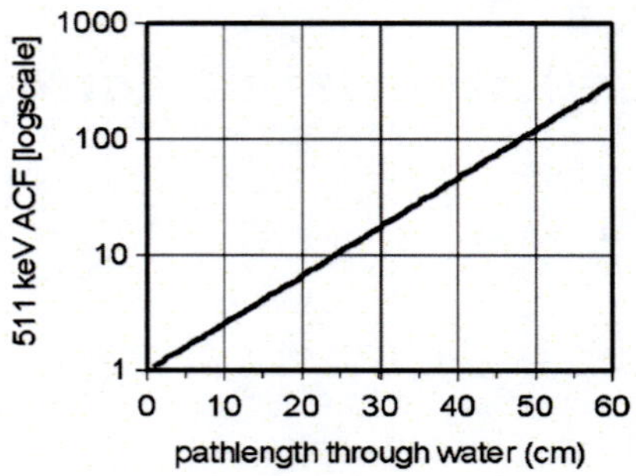

Fig. 4.2 The attenuation correction factors (ACFs) for 511 keV photons as a function of the pathlength through water, giving an indication of the typical ACFs encountered in whole-body PET imaging. ACFs for pathlengths of approximately 50 cm or greater, corresponding to lines of response through the center of large patients, are in the hundreds

Equation 4.2 gives the probability for events along a given line of response not being available for measurement and the multiplicative attenuation correction factor (ACF) for the line of response is precisely the inverse of this probability

$$\mathrm{ACF(LOR)} = e^{\int_{\mathrm{LOR}} \mu(x)_{511\,\mathrm{keV}}\, dx}. \tag{4.3}$$

In order to perform attenuation correction what is needed is the set of line integrals through the linear attenuation map at 511 keV corresponding to the geometry of the acquired PET data. The fundamental step in CT-based attenuation correction is to use the CT images to generate the linear attenuation map at 511 keV.

Figure 4.2 shows the PET attenuation correction factors (ACFs) for pathlengths through water as a function of the pathlength, which are indicative of the values typically encountered in clinical PET imaging. For a pathlength of 20 cm the ACF is approximately 7, providing a rough upper limit on the values encountered in brain imaging. In the case of whole-body imaging the maximum ACFs are much larger, and for pathlengths of 50 cm or more, typical of pathlengths through the center of large patients, the ACFs are in the hundreds. This implies that less than 1 out of 100 annihilation events occurring in the center of very large patients that would be detectable are actually detected due to subsequent interaction with the body. Figure 4.3 shows coronal PET images of the same PET-CT study reconstructed with (*left*) and without (*right*) attenuation correction applied. Particular features seen in the image without attenuation correction are the "hot lungs" and the relatively high uptake near the body contour as compared to the body interior. For example, the uptake in normal liver tissue, seen to be fairly homogeneous in the attenuation corrected image, sharply increases in going from the body interior toward the body contour. All these features are related to the relative degree of attenuation associated with lines of response passing through those regions. Attenuation correction is routinely performed in PET-CT studies and the use of pseudoquantitative measures such as the standard uptake value (SUV), used to evaluate malignancies in FDG oncologic studies [4, 5], requires attenuation corrected images.

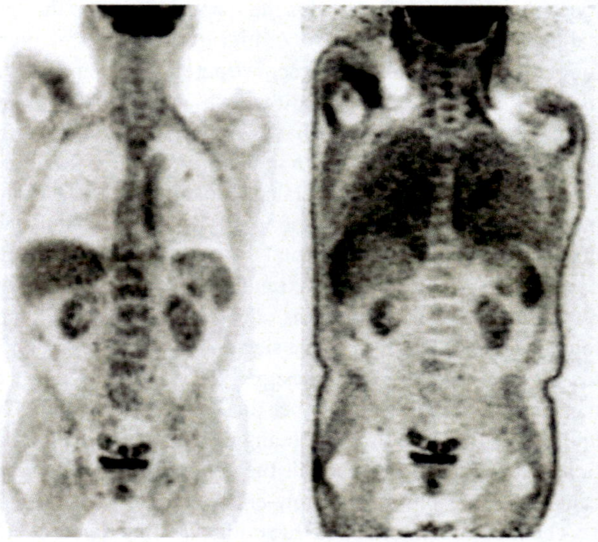

Fig. 4.3 Coronal PET images of the same FDG PET/CT clinical study reconstructed with (*left*) and without (*right*) attenuation correction applied

Transforming the CT Images

In CT the spatial distribution of the linear attenuation μ^{CT} is reconstructed, as measured by the CT x-ray beam. Unlike the case of PET imaging, there is no unique photon energy. The x-ray beam is a polychromatic spectrum of photon energies ranging up to the tube voltage energy, which is the maximum allowable energy. Clinical CT scanners provide a discrete set of selectable tube voltages, typically ranging from approximately 80 to approximately 140 kVp, though values around approximately 120 kVp are generally employed for most studies. Since the underlying attenuating processes are highly energy dependent and the CT spectrum is both polychromatic and dependent on the tube voltage setting, this makes direct interpretation of the computed μ^{CT} values difficult. Therefore CT images are instead presented in terms of Hounsfield units (HU)

$$HU = 1000 \cdot \left(\frac{\mu^{CT} - \mu^{CT}_{water}}{\mu^{CT}_{water}} \right), \quad (4.4)$$

where μ^{CT} is the linear attenuation as measured by the x-ray beam and μ^{CT}_{water} is the linear attenuation value obtained for water at the same tube voltage setting during the CT calibration procedure [6]. The Hounsfield unit for water is 0 HU by definition, and air, which can be approximated as having no attenuation, has a value of –1,000 HU. Bone tissue, being more attenuating than water, will have HU greater than 0, with values of up to approximately 1,500 HU typical of dense cortical bone.

In order to understand the transformation from Hounsfield units to 511-keV linear attenuation values it is instructive to look at the linear attenuation coefficient as a function of energy for the types of material that comprise the human body. The linear attenuation coefficient for a material is the linear attenuation (which is density dependent) divided by the density to isolate the energy dependence [3]. Figure 4.4 shows the linear attenuation coefficient as a function of energy for water/soft tissue and dense bone based on the tabulation by Hubbell and Seltzer [7]. Also shown is the result for atomic iodine, which is used in CT contrast agents that are administered to enhance structures in the CT images. The energy scale shown includes the PET photon energy of 511 keV and the range of energies relevant to CT (~40–140 keV). All materials have a similar linear attenuation coefficient at the PET energy, and differences in their linear attenuation at this energy are attributable to their different densities. All have higher linear attenuation coefficients at the lower CT energies; however, bone has a relatively higher value at CT energies than water does, and iodine has a very high value that is off the displayed scale. Therefore different multiplicative scale factors are needed to transform the linear attenuation coefficients at CT energies to the corresponding values at 511 keV. Bone requires a lower scale factor than water, and iodine requires a much lower scale factor. The transformations used in clinical PET-CT scanners convert the measured Hounsfield units into 511-keV linear attenuation values through a one-to-one bilinear mapping. Here we describe two such transformations that are used. In Ref. [8] a threshold is used to segment soft tissue from bone tissue, and a different scale factor is used for each type of tissue. In Ref. [9] a mixing model is adopted in which pixels with HU>0 are interpreted as a mixture of bone and water and transformed accordingly.

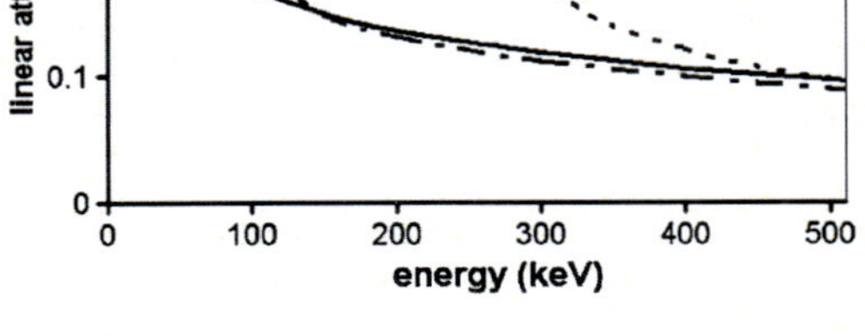

Fig. 4.4 The photon linear attenuation coefficient as a function of energy for water and soft tissue (*solid line*), dense bone (*long-short dashes*), and atomic iodine (*short dashes*). The energy range shown includes the PET energy of 511 keV and the range of energies relevant to CT (~40–140 keV)

Equation 4.4 may be inverted to give the computed linear attenuation in terms of the reported HU and the measured linear attenuation value for water

$$\mu^{CT} = \left(1 + \frac{HU}{1000}\right) \mu^{CT}_{water}. \quad (4.5)$$

In the threshold model it is assumed that tissues can be classified into distinct types by Hounsfield unit and transformed using a single scale factor for each type

$$\mu^{PET} = SF \cdot \mu^{CT} \quad (4.6)$$

In Ref. [8] tissues are classified as either soft tissue (HU<300) or bone tissue (HU>300) and the ratio of the CT linear attenuation to the PET linear attenuation is taken to be 1.90 for water and soft tissue, and 2.26 for bone tissue. In order to determine these ratios, an effective CT energy is assumed to describe the x-ray beam, typically in the range 50–80 keV. Since the narrow-beam value for the linear attenuation of water at 511 keV is 0.096 cm^{-1}, μ^{CT}_{water} is defined by the scale factor and the resulting transformation is:

$$\mu^{PET} = 0.096\ \text{cm}^{-1}\left(1 + \frac{HU}{1000}\right) \quad \text{for} \quad HU < 300, \quad (4.7)$$

$$\mu^{PET} = 0.081\ \text{cm}^{-1}\left(1 + \frac{HU}{1000}\right) \quad \text{for} \quad HU > 300. \quad (4.8)$$

By definition air corresponds to –1,000 HU and water corresponds to 0 HU, and the 511-keV linear attenuation values for these materials are known. This implies that the transformation is uniquely defined in a linear model over the range –1,000 to 0 HU. The mixing model differs from the above transformation in that pixels with HU > 0 are assumed to be a variable mixture of water and dense bone, rather than one distinct class of tissue of varying density. In this approach the transformation for HU < 0 is identical to Eq. 4.7 above, and for HU > 0 the transformation is

$$\mu^{\mathrm{PET}} = \mu^{\mathrm{PET}}_{\mathrm{water}} + \mu^{\mathrm{CT}}_{\mathrm{water}} \left(\frac{\mathrm{HU}}{1000}\right)\left(\frac{\mu^{\mathrm{PET}}_{\mathrm{bone}} - \mu^{\mathrm{PET}}_{\mathrm{water}}}{\mu^{\mathrm{CT}}_{\mathrm{bone}} - \mu^{\mathrm{CT}}_{\mathrm{water}}}\right), \quad (4.9)$$

where the following values taken from Ref. [9] are based on the tabulation by Hubbell and Seltzer [7], assuming a CT effective energy of 80 keV

$$\mu^{\mathrm{PET}}_{\mathrm{water}} = 0.096\ \mathrm{cm}^{-1}, \quad \mu^{\mathrm{PET}}_{\mathrm{bone}} = 0.172\ \mathrm{cm}^{-1},$$
$$\mu^{\mathrm{CT}}_{\mathrm{water}} = 0.184\ \mathrm{cm}^{-1}, \quad \mu^{\mathrm{CT}}_{\mathrm{bone}} = 0.428\ \mathrm{cm}^{-1}. \quad (4.10)$$

Figure 4.5 shows the transformation based on the threshold model (*solid line*) described in Ref. [8] and the mixing model (*dashed line*) described in Ref. [9]. These transformations are used to convert the CT images of the patient into a 511-keV linear attenuation image volume. The image volume is typically down-sampled and smoothed to correspond more closely to the PET scanner resolution. This lower resolution smoothed image volume of the linear attenuation distribution is reprojected according to the PET data acquisition geometry to give the line integrals that determine the attenuation correction factors through Eq. 4.3.

The above transformations suffer from the problem that they are not simultaneously optimized for all the possible kVp settings available on CT scanners. Since most studies are performed with a tube voltage setting of approximately 120 kVp this is not generally an issue as the methods [8, 9] are optimized for these settings. One approach to obtaining a more generally valid transformation is to use a dual-energy CT scan, in which two CT scans are performed at different kVp settings. The dual-energy approach allows for the decomposition of the measured CT linear attenuation values into the Compton scattering and photoelectric components, allowing for detailed information regarding the composition of the imaged material to be obtained [10]. However, the use of dual-energy CT scans solely for the purpose of accurate attenuation correction in PET-CT imaging is unlikely to become a routine imaging protocol. The second scan involves extra dose to the patient, and there may be significant problems in registering the two scans due to patient motion effects. Another approach is to adopt a calibrated transformation at all possible kVp settings. Similar methods have been used to transform CT images into electron density maps for radiotherapy treatment planning [11]. A mixing model transformation for attenuation correction in a PET-CT that takes account of the different kVp settings on a Philips CT AURA system was considered [12]. Figure 4.6 shows the 511-keV linear attenuation values for all reference tissues of a Gammex 467 electron density CT phantom as a function of the measured HU obtained on a Siemens Sensation 16-slice CT scanner. Results are shown for all possible kVp settings that were available, ranging from 80 to 140 keV. A bilinear fit is made at each kVp setting, defined by a linear fit to the air and water points and a separate fit to the three densest bone references tissues. The differences seen in Fig. 4.6 indicate a kVp-dependent transformation may be preferable when using the lower kVp settings.

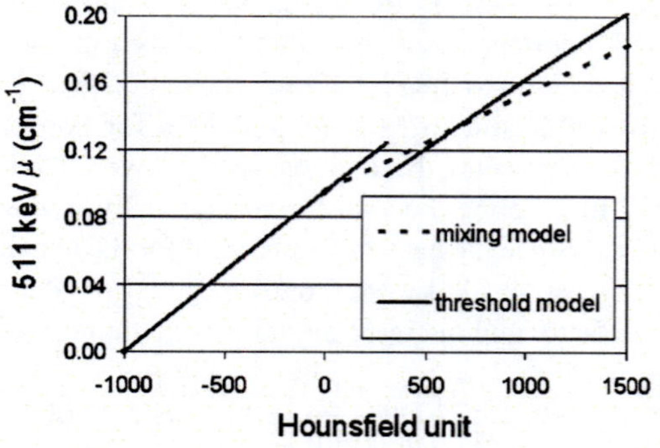

Fig. 4.5 Transformation schemes typically used to convert Hounsfield units into 511 keV linear attenuation values for attenuation correction in PET. The threshold model (*solid line*) is described in Ref. [8], and the mixing model (*dashed line*) is described in Ref. [9]

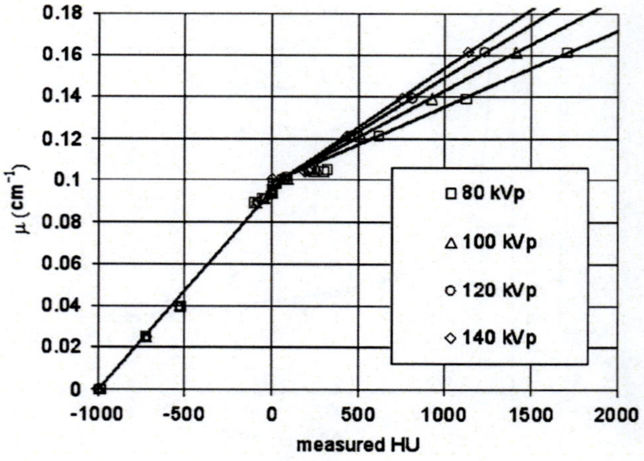

Fig. 4.6 A kVp-dependent transformation for attenuation correction based on a calibration scan of an electron density phantom at all possible kVp settings on a 16-slice PET/CT. A bilinear transformation is defined by linear fits to the air and water measurements, and to the three highest density bone reference measurements

Benefits of CT-Based Attenuation Correction

Prior to the advent of PET-CT, attenuation correction in PET scanners could only be achieved by means of a transmission scan [13]. One or more sources rotate around the patient and the transmitted signal is measured. Since the source strength is generally not known, a blank scan with the gantry empty is also necessary to determine the lines integrals in Eq. 4.3. The ratio of the blank scan to the transmission scan provides a direct measurement of the needed attenuation correction factors in the case that a 511-keV source is used. The duration of the transmission scan is significant, with the optimum time spent performing the transmission acquisition being almost half of the total scan time [14]. In order to reduce the effects of noise in the transmission measurements, the 511 keV spatial linear attenuation map may be reconstructed. This image is smoothed and may be segmented and substituted for known values before being reprojected to obtain the attenuation correction factors [15, 16]. Nevertheless, the contribution of noise in the attenuation corrections factors to the final reconstructed PET image is generally significant [17–19].

Figure 4.7 schematically illustrates the transmission scan and CT-based methods for performing attenuation correction. The CT-based method is used exclusively for attenuation correction in PET-CT studies and current PET-CT scanners no longer incorporate transmission sources other than CT. The benefits of CT-based attenuation correction are twofold: (1) By using the CT images for attenuation correction, the requirement of a transmission scan is eliminated, and the overall scan time is much shorter, by almost a factor of two. Since the CT images are available almost immediately the PET reconstruction workflow is unchanged. (2) In CT the fluxes encountered are so high as compared to PET, by a factor of approximately 1,000 or more, that the 511-keV linear attenuation maps generated from the CT images are effectively noiseless from the perspective of the PET reconstruction, though there remains the possibility of bias being introduced into the PET image dues to artifacts in the CT images, or incorrect energy scaling of the CT images, as discussed below.

Metal Artifacts and Contrast Agents

The transformations previously described are intended to transform the measured Hounsfield units for human tissues into the correct 511-keV linear attenuation values. Objects such as metals that are especially x-ray dense have linear attenuation coefficients at CT energies that are much higher relative to their values at the PET energy than is the case for human tissues, even for dense cortical bone. This was seen in Fig. 4.4 for the case of atomic iodine, which, like metals, is very x-ray dense in sufficient concentrations. Transformation schemes appropriate only for human tissue will overestimate the 511-keV linear attenuation of contrast-enhanced structures or metal

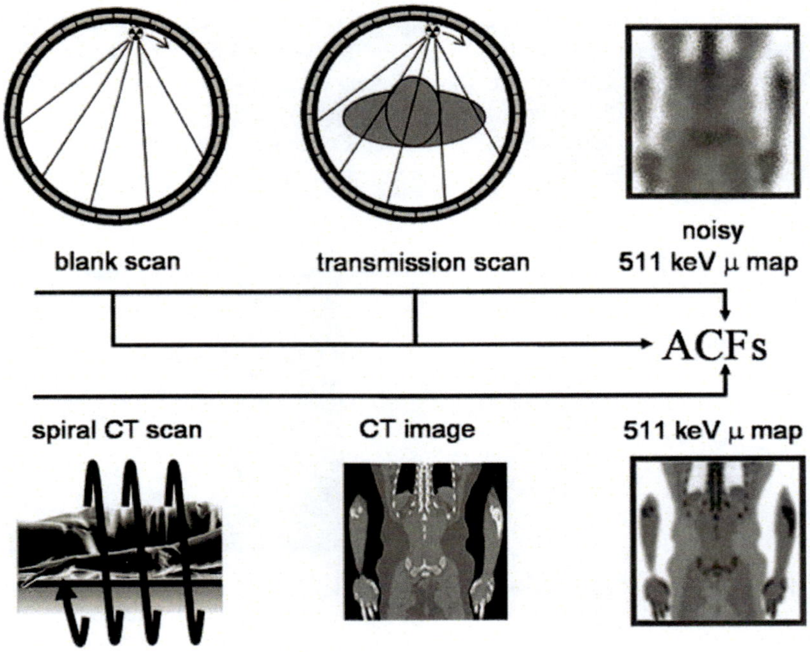

Fig. 4.7 Schematic illustration comparing the transmission scan method for attenuation correction with CT-based attenuation correction

objects. Furthermore, there may be substantial artifacts in the CT image due to the presence of metal, leading to elevated HU values over a large area. The overestimation of the 511-keV linear attenuation leads, through the attenuation correction procedure, to artifactually elevated uptake in the PET image, in some cases to such an extent that a spurious focus is clearly apparent in the attenuation corrected PET image.

This is the case in Fig. 4.8, which shows a FDG PET-CT study in which the patient had a subcutaneous chemotherapy port placed in an abdominal pocket. Since these ports have a titanium lining they are extremely x-ray dense, leading to very high HU in the CT image (*center*). Though there is no FDG activity in the port itself there is a large focus apparent in the attenuation corrected PET image at the location of the port, in addition to the multiple foci seen elsewhere (*left*). Such an artifact may be seen at the location of any metal object, such as hip prostheses [20] and dental implants [21], as well as at the location of a concentrated bolus of intravenous CT contrast agent in the subclavian vein [22]. Though these artifactual foci are present they typically do not confound interpretation of the PET image as the suspicious focus is clearly correlated with the metal object or contrast bolus in the fused image display. If necessary, further confirmation of artifact comes from reviewing the PET images without attenuation correction where it is seen that there is an absence of activity at the location of the suspicious focus, indicative of artifact, whereas the adjacent foci are all still apparent in the PET image without attenuation correction (*right*).

CT contrast agent may be given as part of the PET-CT protocol, either orally to opacify the bowel loops, or intravenously to enhance vascular structure. The degree of enhancement may be in the tens of HU for intravenous contrast or in the hundreds of HU for oral contrast, though as noted above an intravenous contrast bolus may have much higher HU. The contrast enhanced structures cannot be correctly accounted for using a one-to-one mapping since they may have the same HU as bone tissues, but not the same 511-keV linear attenuation values. Nevertheless, contrast agents are routinely administered as part of PET-CT protocols and any bias that is introduced does not appear to be clinically significant.

Regarding the magnitude of the bias in the case of oral contrast agent Carney et al. [23] observed a 20% effect in initial studies, where activity was overestimated in the ascending colon. Visvikis et al. [24] reported a maximum expected bias of 27% associated with oral contrast agent seen in both phantom and patient studies when comparing CT-based attenuation correction with segmented transmission image based attenuation correction, which is very similar to the maximum 26% bias observed by Dizendorf et al. [25]. Larger overestimations in the pelvic region (~100%) have been reported by Nehmeh et al. [26], but in this case, in addition to oral contrast agent, 15 mL of 98% $BaSO_4$ was administered in an enema, which presumably accounted for most of the effect, so this result is not representative of typical PET-CT protocols. Dizendorf et al. [27] compared two patient groups, with and without administration of oral contrast, and were only able to discern a difference in the ascending colon, with higher uptake being associated with the use of oral contrast. Note that such comparisons cannot distinguish between increased artifactual uptake due to bias, and true increased physiologic uptake due to the presence of the oral contrast agent. As pointed out in Ref. [27], Gastrografin, an iodine-based contrast agent used in that study and the cases presented herein, is known to stimulate peristalsis, leading to increased muscular uptake in the bowel wall. Studies of the case of intravenous contrast agent also suggest that there is no clinically significant bias, though a small global increase in uptake values is observed [28]. The exception to this is the case of the intravenous contrast bolus mentioned above, but this artifact is well understood, and may be avoided by suitably modifying the CT protocol to use a postinjection saline flush.

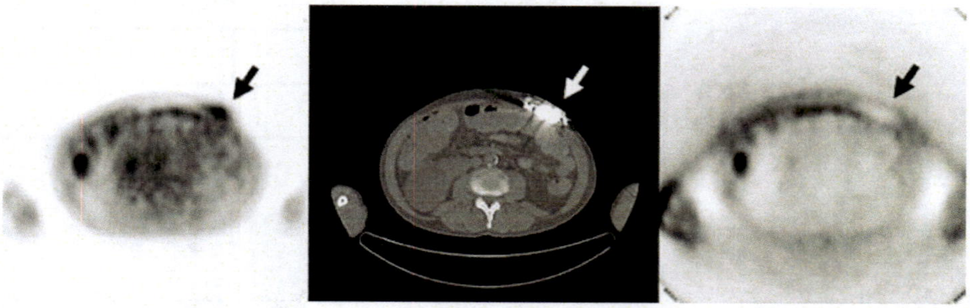

Fig. 4.8 *Center:* CT image showing a metal artifact at the location of a subcutaneous chemotherapy port. *Left:* Attenuation corrected PET image showing multiple foci, including a large focus at the location of the artifact. *Right:* PET image without attenuation correction shows the same foci except at the location of the port, confirming that the uptake there is an artifact of the attenuation correction procedure

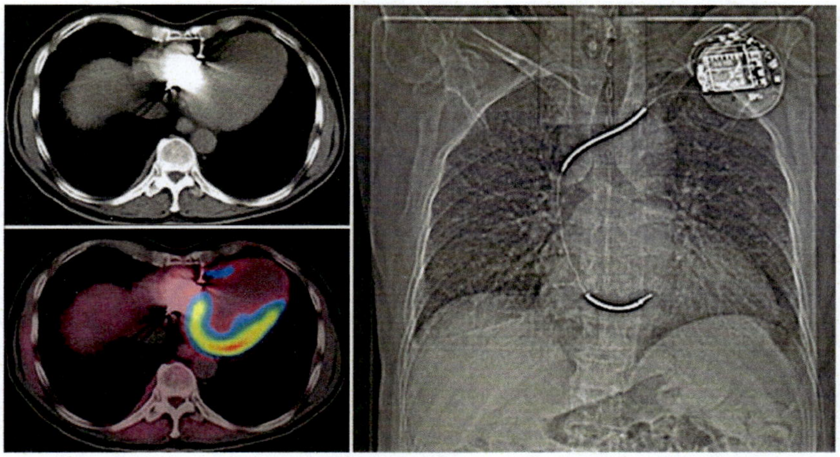

Fig. 4.9 *Right:* Topogram showing an implanted cardiac defibrillator and the leads containing the x-ray dense shocking coils. *Upper left:* CT image showing a severe artifact in the vicinity of the shocking coil. *Lower left:* Fused FDG PET/CT image. Significant artifacts at the level of tens of percent in the myocardial uptake are possible

Cardiac Applications

The use of PET-CT for cardiac applications, whether assessing myocardial viability or performing perfusion studies, requires a special consideration of the role of CT-based attenuation correction. Accurate attenuation correction is needed for cardiac PET studies as relative uptake in different areas of the myocardium is interpreted. The need for precise attenuation correction in cardiac applications is greater than in oncologic applications, since even small differences from normal cardiac uptake patterns can have clinical significance. Cardiac studies may involve implanted devices such as cardiac defibrillators which are becoming more prevalent [29, 30]. It is well known from oncology PET-CT studies that metal objects can lead to artifacts in the attenuation-corrected PET images [20, 21]. DiFilippo and Brunken [31] have characterized the corresponding artifact in cardiac PET-CT studies associated with implanted cardiac defibrillator (ICD) leads. As discussed in Ref. [31], it is specifically the shocking coils in implanted cardiac defibrillators that can cause substantial artifacts in the CT images leading to artifactually elevated uptake in the attenuation corrected PET image. The remainder of the leads do not appear to be sufficiently x-ray dense to cause a serious artifact in CT images, as is also the case for regular pacemaker leads or heart valves.

Figure 4.9 shows a FDG PET-CT study to evaluate myocardial viability in a patient with an implanted cardiac defibrillator. The defibrillator unit is seen in the topogram (*right*) as are the leads containing the x-ray dense shocking coils. In the CT image (*upper left*) there is a severe artifact in the vicinity of the shocking coil. The fused FDG PET-CT image is also shown (*lower left*). Significant artifacts at the level of tens of percent in the myocardial uptake are possible. Preprocessing of the CT images to minimize the bias introduced into the PET image may be necessary for accurate quantification in cardiac studies. In Ref. [31] a low-dose "slow" CT protocol was adopted which averaged over the cardiac motions and proved to be the most robust protocol for performing attenuation correction. However, as the use of PET-CT in the cardiac field increases, the use of cardiac CT protocols, such as CT cardiac angiography protocols, may be desirable to gain the full benefit of both modalities. How to best perform CT-based attenuation correction in PET-CT studies using these protocols will doubtless be the subject of further investigation [32–34].

References

1. Levin CS, Hoffman EJ. Calculation of positron range and its effect on the fundamental limit of positron emission tomography spatial resolution. Phys Med Biol 1999;44:781–799.
2. Tarantola G, Zito F, Gerundini P. PET instrumentation and reconstruction algorithms in whole-body applications. J Nucl Med 2003;44:756–769.
3. Hubbell JH. Review of photon interaction cross section data in the medical and biological context. Phys Med Biol 1999;44:R1–R22.
4. Keyes JW Jr. SUV: standard uptake value or silly useless value? J Nucl Med 1995;36:1836–1839.
5. Zasadny KR, Wahl RL. Standardized uptake values of normal tissues at PET with 2-(fluorine-18)-fluoro-2-deoxy-D-glucose: variations with body weight and a method for correction. Radiology 1993;189:847–850.
6. Kalender WA. Computed Tomography, 1st edn. Munich: Publicis MCD Verlag, 2000.
7. Hubbell JH, Seltzer SM. Tables of x-ray mass attenuation coefficients and mass energy-absorption coefficients from 1 keV to 20 MeV for elements Z = 1 to 92 and 48 additional substances of dosimetric interest. Natl Inst Stand Technol Rpt NISTIR 5632, 1995.
8. Kinahan PE, Townsend DW, Beyer T, et al. Attenuation correction for a combined 3D PET/CT scanner. Med Phys 1998;25: 2046–2053.
9. Burger C, Goerres G, Schoenes S, et al. PET attenuation coefficients from CT images: experimental evaluation of the transformation of CT into PET 511-keV attenuation coefficients. Eur J Nucl Med 2002;29:922-927.

10. Heismann BJ, Leppert J, Stierstorfer K. Density and atomic number measurements with spectral x-ray attenuation method. J Appl Phys 2003;94:2073–2079.
11. Schneider U, Pedroni E, Lomax A. The calibration of CT Hounsfield units for radiotherapy treatment planning. Phys Med Biol 1996;41:111–124.
12. Bai C, Shao L, Da Silva AJ, et al. A generalized model for the conversion from CT numbers to linear attenuation coefficients. IEEE Trans Nucl Sci 2003;50:1510–1515.
13. Bailey DL. Transmission scanning in emission tomography. Eur J Nucl Med 1998;25:1–14.
14. Beyer T, Kinahan PE, Townsend DW. Optimization of transmission and emission scan duration in 3D whole-body PET. IEEE Trans Nucl Sci 1997;44:2400–2407.
15. Meikle SR, Dahlbom M, Cherry SR. Attenuation correction using count-limited transmission data in positron emission tomography. J Nucl Med 1993;34:143–150.
16. Zaidi H, Diaz-Gomez M, Boudraa A, et al. Fuzzy clustering-based segmented attenuation correction in whole-body PET imaging. Phys Med Biol 2002;47:1143–1160.
17. Holm S, Toft P, Jensen M. Estimation of the noise contributions from blank, transmission and emission scans in PET. IEEE Trans Nucl Sci 1996;43:2285–2291.
18. Hsiao I-T, Gindi G. Noise propagation from attenuation correction into PET reconstructions. IEEE Trans Nucl Sci 2002;49:90–97.
19. Dahlbom M, Hoffman EJ. Problems in signal-to-noise ratio for attenuation correction in high resolution PET. IEEE Trans Nucl Sci 1987;34:288–293.
20. Goerres GW, Ziegler SI, Burger C, et al. Artifacts at PET and PET/CT caused by metallic hip prosthetic material. Radiology 2003; 226:577–584.
21. Kamel EM, Burger C, Buck A, et al. Impact of metallic dental implants on CT-based attenuation correction in a combined PET/CT scanner. Eur Radiol 2003;13:724–728.
22. Antoch G, Freudenberg LS, Egelhof T, et al. Focal tracer uptake: a potential artifact in contrast-enhanced dual-modality PET/CT scans. J Nucl Med 2002;43:1339–1342.
23. Carney JPJ, Beyer T, Brasse D, et al. CT-based attenuation correction for PET/CT scanners in the presence of contrast agent. 2002 IEEE Nuclear Science Symposium Conference Record 2003;3: 1443–1446.
24. Visvikis D, Costa DC, Croasdale I, et al. CT-based attenuation correction in the calculation of semi-quantitative indices of [18F]FDG uptake in PET. Eur J Nucl Med 2003;30:344–353.
25. Dizendorf E, Hany TF, Buck A, et al. Cause and magnitude of the error induced by oral CT contrast agent in CT-based attenuation correction of PET emission studies. J Nucl Med 2003;44:732–738.
26. Nehmeh SA, Yusuf EE, Kalaigian H, et al. Correction for oral contrast artifacts in CT attenuation-corrected PET Images obtained by combined PET/CT. J Nucl Med 2003;44:1940–1944.
27. Dizendorf EV, Treyer V, von Schulthess GK, et al. Application of oral contrast media in coregistered positron emission tomography-CT. Am J Roentgenol 2002;179:477–481.
28. Yau YY, Chan WS, Tam YM, et al. Application of intravenous contrast in PET/CT: does it really introduce significant attenuation correction error? J Nucl Med 2005;46:283–291.
29. Bigger JT. Expanding indications for implantable cardiac defibrillators. N Engl J Med 2002;346:931–933.
30. Moss A, Zareba W, Hall W, et al.; Multicenter Automatic Defibrillator Implantation Trial II Investigators. Prophylactic implantation of a defibrillator in patients with myocardial infarction and reduced ejection fraction. N Engl J Med 2002;346:877–883.
31. DiFilippo FP, Brunken RC. Do implanted pacemaker leads and ICD leads cause metal-related artifact in cardiac PET/CT? J Nucl Med 2005;46:436–443.
32. Wilson JW, Wong TZ, Borges-Neto S, et al. An algorithm for correction of PET/CT mismatch induced cardiac attenuation correction artifacts. J Nucl Med 2005;46S(2):55P–56P.
33. Pan T, Mawlawi O, Nehmeh SA, et al. Attenuation correction of PET emission data with average CT for PET/CT. J Nucl Med 2005;46S(2):113P.
34. Hamill JJ, Carney JPJ, Faul DD, et al. Reduction of PET/CT attenuation correction artifacts due to implanted defibrillators. J Nucl Med 2005;46S(2):55P.

Chapter 5
Technical Artifacts in PET-CT Imaging

Thomas Beyer

Introduction

Good-practice patient management mandates accurate diagnostic imaging. However, artifacts may arise from technical or methodologic issues and affect the accuracy of diagnostic imaging. These artifacts can be interpreted as structures in the images that are not really present but that are produced by an external agency or action. For an individual imaging modality, artifacts can be separated into image distortions arising from an intrinsic problem with the imaging system (Fig. 5.1a) and artifacts arising from an external source (Fig. 5.1b).

In combined imaging modalities, artifacts can arise also from the cross-talk of the two modalities in addition to the artifacts from each individual component. With PET-CT in particular, CT is used not only for coregistered anatomic-functional imaging, but also for attenuation correction of the corresponding emission data [1], and therefore a range of serious image distortions can arise [2].

This chapter assists in the recognition and interpretation of artifacts specific to clinical PET-CT imaging. Possible retrospective corrections are discussed and prospective measures are suggested to avoid or reduce PET-CT image artifacts, and thus potentially improve the diagnostic quality of combined PET-CT examinations.

PET-CT and CT-Based Attenuation Correction

In addition to acquiring coregistered anatomical and functional images, in combined PET-CT imaging the CT images can potentially be used for attenuation correction of the PET emission data [1, 3]. In PET-CT imaging, the time for the acquisition of the transmission data (i.e., attenuation coefficients) can be reduced to 1 min or less by substituting the conventional PET transmission measurement with the CT transmission scan, leading to a 30% reduction in total scan time compared with standard PET imaging [4]. Other advantages of CT-based attenuation correction include the option to acquire transmission data routinely in postinjection mode without correcting for emission contamination of the transmission data, as well as the essentially noiseless CT attenuation correction factors that limit noise propagation in the corrected emission images. Further information can be found elsewhere in this book (see Chap. 4).

Most image distortions in PET-CT images can be associated with distortions of the CT images, which propagate into the PET images through the use of CT-based attenuation correction. Similarly, pitfalls arise from the limitations of the standard approach to CT-based attenuation correction, which does not account for the presence of artificial implants or CT contrast agents [3]. Furthermore, misalignment effects between the CT and PET acquisitions may create biases in the reconstructed PET images.

The standard method of CT-based attenuation correction is described in detail in Chap. 4. In brief, the CT images are first segmented into bone tissue and non-bone (i.e., soft) tissue [1]. It is then assumed that the attenuation coefficients of soft tissue and bone at CT energies can be represented by monoenergetic attenuation coefficients at some effective CT energy (~70 keV). Further, it is assumed that at that energy only Compton effects contribute to the attenuation of the x-ray photons. Then the attenuation coefficients at the PET energy (511 keV) can be derived by scaling bone and soft tissue pixels with their respective scale factor calculated from the ratio of the mass attenuation coefficient at 511 keV and that of the effective CT energy. This scaling approach is based on previous work by LaCroix and Tang, who have shown that attenuation correction factors for SPECT emission data can be derived from the corresponding CT images [5, 6].

T. Beyer (✉)
Department of Nuclear Medicine,
University Hospital Essen,
Hufelandstr 55, D 45122, Essen, Germany
and
cmi-experts GmbH, Pestalozzistr 3,
CH-8032, Zürich, Switzerland
e-mail: thomas.beyer@cmi-experts.com

P. Shreve and D.W. Townsend (eds.), *Clinical PET-CT in Radiology: Integrated Imaging in Oncology*,
DOI 10.1007/978-0-387-48902-5_5,

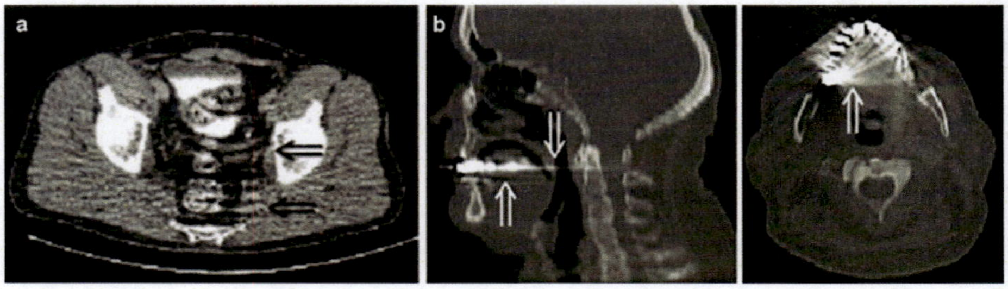

Fig. 5.1 (**a**) Non-calibrated detector responses in CT may lead to ring structures in the reconstructed images (*arrows*). (**b**) Streak artifacts in sagittal (*left*) and axial (*right*) CT images arising from a metal implant (*arrows*)

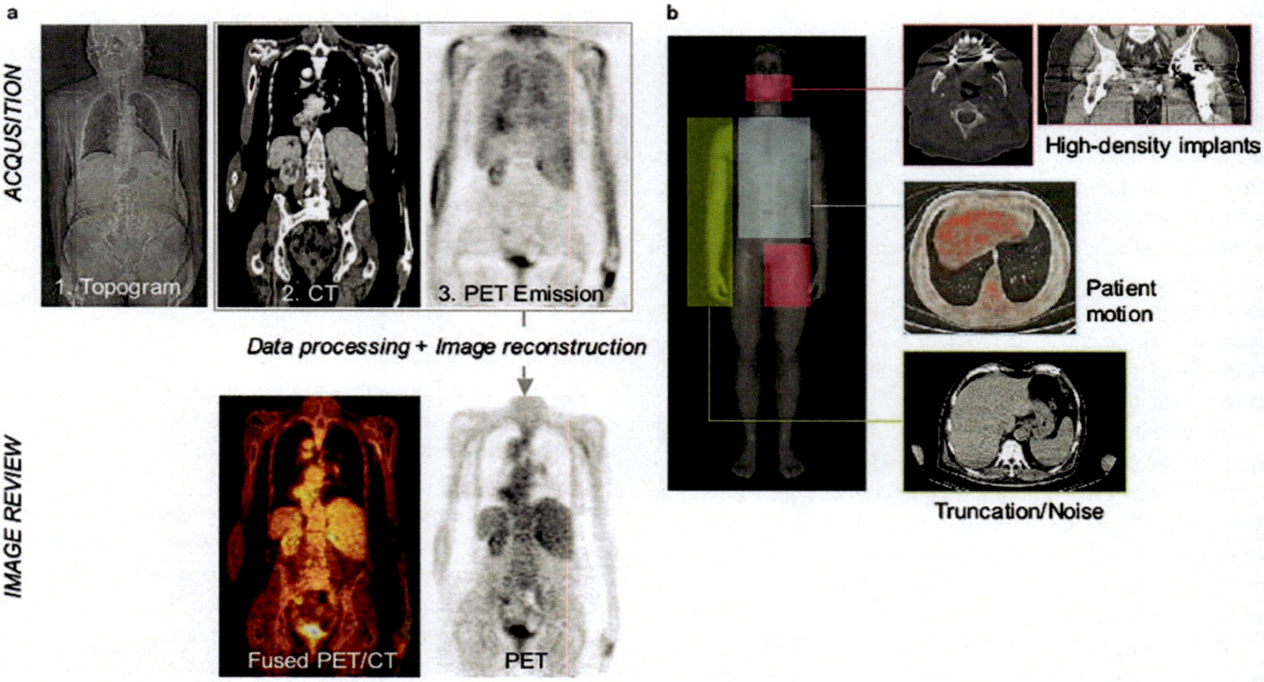

Fig. 5.2 Whole-body PET-CT imaging protocol. (**a**) First, a topogram is acquired to define the coaxial imaging range, second, a CT scan and an emission scan follow, covering the predefined imaging range. The CT data are used to correct the emission data for attenuation. Fused PET-CT images are available for review almost immediately after finishing the PET data acquisition. Several sources for potential image artifacts exist in PET-CT imaging (**b**), which relate to implants and artificial agents, patient motion, as well as patient setup and positioning

Today bilinear scaling methods [1, 7] are widely accepted for clinical PET-CT imaging3 and are, with minor modifications, used routinely for CT-based attenuation correction of the PET emission data (Fig. 5.2a) [8, 9]. While in principle the CT-based attenuation coefficients are unbiased and essentially noiseless, a number of practical limitations exist, which are discussed in detail in the next sections (Fig. 5.2b). Although these artifacts can generally be recognized on the CT and, thus, on the fused PET-CT images, they are harder to detect on the attenuation-corrected PET alone. It is therefore recommended that not only the corrected PET and fused PET-CT images be reviewed, but also the uncorrected PET images, to identify any methodology-based image distortions [10–12].

Artifacts: Origins, Presence, and Corrections

Although CT transmission and PET emission data are acquired independently as part of a state-of-the-art PET-CT exam, artifacts from CT may propagate into the PET images whenever CT is used for attenuation correction of the PET data (see Fig. 5.2b). No image degradation in clinical PET-CT is known that is caused by cross-talk effects [13] between the CT and PET hardware components.

For the purpose of this review, the sources of artifacts in clinical PET-CT imaging are categorized as: (1) patient motion, (2) high-density agents and objects, and (3) patient setup. Such artifacts can arise directly or be complementary to other effects, thus leading to a wide range of possible artifacts on the CT images and on the corrected PET images.

Motion Artifacts

Respiration-Induced Mismatch

Several PET-CT groups have described respiratory motion and the resulting misalignment of the spatial information between CT and PET as a source of potential artifacts in corrected emission images after CT-based attenuation correction [14–16]. These artifacts dominate when full-inspiration breath-hold protocols from clinical CT are implemented without further modifications for combined PET-CT studies (Fig. 5.3) [17].

In the absence of routinely available respiratory gating options, the anatomy of the patient captured from the CT scan must be matched to the PET images acquired over the course of multiple breathing cycles. Reasonable registration accuracy can be obtained, for example, with the spiral CT scan acquired during shallow breathing [15, 18, 19]. Nevertheless, in PET-CT imaging with single- or dual-row spiral CT scanners, significant mismatches between anatomy and function may still be observed, particularly in regions of the upper diaphragm (Fig. 5.4a and b), which become less apparent and less frequent in PET-CT systems with state-of-the-art CT scanners with more detector rows [20].

Currently, most PET-CT users adopt a breath-hold protocol, which requires patients to hold their breath in normal expiration either for a portion of the spiral CT only [21] or for the complete whole-body CT scan [15]. Limited breath-hold protocols are feasible routinely and have been shown to reduce respiration-induced artifacts in single- or dual-row PET-CT systems (see Fig. 5.4c) [21].

Cardiac Motion

With the introduction of multi-slice CT technology into combined PET-CT tomograph designs, cardiac applications of PET-CT imaging have come under consideration in addition to standard oncology applications [22, 23]. As for oncology studies, the CT is also used for attenuation correction [24] and for providing anatomical localization. However, accurate attenuation correction demands good volumetric registration of the emission and transmission data [25]. Since the motion of the heart is affected by respiration in addition to the cardiac cycle, accurate coregistration of CT and PET

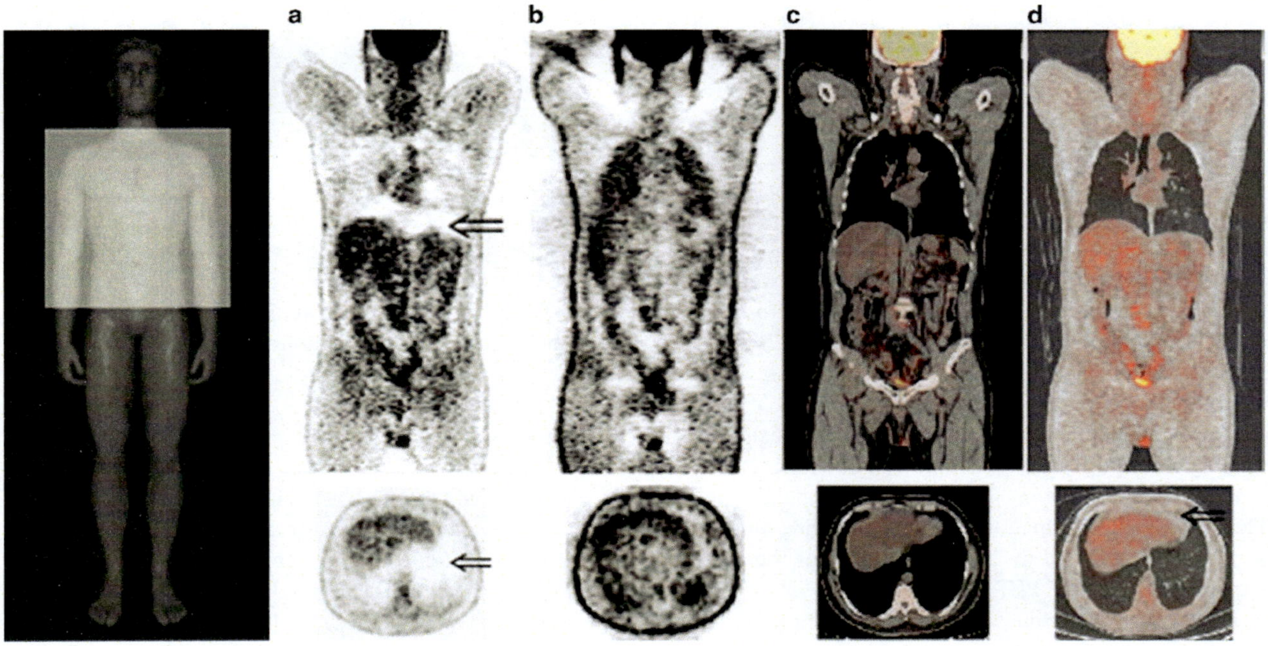

Fig. 5.3 Respiration-induced artifact on FDG-PET-CT may occur as photopenic area (*arrow*) above the upper diaphragm on attenuation-corrected PET (**a**). By comparison, the metabolic activity in the lungs and abdomen appears normal in the uncorrected emission images (**b**). PET-CT image fusion after (**c**) and prior to (**d**) attenuation correction indicates that the lungs were inflated (likely in full-inspiration) during the CT scan, thus leading to a mismatch of anatomical and functional information. This mismatch translates into an underestimation of the emission activity in the region of maximum respiratory mobility (**a**)

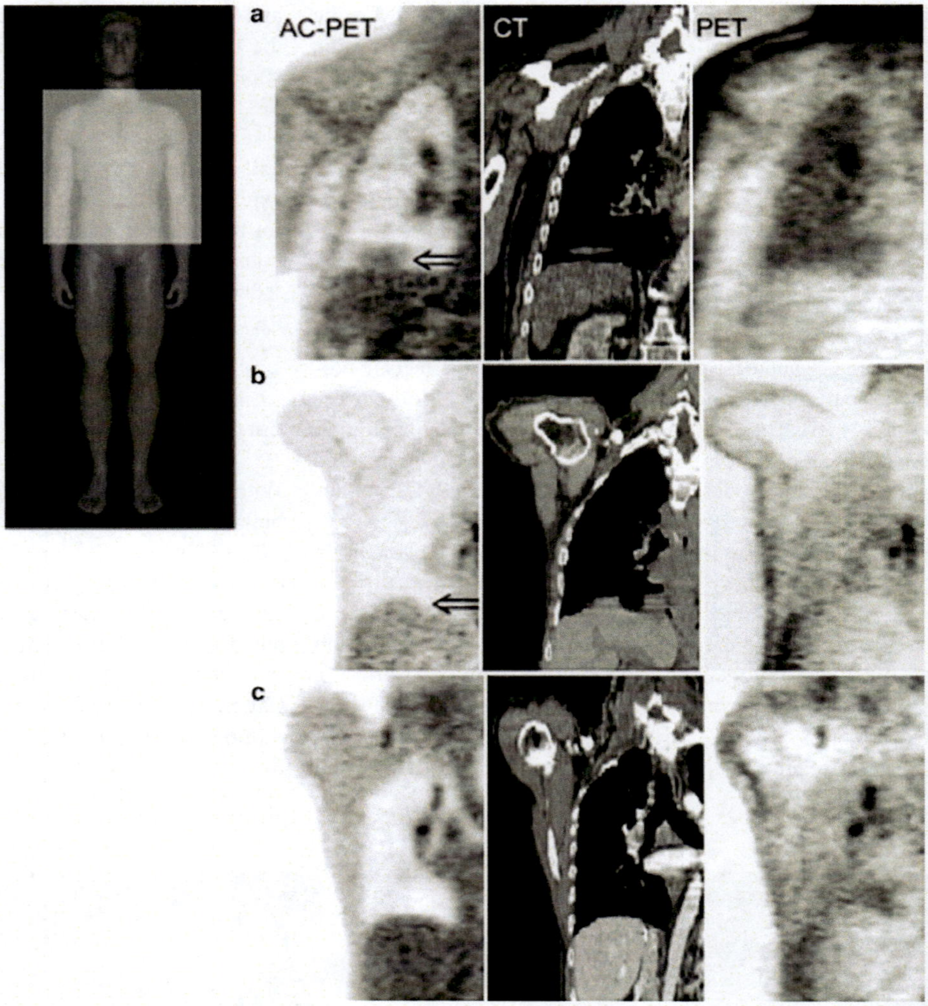

Fig. 5.4 Mild respiration-induced artifacts (*arrow*) in whole-body PET-CT imaging using a single-slice CT (**a**) and a multi-slice ($n=8$) CT (**b**). These artifacts arise from a local mismatch of anatomical (CT) and functional (PET) information, and can be identified on the corrected PET (AC-PET) and confirmed by the CT and the corresponding uncorrected PET (PET). The frequency and magnitude of these artifacts decreases with the use of multi-slice CT in PET-CT systems (**b**). Alternatively, breath-hold protocols may help reduce respiration-induced mismatches and artifacts in the area of the diaphragm even for PET-CT studies with either a single- or dual-slice CT (**c**)

images from combined studies is challenging. One simple approach is to retrospectively align CT transmission data and emission images and alter the shape of the myocardium so as to represent an average density distribution across several breathing cycles [26]. Alternatively, "slow CT" scans have been suggested for combined PET-CT studies, so as to improve the alignment of the complementary exams for unbiased attenuation correction [24]. Slow CT scanning corresponds to a spiral CT acquisition with a pitch <<1 and with a minimum tube current setting to limit patient exposure. The attenuation information of the heart is then blurred in a way that is similar to the averaging effect of the emission acquisition during the PET scan.

However, with a reduced acquisition speed, the CT scan may be susceptible to involuntary movement, such as the physical motion of the heart (thorax) arising from irregular breathing patterns. The resulting misalignment effects may lead to pseudo-defects in the assessment of the myocardial wall, as shown in Fig. 5.5.

Alternatively, both the CT and the PET scan could be acquired in gated mode at the expense of much increased patient exposure. Studies are currently ongoing to optimize alignment in cardiac PET-CT studies through the use of cardiac and respiratory gating options.

Muscle Relaxation

During a typical whole-body PET-CT exam (see Fig. 5.2a), a CT scan is acquired in the craniocaudal direction and followed by a multi-bed PET emission scan in the same direction [27], whereby the total scan time may be anywhere from 20 to 40 min [27, 28]. Therefore, the head and neck has the largest time difference between the PET and CT exams, and the likelihood for neck muscle relaxation within that time difference is rather high [29], leading to spatial misalignment of the CT and PET images (Fig. 5.6a to c). The likelihood for muscle relaxation further increases

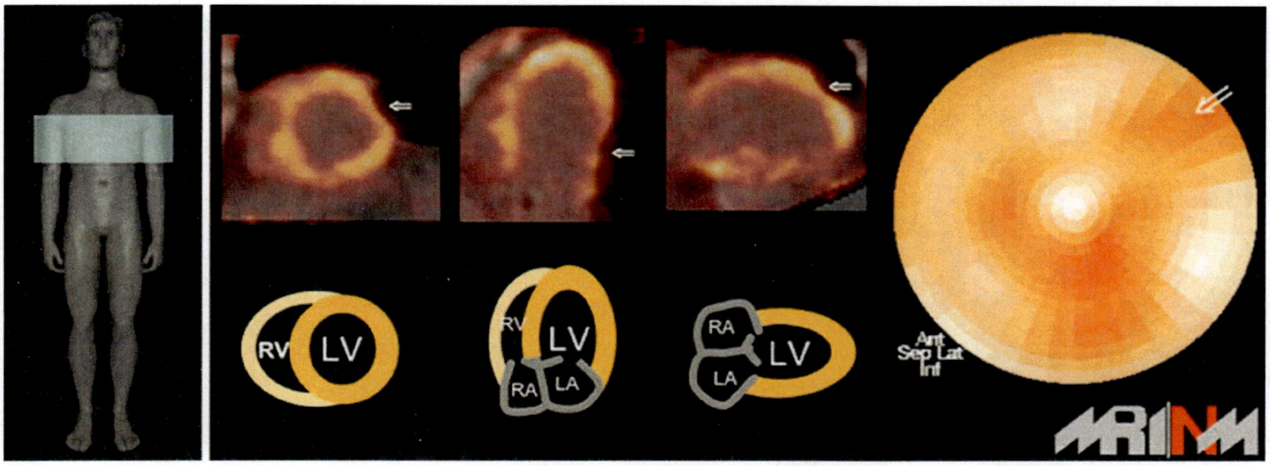

Fig. 5.5 Cardiac FDG-PET-CT imaging using a slow CT protocol (i.e., multiple breathing cycles at minimum CT dose settings). The patient suddenly breathed much more heavily while the central heart was in the active CT field-of-view. This resulted in a local misalignment of the CT and PET information in the anterolateral wall (*arrow*), which propagated through CT-based attenuation correction into the corrected emission images. As a result the bull's eye plot indicates a pseudo-defect (*arrow*) (Courtesy of Stephan Nekolla, Munich, Germany)

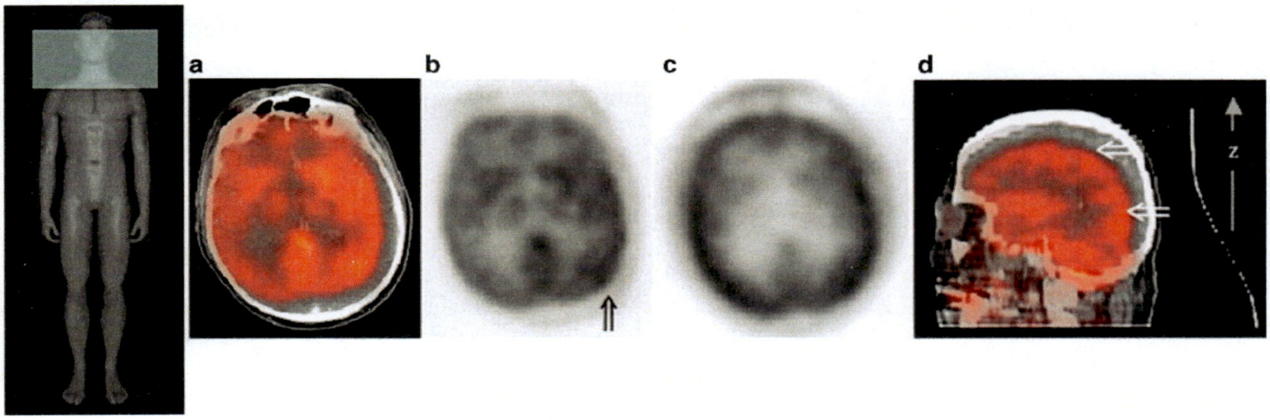

Fig. 5.6 Whole-body FDG-PET-CT study with motion artifact in the head and neck region. Fused PET-CT images indicate a significant misalignment of the PET activity and the CT anatomy (**a**). The attenuation-corrected PET images demonstrate an asymmetry of PET activity (**b**, *arrow*) after CT-based attenuation correction using the misaligned transmission data. The uncorrected PET images (**c**) appear normal and no asymmetric metabolic activity can be seen. The sagittal view of the fused PET-CT images (**d**) shows the magnitude of the misalignment along the main z-axis when adequate patient restraints are not used

with the emission scan time, and therefore longer scan protocols (for example, because of the use of less radioactivity or longer scan times) suggest a higher likelihood for image artifacts. Furthermore, inadequate restraint of the patient may lead to particularly large misalignment effects and can invalidate the fusion of the resulting PET-CT images (Fig. 5.6d).

Recent studies have shown that rigid positioning aids, such as foam molds, or vacuum bean bags are effective in reducing the average motion of the head/neck in whole-body PET-CT exams [29]. While subject-tailored foam molds in combination with an appropriate head holder seem ideal for restraining the head and neck, a standard vacuum packaging bag is preferable since it is reusable, is faster to adapt, and has no smell.

Global Patient Motion

Despite careful patient instruction and preparation prior to the PET-CT exam, more serious motion artifacts may occur (Fig. 5.7). Patients may attempt to shift their bodies into a different position during the PET-CT exam if they feel discomfort, or if the scan procedure is too lengthy.

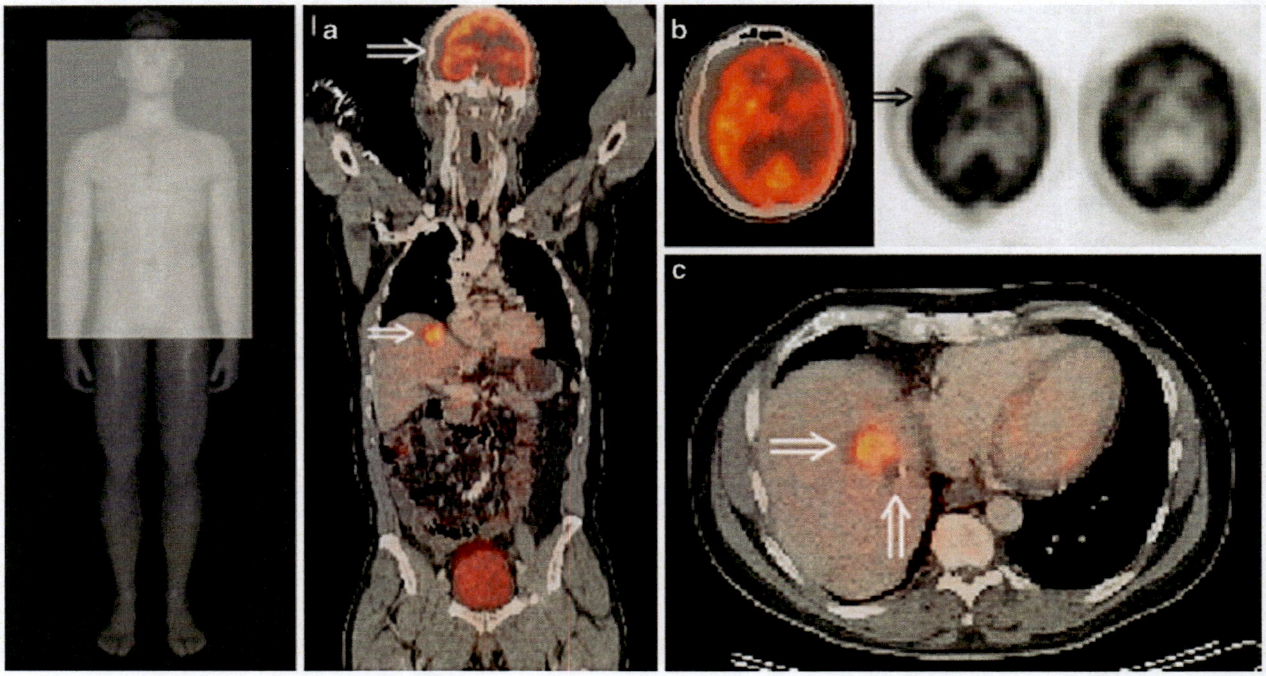

Fig. 5.7 Extensive patient motion between the CT and PET portion of a combined FDG-PET-CT scan was noticeable in this case through a misalignment of the anatomic and functional information in the head and neck region (**a**, *arrow*). The resulting distortion of the metabolic activity pattern on the attenuation-corrected PET (**b**, *left and middle*) is clearly visualized. The uncorrected emission images (**b**, *right*) suggest further patient motion during the emission scan (blurring of the emission data). This patient was scanned during followup after hemi-hepatectomy and intraoperative thermoablation of a right liver lesion (**c**). In view of the expected effects of patient motion, the differentiation of residual tumor and tumor recurrence (*arrows*) based on this PET-CT study alone was not possible

This motion is in addition to any motion from muscle relaxation, and sometimes may cause extensive, rather than local, misregistration of functional and anatomical information (see Fig. 5.7).

High-Density Artifacts

Metal Implants

High-density implants, such as dental fillings, pacemakers, prostheses, or chemotherapy infusion ports may seriously distort the CT images [30, 31]. CT artifacts have been shown to propagate through CT-based attenuation correction into the corrected PET emission images where artificially increased tracer uptake patterns may then be generated [12, 32–35]. The bilinear segmentation-scaling approach to CT-based attenuation correction is valid only for soft tissue and bone (see Chap. 4). In the presence of higher-density implants, the bilinear algorithm will overestimate the attenuation of the implants and thus lead to an overestimated tracer concentration in the vicinity of these implants.

Figures 5.8, 5.9, and 5.10 illustrate the effects of metal implants on combined PET-CT imaging. In head and neck imaging, increased FDG uptake may result in the vicinity of dental fillings (see Fig. 5.8). These uptake patterns are more pronounced when patients move between the CT and the PET (see Fig. 5.8a). Large studies of potentially degraded diagnostic quality of PET-CT studies with dental implants and fillings have yet to be performed [33], but preliminary data suggest that despite the metal-induced alterations of the FDG uptake, primary lesions in the head and neck can be identified [36].

In our experience with PET-CT imaging, patients with hip prostheses or orthopedic fixation (see Fig. 5.9) are less frequent than patients with dental implants. Nevertheless, the patterns of image distortion are similar [32]. As in the case of head and neck imaging, the magnitude of the artifacts increases when the patient has moved between the CT and PET scan [12], and viewing the uncorrected emission images may help in the discrimination of artifactual and true tracer uptake patterns.

Some oncology patients who are referred for a PET-CT scanning during therapy present with chemotherapy ports. These ports are small and have a high density, thus leading to

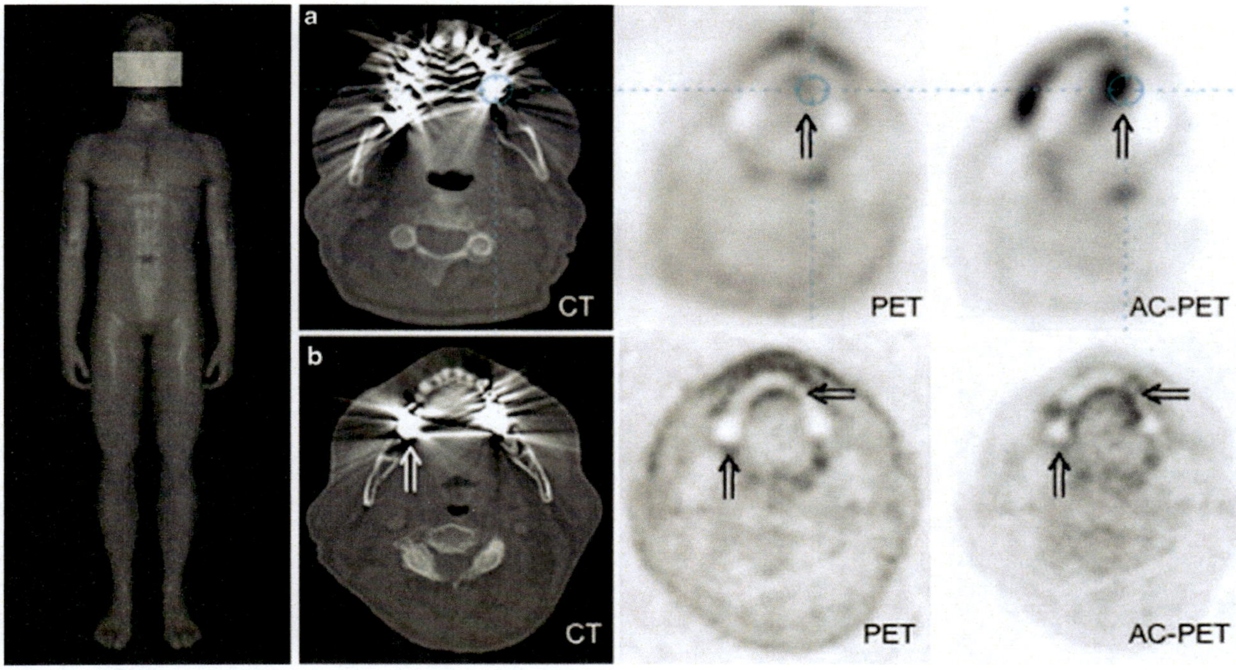

Fig. 5.8 Tracer uptake patterns in the vicinity of metal implants are difficult to interpret correctly on PET-CT images when the CT was used for attenuation correction. If the patient moved between the CT and the PET **(a)** a significantly biased tracer distribution is seen on the corrected PET (AC-PET, *arrow*), which does not correspond to the original tracer distribution from the uncorrected emission image (PET, *arrow*). With sufficient restraints of the head and neck (e.g., VacLock bag) the distortion from dental implants can be limited **(b)**, and photopenic areas remain photopenic on the corrected PET

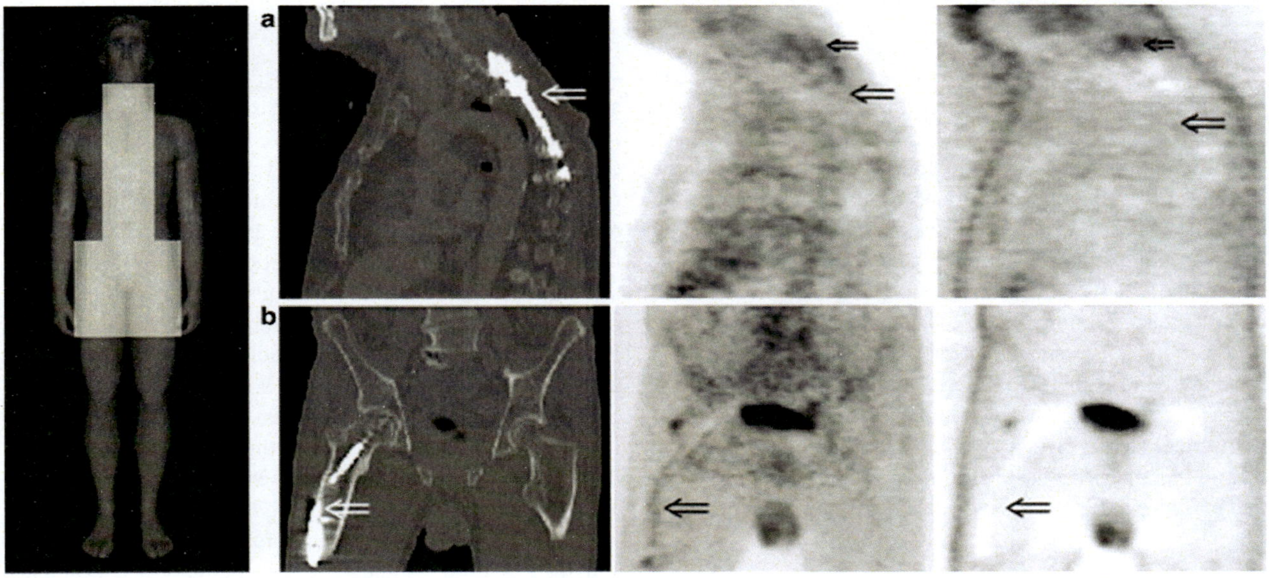

Fig. 5.9 FDG-PET-CT image artifacts from an orthopedic brace (*top*) and a titanium-made hip implant (bottom). The CT images (**a**) are shown in the bone window. The attenuation-corrected PET (**b**) demonstrate pseudo hypermetabolism (*large arrows*). This uptake correlates well with the metal implants on CT, but not with the uptake pattern on the uncorrected PET images (**c**). Note also the presence of hypermetabolism in the vicinity of the spinal fixation due to inflammatory reaction (*small arrow*)

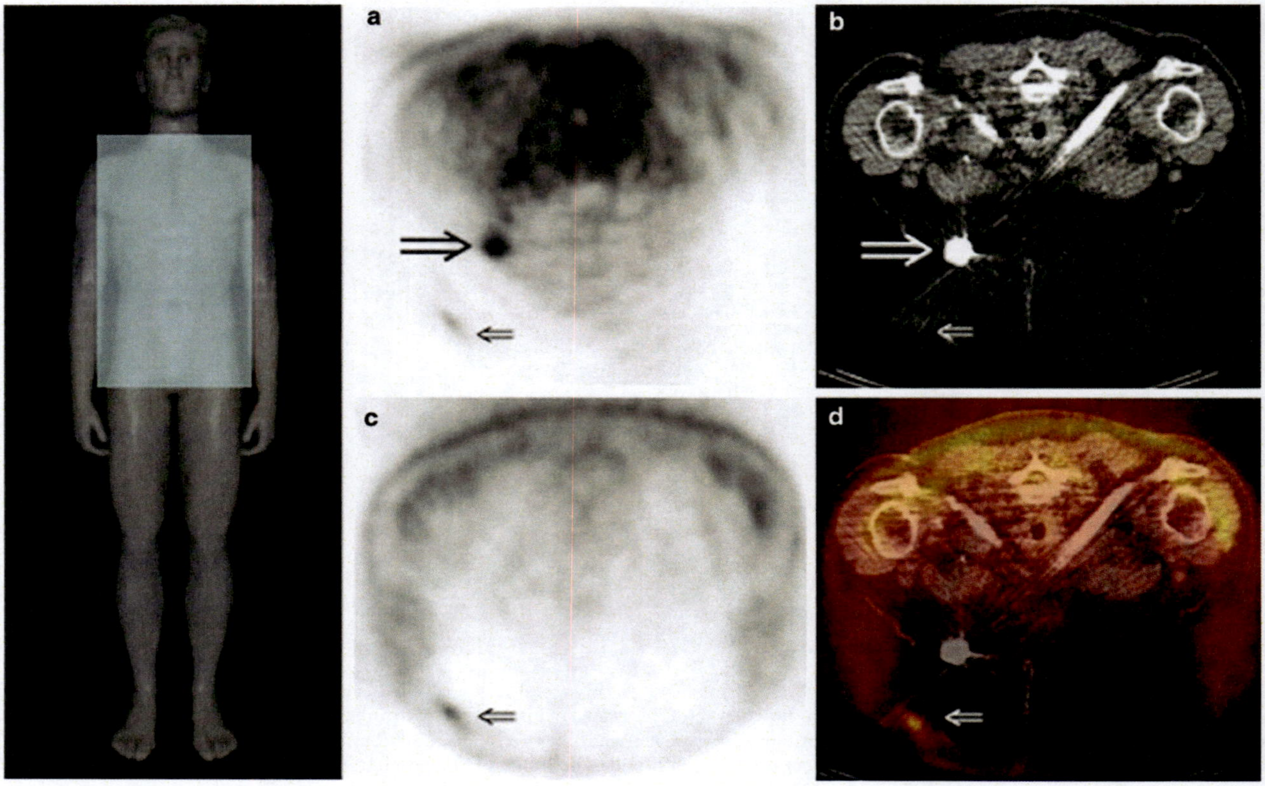

Fig. 5.10 A large breast cancer patient was scanned in head first prone mode for a single bed position covering the breast and axilla. The attenuation-corrected PET demonstrates a hypermetabolic focus (**a**, *large arrow*) and a second faint focal uptake (**a**, *small arrow*) in the right breast. On the corresponding CT (**b**) the larger uptake pattern corresponds to a chemotherapy port and is not seen on the uncorrected image (**c**), while the faint uptake corresponds to an active node in the right breast (**b**) and is confirmed on the uncorrected PET (**c**), and PET-CT (**d**)

a focal overestimation of the attenuation properties, which in turn may introduce a focal hot spot of tracer activity (see Fig. 5.10).

In summary, metal implants can easily be identified on the topogram (localizer scan) prior to the PET-CT acquisition, thus allowing the operator to define, if possible, a coaxial imaging range that does not cover these implants. The reconstruction of the images should include both the corrected and uncorrected emission images. When available, alternative transmission sources can be used to acquire attenuation data for body regions that are affected by metal agents, although some reports suggest that artifactual tracer uptake may occur with metal implants in standard PET imaging [33]. In the future, metal artifact correction may become standard practice to improve PET-CT image quality [37].

CT Contrast Agents

Clinical CT and PET-CT scans are acquired with intravenous (IV) contrast and/or oral contrast (see Chap. 9) to enhance the visualization of structures such as the vascular system or the digestive tract [38]. CT contrast media use substances with high atomic number such as iodine to increase the attenuation of the vessels, bowel, and intestines. In case of IV contrast, soft tissue enhancement of up to 2,000 HU can be observed routinely [39]. While the use of positive oral contrast leads to an average enhancement of no more than 1,000 HU, it is potentially more problematic as it collects in larger-volume structures (e.g., intestines) and in a wider range of concentrations. In the presence of CT contrast agents, the routine CT-based attenuation correction algorithm [1] will incorrectly segment and scale the enhanced structures above the threshold of, for example, 0 HU (Fig. 5.11a), thus resulting in a bias in the attenuation factors. Such biases could potentially generate artefacts in the corrected PET images when the contrast-enhanced CT scan is acquired before the PET scan and then is used to generate the attenuation coefficients (see Fig. 5.11b and c) [39, 40]. An extreme imaging situation is illustrated in Fig. 5.12 in which both the abdominal CT and PET images were degraded in diagnostic quality. The PET images demonstrated an extensive hypermetabolism, which, based on the fused PET-CT, was interpreted as

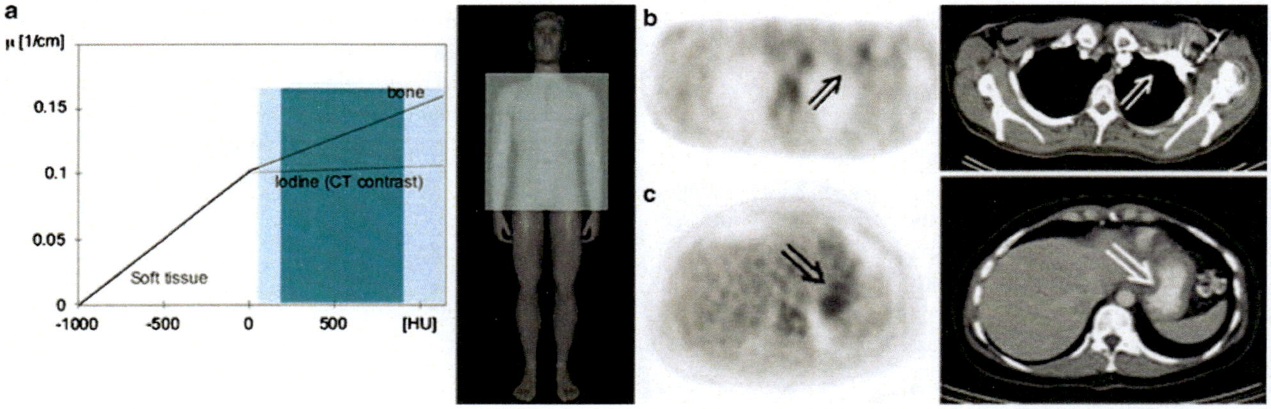

Fig. 5.11 Example of a look-up table to translate CT attenuation values (HU) into attenuation values at 511 keV (**a**). The bi-linear approach accounts for soft tissues and bone. The theoretical transformation for iodinated contrast agents is also shown. The range of CT attenuation values for IV contrast (*light blue*) and positive oral contrast (*blue*) is also indicated. It is clear from this look-up table that contrast-enhanced pixel values are overestimated from the bilinear scaling approach. In practice, this may lead to an artificially increased uptake patterns on attenuation-corrected PET when the contrast-enhanced CT scan is used: (**b**) mono-phase IV contrast (300 mg iodine/mL), (**c**) positive oral contrast

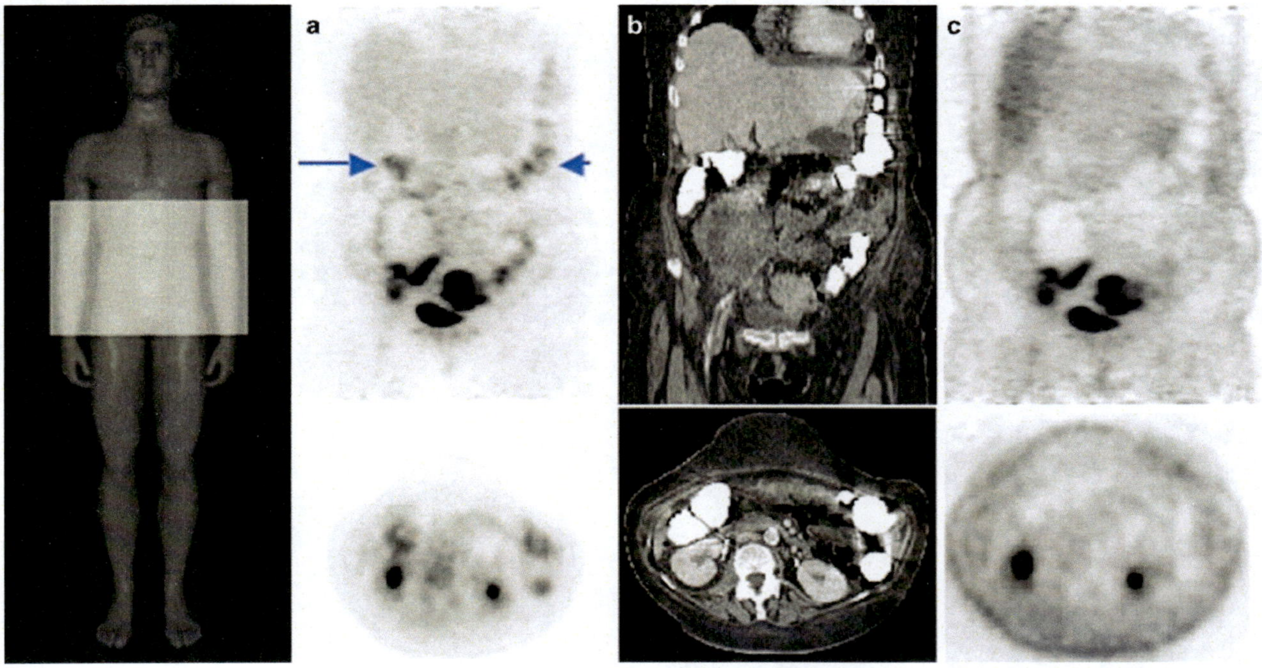

Fig. 5.12 Extensive hypermetabolism in attenuation-corrected FDG-PET (**a**) corresponding to excessive CT attenuation in Barium-filled colon (**b**) from previous barium enema study of this patient. The uncorrected emission images are photopenic in the area of the contrast-filled colon (**c**). The amount of overestimation varies with the local CT attenuation values, thus resulting in a selected increase in apparent metabolic activity on the corrected PET. *Top row:* Coronal views. *Bottom row:* Axial view plane as indicated by arrows in (**a**)

contrast enhancement from a previous barium enema study of that patient.

The use of CT contrast in PET-CT imaging is a subject of debate [38] primarily because of the associated image distortions. However, since most of these distortions relate to contrast administration protocols that were adopted without modification from standard radiology practice, careful revision and optimization of these contrast protocols may help to reduce the likelihood and magnitude of associated image distortion while maintaining diagnostic quality [41–43].

Patient Setup Considerations

Arm Position and Beam Hardening

When whole-body PET-CT imaging protocols are based on standard PET-only imaging protocols, patients are positioned with their arms down alongside the body. This is a different procedure from CT imaging of extracranial body regions in which patients have their arms above their heads for the duration of the scans. If the CT is acquired with the arms down, beam hardening and scatter effects are more pronounced and cause well-known streak artifacts that degrade the CT image quality (Fig. 5.13a). Thus, the quality of fused PET-CT images is significantly degraded, and the identification and localization of smaller lesions is challenging (see Fig. 5.13d to f). Such effects are still under investigation for PET-CT imaging [44].

Truncation Effects

Positioning patients with their arms down may also lead to truncation artifacts (Fig. 5.14) that occur when the patient

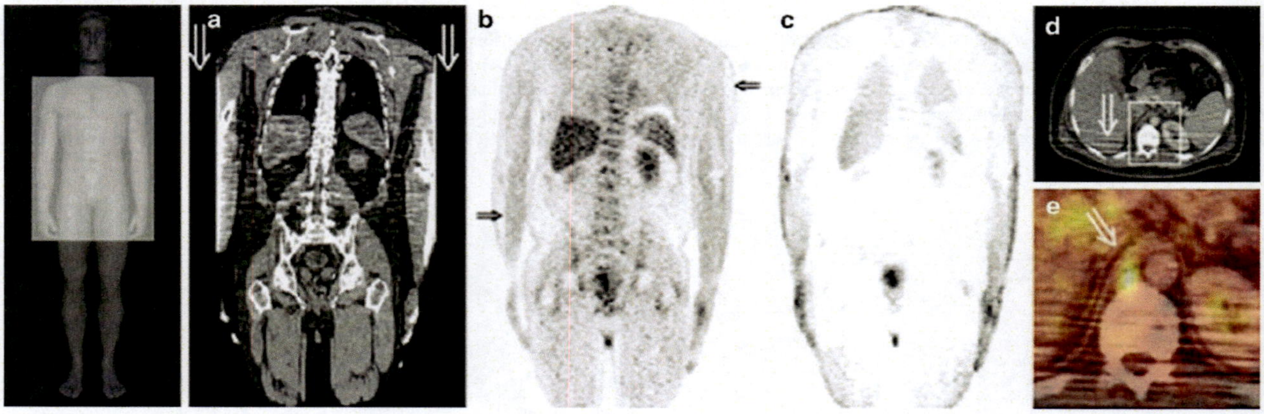

Fig. 5.13 Patient setup with arms down may lead to a variety of image distortions in whole-PET-CT exams. CT truncation artifacts occur when the patient exceeds the maximum transverse field-of-view of the CT (**a**). Subsequently the CT appears to mask the activity on the corrected PET (**b**), thus leading to a gradient in the recovered tracer activity (*arrows*) in regions that are covered by the PET (**c**) but not by the CT (**a**). In addition, streak artifacts arising from x-ray beam hardening and scatter effects are more pronounced (**d**), potentially making the localization and interpretation of small focal uptake patterns more challenging (**e**, zoom-in box)

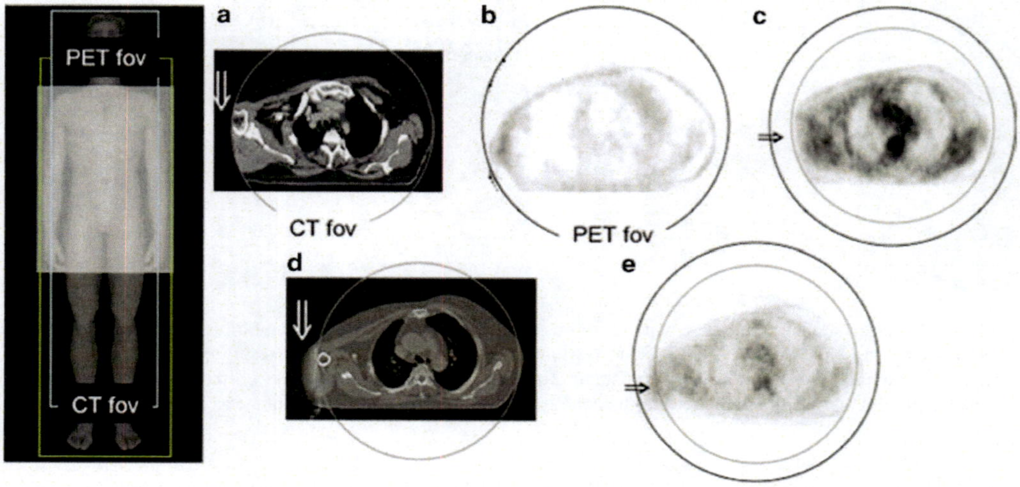

Fig. 5.14 Truncation artifacts occur when the patient imaged exceeds the transverse field-of-view (*fov*) of the CT, which is typically 5–10 cm less than that of PET. Truncation artifacts propagate from the CT (**a**) into the corrected PET (**c**) where the recovered activity distribution appears masked compared to the activity outline in the uncorrected emission images (**b**). Recently, algorithms have become available that artificially extend the truncated areas using the lateral projections (**d**). If these CT data are used for attenuation correction the tracer activity can be recovered to within 5–10% of the actual value in these regions (**e**)

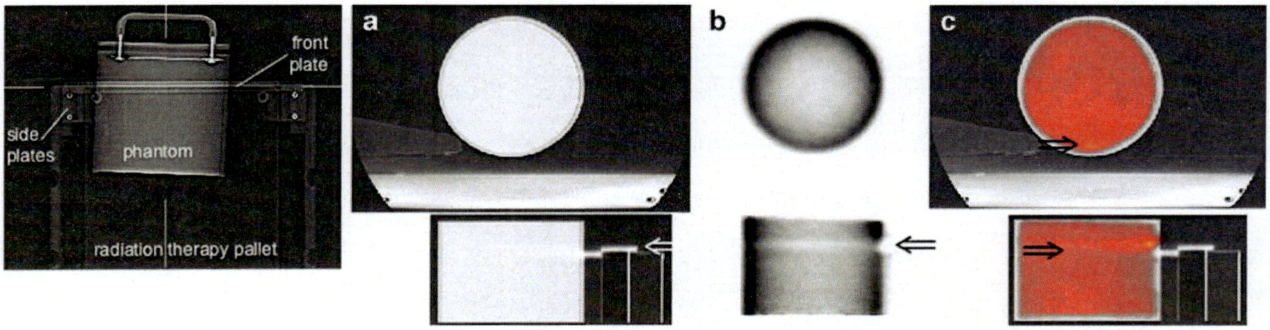

Fig. 5.15 Image artifacts in PET-CT imaging (phantom study, FDG) arising from parts of additional positioning equipment. A radiation therapy pallet was mounted to the top of a PET-CT bed. A carbon fiber front plate prevents the pallet from sliding in the main scanner axis and sideways (**a**). When a uniformly active object is placed in the vicinity of this front plate, attenuation and scatter cause a nonuniform activity distribution (**b**), which is further exaggerated by streak artifacts on CT (**c**)

exceeds the transverse field-of-view of the CT. These artifacts [45] lead to a systematic bias of the recovered tracer distribution and often occur when scanning obese patients, or when imaging larger patients with their arms down. If uncorrected, truncated CT images mask the reconstructed emission data such that the tracer distribution is only partially recovered outside the measured CT field-of-view (see Figs. 5.13 and 5.14).

To reduce the amount of truncation on CT and minimize the frequency of the artifacts, whole-body or thoracic patients should be positioned according to CT practice with their arms raised above their heads. By keeping the arms outside the field-of-view, the amount of scatter [45] and patient exposure are much reduced. Given the short acquisition times of modern PET-CT scanners, most patients tolerate having their arms raised for the duration of the combined exam. In addition, a number of algorithms have been suggested that mathematically extend the truncated CT projections and recover the truncated parts of the measured attenuation map [46]. When applied to the CT images prior to CT-based attenuation correction, these algorithms help to accurately recover the PET tracer distribution [47–49]. Similar algorithms are now routinely available for clinical applications.

Positioning Aids

Dedicated PET-CT examinations frequently require the use of additional positioning devices to hold the patient in a particular position and to restrict the patient, or a specific body region, from moving during the acquisition. In PET-CT-guided radiotherapy planning, a flat table top is mounted to the patient handling system of the PET-CT to which additional positioning aids can be attached, such as a breast board, or an abdominal cast. Figure 5.15 illustrates an image distortion that can occur in the vicinity of the edges or in particularly dense regions of a positioning aid. For illustration purposes a uniform phantom has been used, but such artifacts can also be observed in patient studies. Generally, patients should be positioned such that the primary area of interest (e.g., planning volume) does not coincide with peripheral regions of the additional positioning aids in order to avoid any bias from streak artifacts, such as is seen in Fig. 5.15b and c.

Conclusion

By following the daily QC procedures for both the CT and the PET components of the combined PET-CT systems, the likelihood for artifacts intrinsic to PET-CT hardware can be reduced. If technical problems are detected during the QC, immediate action can help to avoid poor-quality exams.

The methodologic origins of PET-CT imaging artifacts are generally understood and corrections exist for most of them (Table 5.1). Nevertheless, prospective measures, such as accurate patient positioning, optimized contrast administration protocols, and breath-hold instructions help reduce the magnitude and frequency of image artifacts in PET-CT. Limiting patient motion prospectively is even more important when using tracers that are more specific than FDG and therefore offer little, if any, anatomic information from the PET alone. Retrospective image fusion cannot serve as a surrogate quality check in these cases, and therefore monitoring patient motion or gating options may become essential in preventing serious image distortion.

Finally, the importance of carefully reviewing fused CT and PET images, with and without attenuation correction, must be stressed. Even when operating the PET-CT as a "Fast-PET" without adhering to radiology standards of CT

Table 5.1 Categorization of technical artifacts in clinical PET-CT imaging

Category	Source of artifacts	Pitfalls	Importance	Consequence	Practical solutions
Patient motion	Respiration	PET-CT misalignment	More prominent for PET-CT with $n \leq 4$	Mis-registration	Normal expiration ($n \geq 8$)
		Image artifacts on CT	Bias in corrected PET	Bias in corrected PET	Breath-hold protocols
	Cardiac motion	Local misalignment	In all non-gated studies	Mis-registration	Gating
		Image distortions on CT		Bias in corrected PET	Heavy smoothing
	Motion of trunk and extremities	Local and global PET-CT misalignment	Not predictable, somewhat reduced by proper patient preparation	Mis-registration Bias in corrected PET	Careful patient instructions. Patient monitoring. Use of positioning aids.
High-density agents and implants	High-density implants	CT artifacts (streaks)	In all imaging scenarios	Mis-registration Bias in corrected PET	Use alternative TX sources, review non-AC images, eliminate patient motion, employ metal artifact corrections
	Positive CT contrast	Focal artifacts (IV) Extended artifacts (oral, Barium)	In all imaging scenarios	Local overestimation of tracer activity	Acquire separate CT scan without contrast. Optimize CT contrast administration.
Patient setup	Patient setup, arms	Streak artifacts on CT	In all imaging scenarios	Degrade diagnostic quality, truncation effects	Position patient with arms up, use positioning devices, employ corrections
	Positioning devices	Streak artifacts on CT	Positioning for RTP	Distorted tracer uptake	Check positioning devices and position patient carefully

AC Attenuation correction, *n* number of CT detector rows

imaging, PET and CT images should be reviewed jointly to avoid potential diagnostic pitfalls on attenuation-corrected PET alone.

References

1. Kinahan PE, et al. Attenuation correction for a combined 3D PET/CT scanner. Med Phys 1998;25(10):2046–2053.
2. Beyer T, et al. Acquisition schemes for combined F-18-FDG-PET/CT imaging. A European perspective. In: Czernin J, et al. (ed.). Atlas of PET/CT Imaging in Oncology, New York: Springer, 2004: 30–45.
3. Kinahan P, Hasegawa B, Beyer T. X-ray based attenuation correction for PET/CT scanners. Semin Nucl Med 2003;33(3):166–179.
4. Schulthess GKV. Cost considerations regarding an integrated CT-PET system. Eur Radiol 2000;10(Suppl 3):S377–S380.
5. LaCroix KJ, et al. Investigation of the use of X-ray CT images for attenuation correction in SPECT. IEEE Trans Nucl Sci 1994;41: 2793–2799.
6. Tang HR, et al. Implementation of a combined X-ray CT scintillation camera imaging system for localizing and measuring radionuclide uptake: Experiments in phantoms and patients. IEEE Trans Nucl Sci 1999;46(3):551–557.
7. Fleming JS. A technique for using CT images in attenuation correction and quantification in SPECT. Nucl Med Commun 1989;10:83–97.
8. Beyer T, Townsend D, Blodgett T. Dual-modality PET/CT tomography for clinical oncology. Q J Nucl Med 2002;46(1):24–34.
9. Burger C, et al. PET attenuation coefficients from CT images: experimental evaluation of the transformation of CT into PET 511-keV attenuation coefficients. Eur J Nucl Med 2002;29(7): 922–927.
10. Goerres GW, et al. Head and neck imaging with PET and PET/CT: artefacts from dental metallic implants. Eur J Nucl Med 2002;29(3): 367–370.
11. Osman MM, et al. Clinically significant inaccurate localization of lesions with PET/CT: frequency in 300 patients. J Nucl Med 2003;44(2):240–243.
12. Goerres GW, et al. Artifacts at PET and PET/CT caused by metallic hip prosthetic material. Radiology 2003;226(2):577–584.
13. Beyer T. Design, construction, and validation of a combined PET/CT tomograph for clinical oncology, in Department of Physics. Surrey, UK: University of Surrey, 2000:303.
14. Beyer T, et al. Combined PET/CT imaging using a single, dual-modality tomograph: a promising approach to clinical oncology of the future. In: Wieler HJ, Coleman E (eds.). PET in Clinical Oncology. Darmstadt: Steinkopff, 2000:101–124.
15. Goerres GW, et al. PET-CT image co-registration in the thorax: influence of respiration. Eur J Nucl Med 2002;29(3):351–360.
16. Osman MM, et al. Respiratory motion artifacts on PET emission images obtained using CT attenuation correction on PET-CT. Eur J Nucl Med Mol Imaging 2003;30(4):603–606.
17. Townsend DW, Beyer T. Integrated structure/function imaging with X-ray CT and PET. In: Valk PE, et al. (eds.). Positron Emission Tomography: Basic Science and Clinical Practice. London: Springer, 2003.
18. Goerres GW, et al. Accuracy of image coregistration of pulmonary lesions in patients with non-small cell lung cancer using an integrated PET/CT system. J Nucl Med 2002;43(11):1469–1475.

19. Goerres GW, et al. PET/CT of the abdomen: optimizing the patient breathing pattern. Eur Radiol 2003;13:734–739.
20. Beyer T, et al. Respiration artifacts in whole-body 18F-FDG PET/CT studies with combined PET/CT tomographs employing spiral CT technology with 1 to 16 detector rows. Eur J Nucl Med Mol Imaging 2005;32(12):1429–1439.
21. Beyer T, et al. Dual-modality PET/CT imaging: the effect of respiratory motion on combined image quality in clinical oncology. Eur J Nucl Med 2003;30(4):588–596.
22. Namdar M, et al. Improved CAD assessment using a combined PET/CT scanner. J Nucl Med 2004;45(5):117P–118P.
23. DiFilippo F, et al. Initial clinical experience with 82Rb cardiac PET imaging on a PET/CT system. J Nucl Med 2004;45(5):117P.
24. Koepfl P, et al. CT attenuation correction for myocardial perfusion quantification using a PET/CT hybrid scanner. J Nucl Med 527; 45(4):537–542.
25. Meikle SR, Dahlbom M, Cherry SR. Attenuation correction using count-limited transmission data in positron emission tomography. J Nucl Med 1993;34:143–150.
26. Martinez-Möller A, et al. Artifacts from Misaligned CT in cardiac perfusion PET/CT studies: frequency, effects, and potential solutions. J Nucl Med 2007;48(2):188–193.
27. Beyer T, et al. Considerations on FDG-PET/CT imaging protocols. J Nucl Med 2004;45(Suppl 1):25S–35S.
28. Halpern BS, et al. Impact of patient weight and emission scan time duration on PET/CT image quality and lesion detectability. J Nucl Med 2004;45(5):797–801.
29. Beyer T, et al. On the use of positioning aids to reduce misregistration in the head/neck region of whole-body PET/CT studies. J Nucl Med 2005;46(4):596–602.
30. Duerinckx AJ, Macovski A. Polychromatic streak artifacts in computed tomography images. J Comput Assist Tomogr 1978;2(4): 481–487.
31. deMan B, et al. Metal streak artifacts in x-ray computed tomography: a simulation study. IEEE Trans Nucl Sci 1999;46(3):691–696.
32. Bujenovic S, et al. Artifactual 2-deoxy-2-[18F]fluoro-D-glucose localization surrounding metallic objects in a PET/CT scanner using CT-based attenuation correction. Mol Imag Biol 2003;5(1):20–22.
33. Kamel EM, et al. Impact of metallic dental implants on CT-based attenuation correction in a combined PET/CT scanner. Eur Radiol 2002;13:724–728.
34. DiFilippo FP, Brunken RC. Do implanted pacemakers leads and ICD leads cause metal-related artifact in caridac PET/CT? J Nucl Med 2005;46(3):436–443.
35. Schäfers K, Raupach R, Beyer T. Combined 18F-FDG-PET/CT imaging of the head and neck. An approach to metal artifact correction. Nuklearmedizin 2006;45:219–222.
36. Goerres G, Schmid D, Eyrich G. Do hardware artefacts influence the performance of head and neck PET scans in patients with oral cavity squamous cell cancer? Dentomaxillofacial Radiol 200;32: 365–371.
37. Mahnken AH, et al. A new algorithm for metal artifact reduction in computed tomography. In vitro and in vivo evaluation after total hip replacement. Invest Radiol 2003;38(12):769–775.
38. Antoch G, et al. To enhance or not to enhance? 18F-FDG and CT contrast agents in dual-modality 18F-FDG PET/CT. J Nucl Med 2004;45(90010):56S–65S.
39. Antoch G, et al. Focal tracer uptake: a potential artifact in contrast-enhanced dual-modality PET/CT scans. J Nucl Med 2002;43(10): 1339–1342.
40. Dizendorf E, et al. Cause and magnitude of the error induced by oral CT contrast agent in CT-based attenuation correction of PET emission studies. J Nucl Med 2003;44(5):732–738.
41. Antoch G, et al. Introduction and evaluation of a negative oral contrast agent to avoid contrast-induced artefacts in dual-modality PET/CT imaging. Radiology 2004;230:879–885.
42. Beyer T, et al. Optimized IV contrast administration protocols for diagnostic PET/CT imaging. J Nucl Med 2005;46(3):429–435.
43. Brechtel K, et al. Optimized contrast enhanced CT protocols for diagnostic whole-body 18F-FDG PET/CT: single-phase versus multi-phase CT imaging. J Nucl Med 2006;47(3):470–476.
44. Hapdey S, et al. Characterization of noise induced by CT-based attenuation correction in PET/CT images. J Nucl Med 2004;45(5): 413P.
45. Carney JP, et al. CT-based attenuation correction: The effects of imaging with the arms in the field of view. J Nucl Med 2001;42(5):56–57P.
46. Ohnesorge B, et al. Efficient correction for CT image arifacts caused by objects extending oustide the scan field-of-view. Med Phys 2000;27(1):39–46.
47. Schaller S, et al. An algorithm for virtual extension of the CT field of measurement for application in combined PET/CT scanners. Radiology 2002;225(Suppl):497.
48. Beyer T, et al. PET/CT imaging in the presence of truncation artifacts from scanning large patients beyond the smaller CT field-of-view. Radiology 2004;227(P):400.
49. Beyer T, et al. Whole-body 18F-FDG PET/CT in the presence of truncation artifacts. J Nucl Med 2006;47(1):91–99.

Chapter 6
Quantitation of PET Data in Clinical Practice

Michael M. Graham

Visual inspection of FDG PET images is usually sufficient to be able to determine if a region of increased uptake is benign or malignant. This requires significant knowledge of the normal and abnormal distribution of FDG uptake, as well as experience in interpreting these images. Quantitative assessment of uptake can be used to augment visual assessment. Two major situations when quantitative assessment is useful are in visually equivocal sites of increased uptake, to help in determining the probability of malignancy, and in assessing response to therapy by comparing pretherapy uptake with posttherapy uptake.

Prior to clinical use, when PET imaging was a research tool, most studies were acquired with dynamic imaging and blood sampling and the data were analyzed quantitatively using relatively complex kinetic models expressed as differential equations along with a parameter optimization program. As PET imaging began to be used as a clinical tool and patient throughput became an issue, it became clear that both data acquisition and processing had to be simplified. Today, almost all clinical FDG PET imaging is performed in a single imaging session and any quantitation has to be based on the single set of images.

The most commonly used measure of FDG uptake is the standard uptake value (SUV). Other synonymous terms for SUV in the literature are DUR (dose uptake ratio) or SUR (standard uptake ratio). The definition of SUV is tissue uptake (μCi/mL) divided by whole body administered activity, normalized for body weight (mCi/kg).

$$\text{SUV} = \frac{\text{Tissue uptake } (\mu\text{Ci/mL})}{\text{Administered activity (mCi/kg)}}$$

Both activities must be decay corrected to the same point in time. SUV has the dimensions of density (g/mL), but because most of the body has density close to 1.0, the units are usually ignored and SUV is regarded as unitless. It can be viewed as the degree of concentration that has occurred in a particular tissue, since the average whole body SUV would be 1.0 if the activity was uniformly distributed without excretion.

Although SUV is a simple, straightforward concept, there are significant problems with using it as a reliable index of tissue glucose metabolic rate [1–3]. There is an excellent recent review by Thie [4] of many of the problems encountered with SUV. These problems are discussed at length below.

Time Dependence

In the first few minutes after injection of FDG, activity is relatively uniformly distributed throughout the body and the mean SUV in most soft tissues is close to 1.0. As glucose metabolism occurs, FDG is taken up, phosphorylated, and retained to a greater extent in metabolically active tissues. As long as FDG is circulating in the bloodstream, metabolically active tissue will continue to take up FDG and retain it. This means tumor SUV will rise rapidly initially and continue to rise over at least several hours [5]. This means SUV is not constant, and that makes it problematic to compare SUVs from one study to another if the time of imaging is different or not stated.

Most PET centers begin imaging at approximately 1 h after injection. It is inadvisable to image earlier than 1 h for oncology studies because tumor uptake is lower and nonspecific background uptake is higher. There is no widespread agreement on the optimum time to image, and it is likely the optimal time will depend on the type of tumor being studied [6]. One paper suggests that it is optimal to image as early as 50 min for lung cancer [5], while another states that 3 h is the optimal time for breast cancer [7]. Several institutions, including the University of Iowa, routinely image at 90 min. When reading the literature regarding SUV, it is important to pay attention to the time of imaging since this can have a significant impact on the conclusions as well as how the results can be applied at another institution.

M.M. Graham (✉)
Department of Radiology-Nuclear Medicine, University of Iowa, 200 Hawkins Dr., Room 3863JPP, Iowa City, IA 52242, USA
e-mail: michael-graham@uiowa.edu

P. Shreve and D.W. Townsend (eds.), *Clinical PET-CT in Radiology: Integrated Imaging in Oncology*,
DOI 10.1007/978-0-387-48902-5_6,

SUVmax

Most PET centers report the highest SUV found in a focus of increased uptake. This is often referred to as SUVmax. The rationale for this approach is both biologic and methodologic. The most metabolically active part of a tumor is likely to be the most important in terms of prognosis. SUVmax is more reproducible than average SUV because of interobserver variation in defining the border of the tumor [8, 9]. It is important to recognize that SUVmax depends on the reconstructed resolution of the image, as well as the noise level in the image. Because of partial volume effect, a smoother, lower resolution image will have lower SUVmax than a higher resolution image. Resolution depends primarily on the intrinsic resolution of the tomograph, reconstruction filtering, and reconstruction matrix size. It is typically around 10–12 mm for most modern PET systems. Note that it is not around 5 mm, which is the intrinsic resolution for these systems. SUVmax values are less reliable in noisy images since, simply by chance a voxel in the region of interest may have a spurious high value. Similar to the requirement for consistency regarding imaging at a particular time after injection, it is important that image reconstruction be done in a consistent manner to be able to compare tumor SUVmax over time and between different institutions.

Glucose and Insulin Levels

FDG and glucose are taken up into tissue by the same facilitated transport system. This means that high levels of glucose will compete with FDG and inhibit FDG uptake into tissue. FDG images of patients with high glucose levels will show generalized nonspecific uptake and variable uptake in insulin-sensitive tissues such as heart, muscle, and gut. Tumors are not usually insulin sensitive, which means there will be relatively less uptake in tumors if glucose levels are high. There is a high risk that tumors will not be visualized if serum glucose is greater than 200 mg/dl and most PET centers will not study such patients. Some centers use a small amount of IV regular insulin to lower glucose levels and wait at least one hour for insulin levels to drop back toward baseline.

Because of the competition between FDG and glucose, SUV values will be lower if glucose levels are higher, although attempts to correct SUV for glucose level (by dividing by the glucose level) do not seem to help improve diagnostic accuracy [10]. The best policy is to check glucose levels on all patients and be aware that SUV is sensitive to glucose levels. If SUV is being used to assess response to therapy, ideally glucose levels should be the same at each study.

Body Weight

FDG does not distribute uniformly. In particular, it is not taken up very well in adipose tissue. This means that in obese patients there is relatively more FDG available for uptake into tumors. Because of this, SUV tumor values can be artifactually elevated in obese patients. Various attempts have been made to correct for this problem. Early investigators showed that replacing true body weight with calculated lean body mass eliminated the correlation of SUV with weight [11]; however, more recent studies have shown no advantage to this approach [6, 10, 12].

As is the case with other factors that can affect SUV, it is important to be aware of this potential problem and to take it into account when imaging obese patients, or if weight changes significantly between repeated PET studies.

Partial Volume

Because of the limited resolution of PET systems, small objects appear to have less than their true intensity. The precise term used to describe this problem quantitatively is *recovery coefficient*. If the recovery coefficient is 1.0, then the displayed activity/cc or counts per pixel is correct. If it is 0.5, then the displayed activity is only 50% of true. Since SUVmax is usually reported, the recovery coefficient (RC) of interest is the maximum RC in the object. Figure 6.1 shows the relationship between RC and object size for a hot sphere in a warm background. Note that for a 1-cm sphere

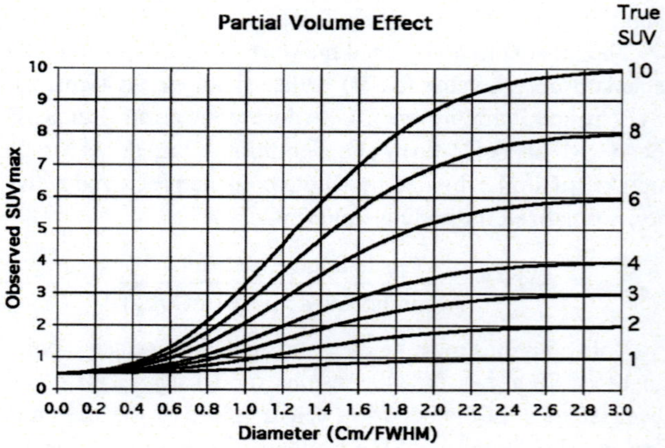

Fig. 6.1 Partial volume effect for spheres with uniform activity imaged in a positron tomograph with reconstructed image resolution of 10 mm full width half maximum. Surrounding tissue background has an SUV of 0.5. The curves were calculated from hot and cold sphere recovery coefficients reported by Hoffman [26]. The true uniform activity is shown on the right. For instance, a 1 cm sphere with a true uniform SUV of 10 would have a measured SUV_{max} of only 3.3

with a true uniform SUV of 6.0 the measured SUVmax is only 2.1. It is feasible to use simple correction using tables or figures such as Fig. 6.1, however, such correction is not commonly done. The PET images cannot be used to estimate tumor size because of limited resolution. However, CT images acquired independently, or as part of PET-CT imaging, can be used to measure tumor size. Because most tumors do not closely approximate a sphere, such correction may not be accurate. More elaborate whole-image partial volume correction schemes are being developed and may become part of clinically available software in the future [13]. Like many of the other problems with determination of FDG uptake, it is essential that the physician is aware of the partial volume effect. Such awareness is important in comparing uptake in different nodules or in attempting to assess if uptake has changed in time, when the nodule has also changed in size [8].

Table 6.1 SUV_{max} values for normal structures in the head and neck[a]

Normal H & N tissues	Maximum and percentile SUVs					
	N	Max	95	90	80	50
Sternocleidomastoid	142	7.14	4.10	3.53	3.12	2.30
Adenoid tonsils	71	8.71	4.10	3.68	3.27	2.61
Palatine tonsils	95	7.32	5.36	4.95	4.41	3.44
Base of tongue	67	7.90	4.69	4.35	4.03	3.36
Palatine mucosa	76	5.71	4.81	4.33	3.86	3.05
Larynx	58	6.56	4.59	4.10	3.67	2.93
Parotid	147	3.75	2.99	2.75	2.48	1.96
Submandibular	140	3.80	3.21	2.96	2.68	2.17
Sublingual/genioglossus	118	8.90	5.78	5.01	3.41	2.58
Occipital muscle	111	2.50	2.08	1.87	1.65	1.28

[a]These values were determined in patients with head and neck malignancy. The structures included were all documented to be unaffected by tumor. Distributions of SUV were determined for all structures and the various percentiles were calculated. This should be regarded as a rough guideline indicating the range of values in normal structures. It is not intended to provide a threshold for determination of malignancy. Indeed, attempts to set such a threshold in the head and neck have not performed well

Nonmalignant FDG Uptake

All regions of relatively increased FDG uptake are not malignant. Many normal tissues, particularly the heart and brain, can show relatively high uptake of FDG [14]. Heart uptake is variable, depending on how long the subject has fasted, insulin levels, and other factors that have not been defined. Brain uptake is consistently high and should have an average SUV in gray matter of 6–8. This can be a useful standard SUV to check the calibration of your PET images. If brain SUV falls well outside this range, it is likely the entire image set is miscalibrated and all SUVs will be in error. Usually this is due to an error in data entry (weight, dose, time after injection, etc.) and can easily be corrected. Liver also provides a useful calibration SUV. The average SUV of liver should be in the range of 2–3.

Uptake in other normal tissue is more variable. The most problematic are intestine and the tissues in the head and neck. In the abdomen, it is usually possible to identify benign intestinal uptake by viewing in the three orthogonal planes and scrolling through the images. Benign uptake usually extends along several centimeters of intestine, while malignant uptake is usually more focal. SUV assessment is generally not useful in differentiating benign from malignant intestinal uptake.

Uptake in the head and neck tissues can be relatively high (Table 6.1). Most squamous cell tumors of the head and neck have an SUVmax of 8–12, somewhat higher than the maximum SUVmax for normal structures. Unfortunately, there is no reliable threshold SUVmax to distinguish benign from malignant foci in the head and neck. Many tumors or lymph nodes are relatively small and their SUVmax is markedly reduced due to partial volume effect. Postsurgical inflammation, radiation-induced inflammation, and infection can all look identical to tumor and have elevated, worrisome SUVmax. The best approach for distinguishing benign from malignant uptake in the posttherapy setting is to obtain appropriate history, particularly regarding surgery that might account for the observed asymmetry, and the time from treatment to imaging. Radiotherapy can be particularly problematic. In the first weeks after radiotherapy there is an inflammatory phase that can cause an increase of SUV in both normal tissues and tumors. It is often useful to perform repeat imaging in this setting. If SUVmax in a suspected lesion drops in images acquired 1–2 months apart, it is most likely benign and vice versa.

Threshold Concept

In 1998, Lowe et al. [15] published a multi-institutional study on FDG uptake in solitary pulmonary nodules. They found a sensitivity of 92% and a specificity of 90% when an average SUV threshold value of 2.5 was used to distinguish malignant from benign nodules. Note that their measurement of SUV was the *average SUV*, determined from a circular region of interest drawn "within the visible margins of uptake." This point has been overlooked by most practitioners and it is often assumed incorrectly that the threshold of 2.5 applies to SUVmax. The correct threshold for SUVmax is necessarily higher since SUVmax is always higher than average SUV. In a study of 124 patients with solitary pulmonary nodules at the University of Iowa, we found the threshold for SUVmax should be set at 2.75 (Fig. 6.2).

It is important to recognize that distinguishing malignant from benign tissue is not simply determining if the SUV is greater than or less than 2.5. The observations by Lowe et al.

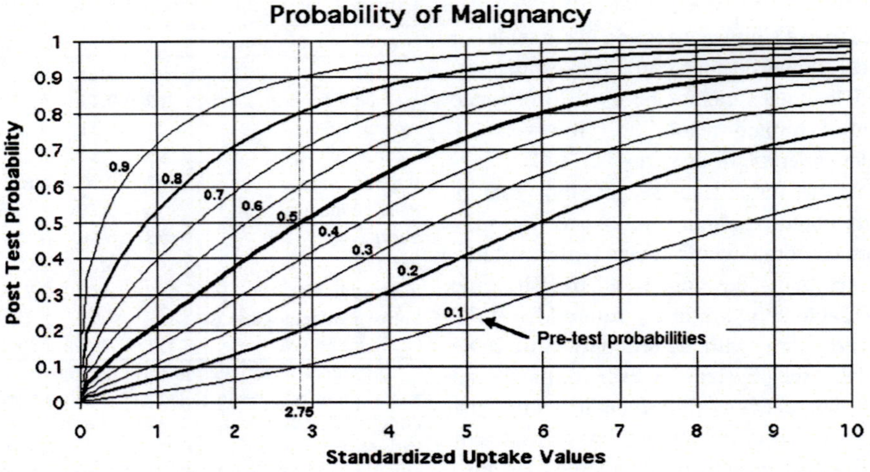

Fig. 6.2 Calculated posttest probabilities for malignancy in solitary pulmonary nodules based on 124 nodules (33 benign, 91 malignant) imaged at the University of Iowa. The curves are constructed after determination of the distribution of SUV_{max} in each group. Note that at an SUV_{max} of 2.75 there is no change in probability. Pretest probability can be estimated using web-based tools such as described by Gurney [27]. There is no abrupt change in probability at an SUV_{max} of 2.75. For example, if the pretest probability of malignancy is 50% and a nodule SUV_{max} is found to be 9.0, the posttest probability of malignancy is 90%. Note that this graph was calculated for a specific set of patients in Iowa. It may be slightly different for patients in other parts of the country because of different distributions of SUV in the benign population

apply only to solitary pulmonary nodules. The concept is not directly extensible to mediastinal disease, head and neck, or the abdomen. Similar threshold values may be determined for other settings but none are widely accepted currently. The optimal threshold depends on the patient population and should be somewhat higher in regions of the country with high incidence of granulomatous disease such as histoplasmosis or coccidiomycosis.

It is also important to recognize that there is no abrupt change in the probability of malignancy at a threshold value. Rather the probability of malignancy rises as the SUVmax exceeds the threshold and decreases as the SUVmax drops below the threshold. This gradual change in probability is shown in Fig. 6.2.

The effect of partial volume complicates the threshold concept. The original work by Lowe et al. included a specific size distribution of nodules. They found lower accuracy for smaller nodules. In general, larger nodules have a higher probability of being malignant. Smaller nodules have more partial volume effect. These two effects together result in a relatively balanced diagnostic accuracy over a range of nodule sizes. In view of this, it is not clear that partial volume correction will actually result in increased diagnostic accuracy.

Target to Background Ratio

Another, somewhat simpler approach to quantitation of tissue uptake is to determine the ratio of uptake of one site relative to another. An example of this might be SUVmax (or maximum counts per pixel) of a solitary pulmonary nodule divided by the average SUV (or average counts per pixel) in the mediastinum. Visual assessment often uses this approach of comparison of uptake with nearby structures. A commonly used visual guideline for assessing solitary pulmonary nodules is to compare the nodule to the mediastinum. If uptake is assessed as greater than mediastinum (i.e., uptake ratio >1.0), then the nodule is likely to be malignant.

Lowe et al. [16] looked at the ratio concept and found tumor to mediastinum ratio performed as well as SUV alone in differentiating benign from malignant nodules. Their paper does not provide any guideline on the optimum ratio to select.

We have explored this approach at the University of Iowa and found essentially identical performance of nodule SUVmax : average mediastinal SUV ratio to the performance of SUVmax alone. In this population, with a relatively high incidence of histoplasmosis, SUVmax threshold of 2.25 yields sensitivity of 83% and specificity of 76%. Nodule SUVmax : average mediastinal SUV ratio of 1.2 yields a sensitivity of 85% and a specificity of 76%.

Target to normal tissue ratio can be used in the same way as SUV and suffer from the same problems, including partial volume effect, time dependence, and competition with glucose level. These ratios can be used to assess response to treatment and to help distinguish posttherapy inflammation from recurrent tumor. One important caveat with regard to assessing change in uptake from one study to the next, is that normal tissues can be affected also. This is particularly true of radiation, but chemotherapy and postsurgical inflammation can also affect normal tissues. This suggests that considerable care must be taken in selecting the normal comparison tissue.

Assessment of Response to Therapy

The conventional approach to determine if a tumor is responding to chemotherapy or radiotherapy is to measure the physical size with CT or MRI and see if the tumor is decreasing or increasing in size. It is apparent that metabolic changes must precede changes in tumor size. Quantitative measures of FDG uptake are beginning to be used as a way to assess response to therapy [17, 18]. FDG has been shown to be an apparently valid method to assess response to therapy in esophageal carcinoma [19], gastric cancer [6], rectal cancer [20], pancreatic cancer [21], colorectal cancer [22], breast cancer [23], and non-small cell lung cancer [24]. It is likely SUV will become an important measure of response to therapy that will be combined with other parameters such as circulating tumor markers and size measured with CT or MRI.

The major questions in using FDG PET to assess response to therapy are when to image and how much change is needed to indicate a response. The answers are likely to be different for each tumor and each treatment modality. Several clinical trials are underway that will help define the approach that should be used in each setting. General guidelines are to wait 2–3 weeks after chemotherapy, 1 month after surgery, and 3–4 months after radiotherapy.

Reproducibility of SUV Measurements

Since the central issue in using SUV to assess response to therapy is the degree of change in SUV, it is important to consider the reproducibility of the measurement. Imaging methodology must be essentially identical for both studies to be able to compare SUVs. The most important parameter is time after injection, but in addition care should be taken that the plasma glucose levels are not markedly different, similar doses are administered, patient preparation and sedation are similar, and the images are reconstructed and processed in the same way for both studies. If this is done carefully the coefficient of variation for SUVs between two studies is 10–13% [10, 25]. Thus if the pretherapy SUV of a tumor is 10, and the posttherapy study shows an SUV of 9, it is not possible to state with any assurance that it has changed. However, if the posttherapy SUV is 8, then it has changed by approximately 2 standard deviations and it is 95% certain that it has actually decreased. This provides guidance in how to interpret change in SUV, but since the criteria for response for each tumor and setting are likely to be different, it is not a rule to determine definite response to therapy. For different types of therapy (i.e., surgery, radiotherapy, and/or chemotherapy) the timing of the second study is important and at some times the change in SUV can be very misleading.

Conclusion

Quantitation of FDG uptake using SUV is a simple and robust measure of the degree of uptake and thus the metabolic rate of a tumor. It is useful for assessing the probability that a mass is malignant or that a known tumor is responding to therapy. In both of these situations it should not be the only parameter used, but needs to be augmented by considerable common sense. It is important to remember that SUV measurements are a continuum and there is no abrupt change in probability of malignancy or probability that a tumor is responding to therapy. However, when used together with visual assessment and other clinical information, it is a valuable tool that should be used on a regular basis to assist in the interpretation of FDG PET studies.

References

1. Keyes JW Jr. SUV: standard uptake or silly useless value? J Nucl Med 1995;36(10):1836–1839.
2. Hamberg LM, Hunter GJ, Alpert NM, Choi NC, Babich JW, Fischman AJ. The dose uptake ratio as an index of glucose metabolism: useful parameter or oversimplification? J Nucl Med 1994;35(8):1308–1312.
3. Graham MM, Peterson LM, Hayward RM. Comparison of simplified quantitative analyses of FDG uptake. Nucl Med Biol 2000;27(7):647–655.
4. Thie JA. Understanding the standardized uptake value, its methods, and implications for usage. J Nucl Med 2004;45(9):1431–144.
5. Lowe VJ, DeLong DM, Hoffman JM, Coleman RE. Optimum scanning protocol for FDG-PET evaluation of pulmonary malignancy. J Nucl Med 1995;36(5):883–887.
6. Stahl A, Ott K, Schwaiger M, Weber WA. Comparison of different SUV-based methods for monitoring cytotoxic therapy with FDG PET. Eur J Nucl Med Mol Imaging 2004;31(11):1471–1478.
7. Boerner AR, Weckesser M, Herzog H, Schmitz T, Audretsch W, Nitz U, Bender HG, Mueller-Gaertner HW. Optimal scan time for fluorine-18 fluorodeoxyglucose positron emission tomography in breast cancer. Eur J Nucl Med 1999;26(3):226–230.
8. Boellaard R, Krak NC, Hoekstra OS, Lammertsma AA. Effects of noise, image resolution, and ROI definition on the accuracy of standard uptake values: a simulation study. J Nucl Med 2004;45(9): 1519–1527.
9. Lee JR, Madsen MT, Bushnell D, Menda Y. A threshold method to improve standardized uptake value reproducibility. Nucl Med Commun 2000;21(7):685–690.
10. Paquet N, Albert A, Foidart J, Hustinx R. Within-patient variability of (18)F-FDG: standardized uptake values in normal tissues. J Nucl Med 2004;45(5):784–788.
11. Zasadny KR, Wahl RL. Standardized uptake values of normal tissues at PET with 2-[fluorine-18]-fluoro-2-deoxy-D-glucose: variations with body weight and a method for correction. Radiology 1993;189(3):847–850.
12. Menda Y, Bushnell DL, Madsen MT, McLaughlin K, Kahn D, Kernstine KH. Evaluation of various corrections to the standardized uptake value for diagnosis of pulmonary malignancy. Nucl Med Commun 2001;22(10):1077–1081.
13. Bencherif B, Stumpf MJ, Links JM, Frost JJ. Application of MRI-based partial-volume correction to the analysis of PET images of

mu-opioid receptors using statistical parametric mapping. J Nucl Med 2004;45(3):402–408.
14. Ramos CD, Erdi YE, Gonen M, Riedel E, Yeung HW, Macapinlac HA, Chisin R, Larson SM. FDG-PET standardized uptake values in normal anatomical structures using iterative reconstruction segmented attenuation correction and filtered back-projection. Eur J Nucl Med 2001;28(2):155–164.
15. Lowe VJ, Fletcher JW, Gobar L, Lawson M, Kirchner P, Valk P, Karis J, Hubner K, Delbeke D, Heiberg EV, Patz EF, Coleman RE. Prospective investigation of positron emission tomography in lung nodules. J Clin Oncol 1998;16(3):1075–1084.
16. Lowe VJ, Hoffman JM, DeLong DM, Patz EF, Coleman RE. Semiquantitative and visual analysis of FDG-PET images in pulmonary abnormalities. J Nucl Med 1994;35(11):1771–1776.
17. Hoekstra CJ, Paglianiti I, Hoekstra OS, Smit EF, Postmus PE, Teule GJ, Lammertsma AA. Monitoring response to therapy in cancer using [18F]-2-fluoro-2-deoxy-D-glucose and positron emission tomography: an overview of different analytical methods. Eur J Nucl Med 2000;27(6):731–743.
18. Graham MM. Is quantitation necessary for oncological PET studies? Eur J Nucl Med Mol Imaging 2002;29(1):135–138.
19. Swisher SG, Erasmus J, Maish M, Correa AM, Macapinlac H, Ajani JA, Cox JD, Komaki RR, Hong D, Lee HK, Putnam JB Jr, Rice DC, Smythe WR, Thai L, Vaporciyan AA, Walsh GL, Wu TT, Roth JA. 2-Fluoro-2-deoxy-D-glucose positron emission tomography imaging is predictive of pathologic response and survival after preoperative chemoradiation in patients with esophageal carcinoma. Cancer 2004;101(8):1776–1785.
20. Guillem JG, Moore HG, Akhurst T, Klimstra DS, Ruo L, Mazumdar M, Minsky BD, Saltz L, Wong WD, Larson S. Sequential preoperative fluorodeoxyglucose-positron emission tomography assessment of response to preoperative chemoradiation: a means for determining longterm outcomes of rectal cancer. J Am Coll Surg 2004;199(1):1–7.
21. Yoshioka M, Sato T, Furuya T, Shibata S, Andoh H, Asanuma Y, Hatazawa J, Shimosegawa E, Koyama K, Yamamoto Y. Role of positron emission tomography with 2-deoxy-2-[18F]fluoro-D-glucose in evaluating the effects of arterial infusion chemotherapy and radiotherapy on pancreatic cancer. J Gastroenterol 2004;39(1):50–55.
22. Dimitrakopoulou-Strauss A, Strauss LG, Rudi J. PET-FDG as predictor of therapy response in patients with colorectal carcinoma. Q J Nucl Med 2003;47(1):8–13.
23. Biersack HJ, Bender H, Palmedo H. FDG-PET in monitoring therapy of breast cancer. Eur J Nucl Med Mol Imaging 2004;31(Suppl 1):S112–117.
24. Weber WA, Petersen V, Schmidt B, Tyndale-Hines L, Link T, Peschel C, Schwaiger M. Positron emission tomography in non-small-cell lung cancer: prediction of response to chemotherapy by quantitative assessment of glucose use. J Clin Oncol 2003;21(14):2651–2657.
25. Minn H, Zasadny KR, Quint LE, Wahl RL. Lung cancer: reproducibility of quantitative measurements for evaluating 2-[F-18]-fluoro-2-deoxy-D-glucose uptake at PET. Radiology 1995;196(1):167–173.
26. Hoffman EJ, Huang, SC, Phelps ME. Quantitation in positron emission computed tomography: 1. Effect of object size. J Comput Assist Tomogr 1979;3(3):299–308.
27. Gurney JW, Swensen SJ. Solitary pulmonary nodules: determining the likelihood of malignancy with neural network analysis. Radiology 1995;196(3):823–829.

Chapter 7
Patient Preparation and Management

Nancy M. Swanston and Paul Shreve

Scheduling

Scheduling PET-CT examinations is an important part of the process to guarantee patients have appointments at the appropriate time, minimize radiopharmaceutical waste, maximize scanner capacity, and optimize staff utilization. The patient's schedule should be reviewed before making appointments for PET-CT scanning to make certain other planned examinations or procedures do not conflict. For example, it is best to avoid scheduling a PET-CT examination after an appointment requiring the patient to undergo an observation and recovery period. Appointments of this nature can be unpredictable, and patients tend to experience delays or feel unable to tolerate another procedure, which could result in their being late for the PET-CT exam. Typically, the radiopharmaceutical for this exam, ^{18}F-fluorodeoxyglucose (^{18}FDG), is ordered as a unit dose and calibrated for a specific time. If the calibrated time is exceeded, there may not be sufficient activity remaining to perform the exam, the exam will be performed with a suboptimal dose, or the examination may have to be canceled. This can lead to patient dissatisfaction and radiopharmaceutical waste, or poor image quality due to low counting statistics. Radiopharmaceutical waste can also occur if appointments are not canceled in a timely fashion. Instituting a policy of asking referring physicians to change or cancel exams at least 24 h prior to the appointment time, or at least the close of the day preceding the scheduled examination can give personnel adequate time to call the radiopharmacy or cyclotron facility and alter the radiopharmaceutical order.

If patients also need procedures performed in general nuclear medicine, the study sequencing should be reviewed. For example, patients cannot have a PET-CT examination with a 511-keV radionuclide in the morning and then present to the general nuclear medicine area in the afternoon for a pulmonary function test utilizing ^{133}Xe or a bone scan with a ^{99m}Tc phosphate compound because of the lower photon energy levels of these radionuclides. However, the reverse is possible and can be quite convenient for patients. For example, many lymphoma patients need both a radionuclide ventriculogram to evaluate left ventricular ejection fraction (LVEF) and a PET-CT scan. For these patients, appointments can be scheduled in general nuclear medicine in the morning and PET-CT in the early afternoon.

A patient's schedule should also be reviewed for recent imaging examinations involving intravenous contrast material. Heart catheterizations or vascular/interventional radiology procedures, as well as CT scans, employ intravenous contrast material, and the total iodine load to the kidneys should be taken into account allowing for patient age and known renal status and function before scheduling a PET-CT examination also employing intravenous contrast material. Generally a minimum of 48 h should be allowed between examinations involving a typical dose of iodinated intravenous contrast material (100–150 mL of 270–350 mg I/mL) in patients with normal renal function, while elderly patients and those with compromised renal function may need a minimum of 5 days between examinations [1]. Trends in renal function must also be taken into account, as worsening renal function can be a relative contraindication to use of intravenous contrast material [2].

In addition to radiologic examinations involving intravenous contrast material, the patient's schedule should be reviewed for barium upper or lower gastrointestinal radiologic examinations, including feeding tube studies which involve use of barium contrast. The density of barium used in these studies can cause beam-hardening artifacts on the CT images and attenuation related artifacts on the attenuation corrected PET images. The barium can remain hyperconcentrated in the colon for days or even weeks in some patients, potentially degrading PET and CT image quality of the abdomen and pelvis. If at all possible, such studies should be scheduled after the PET-CT examination. In some instances, such as inpatients to be scheduled for a PET-CT shortly after a radiologic study involving barium, a single abdominal radiograph on the day preceding the PET-CT exam may be employed to verify that significant residual

N.M. Swanston (✉)
Division of Diagnostic Imaging, The University of Texas M.D. Anderson Cancer Center, Houston, TX, USA
e-mail: nswanston@mdanderson.org

P. Shreve and D.W. Townsend (eds.), *Clinical PET-CT in Radiology: Integrated Imaging in Oncology*,
DOI 10.1007/978-0-387-48902-5_7,

colonic barium is not present. The barium-based oral contrast material used in CT examinations is of much lower density than barium used in radiographic examinations, but can become hyperconcentrated in colon and potentially degrade a PET-CT examination [3].

It is beneficial to maintain patient databases to evaluate trends in the causes of cancelations, which can include improper patient preparation, patient inability to tolerate the procedure, elevated blood glucose levels, or broken appointments. Patient education and consultation policies and procedures can then be reviewed and revised to continue the quality improvement process.

With the advent of combined PET-CT scanners, total scanning time for a whole torso PET examination can be reduced to as little as 20 min or less. Radiopharmaceutical uptake time for a body oncology FDG-PET study ranges from 1 to 2 h or more, and due to the high energy annihilation photons patients need to be isolated from the technologist and ancillary personnel during the uptake period. In a busy PET-CT facility this can result in complex sequencing of as many as five patients simultaneously through the initial consultation, placement of intravenous line, serum glucose assay, radiopharmaceutical injection, monitored uptake period, PET-CT scan acquisition, and finally the postimaging routine. Scheduling becomes critically important for patients requiring extra preparation time or extended scanning protocols. If not taken into account the extended times can, disrupt the efficient sequencing of patients through the facility and overtax technologists and ancillary personnel (Table 7.1).

In a facility performing only combined PET-CT examinations, scheduling of patients must account for the varying time sequence and requirements of different patients. Sufficient shielded and monitored space for patients during the FDG uptake phase must be maintained in the facility. In facilities which use the CT component of the PET-CT scanner additionally for CT only scans, the schedule can be modified to space the PET-CT patients out using CT only exam patients, and reducing facility requirements for shielded and monitored space for the PET-CT patients. An example of appointment schedules is shown in Table 7.2 detailing a combined PET-CT examination only facility a full schedule of PET-CT patients with ample space for injected patients, and a facility, with a limited number of PET-CT patients using the PET-CT scanner for both combined PET-CT examinations and CT only examinations.

Personnel in a PET-CT facility must be trained to accommodate the different patient needs arising in the operation of the facility, and management should have a clear understanding of the time it takes to perform various operations in the PET-CT center, particularly in light of the patient population served, so that the staffing plan is effective and the scanner use is optimized. Patient needs, employee work shifts, referral patterns, hours of operation, and appointment durations should be continually evaluated so appointment

Table 7.1 Typical time involved in procedures performed in a PET/CT facility for typical patients and patients requiring additional time commitments[a]

Appointment time	Injection	Scan time	Patient name	Indication	PET-CT scan	Age	Weight	Dose	Comments
7:00	7:20	8:20	Patient 1	Pulmonary Nodule	Limited Nodule – C	68	84 kg	500 MBq	needs oxygen
7:10	7:30	9:00	Patient 2	Breast Cancer Re-Staging	Whole Torso + C	52	68 kg	500 MBq	
7:50	8:10	9:40	Patient 3	Lung Cancer Staging	Whole Torso + C	76	92 kg	500 MBq	
9:40	10:00	11:30	Patient 4	Lymphoma Re-Staging	Whole Torso – C	28	76 kg	500 MBq	contrast allergy
9:15	9:40	11:10	Patient 5	Cervical Re-Staging	Whole Torso + C	43	65 kg	500 MBq	Lasix/hydration
10:00	10:20	11:50	Patient 6	Head and Neck Ca Staging/RT	Limited Neck for RT + C	56	84 kg	500 MBq	RT planning
11:00	11:20	12:50	Patient 7	Colorectal Cancer Re-Staging	Whole Torso + C	62	78 kg	500 MBq	rectal positive contrast
11:40	12:00	13:30	Patient 8	Esophageal Ca Re-Staging	Whole Torso – C	83	68 kg	500 MBq	
12:20	12:40	14:10	Patient 9	Lymphoma Staging	Whole Torso + C	12	42 kg	350 MBq	peds no sedation
13:20	13:40	15:10	Patient 10	Melanoma Staging	Whole Body + C	38	75 kg	500 MBq	tall
14:20	14:40	16:10	Patient 11	Lung Cancer Restaging	Whole Torso + C	75	82 kg	500 MBq	
15:00	15:20	16:50	Patient 12	Breast Cancer Staging	Whole Torso + C	46	62 kg	500 MBq	
15:40	16:00	17:30	Patient 13	Pulmonary Nodule	Limited Nodule – C	78	65 kg	500 MBq	

[a]Demands on technologist and ancillary personnel will be greater during the FDG uptake period (localization) and image acquisition (scanning) with patients requiring close monitoring even though the time allotment is the same as routine patients

Table 7.2 Example of a daily patient appointment schedule at a facility performing only PET-CT exams and a facility performing a mix of PET-CT and CT only exams[a]

7:30	8:00	9:30	PET-CT patient 1	Lung cancer staging	Whole torso PET-CT+C	66	84 kg	500 MBq	
8:00		8:20	CT Patient 1	Head Pain	Head CT−C	45	66 kg		
8:20		8:40	CT Patient 2	Abdominal Pain	Ab/Pelvis CT+C	62	75 kg		
8:40		9:00	CT Patient 3	Chronic Neck Pain	C-spine CT−C	45	80 kg		
		9:30	PET-CT Patient 1	Scanning PET-CT 1					
10:10		10:30	CT Patient 4	Shortness of Breath	Chest CT−C	64	79 kg		Interstitial lung disease proto
10:40		10:50	CT Patient 5	Head Pain	Head CT−C	39	65 kg		
		11:10	CT Patient 6						
11:15	11:45	13:15	PET-CT Patient 2	Lymphoma Re-Staging	Whole Torso PET-CT-C	32	82 kg	500 MBq	Positive oral contrast
			12:00–1:00 lunch break						
		13:15	PET-CT Patient 2	Scanning PET-CT 2					
		14:10	CT Patient 7	Abdomen Pain	Ab/Pelvis CT+C	35	74 kg		
		14:30	CT Patient 8	Chest Pain	Chest CT+C	56	80 kg		PE protocol
		14:40	CT open for add on						
13:00	13:30	15:00	PET-CT patient 3	Breast Cancer Re-Staging	Whole Torso PET-CT+C	49	64 kg	500 MBq	
15:40		16:00	CT Patient 9	Cough	Chest CT+C	67	84 kg		
16:00		16:20	CT Patient 10	Follow-up lung nodule	Chest CT−C	56	78 kg		
16:20		16:40	CT open for add on						

[a]Different diagnoses and specific patient needs require additional time allotments in the schedule for preparation and scanning times. The workday for (a), a busy PET-CT service, is begins at 6:30 A.M., and ends by 7 P.M. using at least three technologists. The workday for (b), an outpatient imaging facility or mobile PET-CT service with limited PET-CT patients, begins at 7:30 A.M. and ends at 5 P.M. using two technologists

templates can be adapted to changing needs of the patient population and staff.

Support Services

While payment for PET and PET-CT examinations is becoming more common from government programs and health insurance plans, coverage of PET-CT examinations is not yet fully routine or transparent. Depending on the operational setting of a PET-CT facility, it may be advantageous to have an individual on staff to serve as a liaison between the patient, the healthcare providers, and the payers of healthcare. This individual can help certify that the facility receives payment for services rendered and also improve patient satisfaction with the health coverage and medical billing process. This person can insure compliance with specific study protocols involved in payments of indications not routinely covered by government programs or private health plans. Patients should be informed of the likelihood of coverage of all or portions of the PET-CT study prior to their appointment time so that the appointment can be rescheduled or canceled if necessary. It is helpful to keep, in a binder or database, information detailing the payment guidelines for PET-CT by government programs and private commercial payers.

Patient Preparation

Preappointment Communication and Consultation

Communication and education of patients prior to the PET-CT scan appointment is an essential component of patient preparation. An overview of the PET-CT procedure should be mailed to the patient, sent electronically, or made available through web sites, posters, or brochures (Table 7.3). Then, the patient's understanding of the information provided should be verified by a telephone conversation or during a clinic visit prior to the PET-CT scan appointment. At that time the patient's appointment time and directions to the PET-CT facility can be confirmed in an effort to minimize missed or late appointments.

Among the information that should be communicated to the patient are the PET-CT center's recommendations for diet, hydration, and exercise. Moreover, discussions about claustrophobia, pain management, diabetes, renal function, and potential allergies to contrast material should occur prior to the PET-CT appointment so that the patient is prepared appropriately. In addition to the patient's name, identification number, date of birth, weight, and gender, Table 7.4 details information that should be included in a preconsultation worksheet to help

Table 7.3 Example of information contained in a brochure sent to patients prior to their PET-CT appointment

The PET-CT scan

PET (positron emission tomography) and CT (computed tomography) are both important diagnostic tools that physicians use to pinpoint disease states in the body for better management.

The PET scan demonstrates the biological function of the body's tissues, while the CT scan provides information about the body's anatomy such as size, shape, and location. By combining these two technologies, physicians can more accurately diagnose and monitor diseases such as cancer, heart disease, and certain brain disorders.

How the procedure works

To begin the procedure, a small amount of radioactive glucose is injected into your bloodstream through a small catheter (tube) in an arm vein. There is no danger to you from this injection. Glucose (also known as sugar) is a common substance every cell in your body needs in order to function. After the injection, you will wait approximately 90 min in a private waiting room while the injected material is distributed through your body. You may be asked to drink water and oral contrast material during the waiting period.

After the distribution time is complete, you will be asked to lie on a table, which passes slowly through the scanner. The first part of the scan is the CT scan which shows the body's structure. There may be an injection of contrast material into the arm vein through the catheter already placed during this part of the exam. This is routine with most CT scans. The second part of the scan is the PET scan where you will continue to lie on the table which slowly moves through the scanner.

How to prepare for your exam

Typically, you will be asked not to eat or drink anything after midnight the night before your scan except tap or bottled water. You should eat a high protein meal the day before the exam. If you are diabetic, you may have special instructions.

For your comfort and peace of mind, please:

- Tell your doctor if you are pregnant or think that you might be.
- Wear comfortable clothing with no metal buttons or buckles.
- Take any prescribed medication on the day or your exam, unless instructed not to do so.
- Ask your doctor if you can eat after midnight on the day, prior to your exam.
- Avoid all beverages with sugar the day before the exam.

You can expect to be in the PET center for 3–3½ h. The actual scan averages 30–60 min.

Rescheduling your exam

A 24-h notice is required to reschedule a procedure. The injection required for your exam is ordered specifically for you and expires very quickly.

Table 7.4 A preconsultation worksheet to assist PET-CT facility personnel

1. Is the patient and inpatient or an outpatient?
2. Is there a language barrier?
3. Is the patient a diabetic?
4. Is the patient able to lie flat and motionless for a period of time?
5. Does the patient suffer from claustrophobia?
6. Is the patient currently receiving therapy?
7. Was the patient instructed to fast prior to the exam?
8. Did the patient receive hydration instructions?
9. Was the patient educated not to exercise prior to the appointment?
10. Is the patient aware of the duration of the exam?
11. Has the patient had a PET exam previously?
12. Does the patient need a driver after the procedure because of administration of anxiolytic medications?
13. Have the medications that the patient is currently taken been identified?
14. Does the patient have any questions or concerns?

guarantee that a consistent level of communication, preparation, and patient education is achieved.

In outpatient imaging centers it is important to assure patients have adequate directions to the facility and understand the importance of keeping appoint time, and informing the facility of canceled or late appointments. Special needs, including transportation, and medications for pain, anxiety, claustrophobia, or general sedation need to be reviewed. Patients receiving pain, sedative, or anxiolytic medication require a driver after the PET-CT examination. It is crucial to re-emphasize the importance of no sugar or carbohydrate intake of any kind within 6 h prior to the appointment, including any drinks other than tap or unflavored bottled water.

In hospital-based settings, it is imperative to know in advance whether the patient is being treated prior to the appointment. This will assist in eliminating problems associated with transporting the patient throughout the hospital, the patient's diet or intake of fluids, or patient condition. Timing is important when working with a radionuclide with a half-life of less than 2 h. Valuable time could be lost if personnel or a wheelchair, stretcher, or oxygen tank had to be found at the last minute to transport the patient. It is also important with inpatients to know orders the patient's diet and fluid intake. If the patient is receiving dextrose solution or total parenteral nutrition, it should be discontinued 6–8 h prior to the injection of the ^{18}FDG to avoid elevated endogenous insulin levels, just as with routine fasting of outpatients. Inpatients should also be assessed to confirm that they can tolerate the procedure. PET-CT imaging in oncology is generally not considered an emergency procedure, so if a patient needs time to recover from other procedures or feels he or she remaining still during imaging to achieve optimal results, the appointment can be rescheduled.

Barriers to communication such as language, learning skills, or hearing should, when possible, be assessed prior to the patient's arrival at the PET-CT center. For example, if a patient does not speak English or is hearing impaired, the facility may need to arrange for language assistance from an interpreter, a sign language professional, or one of the patient's family members.

Table 7.5 Common insulin types and typical half-lives and effective lives per routes of administration

Insulin type	Onset	Peak activity	Duration
Regular insulin IV	5 min	15–30 min	45 min
Insulin Humalog SC (insulin lispro)	10 min	30–90 min	4 h
Regular insulin SC	30–60 min	2–3 h	6 h
Insulin NPH SC	2–4 h	4–10 h	16 h
Lente Insulin SC	3–4 h	4–12 h	18 h
Ultralente insulin SC	6–10 h	8–18 h	20 h

IV Intravenous, *SC* subcutaneous

Managing Patients with Diabetes

Patients with insulin requiring diabetes require special attention to insure serum glucose and insulin levels are in an acceptable range for ^{18}FDG imaging at the time of the appointment. Glucose does compete with ^{18}FDG, and high levels of serum glucose have been shown to reduce tumor ^{18}FDG uptake and degrade overall PET scan quality due to persistent blood pool tracer activity [4]. Generally, the patient's serum glucose level should be less than 150 mg/dL at the time of ^{18}FDG infusion. Elevated endogenous insulin levels elevate liver and muscle glucose transport, also degrading FDG PET image quality, and in fact the fasting prior to FDG PET imaging is primarily to insure endogenous insulin levels are not elevated at the time of ^{18}FDG infusion, as normally serum glucose levels are maintained well under 150 mg/dL. Many PET centers will generally accept serum glucose levels between 150 and 200 mg/dL at the time of the appointment, although in such instances the supervising physician usually decides on a case-by-case basis whether the PET appointment should proceed. This decision is based on the patient's history and disease process, prior imaging studies, and the patient's ability to manage their serum glucose levels.

Attempts to lower serum glucose in an insulin requiring diabetic at the time of the PET-CT appointment is generally not recommended, since the goal is to have only basal levels of insulin present during the ^{18}FDG uptake phase. Depending on the type of insulin and route, it may require anywhere from about 30 min (IV regular insulin) to over 8 h (subcutaneous intermediate insulin) or even longer before exogenously administered insulin has reached acceptably low levels (Table 7.5). Attempts to titrate serum glucose levels with short-acting intravenous insulin can easily become time consuming for the PET-CT facility personnel. It is usually best for these patients to be rescheduled, in close consultation with the patient and their physician, and ensure that the fast and insulin regimen prior to the rescheduled PET-CT appointment is carefully planned to assure an acceptable serum glucose level at the time of the exam. It is also important to be aware of any insulin administered by a patient prior to the PET-CT appointment to be sure the exogenously administered insulin has reached basal levels at the time of the ^{18}FDG administration.

It is not uncommon for patients to present with low serum glucose levels due to the prolonged fast properly undergone prior to the exam appointment. Serum glucose levels just under 80 mg/dL are generally not of concern if the patient is entirely without symptoms of hypoglycemia. In these patients, however, a source of sugar such as juice (for example, 200 mL fruit juice) can be given after the FDG uptake phase is nearly complete to insure symptoms of hypoglycemia do not occur during the PET-CT imaging acquisition. In patients with serum glucose levels well under 80 mg/dL, a decision must be made whether to proceed with the examination. Patients without symptoms of hypoglycemia can proceed with the intention of supplying an oral source of sugar toward the end of the FDG uptake period. Although the acceptable time interval prior to oral administration of a source of sugar has not been systematically determined, much of the FDG uptake has occurred within 30 min of tracer administration, and many centers have found a ready source of sugar, such as juice, can be given after 30 min without evidence of elevated endogenous insulin levels on the subsequent FDG PET scan. In these patients, however, serum glucose should be monitored prior to the scan acquisition to verify the serum glucose has risen into a normal range and the patient's hypoglycemic symptoms have abated. An oral source of sugar such as fruit juice does not potentially compromise FDG PET image quality due to competition from the glucose as serum glucose levels will not rise out of the acceptable range during the FDG uptake period. Patients with serum glucose below 40 mg/dL, even those without overt symptoms of hypoglycemia, generally should not proceed with the PET-CT examination, but rather receive an oral source of sugar immediately and have their serum glucose monitored until euglycemic serum glucose levels are achieved. These patients can be rescheduled, sometimes simply later in the day, using a shortened fast such as 3–4 h to minimize hypoglycemia. Patients with low serum glucose that have undergone the PET-CT examination should have their serum glucose measured after the scan acquisition, prior to leaving the PET-CT facility, to document a normal range of serum glucose.

Imaging professionals should familiarize themselves with diabetes and appropriate serum glucose levels so they can make informed decisions regarding patients with diabetes who have appointments in the facility. A protocol should be put into place listing the steps that should be taken in the event a patient's serum glucose level is found to be extremely high or low at the time of the PET-CT appointment. Most centers will proceed with the scan if the patient's serum glucose is below 200 mg/dL. If on initial assessment of serum glucose the level is above 200 mg/dL, some centers will have the patient walk around (if they are ambulatory) for 10–20 min and reassess serum glucose. Patients with very high serum glucose (>300 mg/dL) should generally not proceed with FDG tracer injection and the supervising physician should be consulted. Likewise, for very low serum glucose (<60 mg/dL) a physician or nurse should be consulted to examine the patient for signs of hypoglycemia and decide whether to proceed with FDG injection and follow with supplemental fruit juice after 30 min of FDG uptake time or cancel the exam and supplement with a glucose source immediately. It is fairly common for a PET-CT center regularly checking blood glucose levels to discover unknown cases of diabetes. A policy should be in place to deal with these types of patients also. The PET center staff also needs to recognize that certain drugs such as cortisone preparations, diuretics, and anesthetics taken as part of a daily regimen can cause patients to have increased blood sugar levels (Table 7.6).

It can be particularly helpful if, when calling patients to confirm appointment times, PET facility personnel engage them in a thorough discussion of their diabetic status. Patients with diet-controlled diabetes should be asked the history and trends in their blood sugar maintenance to find out when their blood sugar levels are optimal for PET imaging. In many instances, patients with diet-controlled diabetes do not serially check their blood sugar levels in 30 minute intervals, so this may need to be recommended and tracked. In this manner, they can ascertain at what time of the day the patient's blood sugar level is optimal for FDG-PET imaging to determine the most appropriate appointment time. In general, it is also beneficial to develop some general practices such as asking all noninsulin-requiring diabetes mellitus patients to schedule appointments in the afternoon so that they can eat a light breakfast, take their oral medications, start their fast, and present to the PET facility. In contrast, insulin-requiring diabetes mellitus patients can have appointments scheduled early in the morning, so that an overnight fast is utilized, and when they finish the appointment, they can proceed with their normal regimen of insulin injections and eating. Patients with diabetes should always be instructed to bring their medications to the facility in the event that they need them.

Table 7.6 Commonly encountered drugs that can elevate serum glucose

Common or generic	Representative names
Glucocorticoids	Decadron
Phenothiazines	Thorazine, Mellaril, Compazine
Lithium	Eskalith, Lithobid
Tricyclic antidepressants	Elavil, Tofranil, Anafranil
Diphenylhydantoin	Dilantin
Thiazide diuretics	Dyazide
Isoniazid	INH, Nydrazid
Rifampin	Rifadin, Rimactane

Normal fasting serum glucose: <126 mg/dL
Abnormal serum glucose at any time: >200 mg/dL

Managing Patients with Pain, Claustrophobia, or Anxiety

For the PET-CT image acquisition, a patient is required to remain motionless for 10–25 min depending on required axial coverage and particular scan acquisition parameters (cf, PET emission acquisition time). It is particularly important no gross body movement occur between the CT acquisition(s) and the subsequent PET emission acquisitions to promote a correct attenuation correction mapping and accurate coregistration of the reconstructed PET and CT images. Requirements for management of patient pain, claustrophobia, and anxiety during a PET-CT imaging acquisition are similar to that for an MRI in a closed MRI scanner, although the claustrophobia experienced in PET-CT tomographs is usually less than with closed MRI scanners.

Some patients may not be able to lie motionless throughout the imaging sequence because of pain. Medications can help manage the pain and alternative methods of positioning for the imaging acquisition can be pursued (e.g., positioning the patient prone vs. supine to alleviate pressure on areas of the body where the pain originates). If the patient undergoes a PET-CT examination for radiation therapy planning, a flat pallet and immobilization devices will typically be required, exacerbating potential for intolerable pain during the imaging acquisition. For radiation therapy planning, fluctuations in position of relevant body parts are stringently limited, making pain medications even more critical to managing the patient's comfort and ensuring an optimal imaging examination.

Some patients cannot tolerate being inside the scanner gantry due to claustrophobia or anxiety. Even with the increasing bore diameter of contemporary PET-CT systems (70 cm or more), the long bore length can be intimidating. If patients have had bad imaging experiences previously – and even after explanation and education cannot delineate the differences between PET-CT and MRI, CT, or other diagnostic imaging modalities – they may need medication to relieve claustrophobia and help them relax before and during the procedure. Depression and related anxiety are also common among cancer patients, particularly those with oropharyngeal, breast,

Table 7.7 Commonly used medications for anxiety, claustrophobia, and pain during PET-CT imaging

Drug	Indication	Onset, peak, and duration	Dose
Alprazolam (Xanax) oral	Anxiety and Claustrophobia	30 min, 1–2 h, 4–6 h	0.25–0.50 mg for mild claustrophobia 0.5–1.0 mg for moderate claustrophobia 1.0–2.0 mg for severe claustrophobia
Diazepam (Valium) oral	Anxiety	30–60 min, 1–2 h, 3 h	5–10 mg
Lorazepam (Ativan) oral	Anxiety	15–30 min, 1–6 h, 12–24 h	2–6 mg
Midazolam (Versed) IV	Sedation and anxiety	3–5 min, 30 min, 2–6 h	1–2.5 mg intravenous initial dose, maintenance dose 25% of initial dose
Fentanyl IV	Pain, often used in combination with midazolam	1–2 min, 0.5–1 h, 2 h	50–150 μg intravenous
Meperidine (Demerol) IM	Pain	10–15 min, 30–60 min, 2–4 h	50–150 mg intramuscular
Morphine IV	Pain	1–2 min, 20 min, 5–6 h	2.5–15 mg

IM Intramuscular, *IV* intravenous

Table 7.8 Sedation levels, assessment, and required monitoring

Sedation level	Physiologic features	Assessment requirements	Monitoring requirements
Level I Minimal Sedation	Normal response to verbal commands Unaffected airway reflexes and ventilatory and cardiovascular functions	Pre- and postprocedure vital signs	None
Level II Moderate Sedation	Depressed consciousness, but Maintained response to verbal/tactile stimulation, and maintained protective airway reflexes and cardiovascular function	Pre procedure review of systems, vital signs, and airway assessment. Postprocedure monitoring of vital signs and mental status	IV access maintained Blood oxygenation monitoring Blood pressure monitoring optional
Level III Deep Sedation	Near unconsciousness to Unconsciousness with poor or absent response to verbal or tactile stimulation. Loss of protective airway reflexes and reduce respiratory drive. Cardiovascular function impairment possible	Preprocedure review of systems, brief physical examination and airway assessment. Postprocedure monitoring of vital signs and mental status.	IV access maintained Blood oxygenation monitoring Blood pressure monitoring Electrocardiographic monitoring Intubation capability immediately available.
Level IV General Anesthesia	Unconsciousness with no response to verbal and minimal or absent response to painful stimulation. Loss of protective airway reflexes and reducedrespiratory drive. Cardiovascular function impairment Possible.	Preprocedure review of systems, physical examination, and complete airway assessment. Postanesthesiarecovery room monitoring.	IV access maintained Blood oxygenation monitoring Blood pressure monitoring Electrocardiographic monitoring Ventilatory support/intubation

Equipment and facilities and properly trained personal for the next higher level of sedation beyond the intended level of sedation must be available on-site

pancreatic, and lung cancers [5], and some PET-CT centers routinely employ anxiolytic medications with these patients (Table 7.7).

Anxiolysis is defined as "a drug-induced state during which patients respond normally to verbal commands. Cognitive function and coordination may be somewhat impaired; yet, ventilation and cardiac functions are unaffected" [6]. Benzodiazepines are commonly used to reduce anxiety or claustrophobia during medical imaging procedures. Pain, however, is not relieved by anxiolytic medications, and some cancer patients may require specific medication for pain control, or an increase in their preexisting pain medication regimen, for their imaging examination. Different levels of sedation are achieved with different classes and doses of medications, and the level of sedation allowed will depend on the facility and available personnel (Table 7.8). Outpatient facilities are usually not allowed intended sedation beyond level II, while properly equipped and staffed hospitals can perform all levels of sedation, including general anesthesia, for medical imaging procedures.

Anxiolytic and pain medications must be prescribed by a physician. The PET-CT staff can request during the preappointment consultation that the patient bring to the appointment medications to control anxiety or pain prescribed by their primary care or referring specialty physician. In some centers the ordering form for the PET-CT exam has provisions for the ordering physician to prescribe an anxiolytic or pain medication. A PET-CT imaging facility may also choose to adopt a policy that would allow for the administration of anxiolytic medications prescribed by the supervising nuclear medicine physician or radiologist for patients with certain indications. Outpatients undergoing sedation with anxiolytic or pain medications to levels I and II need only cursory medical assessment prior to discharge from the facility, but must not themselves drive home from the appointment. Patients intended to undergo sedation level III and higher require a medical assessment prior to sedation as well as postsedation monitoring and more comprehensive predischarge assessment [7], and also must not themselves drive after the appointment. Patients with a history of sleep apnea require special considerations and procedures for sedation [8]. Since PET-CT imaging is regarded as a noninvasive procedure, patients often are not aware that they will need assistance upon completion of the exam. Also, patients will need to sign a disclosure and consent form for sedation, and the procedure should be documented in the patient's record. These aspects of the exam should be explained during the preappointment consultation.

Hydration

Patient hydration prior to the PET-CT exam is important because it promotes blood pool and urinary tract clearance of the FDG radiotracer, reducing urothelial radiation exposure, and reduces the effects of intravenous CT contrast material on renal function. A hydrated patient's veins will be easier to visualize and access for IV placement and injection as well. The patient should be instructed to drink plenty (1.5–2 L) of tap or unflavored bottled water during the 24-h period immediately prior to the PET-CT scan appointment. The patient can be encouraged to continue drinking water until the time of the exam, although it is important to emphasize only simple tap or bottled water be taken within 4 h of the exam appointment, as patients can unwittingly substitute beverages containing sugar such as juice, soft drinks, tea or coffee with added sweeteners, any of which can effectively break the fast by elevating endogenous insulin levels. Intravenous (IV) hydration (using a nondextrose solution) is generally not required and can be cumbersome and perceived by patients as invasive. Some centers use intravenous hydration during the FDG uptake period in combination with intravenous loop diuretics to accelerate clearance of urinary tracer from the bladder prior to the scan acquisition for improved visualization of pelvic structures on the FDG PET.

Physical Activity

In addition to hydration, strenuous exercise should be avoided in the 24-h period prior to the PET-CT exam appointment. Skeletal muscle can demonstrate marked uptake of FDG even hours after heavy use, reflecting restoration of muscle glycogen stores [9]. If patients continue their exercise regimen it should be noted for the interpreting physician what their routine consisted of prior to the PET-CT appointment so involved muscle groups which may be expected to show elevated tracer uptake can be anticipated. Similarly it is also important that patients are reminded to not chew gum prior to their PET-CT appointment.

Diet and Fasting

Patients should be instructed on fasting and diet prior to the PET-CT exam. The patient should be asked to fast for a minimum of 4 h prior to the ^{18}FDG injection. Fasting allows serum glucose and endogenous insulin levels to approach basal levels. Facilities may choose to extend this fasting period to at least 6 h for a best practices protocol. For patients with morning appointments, Personnel should emphasize that this fasting period includes restricting items containing sugar such as gum, mints, cough lozenges or syrups. Some centers advocate that the last meal consumed prior to the fasting period be high in protein with little or no carbohydrates, to facilitate a shift of myocardial metabolism from carbohydrate metabolism to medium chain fatty acid metabolism and consequently reduce myocardial uptake of the radiotracer [10]. However, this aspect of patient preparation is difficult to verify, as even patients who follow the diet prior to the appointment time exhibit variable ^{18}FDG uptake in the myocardium. In general, a sufficiently long fast will result in a shift of myocardial metabolism to fatty acids throughout the myocardium, resulting in soft tissue background level myocardial tracer activity on the FDG PET images, but even overnight fasts do not consistently achieve this.

Bowel Preparations

Physiologic bowel FDG tracer uptake can be confounding in interpretation of FDG PET scans [9], although the anatomic localization of tracer activity and morphologic assessment of bowel now possible with PET-CT has made the physiologic FDG uptake in bowel less problematic. Some centers have advocated isosmotic bowel preparations the evening prior to the PET-CT exam to reduce tracer activity in the bowel [11]; however, the effectiveness of this technique has not been widely experienced and such preparations are not easily tolerated by some cancer patients.

Managing Patients Who Are Pregnant or Nursing

Female patients should be questioned about their last menses to safeguard that they are not pregnant at the time of the exam.

If the patient cannot remember when her last menstrual period was or there is a suspicion of pregnancy, a urine or blood test can be performed to confirm the patient's status. If the patient is found to be pregnant after referral or a pregnant patient is referred for PET imaging, the physician and the patient should discuss the risks and benefits of having a PET-CT procedure during pregnancy. If the woman has recently had a baby and is breastfeeding, instructions need to be given on how to feed the infant after the PET-CT procedure. It is generally recommended that the patient pump enough breast milk to sustain the infant for 18.5 h after injection time. (Multiplying the short radiopharmaceutical half-life of the ^{18}FDG of 110 min by a factor of 10 yields this duration.) Hicks and his colleagues reported that there is little excretion of ^{18}F-FDG in breast milk and that the majority of radiation exposure to the infant occurs because of the "close proximity to the breast (external) rather than the ingestion of the milk (internal)" [12]. It should also be noted that there is substantially greater uptake of FDG in the lactating breast, increasing radiation exposure to breast tissue.

PET-CT Examination Duration

Patients should be given an accurate estimate of the duration of the PET-CT exam. Although the actual scan acquisition is generally 10–25 min, the time for the entire appointment is usually over 3 h (see Table 7.1). It is essential that patients and their families or accompanying persons understand this timeframe. The time the patient spends in the facility depends on the efficiency of the personnel, the reason for the exam, the protocols followed, the type of scanner utilized, and any special needs or protocols, such as radiation therapy planning. The imaging sequence is also affected by the patient's height because PET scan acquisition is acquired in blocks referred to as bed positions. Most PET-CT scanners currently available have an axial field of view of around 15 cm for each bed position, and most patients require 5–7 bed positions for a scan covering the neck, chest, abdomen, and pelvis. Scans for melanomas and sarcomas can require as many as 16 bed positions for tall patients. This extends the appointment as much as 30 min.

Prior Imaging Examinations and Clinical Information

Arrangements should be made prior to the appointment to obtain data for comparison from PET, PET-CT, and CT exams, as well as any other recent imaging studies relevant to the patient's current diagnosis from outside institutions. The requesting physician office and patient should be encouraged to arrange for such images to be sent to the facility. Owing to the resolution and complexity of PET and contemporary CT images, they are increasingly archived on PACs or digital storage media. This means that facilities need to have a standard mechanism to review and transfer images and outside media from various vendors. Another option is to have a file transfer protocol (FTP) in place to send images electronically if this is in compliance with the center's policies and meets the confidentiality criteria outlined by the Health Information Portability and Accountability Act (HIPAA). The outside studies can be viewed on an additional workstation as needed, or if possible, transferred onto the facility PACs system and viewed directly on the PACs workstations or on the dedicated PET-CT workstation. At the very least, the reports of prior PET, PET-CT, and CT exams, as well as recent clinical notes relevant to the patient's current diagnosis, should be obtained prior to the PET-CT appointment date to aid both prescribing the specific PET-CT protocol that will be used to facilitate proper interpretation and reporting of the exam.

Appointment Check-in and Day of Service Clinical Consultation

If the patient has been properly prepared during the preappointment consultation, obtaining the patient's clinical history and conducting the PET-CT exam will be greatly facilitated. The patient questionnaire and assessment should occur in a private place. Lack of privacy can decrease the openness of the patient and the effectiveness of the communication. The patient assessment allows personnel to observe and report any significant patient history or symptom to the interpreting physician. The collection of this information should be systematic and consistent so that each patient receives the same standard of care. The data must be easily accessible to the physician and communicated effectively by the technologist. This methodical gathering of information could include questions listed in Table 7.9. At the time of the PET-CT appointment, the patient will be assessed to determine the need for applying age-specific criteria or fall precautions. Geriatric patients might have sensory or cognitive impairment that needs to be considered. Pediatric patients should have a parent or guardian present during certain portions of the procedure, and age-appropriate language should be used during communication. Pediatric patients may also present other challenges, such as limited intravenous access, the inability to fast, lack of urinary tract clearance, and complex sedation protocols (see Chapter 11).

At each visit to the PET-CT facility, the patient's height and weight should be taken. As discussed earlier, the patient's height effects the duration of the imaging sequence. The patient's true weight at the time of FDG administration is

Table 7.9 Example of a comprehensive patient questionnaire and assessment to be completed by the patient at the time of the PET-CT appointment in consultation with the technologists or other facility personnel

1.	When did you eat last and what did you have?
2.	How many glasses of water did you drink in the last 24 h?
3.	List surgical history.
4.	Where are your incision sites?
5.	Have you had any biopsies recently?
6.	Have you had chemotherapy? If so, when?
7.	Have you had radiation therapy? If so, when and to what area?
8.	Do you have any ostomy sites?
9.	Do you have a CVC line, Port-A-Cath, or any other existing lines?
10.	Do you have any metal objects or prothesis on at present?
11.	Do you have arrhythmia/ pacemaker?
12.	Have you had any recent injuries, areas of inflammation, or infection?
13.	Do you have any chronic conditions?
14.	If female, when was your last menses?
15.	What medications are you currently taking?
16.	Are you taking any blood thinners?
17.	Are you taking herbal supplements?
18.	List your allergies.
19.	Are you allergic to iodine? What symptoms/ reaction did you have?
20.	Do you have any other appointments today after this test?
21.	Did you receive instructions about this test?
22.	Do you have any questions in reference to the procedure?
23.	Have you ever had a PET/CT scan previously?
24.	Rate your current level of pain on a scale of 1 to 10.
25.	Do you have a history of any of the following conditions?
	Angina
	Asthma
	Bronchitis
	Congenital heart defect
	Diabetes
	Heart attack
	High or low blood pressure
	Hypoglycemia
	Kidney disease
	Pheochromocytoma
	Rheumatoid arthritis
	Sarcoidosis
	Toxoplasmosis
	Tuberculosis

needed if semiquantitative standard uptake values (SUV) associated with the patient's images are to be as accurate as possible. Likewise, if the SUVs are to be corrected for lean body mass, an accurate measure of the patient's height is needed. In addition, PET-CT scanners have different weight limits associated with the patient tables. Now, with the larger-bore (78-cm) PET-CT scanners, it is infrequent that a patient's body habitus is restrictive; it is generally their weight that prevents imaging from commencing.

PET-CT facility personnel should always be conscientious about following universal precautions. Good hand hygiene is considered the most important measure in controlling and preventing the spread of infection in health-care facilities [13]. However, some patients have conditions that necessitate adherence to more than standard precautions. Technologists should familiarize themselves with facility policy and review the necessary precautions for the specific isolation system when caring for these patients. If a patient presents to the PET facility with a known source of infection, such as vancomycin-resistant enterococcus, methicillin-resistant *Staphylococcus aureus,* or tuberculosis, other measures of infection control should be followed. These precautions include the use of gloves, gowns, masks, and other personal protective equipment. Moreover, depending on the patient's diagnosis, the scanner may need to be wrapped and patient contact areas disinfected. It is imperative that the technologists understand the reason for the isolation and the mode of transmission. Additionally, infectious conditions need to be documented so that any areas of hypermetabolism on the PET images can be evaluated for correlation with infectious or inflammatory processes. It has been well documented that sites of infection and inflammation are ^{18}F-FDG avid, including less commonly encountered conditions.

Also at the PET-CT appointment, the patient's serum blood glucose level will be measured using a glucometer. Assay of patient serum glucose is frequently a regulated procedure requiring records and oversight of glucometer calibration. Also expiration dates on reagent strips must be routinely checked, as they deteriorate with exposure to air over time. This immediate feedback on the patient's glucose status allows the technologist to determine whether or not to proceed with the appointment, or specific actions that need to be taken (see Table 7.6). Additionally, if a patient is concerned about his or her blood glucose level, the technologist can take serial measurements every 30 min to trend that the levels are not increasing or decreasing too quickly and put the patient at ease. At times, fasting patients may feel weak due to hypoglycemia. Many facilities follow protocols that allow 200 mL of fruit juice 30 min after FDG tracer injection for patients experiencing hypoglycemia. It is also useful at the time of serum glucose measurement to review available records of patient's renal function (serum creatinine, blood urea nitrogen and estimated GFR (we can spell out if it is first mention)) if intravenous contrast is to be used during the PET-CT exam.

FDG Administration and Uptake Phase

Once the FDG has been administered to a patient, they become a source of radiation exposure to those near them. For technologists and ancillary personnel at the PET-CT facility this radiation exposure must be minimized, otherwise their allowable occupational exposure of 5 rem per year will be easily exceeded. Thus special precautions are required for the injection of FDG tracer and management of patients after the FDG has been administered. Due to the high energy (511 keV) of the annihilation gamma radiation associated with PET radiotracers, radiation shielding in a PET-CT facility is much more extensive than for conventional single photon nuclear medicine imaging [14]. Dedicated uptake rooms or areas for each patient are typically needed to provide sufficient isolation and shielding of the patient source of radiation. In addition, such rooms provide a private and quite environment for the patient during the FDG uptake phase. Figure 7.1 shows a typical "uptake room" for patients undergoing FDG PET imaging at a PET-CT facility. Note there is intercom and video monitoring so the technologists can communicate with and monitor the patient during the FDG uptake phase without coming in close proximity to the patient, thus minimizing cumulative radiation exposure. Since the FDG uptake phase can range from a minimum of one hour to two hours or more, it is also common to have audio and video entertainment in each uptake room. Patient family members (although not typically young children) can be present in the uptake room for the duration of the FDG uptake phase as the short exposure is not significant [15].

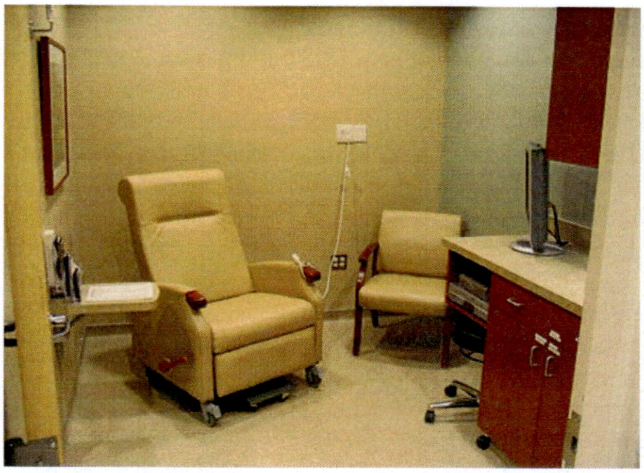

Fig. 7.1 Private patient room for the FDG uptake phase. A comfortable reclining lounge chair minimizes patient muscle tension and movement at the time of the radiopharmaceutical administration and throughout the FDG uptake phase. Room for family members and video and audio entertainment devices are incorporated. A call intercom and video camera monitor allow for constant surveillance and communication while minimizing technologist radiation exposure. The room is extensively shielded with lead to minimize radiation exposure to technologists, ancillary personnel, and nonmonitored workers in the adjoining space

IV Setup and FDG Administration

Once all the patient preparation steps have been completed, the patient is ready to have the IV line set up for the radiopharmaceutical injection. Before it is injected into a patient, two distinct identifiers, such as name and medical record number, should be used to insure the correct dose is administered to the correct patient. FDG should be administered through an intravenous (IV) catheter or butterfly needle set rather than straight needle sticks to reduce the likelihood of radiotracer extravasation at the injection site. If intravenous contrast is to be used for the CT portion of the PET-CT examination, the IV catheter used for the radiopharmaceutical can be used for the subsequent intravenous contrast injection as well. Utilization of an IV catheter or a butterfly set allows the technologist to place and check the IV line using normal saline prior to administering the radiopharmaceutical. This allows techniques which minimize the time handling the dose of radiopharmaceutical at the time of intravenous injection using the heavy shielded syringe sets. The syringe shields used in PET imaging are more substantial than those in general nuclear medicine because of the differences in half value layer (HVL) for 140 vs. 511 keV gamma rays. Some shields crafted of tungsten can weigh as much as 4 kg, therefore making them cumbersome to manage. It is helpful to have a small, wheeled pushcart or tray to transport

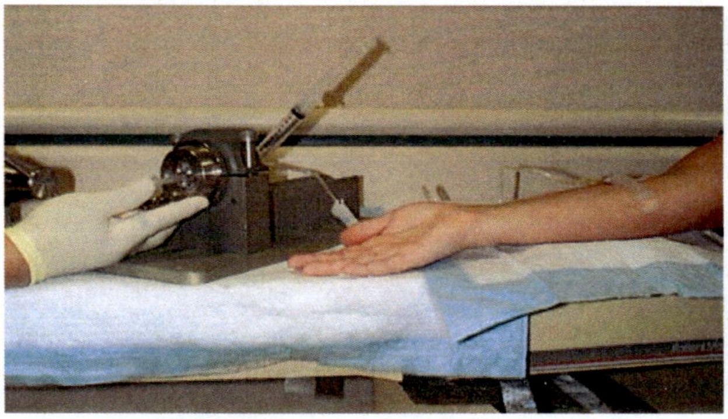

Fig. 7.2 FDG infusion set up on a push cart carrying a heavy shielded syringe set. The intravenous (IV) catheter is placed, and then the shielded syringe set connected for infusion. Note saline flush syringe used to check the IV before FDG infusion and flush the line after radiopharmaceutical infusion

the heavy shielded syringe set from the radiopharmaceutical preparation room ("hot lab") to the patient in the uptake room (Fig. 7.2). Some centers even utilize automated syringe injection devices to further minimize close proximity of the technologist to the patient. In keeping with good practice, single-use items such as tourniquets should be discarded, and all radioactive sharps should be disposed of in a shielded, puncture-resistant box.

Common sites for IV lines to be set include the anterior forearm, dorsal hand, radial aspect of the wrist, and the antecubital space [16]. For some indications in PET imaging, it is necessary for radiopharmaceutical injections to be administered contralaterally or pedally to the disease process. Patients with suspected disease in the axilla or arm should not be injected in the ipsilateral arm, for example. Moreover, breast cancer patients at times have restrictions placed by physicians on sites of injection owing to a history of disease in the area. Technologists need to evaluate the patient's request, questionnaire, and history to determine the best site for administration of the radiopharmaceutical. Integrity of the intravenous line should be checked for blood return and ease of brief normal saline flush. Care should be taken to avoid persistent pooling of blood in the line or catheter hubs, as radiotracer in tiny blood clots can result in artifactual foci of tracer in lungs on subsequent PET imaging due to emboli. Typically, 370–740 MBq (10–20 mCi) of ^{18}FDG is injected when whole-body imaging for oncology is ordered. The exact dose depends on the patient, scanner characteristics, and acquisition mode. After injection of the radiopharmaceutical it is important to always flush with 10–20 cc of normal saline. Any suspicion of extravasation should be noted for the imaging professional and interpreting physician. Residual levels of ^{18}FDG in the injection apparatus (lines and catheters) should be monitored if SUV values are to be used and are to be as accurate as possible. If IV contrast-enhanced CT protocols are used, the IV catheter will remain in use until the completion of the PET-CT imaging acquisition. In this case, residual measurements of the apparatus cannot be performed, so the technologist should be confident that the technique used promotes proper and consistent administration of the radiopharmaceutical.

When intravenous contrast material will be used with the CT portion of the PET-CT scan, an intravenous catheter should be placed which can be used for both the radiopharmaceutical administration and the intravenous contrast material injection. Care must be taken to insure the IV line is inserted at a stable site suitable for rapid injection of contrast material such as the forearm or antecubital fossa. Generally a 22-gauge IV catheter is adequate for intravenous contrast injection of rates of up to 3 mL/sec used in most body oncology CT scanning protocols. For some arterial phase protocols and vascular imaging protocols requiring injection rates of up to 4 mL/sec, a 20-gauge IV catheter is required. Some centers use a 20-gauge IV catheter routinely for most adult patients to reduce to incidence of contrast extravasation incidents at the IV site. Vascular protocols requiring very high rates of intravenous contrast administration up to 5 mL/sec require an 18-gauge IV catheter. A 24-gauge IV catheter, which may be used in small adults and pediatric patients, can be used for intravenous contrast administration rates of 2 mL/sec. When intravenous access is difficult, or in small children, a 24-gauge catheter may be preferred, and the intravenous contrast injection rate used for the CT image acquisition reduced to 1–1.5 mL/sec. When the intravenous access is to be used only for the radiopharmaceutical administration, a 22-gauge IV catheter or butterfly set is preferred for adults, and 24-gauge IV or butterfly set for children. Very difficult intravenous access situations may require use of catheters or butterfly needles sets as small as 25 gauge. If intravenous contrast material will not be used in the PET-CT scan, the IV line can be removed after radiopharmaceutical infusion and saline flush. For patients undergoing sedation using intravenous agents or in those patients requiring continued serum glucose monitoring, IV access should be maintained until completion of the examination.

Central venous catheter (CVC) lines or Port-A-Cath sites should only be used if a peripheral line cannot be established. Radioactivity can adhere to these apparatuses and cause uptake in the area that may impede visualization of disease processes in close proximity to the site. Special procedures are required to maintain sterility when accessing central venous access devices, and heparin flush is required after access to prevent line thrombosis. Technologists should be fully trained in the access and maintenance of central venous access devices, or appropriately trained personnel must be available when central venous access devices must be used. In general, central venous lines should not be used for intravenous contrast administration using a power injector, although hand injection of intravenous contrast can be employed with most nonperipherally inserted central venous lines. Peripherally inserted central venous lines (color-coded purple PICC lines) are now available which are designed to accommodate the pressures encountered when a power injector is employed.

CT Contrast Media

The CT portion of the PET-CT examination will be optimized for a particular patient and indication, and this often involves use of oral and intravenous contrast material. Appropriate intravenous access for injection of intravenous contrast material has been addressed previously. Technologists should be thoroughly familiar with the adverse reactions to intravenous contrast material and appropriate measures for different levels of contrast reaction severity [1, 17]. Oral contrast must be administered prior to the time of scan acquisition to allow for progress of the contrast material through the bowel. If complete opacification of the colon is not required, ingestion of oral contrast during the FDG uptake phase will adequately opacify the small bowel of most patients. Water-soluble contrast will move more quickly through the small bowel than thin barium suspensions, with the terminal ileum reached in as little as 30 min. Generally 750–1,500 mL of positive or negative oral contrast is ingested over the course of the FDG uptake period. Oral contrast is generally more palatable when chilled. If opacification of the colon is desired, the contrast material must be ingested at least 4 h before the PET-CT exam acquisition. If contrast is present in the colon for several hours or longer, both water-soluble and thin barium suspension positive contrast material can become hyperconcentrated in the colon, resulting in degradation of the

CT images due to beam hardening artifact from the radiodense hyperconcentrated contrast and artifactual apparent increased tracer activity on the attenuation corrected PET emission images [3]. In some patients, such as rectal cancer and cervical cancer, per rectal alimentary tract contrast will be administered, usually when the patient is on the scanner table just prior to the imaging procedure.

The FDG Uptake Phase

Once the FDG radiopharmaceutical has been administered intravenously, distribution of the glucose analog can be effected by patient activity due to skeletal muscle uptake. A quiet secure environment must be available for patients during the FDG uptake phase. Anxiety is common among cancer patients, and noise, lack of privacy, lack of security of their possessions, and distractions can additionally increase anxiety in some patients. Anxiety raises muscle tension [13] potentially resulting in increased muscle tracer activity on the PET images. Ideally private rooms, such as shown in Fig. 7.1, should be available for the radiopharmaceutical administration and the entire FDG uptake period. Patients should be instructed not to talk, chew, or move extensively during radiopharmaceutical uptake, especially during the first 30 min of the uptake phase, as skeletal muscle contraction, particularly during the early FDG uptake phase, when serum availability of the tracer is high, can result in ^{18}FDG uptake in the muscle. A reclining chair or supine position on a comfortable couch or bed is preferred to minimize muscle tension, especially neck and back muscles during the FDG uptake phase. For patients with head and neck cancer, special additional maneuvers to minimize FDG tracer uptake in the muscles of vocalization, including a "quiet time" of no talking, swallowing, or chewing for a period prior to the FDG administration, are added at some centers.

Brown adipose tissue can be a source of intense FDG tracer uptake usually in a symmetrical pattern in the neck and adjacent upper thorax and along the paraspinous musculature (see Figs. 16.15 and 28.9). Even in the setting of PET-CT, specious FDG uptake in brown fat can complicate interpretation. Brown adipose tissue functions in thermal regulation, generating heat from elevated glycolytic metabolism in response to sympathetic neural stimulation. Exposure to cold causes sympathetic stimulation of brown adipose tissue, markedly raising glucose uptake in this richly vascularized adipose tissue. Anxiety alone, which raises adrenergic neural activity, can also stimulate brown fat glucose uptake. This is more commonly seen in younger and lean patients, and more commonly encountered when patients are chilled. Immediately before, and during, the FDG uptake phase, patients should be in a warm environment. In addition to keeping FDG uptake rooms at an elevated thermostat setting, some centers additionally provide warmed blankets. Because anxiety alone can cause brown fat FDG uptake, a quiet secure environment, including private uptake rooms, and supportive attitude of technologists, nurses, physicians, and ancillary personnel is helpful in reducing brown fat FDG radiotracer uptake on the PET images. Anxiolytic medications are effective in minimizing spurious brown fat FDG radiotracer uptake and are used routinely at some centers. Beta blocker medications may also reduce cold or anxiety stimulated brown fat FDG tracer uptake by directly blocking the adrenergic stimulation.

During the FDG uptake phase, and immediately prior to imaging, patients should be encouraged to void. This will reduce overall radiation dose to the bladder. Properly hydrated patients typically will need to void more than once, and therefore easy access to a restroom, both from uptake rooms and the scanner room, is an important design feature of a PET-CT facility. It is important to have patients void immediately prior to imaging, as they may not appreciate the effect of hydration (and especially diuretics, if used) or the length of the scan acquisition. Urgency to void during the scan acquisition is a common cause of patient movement, and in some circumstances the urgency to void may require interruption of the scan acquisition.

The time allotted for radiopharmaceutical uptake typically ranges from 1 to 2 h, although research has suggested that even longer localization times may be advantageous in terms of improving tumor to background ratios [18]. However, longer uptake times require an increase in the available uptake rooms in a busy PET-CT facility, so a balance between desired uptake time and capacity of the PET-CT facility must be made. If SUVs are to be used, it is important to strive for consistent uptake time, as the SUV is significantly influenced by the uptake time [19, 20]. Some facilities may opt to specify the uptake time based on tumor type or treatment regimens, using much longer uptake times for cancers, such as breast, pancreatic, or hepatocellular carcinoma, which are not generally highly FDG avid, or for suspected liver metastases [21, 22]. PET is useful in determining response to therapy for some cancer indications, so consistency in technique becomes very important, and if SUVs are to be used, a consistent uptake time, in addition to consistent method of image reconstruction [23], correction for lean body mass and measurement, must be followed (see Chapter 6).

PET-CT Imaging Acquisition

The patient's diagnosis, requesting physician's orders, and the prescribed imaging protocol should be reviewed again immediately prior to the PET-CT imaging procedure to verify that the imaging protocol and reason for the exam are appropriate for the diagnosis. As noted earlier, dense residual barium can substantially degrade the CT images and cause attenuation correction errors on the PET images resulting in unauthentic apparent elevated tracer activity, and this possibility should be addressed during the screening procedure at scheduling and at clinical consultation. The patient should be asked to remove all metal objects and to void as completely as possible just prior to the imaging sequence. Image degradation due to small metallic objects such as zippers, snaps, or small metal hooks are generally negligible, but larger metallic objects such as large belt buckles, pocket change, keys, and the like, can cause significant beam hardening artifact on the CT images and attenuation correction errors on the PET images (Fig. 7.3). For head and neck cancer patients, earrings and detachable metallic dental appliances should be removed.

Before being placed on the scanner table, patients should again be informed of the total time they will have to remain motionless for the complete scan acquisition, and asked if they anticipate any problems with claustrophobia or pain during the procedure. It is sometimes helpful to place the patient on the scanner pallet in the position they will have to assume for the scan and advance the pallet into the scanner gantry as a "dry run." As discussed previously, the total time for the imaging acquisition is largely determined by the PET emission acquisition time, which is determined by the number of bed positions and the emission time allotted to each bed position. The number of bed positions is based on the height of the patient and the required anatomic coverage of the scan. Longer emission acquisition times per bed position improve the PET image quality, but this must be balanced with patient comfort and ability to withstand a longer procedure. Patient movement during both the CT and PET image acquisitions will degrade image quality and can result in image artifacts, negating any gains in statistical image quality. Current PET-CT scanners use PET emission image acquisition times per table position of between 3 and 5 min, although with small and thin patients acquisition time per table position are reduced to 2 min or less at some centers. Similarly, protocols employing 1–2 min per bed position emission acquisition times are used at some centers for patients dealing with extreme pain or claustrophobia.

Patients are generally positioned supine with arms raised above the head for most body oncology indications. To support the patient's comfort and minimize movement during the scan acquisition use positioning devices to support the head and arms and elevate the patient's knees. Dedicated imaging of the head and neck is performed with arms down and usually more secure restraints of the head. Some patients cannot tolerate having their arms raised above their head for a body imaging acquisition, and other instances, for melanomas, sarcomas, and other disease processes potentially involving the upper extremities, patients may be asked to keep their arms down to the side to incorporate the area of interest into the field of view. It is important that the technologist verify on the scout or topogram that the patient is in the field of view and that there is no peripheral truncation observed before proceeding with the CT and PET acquisitions. It is also important when arms are down, they are secured and the patient is reminded to keep arms and hands motionless throughout the scan acquisition, as any movement of the arms or hands between the CT and PET image acquisition can lead to substantial attenuation correction artifacts. In some circumstances a patient cannot tolerate the supine position, but they may tolerate prone positioning. Patients for whom the PET-CT images will be utilized for radiation treatment planning will have to be placed in the exact same position for both procedures, hence the PET-CT imaging acquisition must be performed using the same configuration flat radiation therapy pallet and positioning and immobilization devices, and in addition positioning lasers may need to be used during the patient's exam so that the positioning of the patient is identical to the treatment position.

Because the PET emission data at all table positions is corrected for attenuation by the same single-setting CT

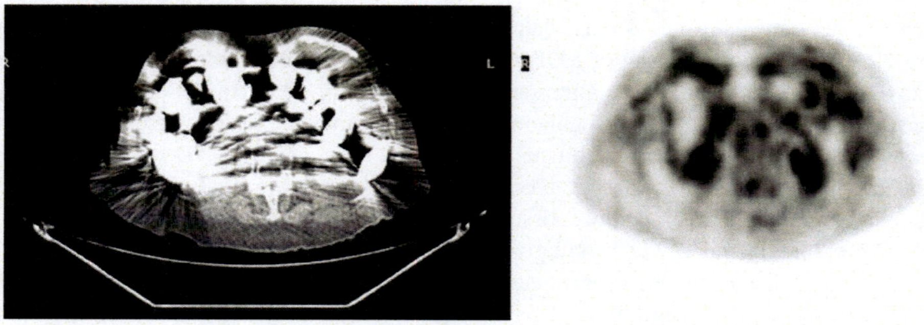

Fig. 7.3 Beam hardening artifacts. High density residual barium from prior radiographic upper GI barium examination (**a**). Note the extent of degradation of the CT images from the beam hardening artifact and extent of apparent "hot" areas on the attenuation corrected FDG PET scan

acquisition, the time between the CT image acquisition and the PET emission image acquisition ranges from 1 to 2 min for the first table position PET acquisition, to over 20 min or more for the last table position PET acquisition. One technique to minimize the possibility of patient movement between the CT used for attenuation correction and the PET emission imaging is to start the PET imaging sequence over the area of interest. For example, lung and esophageal cancer patients would have their PET imaging sequences run craniocaudad. In contrast, ovarian, colorectal, and cervical cancer patients would have their PET imaging sequences start at the pelvis and proceed caudocranial. For lymphoma patients with disease in the neck or chest, a craniocaudad sequence will minimize CT and PET misregistration and attenuation correction errors at the neck, while lymphoma patients with disease at the pelvis, a caudocranial sequence is preferred. The orientation of the CT acquisition is driven by considerations of intravenous contrast and breath-hold as the CT image acquisition of the entire body is accomplished in less than 1 min with contemporary helical CT scanners. Head and neck cancer patients may benefit from a dedicated CT and PET acquisition sequence of the head and neck only, using CT and PET imaging parameters appropriately optimized for the that region of the body, with the rest of the body, when included in the examination, acquired as a separate set of CT and PET acquisitions.

When IV contrast material is employed for the CT portion of the examination, it is important to check the integrity of the IV access with a brief saline flush after the patient has been positioned for scanning. This is easily accomplished using a saline flush syringe, or as part of an integral feature of a dual source power injector. Any undue resistance to flush should raise suspicion of the adequacy of the indwelling IV catheter, although repositioning of the arm is sometimes all that is required to achieve adequate flow. It is also important to remind the patient of the expected sensation of contrast injection, including coolness along the vein and a flushing sensation, and sometimes urinary urgency. Contrast warmers reduce the sensation of coolness along the route of the injected vein and reduce viscosity of the contrast material thus reducing line pressures. While nausea and vomiting are a potential side effect of the contrast material injection which must be conveyed to the patient, it may be best not to overly emphasize this due to the suggestive potential on the sensation of nausea. Cancer patients are, however, more prone to this side effect, and therefore many centers use isotonic nonionic intravenous contrast material exclusively.

Depending on the type of CT scanner and protocol employed in a PET-CT examination, a breath-hold may be required to obtain a fully optimized CT scan of the chest and upper abdomen. Certain radiation therapy protocols require breath-hold CT scans at certain specified inspiratory or expiratory stations. Facilities must develop a consistent way to give patients breathing instructions during the CT acquisition. If a single CT acquisition with breath-hold is to be used for the attenuation correction of the PET emission image data, a mid-expiratory position of breath-hold is required to match the average position of the diaphragm and chest wall expansion of the reconstructed PET images, otherwise there will be misregistration of the PET and CT images. An alternative used by some centers is to simply tell the patient to "stop breathing" as the CT acquisition passes to the upper thorax, and then to resume breathing after the pelvic inlet is passed. Regardless of the breathing technique chosen, it should be practiced with the patient prior to the procedure. This will give the operator an idea of the patient's ability to comply with the requested protocol.

Respiratory gating is another technique that could be used to address the problem of movement during breathing. These devices are particularly useful in the respiratory gating used in advanced IMRT radiotherapy, and are being applied to PET-CT for matching the PET reconstructed images to a particular breath hold position CT acquisition. The real-time position management (RPM) system, for example, monitors the motion of a patient's chest using reflective markers attached to a block positioned on the patient's abdomen and an infrared camera mounted on the end of the patient couch of the PET-CT scanner. The motion of the block is registered to a RPM workstation and the data can be used to gate the PET emission data acquisition for a specific phase of the respiratory cycle.

Patients should be monitored continually throughout imaging acquisition at the very least, by visual observation and verbal communication. Scanner room intercom systems and monitoring cameras are important design features of a PET-CT facility. Patients should be instructed to verbally apprise the technologists of any symptoms of contrast reaction, urgency to void, or increasing anxiety or claustrophobia while in the scanner gantry. Some patients, particularly children, can better tolerate the scanning session if a family member or caretaker is in the scanner room with them. This can be permitted during the PET emission acquisition with few restrictions, while during the CT scan(s) persons in the scanner room should use lead jackets and be positioned at a room site of low exposure. Sedated patients require careful monitoring of respiratory movement, and certain levels of sedation require continuous pulse and blood oxygen monitoring. Observations including gross patient movement, coughing, noncompliance with breathing protocol, etc. should be noted for the interpreting physician. The patient's ability to comply with necessary imaging parameters dictates the need for additional imaging, changes in protocol, or cessation of the exam.

Postimaging Considerations

Before the patient leaves the scanner room, the available images (typically all of the CT images and some PET image reconstructions) of the PET-CT exam should be quickly reviewed to insure appropriate anatomic coverage was obtained and whether any imaging artifacts will require rescanning. Before the IV catheter, if present, is removed, the technologist should assess the patient for signs or symptoms of evolving contrast reaction. Also, if additional serum glucose measurements are needed for diabetic patients or who presented with hypoglycemia, these can be performed using the venous access prior to removal of the IV catheter. Before the patient leaves the PET-CT facility, the entire PET-CT exam should be reviewed by the technologist, with particular attention to image quality and artifacts, with an explanation for artifacts (metallic foreign bodies, excessive patient movement, coughing, noncompliance with breathing protocol, etc.) noted for the interpreting physician. Also, incidental and unexpected clinically significant imaging findings such as deep venous thrombosis, pulmonary embolism, pneumothorax, large pleural effusions, and the like need to be recognized and reported to the radiologist or nuclear medicine physician before an outpatient leaves the PET-CT facility. Outpatients who have undergone level I and II sedation will require a brief medical assessment prior to leaving the PET-CT facility. Outpatients who have undergone level III and higher sedation will require additional postsedation monitoring and more comprehensive assessment prior to leaving the PET-CT facility. All final assessments of sedated patients must be documented. Also, before a patient leaves the PET-CT facility all medical releases of information should be signed if the patient or their physician wishes to have the imaging data sent to another facility for review.

Conclusion

The physician, technologist, and ancillary staff all play valuable roles in the care and management of patients in a PET-CT facility. With the advent of combined scanners such as PET-CT, expertise and skill level of personnel are increasing as they pursue additional knowledge to practice in this modality. PET-CT imaging requires that each member of the team exercises due diligence for their part of the patient's experience. PET-CT is a dynamic, rapidly evolving modality that offers a myriad of opportunities to those who practice in the profession and a wealth of information for the patients and physicians it services.

References

1. Bettmann MA. Frequently asked questions: iodinated contrast agents. RadioGraphics 2004;24:S3–S10.
2. Thomsen HS, Morcos SK. Contrast media and the kidney: European society of urogenital radiology (EUSR) guidelines. Br J Radiol 2003;76:513–518.
3. Beyer T, Antoch G, Muller S, et al. Acquisition protocol considerations for combined PET/CT imaging. J Nucl Med 2004;45:25S–35S.
4. Wahl RL, Henry CA, Ethier SP. Serum glucose: effects on tumor and normal tissue accumulation of 2-[F-18]-fluoro-2-deoxy-D-glucose in rodents with mammary carcinoma. Radiology 1992;183:643–647.
5. Massie MJ. Prevalence of depression in patients with cancer. J Natl Cancer Inst 2004;32:57–71.
6. The University of Texas M.D. Anderson Cancer Center Anxiolysis Policy. 2003. Volume VII.A.1.007.
7. Practice guidelines for sedation and analgesia by non-anesthesiologists. Anethesiology 2002;96:1004–1017.
8. Martin ML, Lennox PH. Sedation and analgesia in the interventional radiology department. J Vasc Interv Radiol 2003;14:1119–1128.
9. Shreve PD, Anzai Y, Wahl RL. FDG PET imaging: physiologic and benign variant pitfalls in oncologic diagnosis. RadioGraphics 1999; 19:61–77.
10. Lum D, Wandell S, Ko J, Coel M. Positron emission tomography of thoracic lesions: reduction of myocardial fluorodeoxyglucose uptake artifacts with carbohydrate restricted diet. Clin Positr Imag 2000;3(4):155.
11. Vesselle HJ, Miraldi FD. FDG PET of the retroperitoneum: normal anatomy, variants, pathologic conditions, and strategies to avoid diagnostic pitfalls. RadioGraphics 1998;18:805–823.
12. Hicks RJ, Binns D, Stabin MG. Pattern of uptake and excretion of ^{18}F-FDG in the lactating breast. J Nucl Med 2001;42:1238–1242.
13. Elkin MK, Perry AG, Potter PA. Nursing Interventions and Clinical Skills, 3 rd edn. St. Louis: Mosby, 2004.
14. Shreve P. Establishing a PET/CT practice. Am J Roentgenol 2005;184:S146–S151.
15. Faasse T, Kloska M, Ploeg M, Shreve P. Radiation exposure levels near patients during FDG uptake phase. Mol Imag Biol 2005;7(Suppl):24.
16. Jensen SC, Peppers MP. Pharmacology and Drug Administration for Imaging Technologists. St. Louis: Mosby, 1998.
17. Koenraad JM, Oliva M-R, Ondategui S, Ros PR, Silverman SG, Universal use of nonionic contrast medium for CT: evaluation of safety in a large urban teaching hospital. Am J Roentgenol 2005;184:31–34.
18. Thie JA, Hubner KF, Smith FT. Optimizing imaging time for improved performances in oncology PET studies. Mol Imag Biol 2002;4:238–244.
19. Keyes JW. SUV: standard uptake or silly useless value? J Nucl Med 1995;36:1836–1839.
20. Beaulieu S, Kinahan P, Tseng J, et al. SUV varies with time after injection in ^{18}F-FDG PET of breast cancer: characterization and method to adjust for time differences. J Nucl Med 2003;44:1044–1050.
21. Torizuka T, Tamaki N, Inokuma T, et al. In vivo assessment of glucose metabolism in hepatocellular carcinoma with FDG-PET. J Nucl Med 1995;36:1811–1817.
22. Tatsuya H, Tsuneo S, Yuji N, et al. Relationship between retention index in dual-phase 18F-FDG PET, and hexokinase-II and glucose transporter-1 expression in pancreatic cancer. J Nucl Med 2002;43:173–180.
23. Jaskowiak CJ, Bianco JA, Perlman SB, Fine JP. Influence of reconstruction iterations on 18-F-FDG PET/CT standardized uptake values. J Nucl Med 2005;46:424–428.

Chapter 8
Radiation Protection of Technologists and Ancillary Personnel

Robert E. Reiman

Introduction

Within a year following the first medical radiographs in early 1896, two things became readily apparent. First, x-rays had the potential to reveal disease in areas of the living human body previously inaccessible to physicians except by invasive techniques. Second, x-rays carried great capacity for harm. Cases of radiation dermatitis in radiologists and patients alike were observed soon after the first publications of the new technique, followed by numerous reports of radiation-induced cancers during the next 2 decades. The isolation and purification of useful amounts of radium demonstrated that radioactive material could be used to treat malignant tumors. However, the unfortunate experience of the radium-illuminated dial painters and other individuals who ingested radium demonstrated that internally deposited radionuclides could induce cancer as well. As the fields of diagnostic imaging and radiation biology developed, it became increasingly apparent that the benefits to society from ionizing radiation came with a price. As a result, the field of medical radiation protection was born. Radiation protection combines the techniques of physicists in measuring radiation exposure and dose with the expertise of biologists, physiologists, and physicians regarding biomedical effects in safeguarding patients and the public against the adverse effects of ionizing radiation.

The Challenges of PET-CT

During the 1960s and 1970s, the simultaneous development of positron-emission tomography (PET) and x-ray computed tomography (CT) enabled physicians to visualize both physiologic function and structural anatomy in patients in three dimensions. Initially, these modalities were implemented asynchronously by radiologists and nuclear medicine physicians. Separate PET and CT procedures on a patient might be performed days or weeks apart, and the correlation of anatomic and functional information was accomplished through side-by-side comparison of film or digital images. Consequently, completely separate regulations and techniques were developed to accommodate the different radiation protection requirements of the two modalities. Radiation safety policies and procedures for PET were based on those developed for traditional nuclear medicine radiopharmaceuticals, while methods for CT were derived from those for existing diagnostic and fluoroscopic x-ray units.

Instruments that simultaneously acquire PET and CT images now permit a correlation of anatomy and physiologic function which is free from the constraints imposed by variations in patient positioning, patient size, image scale, and disease progression between procedures. The marriage of these disparate techniques brings the radiation protection challenges posed by PET and CT into a single imaging suite.

The Principle of ALARA

A guiding tenet of radiation protection is that there be no *unnecessary* exposure to ionizing radiation; that is, every x-ray that is taken and every radiopharmaceutical that is administered should be of benefit to the patient. In addition, radiation exposure to patients, medical personnel and the public should be maintained *as low as reasonably achievable* (ALARA), within the constraints of medical, social, and economic considerations. In this chapter, we will review how the principle of ALARA is applied to PET and CT administratively in the form of governmental regulations. We will also demonstrate how ALARA can be implemented operationally to minimize radiation exposure to the personnel in the PET-CT facility, to the patients who undergo PET-CT imaging, and to the public.

R.E. Reiman (✉)
Radiation Safety Division, Duke University Medical Center,
2214 Elder St., Building E, Durham, NC, 27710, USA
e-mail: robert.reiman@duke.edu

P. Shreve and D.W. Townsend (eds.), *Clinical PET-CT in Radiology: Integrated Imaging in Oncology*,
DOI 10.1007/978-0-387-48902-5_8, © Springer Science+Business Media, LLC 2011

PET-CT Regulations

As a combined imaging modality, PET-CT is subject to state and federal regulations governing the production, transport, and utilization of radioactive material and x-ray producing devices. With the exception of regulations addressing the certification of technologists who perform PET-CT or SPECT/CT studies in California, there are no state or federal regulations that directly address PET-CT.

Regulatory Authority

In the United States, general regulatory authority for the possession and use of reactor byproduct material, source material and special nuclear material is vested in the United States Nuclear Regulatory Commission (NRC). The majority of the specific regulations governing the medical use of byproduct material are contained in Title 10, Parts 20 and 35 of the Code of Federal Regulations (CFR). In general, Part 20 (10 CFR 20) covers the administrative aspects of the possession, use, and disposal of byproduct material, including the requirements for radiation protection programs, radiation dose limits to occupational workers and the public, security and storage of radioactive material, and monitoring radioactive contamination and radiation dose to personnel. Part 35 (10 CFR 35) addresses the medical use of radioactive material, and therefore is of immediate interest to practitioners of nuclear medicine and PET-CT. Part 35 contains provisions for the quality control of instrumentation, the release of patients containing radioactive material, the reporting and documentation of improper administration of radioactive material to patients or inadvertent exposure of an embryo or fetus to radioactive material (so-called medical events), and the storage for decay and disposal of short-lived radioactive material.

Since the radionuclides used to synthesize PET radiopharmaceuticals are typically cyclotron-produced and therefore are not classified as byproduct material, their use has been regulated by the individual states. State regulations governing the use of non-byproduct forms of radioactive material are generally based on NRC regulations, and may contain requirements that are more stringent than those of the NRC. For that reason, the regulations governing the radionuclides used in PET-CT vary from state to state. Regulatory authority over radioactive material may be vested in state agencies that oversee public health or environmental protection. Requirements for the use of CT scanners, including shielding design, x-ray output limits, and operator training, are also provided at the state level. However, it is likely that the NRC will assume oversight of the use of accelerator-produced radioactive material in the future. As a result, changes in state regulations addressing accelerator-produced radioactive material can be expected as the states adapt their rules to new NRC requirements.

The United States Food and Drug Administration (FDA) has oversight of the development and production of PET radiopharmaceuticals in the United States, and the protection of research subjects who participate in studies investigating the biodistribution of new radiotracers. In addition, the Center for Devices and Radiological Health, a branch of the FDA, provides oversight for the production and sale of CT scanners.

Occupational and Public Dose Limits

PET-CT personnel and members of the public are subject to annual radiation dose limits. Dose limits for the United States and the United Kingdom are summarized in Table 8.1. In the United States, PET-CT personnel whose annual occupational doses are expected to exceed 10% of the applicable limits in Table 8.1 must be provided with personal dosimeters to document compliance with the limits. It is recommended that personal dosimeters be changed at monthly intervals to ensure dose limit compliance and assist in maintaining radiation exposure to staff as low as reasonably achievable. Personal dosimeters should be worn according to the vendor's instructions. Nurses will be an integral part of the patient care team if invasive or interventional procedures such as image-guided needle-aspiration biopsies are performed in the PET-CT facility, or patients who require sedation are imaged. Although nurses usually do not dispense radiopharmaceutical doses or handle radioactive material directly, they are exposed to patients and the x-ray beam. For that reason, they should be provided with personal dosimeters.

Pregnant radiation workers are subject to a special occupational limit. The embryo or fetus is limited to a total dose

Table 8.1 Annual radiation dose limits for occupational workers and the public in the USA and UK

	United States			United Kingdom		
Population	Total body	Lens of eye	Extremities	Total body	Lens of eye	Extremities
Occupational Workers	50	150	500	20	150	500
General Public	1	–	–	1	15	50

of 5.0 mSv (500 mrem) during the period of gestation. Regulatory compliance is documented by a dosimeter worn at the level of the waist and under the shielding apron. Fetal dosimeters should be changed monthly to provide documentation of regulatory compliance and permit adequate monitoring consistent with ALARA principles.

Receipt and Disposal of Radioactive Material

Shipments of radioactive material to the PET-CT facility must be inspected for integrity and determined to be free of removable contamination upon arrival. Vials, syringes, intravenous infusion tubing, and other items used in the administration of radiopharmaceuticals must be segregated from the nonradioactive trash and held for decay for at least 10 half-lives (about 20 h for ^{18}F). Following storage for decay, the radioactive waste must be surveyed using a Geiger-Mueller detector or other suitable instrument. If the survey detects no residual activity, the waste may be disposed via the normal waste stream. Patient excreta, if not collected by the facility, may be disposed via the sanitary sewer system without regard to radioactivity content.

Quality Control

In general, calibration of survey instruments that are capable of measuring dose rate must be performed annually. Operational checks must be performed before each use; an instrument that is not functioning properly must be removed from service. Linearity checks and calibration of dose calibrators must be performed at prescribed intervals.

Warning Signs and Shielding Personal Protective Equipment

Signs depicting the standard radiation symbol (a black or magenta tri-blade on a white or yellow background) containing the words "Caution: Radioactive Material" must be posted on doors to the "hot lab," injection rooms, and scanner room. A sign should be posted prominently in the patient waiting area that advises patients that "If You Are Pregnant, or Think You Are Pregnant, Please Inform the Technologist."

Personnel who must be present in the scanner room while the x-ray beam is activated must wear shielding aprons, or shielding vest/skirt combinations that cover the entire front of the trunk. This shielding protective equipment must be constructed using material providing the equivalent shielding capability of a 0.5-mm thickness of lead. Persons performing needle aspiration biopsies in conjunction with CT must not place their hands in the primary x-ray beam unless they are protected by gloves or mitts containing 0.5 mm lead equivalent. Although shielding aprons provide effective protection against x-rays, they afford virtually no protection against the 511-keV annihilation photons from PET radiopharmaceuticals.

Medical Events

The improper administration of a radiopharmaceutical that results in excessive radiation dose to a patient or research subject constitutes a "medical event," as defined in 10 CFR 35. Administration: (a) of the wrong radiopharmaceutical, (b) by the wrong route of administration, (c) to the wrong patient, or (d) in an amount that differs by more than 20% of the prescribed dosage will result in a medical event if the resulting effective dose equivalent exceeds 50 mSv (5.0 rem), or the dose equivalent to any organ or tissue exceeds 0.5 Sv (50 rem). The occurrence of a medical event must be reported to the appropriate regulatory agency within one calendar day, followed by a written report of the event within 15 days. The occurrence of a reportable medical event in the PET-CT setting is unlikely, due to the low radiation doses associated with short-lived PET radiopharmaceuticals. For example, the effective dose equivalent due to ^{18}F FDG is about 0.03 mSv per administered MBq (0.11 rem/mCi). A typical administration of 370 MBq (10 mCi) would result in an effective dose equivalent of only 11 mSv (1.1 rem); an administration of over 1,660 MBq (45 mCi) of ^{18}F FDG would be required to exceed the 50 mSv criterion. Nevertheless, errors in PET radiopharmaceutical administration, even if they do not rise to the level of reportable medical events, must be documented as part of a quality management program. These so-called "recordable events" must be analyzed as to the cause of the event, and what corrective actions were taken to prevent the errors from occurring in the future.

Similarly, the inadvertent administration of a PET-CT radiopharmaceutical that results in a dose equivalent of greater than 50 mSv to a developing embryo or fetus is reportable to the appropriate regulatory agency as a medical event.

Record Retention

In general, records of the receipt and disposal of radioactive material, the results of area surveys for radioactive contamination, documentation of compliance with public dose limits, and records of medical events must be retained in the PET-CT facility for 3 years. Records documenting compliance with occupational dose limits must be retained for the lifetime of the individuals subject to monitoring.

Minimizing Radiation Exposure to Technologists and Physicians

PET-CT technologists and physicians are exposed to radiation during the dispensing and administration of radiopharmaceuticals, while performing interventional or biopsy procedures during CT imaging, and during interactions with radioactive patients. The occupational radiation dose to technologists and physicians from PET-CT can be predicted using data obtained from standard PET and CT fluoroscopic studies [1–4]. These doses are summarized in Table 8.2. Whole body and hand doses from a single PET-CT study during which an interventional procedure is performed are about 0.02 mSv (2 mrem) and 0.15 mSv (15 mrem), respectively.

Simple techniques employing the protective principles of time, distance and shielding can significantly reduce radiation dose to personnel. The total radiation dose incurred by a technologist during a PET-CT study is the product of the dose rate and the exposure time. Limiting exposure time to the minimum necessary to complete a task will minimize radiation dose. Therefore, interactions with vials and syringes containing radiopharmaceuticals, and with the patients following radiopharmaceutical administration, should be performed swiftly and efficiently in order to minimize dose. However, good patient care and safety must not be sacrificed in the interest of speed. Practicing dose dispensing and calibration techniques with nonradioactive material will reduce the chance of error. Substitution of personnel is an effective administrative control in reducing individual occupational doses by limiting the time that staff members spend interacting with patients. If the PET-CT facility is located within a larger nuclear medicine department, staff may be rotated from the PET-CT facility into operations such as general nuclear medicine or nuclear cardiology where the exposure rates encountered are typically lower. Within the PET-CT facility, tasks should be distributed evenly so that no single technologist is consistently working in a high-exposure setting.

Table 8.2 Personnel whole-body and hand doses from FDG PET and CT fluoroscopic examinations

	Radiation dose (mSv) per examination	
Imaging modality	Whole body	Hand
CT, normalized to 250 mAs	0.011[a]	0.085[b]
PET, normalized to 370 MBq (10 mCi)	0.007[c]–0.009[d]	0.069[c]
PET+CT	0.018	0.154

[a] Computed from data by Paulsen EK et al. [1]

[b] Computed from data and review of 9 CT fluoroscopy studies by Buls N et al. [2]

[c] Computed from data by Biran T et al. [3]

[d] Computed from data by Robinson CN et al. [4]

Maintaining the maximum practical distance from a radiation source will dramatically reduce the dose rate to technologists and other personnel. Dose rate is inversely proportional to the square of the distance. For example, a dose rate of 50 μSv/h (5 mrem/h), as measured at a distance of 1 m from an ^{18}F FDG patient, will be reduced to about 12.5 μSv/h (1.25 mrem/h) at 2 m from the patient. Using tongs or long forceps to grasp radiopharmaceutical vials during transfer from holding area to dose calibrator will reduce radiation dose to the fingers and hands. If practical, automation of repetitive tasks can be employed to reduce staff exposure. For example, remote administration of radiopharmaceuticals may be accomplished via infusion pump instead of administration by hand. Similarly, automated dose-dispensing and calibration equipment for use in PET facilities is available commercially.

PET radiopharmaceuticals produce higher radiation dose rates to personnel than standard radiopharmaceuticals labeled with ^{99m}Tc. This is due to the higher exposure rate constants for positron-emitting radionuclides, as well as reduced self-shielding of the highly energetic annihilation photons by the patients' body tissues. For this reason, shielding can play an important role in reducing staff doses in the PET-CT facility. Vials containing PET radiopharmaceuticals should remain in their shielded shipping containers during dose dispensing. A "shadow shield" constructed of commercially available lead shielding bricks can be used to store the radiopharmaceuticals and associated waste vials and syringes, and to protect the lower body of the technologist during dose dispensing. Alternatively, shielded dose calibrators and associated shielded storage cabinets suitable for PET radiopharmaceuticals may be purchased from commercial suppliers. Syringe shields constructed of lead and intended for use with ^{99m}Tc are not effective in reducing hand and body dose incurred during the administration of PET radiopharmaceuticals. Syringe shields capable of reducing hand exposure from the annihilation photons by 95% would be unacceptably bulky if constructed of lead. Tungsten, with a density twice as great as lead, is more effective in absorbing annihilation photons and is a more suitable choice for constructing syringe shields. Tungsten syringe shields are available from commercial suppliers. Similarly, standard shielding aprons, with 0.5 mm lead or equivalent that are designed for use in diagnostic radiology, are not effective in reducing dose rate from PET radiopharmaceuticals. Approximately 90% of the annihilation photons pass through a shielding apron. Although the aprons are ineffective in reducing gamma exposure, their use is still mandatory in cases where staff must be present when the x-ray beam is activated during PET-CT procedures. Lightweight shielding aprons constructed with modern composite materials consisting of tungsten and barium are widely available from commercial suppliers of x-ray shielding equipment. Besides providing ergonomic benefits, these composite materials do not present the waste disposal problems associated with lead.

Standard precautions against blood and body fluids, which are familiar to x-ray technologists and nurses, are highly effective in preventing unnecessary radiation exposure due to inadvertent ingestion or inhalation of radioactive contamination. Eating, drinking, smoking, or applying cosmetics must not be permitted in areas where unsealed radioactive material is in use. Laboratory coats and protective gloves should be worn while dispensing and administering PET radiopharmaceuticals; protective gloves should be changed frequently. Hand washing following the removal of protective gloves is recommended. In addition, fingers should not contact mucus membranes such as those found in the mouth and eyes.

Work surfaces in areas where unsealed radioactive material is present should be covered with absorbent paper to contain spills. Radioactive material that is spilled onto the floor or other unprotected surfaces should be cordoned off and cleaned up immediately to prevent the spread of contamination. Absorbent paper should be placed over small liquid spills to contain the spill. Once most of the spill has been absorbed, the paper should be carefully removed and treated as radioactive waste. Wiping the spill should be confined to the minimum practical area to avoid enlarging the contaminated zone. Wiping should proceed from the outer areas of the contaminated area inward. Successful removal of contamination must be documented by repeat survey with a Geiger-Mueller detector or other suitable instrument.

Because PET radiopharmaceuticals may emit high energy positrons, a spill of a PET radiopharmaceutical onto exposed skin carries the potential for a significant radiation dose to the skin. In the event of a spill onto exposed skin, the affected area should be flushed immediately with lukewarm water, and then washed gently with soap and lukewarm water. Vigorous scrubbing will disrupt the normal dermal barrier and should be avoided. Washing should continue until a survey of the affected area is negative. Stubborn spots may be covered with talcum powder or cornstarch and wrapped with a protective glove or plastic wrap to induce perspiration. Following removal of the wrapping, the affected area is washed and resurveyed.

Minimizing Radiation Exposure to Patients

Based on the ALARA principle, patients must not be exposed to ionizing radiation unless there is a clear benefit to them in terms of diagnosis or treatment of their medical condition. Policies and procedures must be implemented to avoid the occurrence of reportable medical events and other dosing errors. Imaging protocols that yield diagnostically adequate information with as little radiation exposure to patients as possible should be developed and strictly followed. Because PET-CT personnel incur radiation exposure due to annihilation photons from the patients and scattered x-rays from the CT beam, steps to minimize patient dose will have the added benefit of reducing staff dose.

Errors in radiopharmaceutical administration can result in unnecessary radiation exposure to patients. The administration of a PET radiopharmaceutical to the wrong patient is an example of unnecessary radiation exposure. This error may be due to misidentification of the patient by staff, or due to improper self-identification by the patient. In either case, misidentification can be prevented in several ways. First, staff should have the patients assert their identity in an active manner rather than a passive manner. For example, the technologist might ask the patient "What is your name?" instead of "Are you Mr. Smith?" Second, other identifying information available to the technologist, such as birth date, address, telephone number, and so forth, may be used to confirm the patient's identity through active questioning. Finally, armbands bearing unique identifying information may be provided to the patient upon registration in the PET-CT facility. The armband information can act as a final check prior to radiopharmaceutical administration.

Administration of the wrong radiopharmaceutical, or the correct radiopharmaceutical in the wrong amount, is another cause of unnecessary radiation exposure. Errors of this nature can be prevented by maintaining a continuous chain of custody from the receipt of the radiopharmaceutical to its administration, in the form of adhesive labels bearing the radionuclide, chemical form, and radioactivity on vials and syringes. Double-checking labels at every step to verify the content of vials and syringes is crucial in preventing improper administrations.

The effective radiation doses for selected PET radiopharmaceuticals are shown in Table 8.3 [4]. The radiation dose to the patient following the administration of a PET radiopharmaceutical is directly proportional to the amount of radioactivity administered. Therefore, radiation dose to the patient may be decreased by decreasing the administered activity. For static images, activity reduction may be easily accomplished without sacrificing image quality by extending the time during which the image is acquired. Extension of imaging time is subject to several constraints, including the ability of the patient to tolerate the extended imaging time and the requirements of the facility to maintain its patient schedule.

Table 8.3 radiation effective dose equivalent to patients for selected PET-CT radiopharmaceuticals

Radiopharmaceutical	Effective dose equivalent		Clinical indications
	mSv/MBq	rem/mCi	
^{11}C carbon monoxide	0.00649	0.024	Organ/tumor blood volume
^{13}N ammonia	0.00224	0.0083	Myocardial perfusion
^{15}O water	0.00114	0.0042	Organ/tumor blood flow
^{18}F Fluorodeoxyglucose	0.0297	0.11	Tumor localization, Alzheimer's disease, Seizure focus localization
^{18}F Sodium fluoride	0.0270	0.10	Skeletal imaging
^{82}Rb rubidium chloride	0.00116	0.0043	Myocardial perfusion

Data from Stabin MJ, Stubbs JB, and Toohey RE [5]

However, reduction of administered activity and extension of imaging time should be employed whenever possible to maintain patient dose as low as reasonably achievable. If dynamic PET images are required, the choice of frame time and administered activity must be optimized to ensure adequate image quality at the lowest practical patient dose.

The x-ray component of the PET-CT procedure will likely result in effective radiation doses to the patients that exceed those due to the PET radiopharmaceutical. Therefore, additional care must be taken to minimize patient dose from the CT component. The primary determinant of patient dose from x-ray procedures is the time-integrated tube current (mAs). Substantial decreases in patient dose may be achieved without perceptible loss of image quality by reducing total mAs by 50% or more. Each PET-CT facility should develop technique or protocol charts that take into account the higher doses incurred in children and small adults by CT imaging, and reduce mAs accordingly to prevent unwarranted radiation exposure. Advances in multidetector helical CT technology are also contributing to patient dose reduction. These improvements include adaptive filtering for noise reduction at low mAs [6] and real-time optimization of tube current during scanning based on estimations from acquired attenuation data [7]. Finally, the radiation dose to the breast tissue in young women and girls from multidetector helical CT can be reduced by 30% without perceptible loss of image quality by the use of in-plane bismuth shields [8].

Obtaining a complete obstetrical and gynecological history from women of childbearing potential can avoid inadvertent exposure of the embryo or fetus. For studies performed under research protocols, pregnancy exclusion by appropriate blood tests may be required. Under certain circumstances, it may be necessary to study a pregnant patient with PET-CT. The radiation dose to the fetus from PET radiopharmaceuticals is comparable to that from ^{99m}Tc labeled radiopharmaceuticals, and would not be expected to lead to adverse effects on development. Fetal radiation exposure may be minimized by reducing the administered radioactivity, catheterizing the urinary bladder (useful for ^{18}F FDG and ^{13}N ammonia) and shielding the fetus if it is not in the primary x-ray beam.

Minimizing Radiation Exposure to Ancillary Personnel

The staff required to operate a PET-CT facility is not comprised solely of physicians and technologists. Ancillary personnel will include nurses, receptionists, housekeepers, and administrative assistants who may not be expected to incur radiation exposure consequential to their employment. In general, unmonitored ancillary staff must not accrue more than 1.0 mSv (100 mrem) in a year, exclusive of natural background radiation, as a consequence of their employment in the PET-CT facility. In addition, ancillary staff must not accrue more than 20 μSv (2 mrem) in any given hour. Since ancillary personnel will not usually be provided with the means to record occupational radiation exposure, care must taken to ensure that they do not enter areas where unsealed radioactive material is used, and that "public access" areas of the PET-CT facility are adequately shielded from scattered radiation. In general, compliance with the dose limits may be achieved by excluding ancillary personnel from certain areas, either by posting signs or by physically securing the areas. However, there will be instances where additional shielding must be provided. Although a detailed treatment of the design of supplementary shielding for a PET-CT facility is beyond the scope of this chapter, an understanding of the basic considerations of shielding requirements will be helpful in planning the facility.

PET-CT Shielding Considerations

In general, the dose rates due to the annihilation photons from radioactive patients and positron-emitting radiation sources are sufficiently low that detailed preinstallation shielding plans are not required by regulatory agencies. However, this is not true for the CT component. Regulatory agencies in most jurisdictions require an a priori analysis of the expected annual radiation dose in areas accessible to ancillary staff and the public, and require the submission of detailed plans of the construction of shielding that will ensure compliance with the dose limits. Parameters that are required for a shielding design project are: (1) the expected incremental radiation dose per procedure due to scattered radiation per imaging procedure in areas of the PET-CT facility that will be occupied by ancillary personnel; (2) an estimation of the fraction of the operational hours that unmonitored personnel will be present in accessible areas, known as the *occupancy factor*; (3) an estimation of the maximum number of procedures to be performed per day; (4) the number of operational days per calendar year; and (5) the types and thickness of barrier material that are in place or planned within the facility.

To estimate the dose contribution per procedure (d_i) from scattered x-rays at a given location within the facility, it will be necessary to measure the incremental dose at some distance r_0 from the scanner when the x-ray tube is activated (d_{0i}). The inverse square law can be applied to determine the incremental dose at any occupied location:

$$d_i = d_{0i} / (r / r_0)^2$$

where r is the distance from the scanner to the occupied location. Values of d_{0i}, usually measured at $r_0 = 1.0$ m, may be obtained from the CT scanner manufacturer. The annual unshielded dose d_u at r can be calculated from the number of scans per day (n), the occupancy factor (o) and the number of working days per year (a):

$$d_u = (d_i)(n)(o)(a)$$

If d_L is the annual limiting dose, then the required dose reduction factor F that must be provided by shielding is

$$F = d_u / d_L$$

If F is less than 1.0, then no additional shielding is required. If F is greater than 1, then shielding must be interposed between the scanner and the occupied area. This analysis must be applied to each occupied area, including areas on the floors above and below the facility.

For F greater than 1, the types and dimensions of existing or planned barrier material required to reduce the estimated annual dose by a factor of 1/F must be determined during the facility planning stage. Ordinary building materials such as concrete and even sheetrock can provide significant shielding at scattered x-ray energies. Knowledge of the barrier thickness, along with published tables of dose x-ray exposure reduction factors for various materials as a function of material thickness and x-ray energy, may be employed to determine if a reduction of 1/F can be achieved. If not, then supplemental shielding, usually in the form of large sheets of lead placed behind sheetrock, will be required. The thickness of lead that is required can be determined from the tables. It is recommended that conservative values of occupancy factor, daily workload and working days per year be assumed during the planning phase, so that the expected annual dose (and therefore the shielding requirement) is not underestimated. Due to the complex nature of shielding design considerations, it is recommended that planners of a PET-CT facility consult a qualified expert in x-ray shielding calculations before architectural designs are finalized and construction begins. State regulatory agencies maintain lists of individuals who are registered to perform such calculations within their jurisdictions. Once construction is complete and the PET-CT scanner is in place, a radiation survey demonstrating integrity of the shielding and expected compliance with annual dose limits must be performed and submitted to the appropriate state agency within a specified time following the beginning of operation of the facility.

Summary

Because PET-CT employs both radioactive material and x-rays in the same imaging suite, it presents special challenges for radiation protection. Diligent application of the ALARA principle can minimize radiation doses to PET-CT technologists, ancillary personnel, and patients. Specifically, technologists should minimize the time spent in close proximity to patients following the administration of PET radiopharmaceuticals and during interventional CT localization procedures. Shielding PPE must be worn if there is a potential of exposure to scattered x-rays; tungsten-based shielding equipment should be employed to reduce hand and body exposure to annihilation photons during dose calibration and administration. Thorough documentation of standard operating procedures, training, personnel dose monitoring, receipt and disposal of radioactive material, shielding design, and the results of contamination surveys will help ensure regulatory compliance.

References

1. Paulsen EK, Sheafor DH, Enterline DS, et al. CT fluoroscopy-guided interventional procedures: techniques and radiation doses to radiologists. Radiology 2001;220:161–167.
2. Buls N, Pagés J, deMey J, et al. Evaluation of patient and staff doses during various CT fluoroscopy guided interventions. Health Phys 2003;85:165–173.

3. Biran T, Weininger J, Malchi S, et al. Measurements of occupational exposure for a technologist performing ^{18}F FDG PET scans. Health Phys 2004;87:539–544.
4. Robinson CN, Young JG, Wallace AB, Ibbetson VJ. A study of the personal radiation dose received by nuclear medicine technologists working in a dedicated PET center. Health Physics 2005;88(Suppl 1):S17-S21.
5. Stabin MG, Stubbs JB, Toohey RE. Radiation dose estimates for radiopharmaceuticals. Oak Ridge: Oak Ridge Institute for Science and Education, 1996.
6. Kachelreiss, M, Watzke O, Kalender WA. Generalized multi-dimensional adaptive filtering for conventional and spiral single-slice, multi-slice, and cone-beam CT. Med Phys 2001;28: 275–490.
7. Fuchs T, Kachelreiss M, Kalender WA. Technical advances in multi-slice spiral CT. Eur J Radiol 2000;36:69–73.
8. Fricke BL, Donnelly LF, Frush DP, et al. In-plane bismuth breast shields for pediatric CT: effects on radiation dose and image quality using experimental and clinical data. AJR 2003;180: 407–411.

Chapter 9
Application of CT Contrast Agents in PET-CT Imaging

Gerald Antoch, Patrick Veit, Andreas Bockisch, and Hilmar Kuehl

Introduction

Dual-modality positron emission tomography/computed tomography (PET-CT) allows acquisition of accurately aligned functional and morphological data sets within a single session [1]. Advantages over CT are the additional functional information acquired, and combined PET-CT has been shown to increase the diagnostic accuracy when staging different malignant diseases compared with CT alone [2, 3]. This advantage arises from improving both lesion detection and lesion characterization when adding function to morphology. Furthermore, PET-CT offers anatomic information for correlation with PET. With these anatomic data an area of increased tracer uptake may be accurately localized within a specific organ or part of an organ. Thus, the limited morphologic information, which must be considered the major limitation of PET imaging alone, can be overcome. Studies comparing PET with PET-CT have reported a significant advantage of the combined imaging approach over functional images alone [2–5].

When adding CT to PET, what CT image quality is really needed for PET-CT image interpretation? Are low-dose and non-contrast-enhanced CT images sufficient for evaluation or are diagnostic contrast-enhanced CT images required? Does FDG (or other PET tracers) provide adequate lesion-to-background contrast, making it the *new CT contrast agent* and rendering conventional CT contrast agents unnecessary? Does the quality of the CT component affect the diagnostic accuracy of the combined imaging approach? These questions are currently being debated in the PET-CT community [6, 7]. This chapter addresses the issue of CT contrast agents in dual-modality PET-CT imaging and suggests indications for which oral and intravenous (IV) contrast agents will be of benefit over non-contrast-enhanced PET-CT.

G. Antoch (✉)
Department of Radiology, University Hospital Duesseldorf, Moorenstrasse 5, 40225 Duesseldorf, Germany
e-mail: antoch@med.uni-duesseldorf.de

Contrast Agents in CT

Intravenous Contrast Agents

When assessing CT images, all major parenchymal organs, lymph nodes, non-contrast-enhanced blood vessels, and muscles are characterized by similar attenuation values. Based on only minor differences in Hounsfield units (HU) (Fig. 9.1), these structures are visualized in similar shades of gray on the computer monitor. Thus, difficulties may arise when differentiating anatomical structures from one another. Furthermore, lesion detection within parenchymal organs may be hampered if both the lesion and the organ are of comparable density. Early studies have demonstrated that the use of intravenous contrast agents can aid differentiation of adjacent anatomical structures based on differences in contrast enhancement [8–10]. In addition, detection of parenchymal lesions substantially benefits from application of IV contrast agents. Violante et al. [11] have demonstrated an increase from 63% to 90% in the accuracy of detection for small liver lesions with IV contrast agents (Fig. 9.2). Burgener et al. [12] found an increase in accuracy when assessing local growth of pelvic malignancies with contrast-enhanced data sets as compared with nonenhanced images. Furthermore, contrast dynamics including scans in the arterial, portal-venous, and venous phases may be used to characterize a lesion of unknown etiology. This additional information proves valuable when differentiating benign from malignant lesions with CT alone (Fig. 9.3). In summary, application of IV contrast agents in CT imaging provides valuable information for delineation of anatomical structures, detection, and localization of pathologic lesions, and lesion characterization.

IV contrast agents used for CT imaging are mainly nonionic monomers with low osmolarity. These nonionic contrast agents are subclassified according to the amount of iodine in 1 ml of solution. Typical concentrations in clinical use are 240–370 mg/ml. Side effects include acute and delayed allergic reactions (Table 9.1). While acute allergic reactions may be mild, intermediate, or severe, delayed allergic reactions are mostly of mild extent. However, a few cases

P. Shreve and D.W. Townsend (eds.), *Clinical PET-CT in Radiology: Integrated Imaging in Oncology*,
DOI 10.1007/978-0-387-48902-5_9, © Springer Science+Business Media, LLC 2011

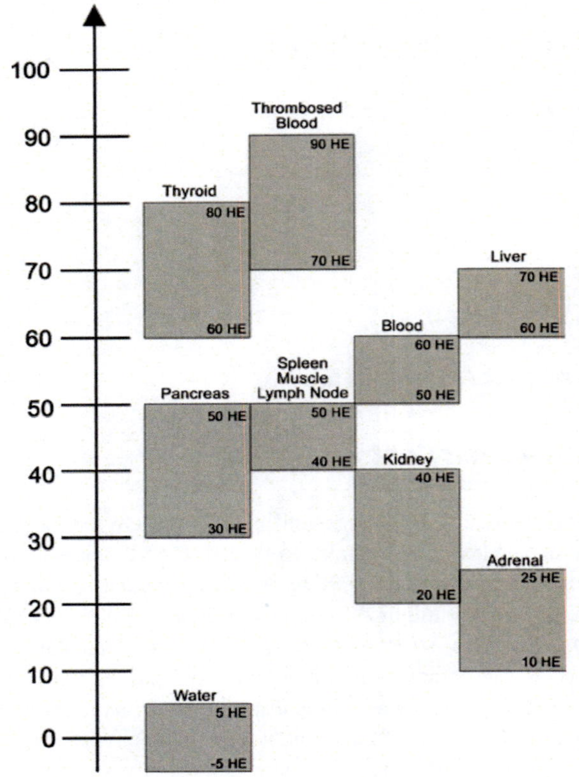

Fig. 9.1 Attenuation of CT x-rays expressed in Hounsfield units for a variety of internal organs and anatomic structures

of severe delayed reactions have been reported after using nonionic dimers. Further adverse reactions to intravenous contrast agents include nephropathy, thyrotoxic shock, and an increased risk of lactic acidosis in patients with diabetes undergoing metformin therapy [13, 14].

Oral Contrast Agents

When imaging the abdomen, intestinal structures must be clearly delineated to avoid misinterpretation of lymph nodes or other pathologic lesions as stomach or bowel loops (Fig. 9.4) [15]. The application of IV contrast agents alone is of limited value in this setting because lymph nodes and the bowel wall may present similar contrast-enhancing characteristics. Oral contrast agents are required for bowel identification. In addition, distention of the intestine by oral contrast agents offers more accurate assessment of intestinal tumors and their potential infiltration of adjacent organs (Fig. 9.5). Furthermore, invasion of the intestinal wall by extraintestinal tumors may be correctly characterized. Thus, the administration of oral contrast agents improves delineation of anatomic structures and detection and localization of pathologic lesions within the lumen, within the bowel wall, or adjacent to the bowel wall.

Oral contrast agents can be divided into two groups, positive and negative oral contrast agents. Iodine and barium are most frequently applied for positive oral contrast. CT attenuation values of the bowel lumen are increased by positive contrast materials leading to bowel opacification. By increasing Hounsfield units, the intestine can be delineated from adjacent structures (Fig. 9.6a). While iodine-based positive oral contrast may also be applied in perioperative patients, barium must not be administered in either patients undergoing surgery of the intestine or those with known or suspected intestinal perforation or obstruction.

Negative oral contrast agents provide delineation of bowel loops by intestinal distension rather than intestinal opacification (Fig. 9.6b). Negative oral contrast agents range from 0 to 20 HU. Water is the most frequently used negative oral contrast agent in CT imaging. However, water alone is absorbed from the intestinal lumen and, thus, frequently renders bowel distention in the distal parts of the jejunum and ileum unsatisfactorily. Thus, different substances (mannitol, sorbitol, locust bean gum, etc.) may be added to prevent intestinal absorption. These solutions are frequently called *water-equivalent* contrast agents.

For CT alone, advantages of negative oral contrast agents are the more accurate assessment of the stomach or bowel wall that can be distinctly delineated from the water-filled lumen. Thus, tumors arising from the intestinal wall will be easily identified. Negative oral contrast agents are mainly used for imaging of the stomach or pancreas (delineation of pancreatic head from distended duodenum) on CT alone. In addition, CT-angiography is frequently performed using negative oral contrast. Positive oral contrast agents are applied in the majority of CT indications. Advantages of positive contrast agents are their general availability, strong bowel opacification, and a certain benefit in patients with centrally necrotic lymph nodes, which may be misinterpreted as water-filled bowel loops when applying negative oral contrast (Fig. 9.6c).

Contrast Agents in PET-CT

Contrast Agents and PET Attenuation Correction

In PET-CT imaging, PET attenuation correction is usually performed based on the CT data. All currently available PET-CT scanners use a two-step scaling algorithm to calculate PET attenuation coefficients at 511 keV [16]. However, with CT-based attenuation correction PET attenuation can be overestimated in the presence of positive contrast agents

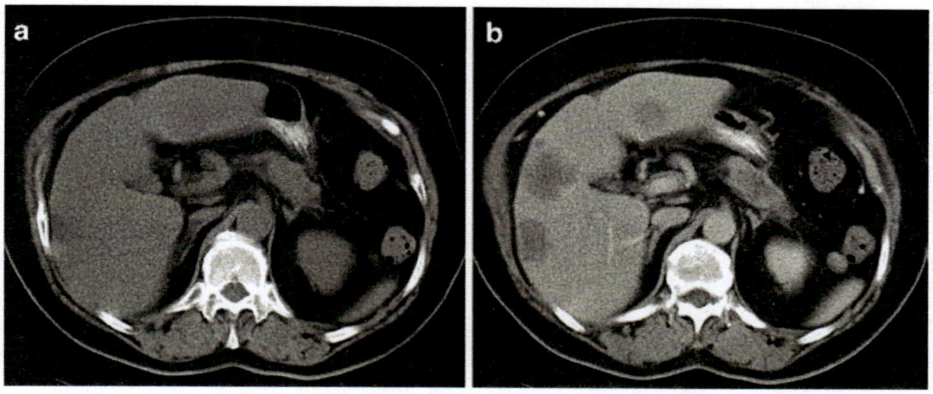

Fig. 9.2 A 67-year-old woman with hepatic metastases from pancreatic carcinoma. On nonenhanced CT the metastatic lesions are barely visible (**a**). When assessing the liver in the portovenous phase the metastases can be clearly visualized (**b**)

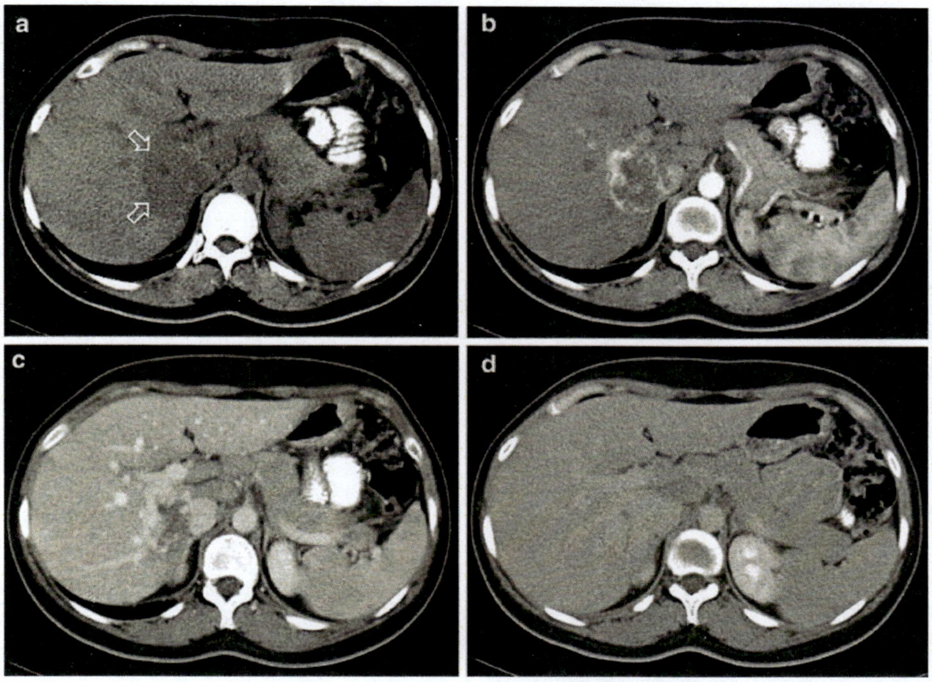

Fig. 9.3 A 28-year-old woman with hypodense hepatic lesion of unknown etiology in the right liver lobe on nonenhanced CT (*arrows in* **a**). After contrast enhancement the lesion demonstrates peripheral nodular enhancement (**b** arterial phase) and centripetal filling (**c** portovenous phase). (**d**) In the late venous phase the lesion shows homogeneous contrast enhancement. Typical radiologic appearance of a hepatic hemangioma

[17, 18]. The overestimation of the attenuation properties may lead to image artifacts on PET appearing as areas of apparently increased glucose metabolism coregistered with regions of high contrast concentration (see Chapter 5) [19]. Furthermore, the quantification of the tracer activity concentration is also affected by overestimation of the attenuation properties in the presence of positive oral contrast agents. Both artifacts and inaccuracies in tracer quantification are strongly correlated with attenuation on the CT images and increase with higher HU.

With intravenous contrast agents, the associated artifacts are limited to thoracic veins carrying undiluted contrast material (Fig. 9.7). These areas of apparently increased tracer uptake usually do not cause interpretative problems as the artifact can be accurately attributed to the underlying vessel. In the presence of positive oral contrast media, artifacts can be identified based on the underlying contrast-enhanced intestinal structure (Fig. 9.8). In cases in which an artifact cannot be differentiated from pathology, non-attenuation-corrected images should also be viewed. Without attenuation

Table 9.1 Adverse allergic reactions to intravenous contrast media

		Symptoms	Incidence
Acute	Minor	Flushing, nausea, arm pain, pruritus, vomiting headache, urticaria	Nonionic: 3% (ionic: up to 15%)
	Intermediate	More serious degrees of the above, moderate hypotension and bronchospasm	Nonionic: 0.04% (ionic: 0.22%)
	Severe	Severe hypotension, severe bronchospasm, convulsions, unconsciousness, laryngeal edema, pulmonary edema, cardiac arrhythmia, cardiac arrest	Nonionic: 0.004% (ionic: 0.04%)
Delayed	Mostly mild	Fever, rash, flushing, dizziness, pruritus, arthralgia, diarrhea, nausea, vomiting, headache, seldom hypotension	2–8%

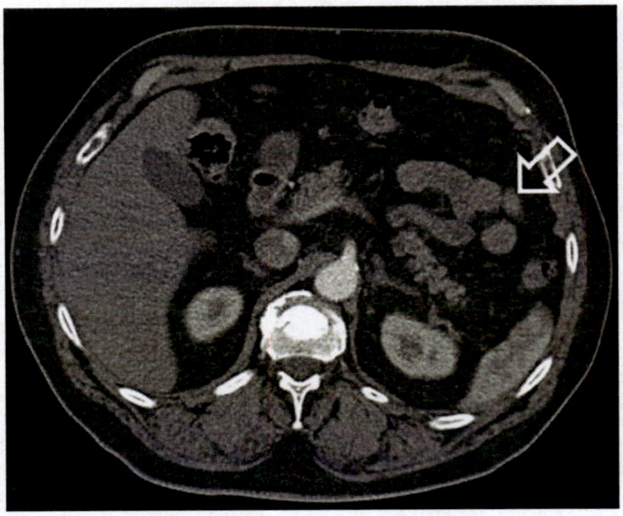

Fig. 9.4 A 54-year-old man with lymphoma. Pathologic mesenteric lymph node (*arrow*) adjacent to small bowel loops. Without oral contrast agents the lymph node cannot be reliably differentiated from non-enhanced and only poorly distended small bowel

correction, PET data should be free of artifacts (Figs. 9.7 and 9.8).

The effect of positive CT contrast agents on PET tracer quantification has been examined extensively. Nakamoto et al. [18] have found a maximum bias of 15% for parenchymal organs when measuring PET activity concentration in the presence of IV contrast agents. Other authors have verified these results [20, 21]. Based on these reports the effect of IV contrast on PET tracer quantification has only a minor effect on the SUV which may be considered clinically insignificant. For clinically used concentrations of oral contrast agents different studies have reported an overestimation of the PET tracer-activity concentration of approximately 20% [22, 23]. This overestimation does not, however, affect the corresponding standard uptake value (SUV) in a clinically relevant manner. Dizendorf et al. [17] reported only a 4% overestimation of the related SUV in the presence of oral contrast agents. Based on these results, the effects of homogeneously distributed oral contrast agents on the SUV can be considered negligible in daily clinical routine. Local accumulation of oral contrast agents caused by gastrointestinal stenoses or compromised gastrointestinal motility may, however, lead to a strong increase in local attenuation, resulting in increased inaccuracy of PET tracer quantification.

While only positive contrast agents are available for intravenous opacification, oral contrast may be achieved by using a negative contrast agent. As explained previously, these substances provide intestinal contrast by bowel distention rather than opacification. Based on low attenuation with HU typically in the range of 0–20, negative oral contrast does not cause artifacts or inaccuracies in PET tracer quantification. However, application of water alone usually does not provide satisfactory bowel distention due to intestinal absorption. We routinely use a combination of 1.5 L of water containing 2.5% mannitol and 0.2% locust bean gum (LBG) for negative/water-equivalent oral contrast. Mannitol has an osmotic property that increases bowel distension, while LBG (gelling action) reduces water absorption [24].

Contrast Protocols

The administration of oral contrast agents has been generally adopted in the PET-CT community to increase the accuracy of lesion localization in the abdomen [26], whereas in most institutions, intravenous contrast agents are not routinely applied for PET-CT imaging. Currently, there are two main imaging protocols used worldwide, summarized in Table 9.2. Protocol 1 uses CT mainly for anatomical correlation and attenuation correction of PET. Oral contrast agents are applied for better delineation of intestinal structures; however, no IV contrast agents are used and the CT is frequently acquired with low-dose radiation. Additional diagnostic CT data are thus required in this setting. Protocol 2 provides state-of-the-art CT with oral and intravenous contrast agents as well as full-dose acquisition. This PET-CT protocol offers whole-body functional and anatomical staging in a single session. An additional CT scan is not needed. The radiation exposure from the CT component amounts to approximately 15–18 mSv when scanning a field of view from head to the

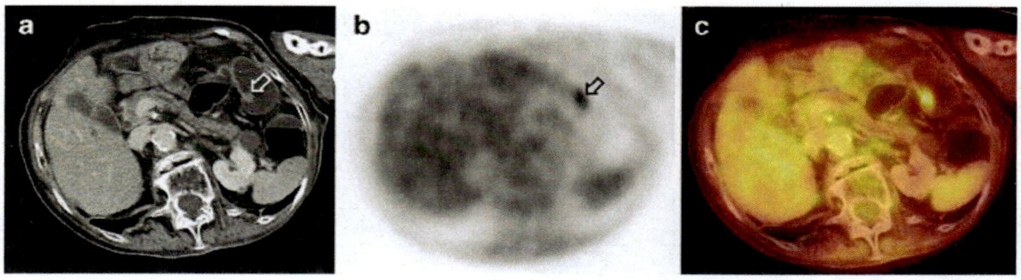

Fig. 9.5 (a–c) FDG-PET-CT colonography in an 82-year-old woman with multifocal colon cancer. The colon was filled with 3 L of water for intestinal distention before positioning the patient on the examination table. A small (9-mm) carcinoma with increased glucose metabolism at the left colonic flexure can be clearly visualized based on good colonic distention

upper thighs. A low-dose protocol using 80 mAs (as frequently applied in protocol 1) leads to a radiation exposure of the patient of approximately 4–5 mSv. Some institutions perform a third variation that consists of protocol 1 with very low-dose CT for attenuation correction followed by a state-of-the-art CT with additional IV contrast immediately following the low-dose protocol. This setting provides diagnostic PET and CT comparable with protocol 2. IV contrast-associated artifacts are avoided as the first low-dose CT is used for PET attenuation correction. This protocol, however, involves additional radiation exposure. According to current data the contrast-enhanced PET-CT can be used for attenuation correction of PET [26].

Oral contrast agents are administered to improve differentiation of bowel loops from adjacent structures and pathology. This applies mainly to the small bowel since the colon can typically be well delineated by its larger size and stool filling. Therefore, the application of oral contrast agents must be timed to provide gastric and small bowel distention and opacification. The exact application depends on the different types of contrast agents and the different amounts used. All patients should be instructed to slowly and steadily ingest the oral contrast agent to provide homogenous distribution. We use 1.5 L of water containing LBG and mannitol [24]. The patient is instructed to ingest 1.3 L over the course of 50 min starting directly after IV administration of the PET-tracer. The remaining 200 ml are administered immediately before positioning the patient on the examination table to ensure gastric distention. Administration of oral contrast agents during the uptake time of the radioactive tracer may cause slightly elevated tracer utilization in the pharyngeal region due to swallowing. From the fused images, this muscular uptake generally does not cause interpretative problems when reading PET-CT images.

The protocol for the administration of IV contrast agents depends on several factors, and the protocols must be adapted to the performance of the CT scanner integrated in the combined PET-CT system. Systems with less CT detector-rows require administration protocols different from 64-slice scanners. In addition, the administration protocol depends on the region of interest scanned with PET-CT. Scans of single body regions, such as the abdomen or the thorax, demand different protocols than those for whole-body examinations. For tumors of the head and neck, our institution uses a protocol that first scans the head and neck, followed by the remainder of the body. Image acquisition can be optimized by using thinner CT slices for the head and neck, with the arms positioned out of the field of view, and with fixation of the head to avoid image misregistration due to patient movement [27]. The rest of the body is scanned following the head and neck protocol. In this setting, IV contrast agents are administered twice to ensure optimal IV contrast in both scans. In addition, for certain tumor types, scanning in a specific contrast phase or multiphase imaging may be required. Hepatocellular carcinoma or neuroendocrine tumors of the gastrointestinal tract, for example, typically enhance in the arterial phase, whereas they may be less well visualized in the portovenous and venous phases. For most tumors, however, the contrast phases shown in Fig. 9.9 are applicable.

To achieve whole-body contrast enhancement as shown in Fig. 9.9, the patient would have to be scanned starting with the thorax and neck in a caudocranial direction, followed by the abdomen and pelvis in a craniocaudal direction, and finally the head. Currently available PET-CT systems do not offer this option but instead require a single CT spiral covering the same field of view as the PET acquisition for the purposes of CT-based attenuation correction. Thus, all imaging protocols for PET-CT will be a compromise for IV contrast administration. We currently use a whole-body protocol acquired in the caudocranial direction (upper thighs to head). Caudocranial imaging has the advantage of avoiding artifacts caused by the passage of the bolus of IV contrast agent in upper thoracic veins. Once the CT reaches the upper thorax, the contrast bolus has passed and the contrast agent is homogeneously distributed throughout the body [28, 29]. A different approach to avoid contrast-associated artifacts in the upper thorax would be the use of a saline flush immediately following the injection of the contrast agent combined with an adequate start delay (typically 40–70 s). By flushing the

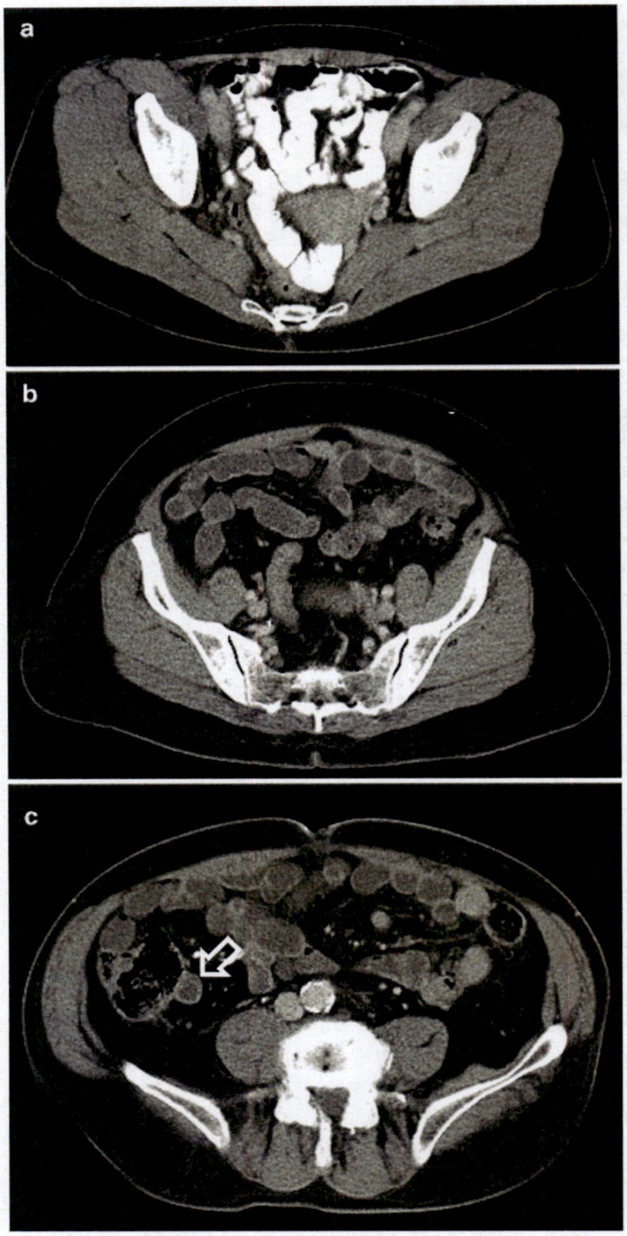

Fig. 9.6 Positive and negative CT contrast agents. The small bowel can be nicely differentiated from adjacent structures in the pelvis after administration of a positive, barium-based CT contrast agent (**a**). Negative oral contrast agents provide identification of bowel loops by bowel distention rather than opacification (**b**). Centrally necrotic lymph nodes may have a similar appearance as distended small bowel loops (*arrow in* **c**) which may hamper their detection when applying negative oral contrast

injection site with saline the upper thoracic veins are cleared of the highly concentrated contrast agent, avoiding the artifact caused by the passage of the bolus. A two-lumen injector is preferable in this setting.

Benefits of CT Contrast Agents in PET-CT

Lesion Detection and Characterization

A number of different studies have reported superior tumor staging results when comparing PET-CT with separate morphologic and functional image acquisition [2, 4, 30, 31]. While some of these studies included contrast-enhanced PET-CT data, others used only nonenhanced CT. Therefore, both contrast-enhanced and nonenhanced PET-CT seem to improve lesion detection and characterization over CT and PET alone. However, some recent studies have detected an advantage of contrast-enhanced PET-CT over nonenhanced PET-CT. Pfannenberg et al. [32] found an increase in the number of correctly assessed TNM-stages in NSCLC by 8% if performing contrast-enhanced PET-CT vs. nonenhanced PET-CT. Setty et al. [33] reported a higher accuracy of contrast-enhanced PET-CT as compared to the nonenhanced protocol for detection of hepatic metastases from colorectal cancer. However, for primary staging of lymphoma no benefit of CT contrast agents has been reported [34]. So the use of IV contrast agents cannot generally be recommended in all PET-CT scans, but seems to, at least partially, depend on the tumor entity in question. Other factors are also of interest: In the case of increased tracer uptake, lesion detection and characterization is mainly based on functional data rather than morphology in combined PET-CT. However, CT contrast agents may add valuable information in patients with PET-negative tumors or those with only slightly increased tracer uptake. By increasing lesion-to-background contrast, intravenous contrast agents enhance lesion detection (Fig. 9.10) [8, 10]. The pattern of contrast enhancement may aid lesion characterization in patients with PET-negative tumors [8, 11, 12, 35]. Oral contrast agents avoid misinterpretation of small abdominal lesions as intestinal structures in the case of a PET-negative result. In our patient population we have determined a benefit of IV contrast enhancement with regard to lesion detection and characterization in approximately one patient in ten.

Lesion Localization

Compared with PET alone, PET-CT offers accurate anatomical localization of areas that demonstrate increased tracer uptake. As explained earlier, lesion localization may be obscured by the similar density of different anatomical structures on nonenhanced CT scans [10, 12]. Inaccuracies in lesion localization may, however, affect the TNM tumor stage [32]. This is the case if an area of focally increased tracer uptake cannot be clearly attributed to either a lymph

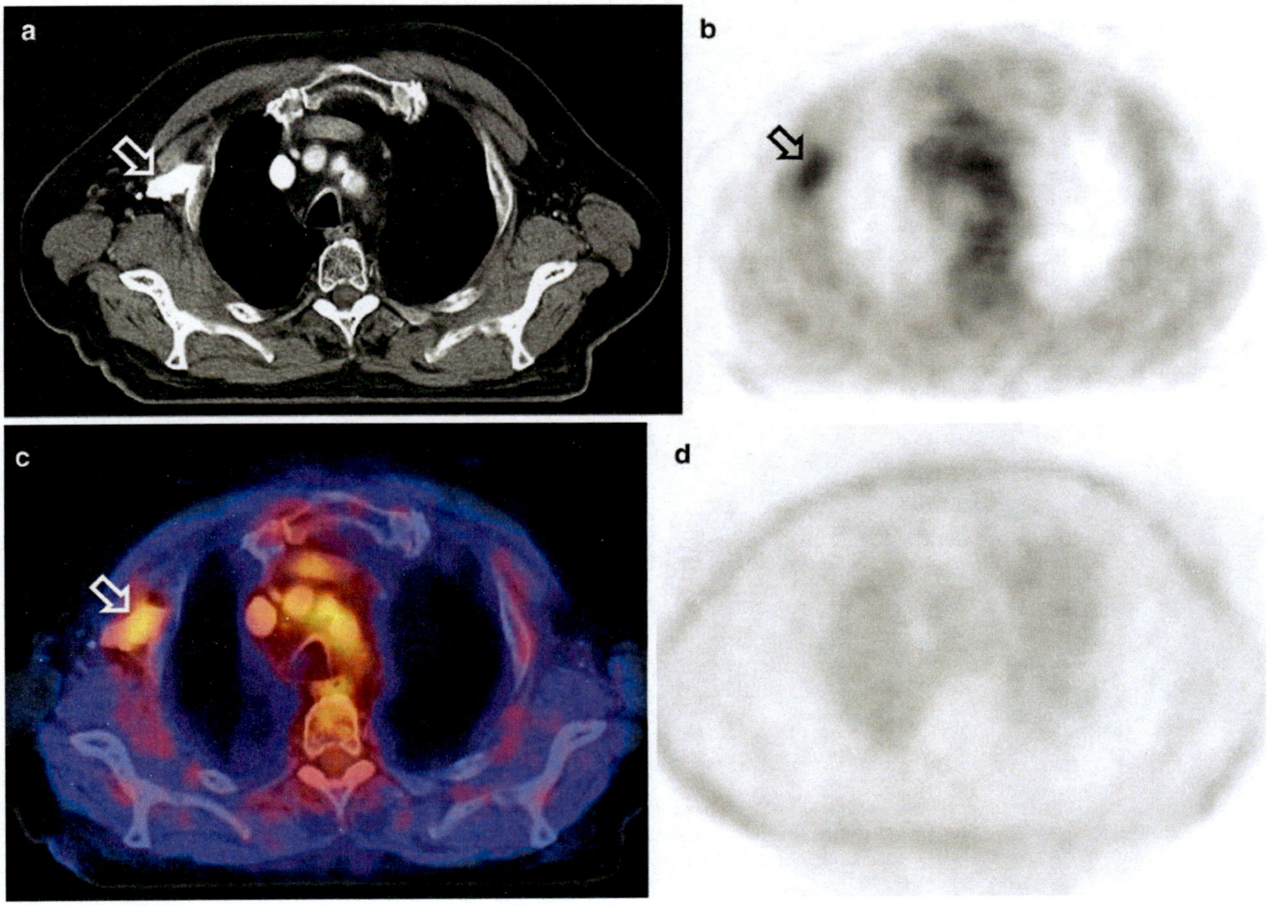

Fig. 9.7 Bolus passage of highly concentrated intravenous contrast agent in left subclavian vein (*arrow in* **a**). Contrast-associated PET artifact showing as an area of apparently increased glucose metabolism (*arrow in* **b**) which can be accurately co-registered with the underlying vessel (**c**). No artifact is visible when reconstructing PET data without attenuation correction (**d**)

node or an internal organ. Furthermore, accurate anatomical data from CT aid interpretation of PET images when differentiating benign from malignant tracer uptake. Increased FDG utilization may be physiologic when coregistered with the bowel or the stomach wall, whereas it may be pathologic if fused with a lymph node. Thus, differentiation of intestinal structures from adjacent lesions is essential for correct image assessment (Fig. 9.11). To address this issue, most PET-CT facilities worldwide have adopted imaging protocols that include application of oral contrast agents, either negative or positive. In addition, small lymph nodes need to be clearly differentiated from surrounding blood vessels (Fig. 9.12).

Lesion localization must also be discussed with regard to other body regions. In the thorax, hilar, and mediastinal lymph nodes need to be differentiated from adjacent blood vessels. When imaging the neck, pathologic lesions may be mistaken for muscle or blood vessels on nonenhanced CT. In patients undergoing PET-CT-guided liver interventions, contrast enhancement is required preinterventionally to clearly visualize all vascular structures that may cause severe bleeding if injured (Fig. 9.13). In these cases, the application of IV contrast agents substantially increases the accuracy of lesion localization based on their contrast-enhancing characteristics. We have determined a benefit of oral and intravenous contrast agents when localizing pathologic lesions to specific structures in 50% of our patient population. Additional clinical contrast-enhanced CT scans are acquired on a different CT scanner and may be correlated with the PET-CT. However, in this setting the patient is repositioned between the PET-CT and the clinical CT scan, which may render image correlation difficult due to organ movement. Another approach, used infrequently, is an additional contrast-enhanced CT immediately following the combined PET-CT in patients with ambiguous findings on nonenhanced PET-CT. This approach requires a physician to be available for image assessment immediately following each PET-CT examination, which makes the procedure impractical in general.

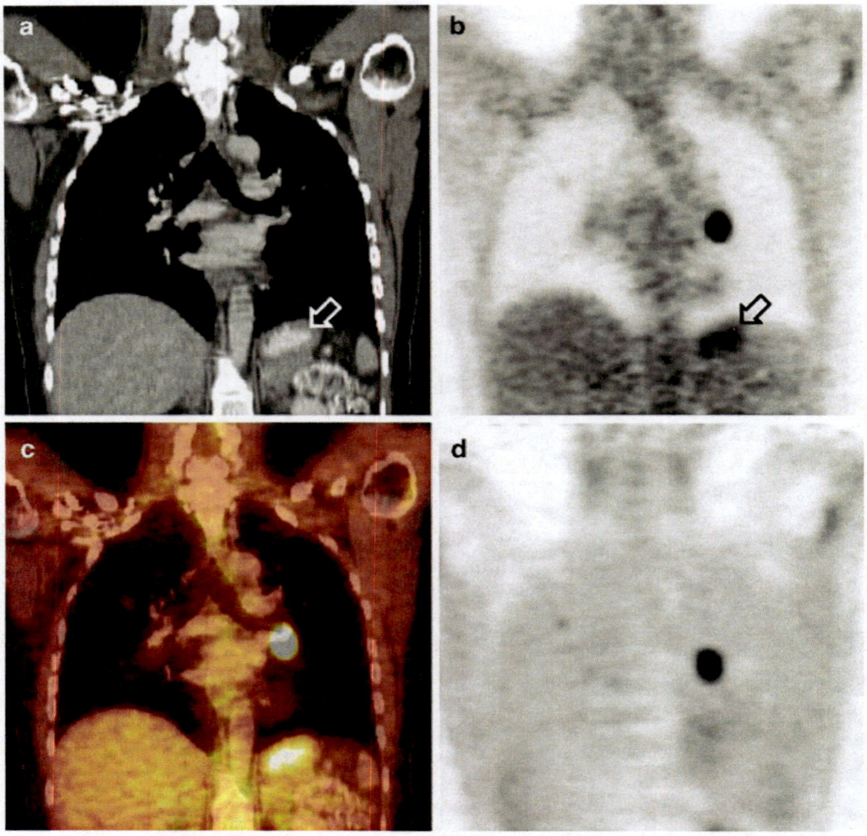

Fig. 9.8 Contrast-enhanced stomach after application of barium as a positive oral contrast agent (*arrow in* **a**). Area of apparently increased tracer uptake on PET (**b**) after CT-based attenuation correction which can be accurately co-registered with underlying contrast-enhanced stomach (**c**). No artifact can be detected on nonattenuation corrected PET (**d**)

Table 9.2 General imaging protocols in PET-CT

Imaging protocol	Clinical demand	Demand on PET	Demand on CT
CT for anatomic correlation of PET	• PET-CT as PET with additional anatomic information • CT for PET attenuation correction • CT with oral contrast for anatomic correlation of PET	High	Low
Diagnostic CT	• PET-CT replaces PET *and* CT • State-of-the-art CT with IV and oral contrast and standard radiation exposure levels • CT for PET attenuation correction	High	High

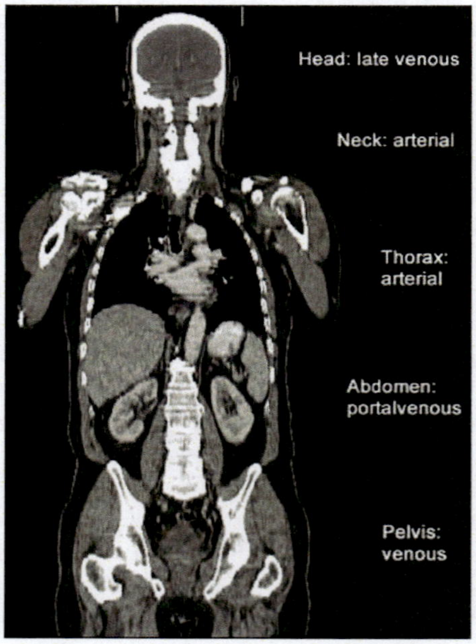

Fig. 9.9 Typical contrast-enhancing phases desirable when staging a patient with CT. Depending on the tumor in question additional abdominal scans in the arterial or late venous phases may be required

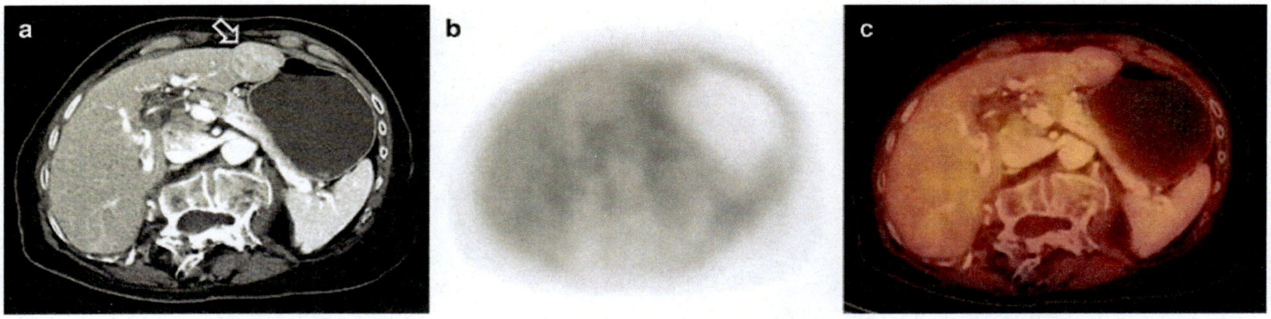

Fig. 9.10 A 66-year-old woman with hepatocellular carcinoma of the left liver lobe (*arrow in* **a**). FDG-PET was found to be negative (**b**). The diagnosis was made with the PET-CT examination based on the CT data

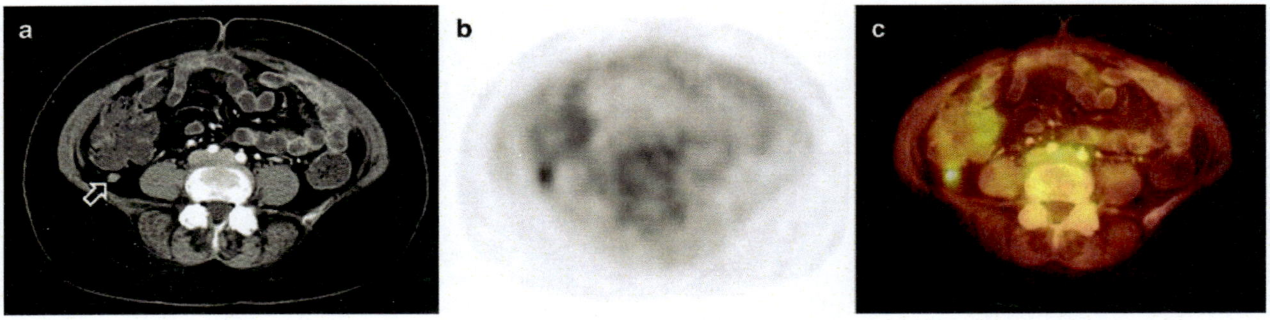

Fig. 9.11 A 56-year-old woman with carcinoma of the uterus. Small contrast-enhancing lymph node which can be differentiated from the colon and ileum which are filled with negative oral contrast (**a**). Increased glucose metabolism on FDG-PET (**b**) and FDG-PET-CT (**c**) suggests malignancy

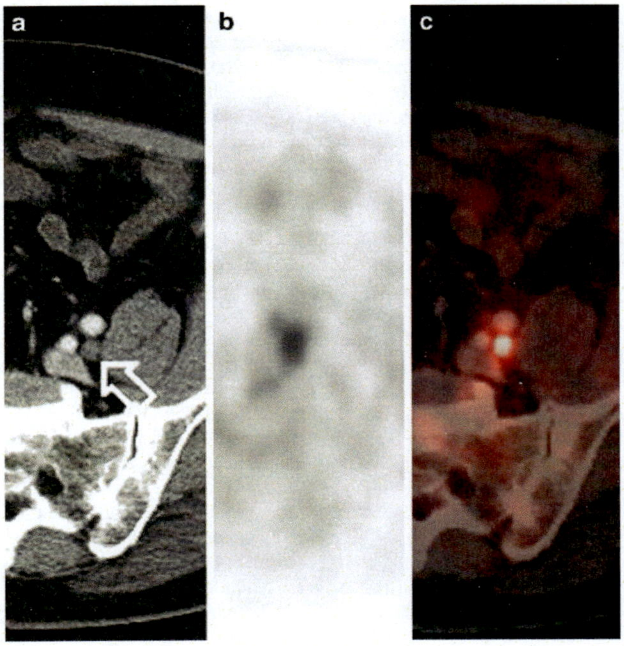

Fig. 9.12 A 46-year-old man with non-Hodgkin's lymphoma. Small lymph node can be clearly differentiated from surrounding blood vessels based on vascular contrast-enhancement (*arrow in* **a**). Increased glucose metabolism on FDG-PET (**b**) and FDG-PET-CT (**c**) indicate malignant disease

Contrast Indications in PET-CT

In view of the advantages for lesion localization, both oral and intravenous contrast agents are indicated in PET-CT examinations (Table 9.3). There are, of course, indications in which nonenhanced CT will be preferable when lesion localization is not the main focus of the examination, primarily in patients undergoing follow-up PET-CT to assess the effects of radiotherapy or chemotherapy. On tumor follow-up, a change in tracer uptake will indicate whether the tumor has responded to therapy. In this setting, accurate lesion localization was ensured for the initial staging PET-CT prior to the start of the therapy. Thus, the follow-up can be acquired without contrast. For patients with a previous contrast-enhanced CT scan, this contrast-enhanced CT may serve as correlation with PET. However, as mentioned previously, organ shift or a suboptimal respiration state for image fusion (CT normally acquired in inspiration breath-hold) may limit image correlation in this clinical scenario. In addition, contrast-enhanced CT data are often only available from a single body region. Patients with lung cancer, for example, may have undergone a CT of the thorax. In this case, contrast agents should be applied in PET-CT imaging if state-of-the-art morphologic data from the other body regions are desired.

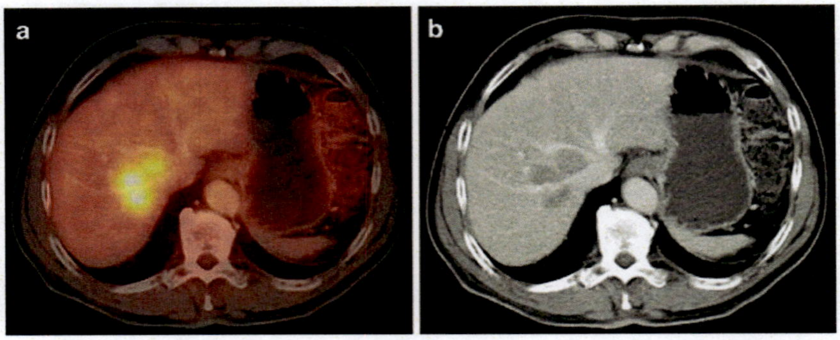

Fig. 9.13 A 70-year-old man patient with three hepatic metastases from colon carcinoma (**a**) scheduled to undergo radiofrequency ablation. Three metastases are visualized in close proximity to liver veins and the inferior vena cava the contrast-enhanced CT data. Without knowledge of the vascular anatomy, severe bleeding may be induced if one of the adjacent blood vessels is injured during the intervention

Table 9.3 Indications for CT contrast agents in PET-CT (Reprinted by permission of the Society of Nuclear Medicine from Ref. [29])

	PET-CT indication	IV/oral contrast	No contrast
Staging	Tumor staging	•	
	Tumor restaging	•	
Therapy Planning	RT-planning: head-and-neck, abdomen, pelvis	•	
	RT-planning: thorax	(•)	•
	Surgery	•	
	Interventions: separate contrast-enhanced CT available		•
	Interventions: no contrast-enhanced CT available	•	
Therapy Control	Therapy control (chemotherapy/irradiation)		•
	Therapy control (surgical/interventional)		•

RT Radiation therapy

• Recommended

(•) Recommended if tumor invasion into the mediastinum or hilar lymph node involvement is suspected

Summary

For a number of indications, a clinical contrast-enhanced CT scan may provide additional information compared with a nonenhanced PET-CT scan. The main benefit of oral and IV contrast is more accurate anatomical correlation with PET. Areas of focally increased tracer uptake may be more precisely localized by differentiation of the lesion from its surrounding structures. In addition, contrast-enhanced CT may provide valuable information for lesion detection and characterization in PET-negative tumors. The effects of positive CT contrast agents on PET attenuation correction can be avoided by using water-equivalent oral contrast and adapting the acquisition protocol after IV contrast administration. CT contrast agents should be considered with PET-CT imaging since they not only enhance the CT image but also enhance the quality of PET-CT.

References

1. Beyer T, Townsend DW, Brun T, et al. A combined PET/CT scanner for clinical oncology. J Nucl Med 2000;41(8):1369–1379.
2. Lardinois D, Weder W, Hany TF, et al. Staging of non-small-cell lung cancer with integrated positron-emission tomography and computed tomography. N Engl J Med 2003;348(25):2500–2507.
3. Antoch G, Saoudi N, Kuehl H, et al. Accuracy of whole-body dual-modality FDG-PET/CT for tumor staging in oncology: comparison with CT and PET. J Clin Oncol 2004;22:4357–4368.
4. Bar-Shalom R, Yefremov N, Guralnik L, et al. Clinical performance of PET/CT in evaluation of cancer: additional value for diagnostic imaging and patient management. J Nucl Med 2003;44(8): 1200–1209.
5. Collins CD. PET/CT in oncology: for which tumours is it the reference standard? Cancer Imaging 2007;7(Spec No A):S77–87.
6. Kuehl H, Antoch G. How much CT do we need for PEt/CT? A radiologist's perspective. Nuklearmedizin 2005;44(Suppl 1):S24–31.
7. Strobel K, Thuerl CM, Hany TF. How much intravenous contrast is needed in FDG-PET/CT? Nuklearmedizin 2005;44(Suppl 1): S32–37.
8. Kormano MJ, Goske MJ, Hamlin DJ. Attenuation and contrast enhancement of gynecologic organs and tumors in CT. Eur J Radiol 1981;1(4):307–311.
9. Alfidi RJ, Haaga JR. Computed body tomography. Radiol Clin North Am 1976;14(3):563–570.
10. Albertyn LE. Rationales for the use of intravenous contrast medium in computed tomography. Australas Radiol 1989;33(1):29–33.
11. Violante MR, Dean PB. Improved detectability of VX2 carcinoma in the rabbit liver with contrast enhancement in computed tomography. Radiology 1980;134(1):237–239.
12. Burgener FA, Hamlin DJ. Intravenous contrast enhancement in computed tomography of pelvic malignancies. ROFO Fortschr Geb Rontgenstr Nuklearmed 1981;134(6):656–661.
13. Morcos SK, Thomsen HS. Adverse reactions to iodinated contrast media. Eur Radiol 2001;11(7):1267–1275.
14. Katayama H, Yamaguchi K, Kozuka T, Takashima T, Seez P, Matsuura K. Adverse reactions to ionic and nonionic contrast media. A report from the Japanese Committee on the Safety of Contrast Media. Radiology 1990;175(3):621–628.
15. Garrett PR, Meshkov SL, Perlmutter GS. Oral contrast agents in CT of the abdomen. Radiology 1984;153(2):545–546.

16. Kinahan PE, Townsend DW, Beyer T, Sashin D. Attenuation correction for a combined 3D PET/CT scanner. Med Phys 1998;25(10): 2046–2053.
17. Dizendorf E, Hany TF, Buck A, Von Schulthess GK, Burger C. Cause and magnitude of the error induced by oral ct contrast agent in CT-based attenuation correction of pet emission studies. J Nucl Med 2003;44(5):732–738.
18. Nakamoto Y, Chin BB, Kraitchman DL, Lawler LP, Wahl RL. Effects of nonionic intraveneous contrast agents at PET/CT imaging: phantom and canine studies. Radiology 2003;227: 817–824.
19. Antoch G, Freudenberg LS, Egelhof T, et al. Focal tracer uptake: a potential artifact in contrast-enhanced dual- modality PET/CT scans. J Nucl Med 2002;43(10):1339–1342.
20. Matsumoto K, Nakamoto Y, Sakamoto S, Murase K, Senda M. Feasibility of diagnostic contrast-enhanced CT for attenuation correction of whole body PET images. Nippon Hoshasen Gijutsu Gakkai Zasshi 2007;63(7):757–765.
21. Mawlawi O, Erasmus JJ, Munden RF, et al. Quantifying the effect of IV contrast media on integrated PET/CT: clinical evaluation. AJR Am J Roentgenol 2006;186(2):308–319.
22. Antoch G, Freudenberg LS, Debatin JF, Kroger K. Images in vascular medicine. Diagnosis of giant cell arteritis with PET/CT. Vasc Med 2003;8(4):281–282.
23. Cohade C, Osman M, Nakamoto Y, et al. Initial experience with oral contrast in PET/CT: phantom and clinical studies. J Nucl Med 2003;44(3):412–416.
24. Antoch G, Kuehl H, Kanja J, et al. Dual-modality PET/CT scanning with negative oral contrast agent to avoid artifacts: introduction and evaluation. Radiology 2004;230(3):879–885.
25. Groves AM, Kayani I, Dickson JC, et al. Oral contrast medium in PET/CT: should you or shouldn't you? Eur J Nucl Med Mol Imaging 2005;32(10):1160–1166.
26. Berthelsen AK, Holm S, Loft A, Klausen TL, Andersen F, Hojgaard L. PET/CT with intravenous contrast can be used for PET attenuation correction in cancer patients. Eur J Nucl Med Mol Imaging 2005;32(10):1167–1175.
27. Beyer T, Antoch G, Muller S, et al. Acquisition protocol considerations for combined PET/CT imaging. J Nucl Med 2004; 45(1 Suppl):25S–35S.
28. Antoch G, Freudenberg LS, Beyer T, Bockisch A, Debatin JF. To enhance or not to enhance? 18F-FDG and CT contrast agents in dual-modality 18F-FDG PET/CT. J Nucl Med 2004;45(Suppl 1): 56S–65S.
29. Kuehl H, Veit P, Rosenbaum SJ, Bockisch A, Antoch G. Can PET/CT replace separate diagnostic CT for cancer imaging? Optimizing CT protocols for imaging cancers of the chest and abdomen. J Nucl Med 2007;48(Suppl 1):45S–57S.
30. Antoch G, Stattaus J, Nemat AT, et al. Non-small cell lung cancer: dual-modality PET/CT in preoperative staging. Radiology 2003; 229(2):526–533.
31. Antoch G, Vogt FM, Freudenberg LS, et al. Whole-body dual-modality PET/CT and whole-body MRI for tumor staging in oncology. J Am Med Assoc 2003;290(24):3199–3206.
32. Pfannenberg AC, Aschoff P, Brechtel K, et al. Low dose non-enhanced CT versus standard dose contrast-enhanced CT in combined PET/CT protocols for staging and therapy planning in non-small cell lung cancer. Eur J Nucl Med Mol Imaging 2007;34(1):36–44.
33. Setty BN, Blake MA, Sahani DV, Holalkere NS, Fischman AJ. Role of Contrast-enhanced CT (CECT) in hybrid PET-CT for liver metastases in patients with colorectal cancer. Paper presented at: RSNA, Chicago, 2005.
34. Rodriguez-Vigil B, Gomez-Leon N, Pinilla I, et al. PET/CT in lymphoma: prospective study of enhanced full-dose PET/CT versus unenhanced low-dose PET/CT. J Nucl Med 2006;47(10): 1643–1648.
35. Alfidi RJ, Haaga J, Meaney TF, et al. Computed tomography of the thorax and abdomen; a preliminary report. Radiology 1975;117(2): 257–264.

Chapter 10
Performance, Interpretation, and Reporting of PET-CT Scans for Body Oncology Imaging

Paul Shreve and Harry Agress Jr.

PET-CT Protocols for Body Oncology Imaging

The intent of PET-CT was to combine clinical FDG PET and clinical CT in a single examination [1]. FDG PET alone applied to body oncology imaging had shortcomings due to the limited spatial resolution and false positive findings caused by inflammation and normal physiologic processes. Consequently FDG PET scans for body oncology applications were typically interpreted in conjunction with body CT scans, with the two modalities providing complimentary information. This co-interpretation of anatomic findings of CT and the metabolic findings of FDG PET was most powerful when the two images sets were accurately registered and aligned, although this was difficult to routinely accomplish when the scan acquisitions were performed on a separate PET scanner and CT scanner at different times. By combining both the PET tomograph and CT scanner into a single device with a common (scanning table), the PET and CT images would be inherently registered and aligned if the patient did not move on the pallet during the two scan acquisitions. Combining the two complimentary modalities into a single scan procedure for body oncology imaging fostered an implicit and routine merging of the interpretation of the PET and CT images as well. During the development of the first PET-CT scanner prototype by Townsend and Nutt, it was determined that CT portion of the exam could provide, with appropriated energy scaling, the attenuation map for the PET image reconstruction replacing the time consuming sealed source transmission scan employed on stand-alone PET scanners. This was an added advantage of the hybrid imaging device, but not the reason for developing the technology [1].

The PET emission acquisition portion of the PET-CT examination is essentially the same as with a stand-alone PET scanner. With PET-CT, however, there is no sealed 511 keV source transmission scan to generate an *attenuation*, or mu, map for *attenuation correction* of the PET emission *projection* data. Since PET-CT scanners have nearly completely replaced stand-alone PET tomographs in the last decade, this difference is largely of historic interest. By eliminating the sealed source transmission scan with the rapidly acquired CT scan in the PET-CT scanner, the total time of performing a PET scan with attenuation correction was reduced by over 30%. The CT-based attenuation map does have the potential for generating artifacts on the attenuation-corrected FDG PET images due to dense structures such as metallic implants of cardiac pacers and orthopedic hardware, as well as very dense contrast material. This is easily verified and accounted for by reviewing the non-attenuation-corrected PET image reconstructions, however.

The CT acquisition portion of the PET-CT examination is also very similar to a CT performed for body oncology indications, particularly a routine CT of the chest, abdomen and pelvis performed for cancer indications. The difficulty of intravenous contrast bolus timing and breath holding during such an extended axial field-of-view acquisition, particularly on the earlier PET-CT scanners with single, dual, or four-slice CT scanner components, was the same as stand-alone CT, and was surmountable with careful attention to scanning protocols. As early as 2002, only 1 year after the introduction of commercial PET-CT scanners, fully optimized contrast enhanced CT exams with breath hold covering the neck, chest, abdomen, and pelvis were obtained on the earliest single slice PET-CT scanners [2]. With the ensuing advancement in multislice CT scanners, which was rapidly incorporated into PET-CT scanners, the ability to perform fully optimized contrast enhanced breath-hold CT of the whole torso or whole body as part of a PET-CT exam has been greatly facilitated, and details of optimal protocol options have been published for some time [3–6]. With contemporary PET-CT scanners whole torso (skull base to upper thighs) scans performed with a single optimized CT acquisition and rapid PET emission acquisitions can be routinely performed in less than 15 min (Fig. 10.1).

A key component of a PET-CT scanner is a pallet that maintains constant deflection as it passes through the in-tandem PET scanner and CT gantry, such that the PET and

P. Shreve (✉)
Advanced Radiology Services, P.C., Grand Rapids, MI, USA
e-mail: pshreve@advancedrad.com

P. Shreve and D.W. Townsend (eds.), *Clinical PET-CT in Radiology: Integrated Imaging in Oncology*,
DOI 10.1007/978-0-387-48902-5_10, © Springer Science+Business Media, LLC 2011

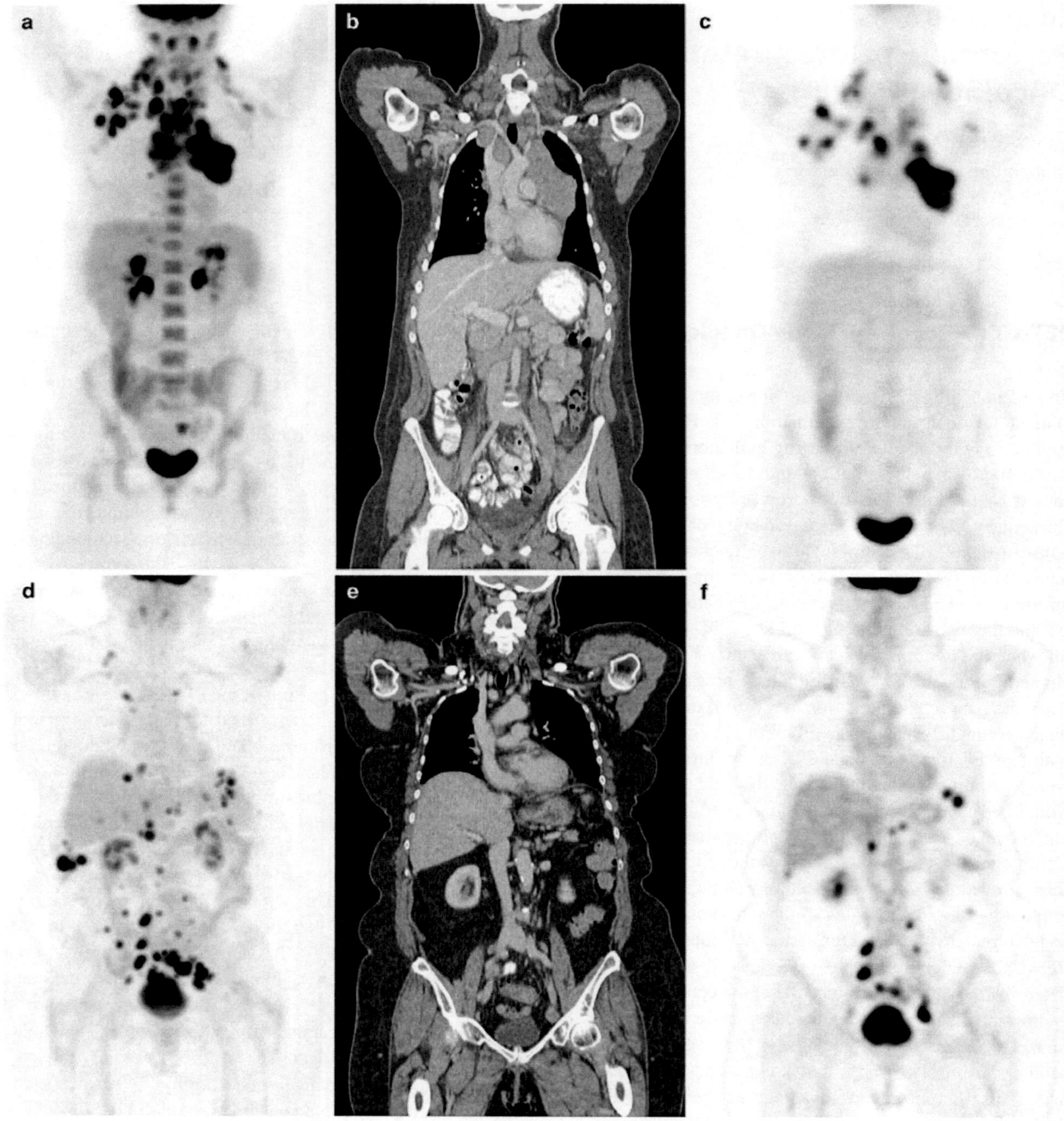

Fig. 10.1 PET-CT scans of the whole torso performed in under 15 min. Anterior maximum intensity projection (MIP) image (**a**), and should be (MIP) image (**a**), coronal CT (**b**) and FDG PET (**c**) image coronal FDG PET (**b**) and CT (**c**) images of a patient with a body mass index (BMI) of 22. PET acquisitions with 1.5 min per bed position for 5 bed positions, CT at 80 mAs with 100 mL intravenous contrast. Another patient with a body mass of 35 is shown (**d, e, f**) acquired with 2.5 min per bed position for 5 bed positions with CT at 120 mAs using 125 mL intravenous contrast. In both cases, FDG uptake time was 90 min and CT was performed as a single acquisition with breath hold

CT images maintain inherent registration. Patients are scanned in the supine position in the cranial-caudal direction, although caudal-cranial direction may be preferred when pathology is expected in the pelvis. For most indications other than head and neck cancer, it is preferred to have the arms positioned over the head to decrease beam-hardening artifact during the CT portion of the exam and arm movement-related artifact during the PET acquisition. As with any

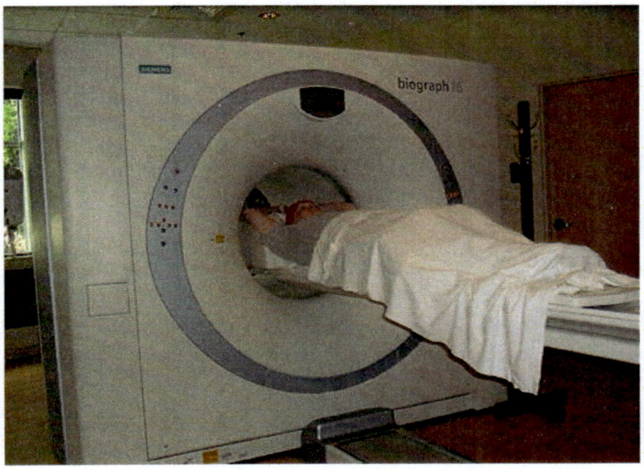

Fig. 10.2 Routine positioning of patient with arms up utilizing a arm support. A support under the knee slightly raises the knees for comfort. Patients must not move portions of the body scanned throughout both sequential CT and PET imaging acquisitions to insure proper registration and alignment of the image sets

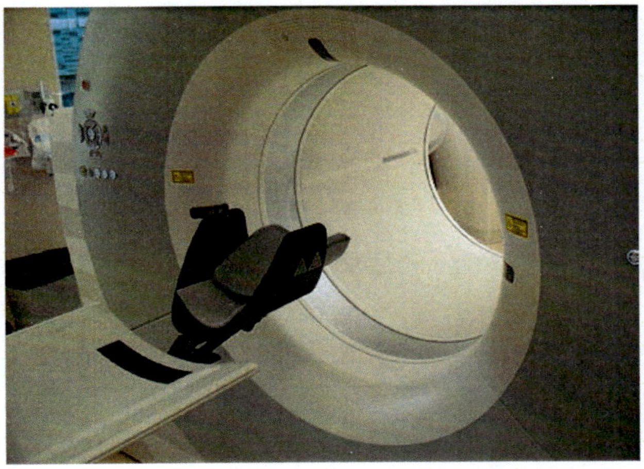

Fig. 10.3 Head support for dedicated head and neck PET-CT scans. For these exams arms are down at the patient's side and the head comfortably secured in the padded restraint. The complex and closely spaced anatomy in the neck mandates special attention to maintaining a stable positioning during the PET and CT scan acquisitions through the neck

imaging technique, one potential limitation is patient motion, and in the case of PET-CT, subsequent misregistration of the PET and CT image sets. It is therefore critical that the patient not move between the two scans and must be as comfortable as possible. To this end supports help keep the arms stable when held above the head (Fig. 10.2). Cushions under the neck and knees are also useful in decreasing muscle tension and back discomfort during the examinations. Likewise, head restraints are also recommended for head and neck studies (Fig. 10.3).

With the advent of PET-CT and advancements in the sensitivity of PET tomographs, the total scan time for an attenuation corrected whole torso FDG PET scan has been reduced from over 40 min to less than 15 min, greatly improving patient comfort and compliance. Nonetheless, medication may be necessary to perform a PET-CT scan in certain clinical situations. If the patient is known to be claustrophobic, anti-anxiety medication may be given prior to the FDG administration. This may also serve to diminish uptake due to muscle spasm and within brown adipose tissue (see Chap. 7). The patient must be accompanied by a driver to take the patient home after the examination. Intravenous Lasix and fluids may also be administered during the FDG uptake period (Fig. 10.4), in order to clear tracer from the kidneys and bladder in patients being evaluated for primary pelvic tumor and/or recurrences (e.g., gynecologic, colon, and bladder cancers).

The typical order of scan acquisition is the CT scan followed by the PET acquisition. The CT scan on contemporary PET-CT scanners is a continuous scan acquisition lasting approximately 10–20 s depending on the axial coverage, while the PET scan is a series of fixed table position acquisitions lasting 1–4 min and typically requiring 5–6 table positions for a typical whole torso exam. The reconstruction of the CT images is nearly instantaneous with the scan acquisition with contemporary scanners, while the attenuation corrected PET images reconstruction using iterative techniques typically can take a few minutes per bed position and requires the CT based attenuation mu map. Hence, with the CT scan performed first, the PET image reconstruction can occur concurrently during the PET emission acquisitions such that the PET image reconstruction is nearly completed for all table positions at the end of the PET acquisition sequence. If the PET scan is performed first followed by the CT portion of the exam, it would not be possible to review the attenuation corrected PET images promptly after complete of the scan. An advantage of this sequence, however, is the PET emission data is obtained at the very least, and any problems with the CT portion of the scan such as contrast reaction do not adversely affect the PET acquisition.

The CT portion of the PET-CT examination provides several different options that will be discussed in detail in this chapter. The two basic CT choices are: (1) a transmission scan for attenuation correction purposes only (typically 10 mAs) and (2) a diagnostic CT scan that utilizes various CT techniques in terms of beam current, breath hold, and use of intravenous and oral contrast. In some instances, for example, in a patient who has had a relatively recent diagnostic CT that is available for direct comparison, or a patient receiving a follow-up scan for certain cancer indications such as lymphoma, in which the PET information is of primary clinical importance and high resolution anatomic CT detail may not be necessary, the CT scan may be performed with

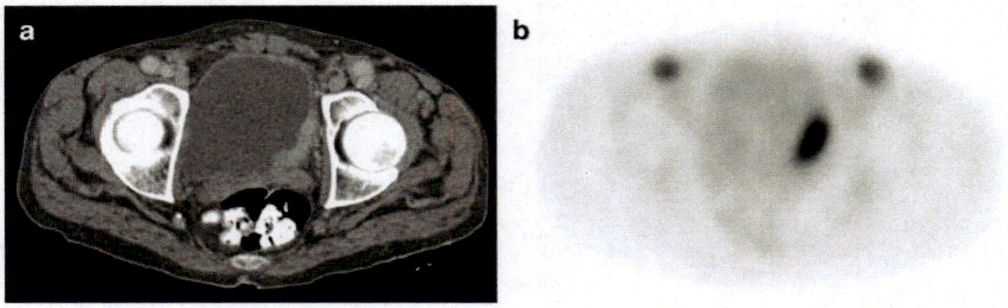

Fig. 10.4 PET-CT scan performed with protocol intended to minimize urinary tracer activity in the urinary bladder. During the FDG uptake phase a total of 1 L intravenous hydration was given and 40 min prior to scan time 40 mg intravenous furosemide, resulting in washout and voiding of the intense urinary tracer activity. Transaxial CT (**a**) and FDG PET (**b**) demonstrate urinary bladder tracer activity slightly greater than soft tissue background, allowing unobscured demonstration of the hypermetabolic urothelial neoplasm at the left bladder wall. Focal inguinal tracer activity bilaterally reflects arterial bypass grafts

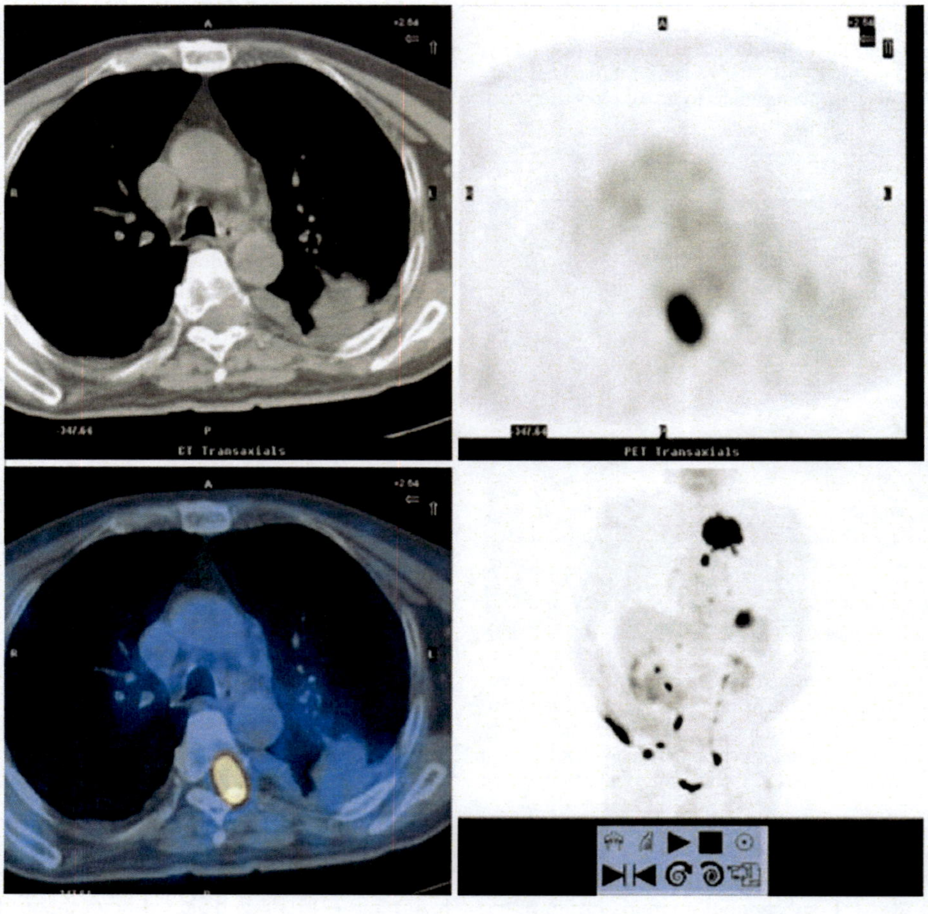

Fig. 10.5 PET-CT performed with CT as a low-dose noncontrast "localization CT." The MIP image (*lower right*) shows the left upper lobe hypermetabolic mass reflecting the primary lung cancer. The transaxial CT (*upper left*), FDG PET (*upper right*), and FDG PET-CT fusion image (*lower left*) demonstrates a focus of abnormal FDG tracer at the spine. While the PET-CT fusion image "localizes" the abnormal tracer activity to the left aspect of the spine, review of the CT image reveals the soft tissue mass with lytic changes at the left pedicle and encroachment on the spinal canal.

relatively lower beam current (40 mAs), no specific breath hold, and no intravenous contrast material (Fig. 10.5). These scans, often referred to as "low dose CT" or "localization CT scans," however, contain a great deal of anatomic information including to a useful degree the extent of tumor for T-staging as well as depiction of significant noncancerous abnormalities such as pneumothorax, small pulmonary nodules, aortic aneurysms, abnormal fluid collections, to name a few, and neoplastic masses that are not FDG avid. These CT scans are in fact diagnostic CT scans requiring full interpretation and integration with the FDG PET findings. The limitations of these so-called "low-dose" CT scans include respiratory motion related artifact at the lower lungs and upper abdomen, limitations in identifying local tissue and organ invasion of primary tumor and metastatic lesions, the inability to identify lesions that are best seen on CT with intravenous contrast, both cancer-related (non-FDG avid cancers in organs, very small hepatic metastases) and certain incidental clinically relevant findings (deep venous thrombus, pulmonary embolism).

The nature of a fully optimized CT ("full diagnostic CT") will depend on the clinical application. Contemporary PET-CT scanners incorporate 16- to 64-channel CT scanners with extended tube heating capacity such that the fan beam collimation is always thin, and slice thickness reconstruction of 3 mm or less is available routinely for all body imaging. Beam current can be set by noise factor and dose modulation applied to limit patient dose, with the tradeoff between image noise and patient dose adjusted for size of the patient, diagnostic intent, and patient age. In the pediatric population beam current is kept very low (40 mAs or less) to minimize radiation exposure, relying on intravenous contrast to compensate for limitations in tissue contrast due to image noise [7]. In young adults similar, but less extreme, reductions in beam current (40–80 mAs) may be employed, especially on follow-up surveillance scans. Otherwise, in adult patients with known or suspected cancer, the beam current should provide sufficient image detail for the anticipated CT diagnosis [8, 9] at the lowest dose reasonably achievable. This can be achieved with beam current in the range of 80–160 mAs for most patients. It should be noted that due to differences in manufacturers and the current rapid advancements in dose reduction in CT, it is not realistic to refer to a CT as a "low dose" CT in contradistinction to a "diagnostic CT"; no line can be drawn between the two in terms of a beam current specification, and even noise factor specification varies depending on particular clinical application or institution or center performing the scans.

Although solutions to performing a whole torso PET-CT using a single breath-hold CT acquisition were available in the published literature from nearly the onset of commercial PET-CT scanners [2–4], many centers have used protocols using two separate CT acquisitions of identical axial coverage: one so-called "CT performed for localization purposes," a diagnostic CT of relatively low beam current at quiet breathing with no intravenous contrast, with an additional diagnostic CT of relatively increased beam current with use of intravenous contrast and breath hold while scanning through the chest and abdomen (Fig. 10.6). This double CT scan acquisition approach simplifies registration issues of the PET image set with a CT image set with respect to respiratory movement, but the "low dose" diagnostic CT image

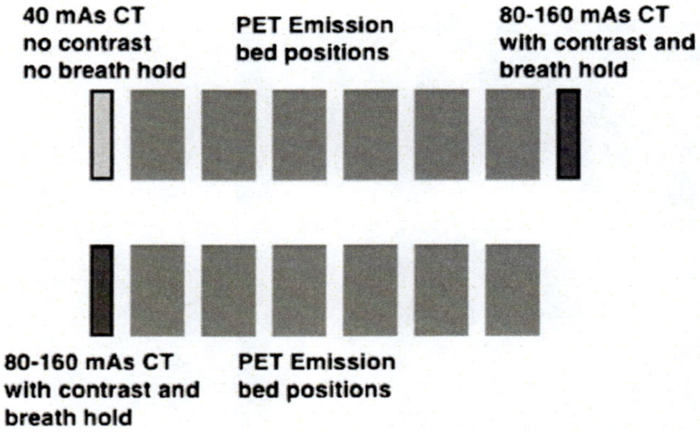

Fig. 10.6 General PET-CT scan sequencing. The upper sequence involves two CT scan acquisitions, with the less optimized diagnostic CT scan registered and aligned with the PET image set, rather than the fully optimized diagnostic CT scan. The lower sequence involves a single fully optimized diagnostic CT scan acquisition that is performed to be registered and aligned with the PET image set

set registered with the PET images is not the fully optimized diagnostic CT image set, which would be the preferred CT image set for interpretation. The two CT scan acquisitions also unnecessarily increase patient radiation dose.

Use of a single diagnostic CT acquisition requires a few refinements in technique, but is easily accomplished with contemporary PET-CT scanners [4–6]. A consequence of using the CT portion of the PET-CT scan for the attenuation, or mu map, needed for attenuation correction of the PET image reconstruction is that dense material such as metallic implants will result in "hot spot" artifact on the attenuation-corrected PET images. Very concentrated intravenous contrast in the precardiac central vein introduction route (cf. subclavian and innominate veins and superior vena cava) can result in such "hot spot" artifacts [10], but the effect is minor, and in fact the image degradation is more of a problem for the CT images than the attenuation corrected FDG PET images (Fig. 10.7). Proper contrast bolus technique, including either caudal cranial CT acquisition [3, 4], or dual contrast-injector saline chase methods eliminates this possible artifact on both the CT and attenuation-corrected PET images (Fig. 10.8). Use of intravenous contrast CT for the attenuation mu map in PET-CT does result in small changes in semi-quantitative Standardized Uptake Value measurements (SUVs) relative to a nonintravenous contrast enhanced CT scan, but the effect is small in soft tissue and tumors and has been shown to be not clinically relevant [11–13]. When every effort to standardize SUVs in a research setting is required, a true CT transmission scan (10 mAs) can be performed separately for the attenuation correction function.

The larger challenge in using a single fully optimized CT acquisition for the attenuation mu map is breathing-related artifact on the CT images and breath-hold registration of the PET and CT image sets. With contemporary PET-CT

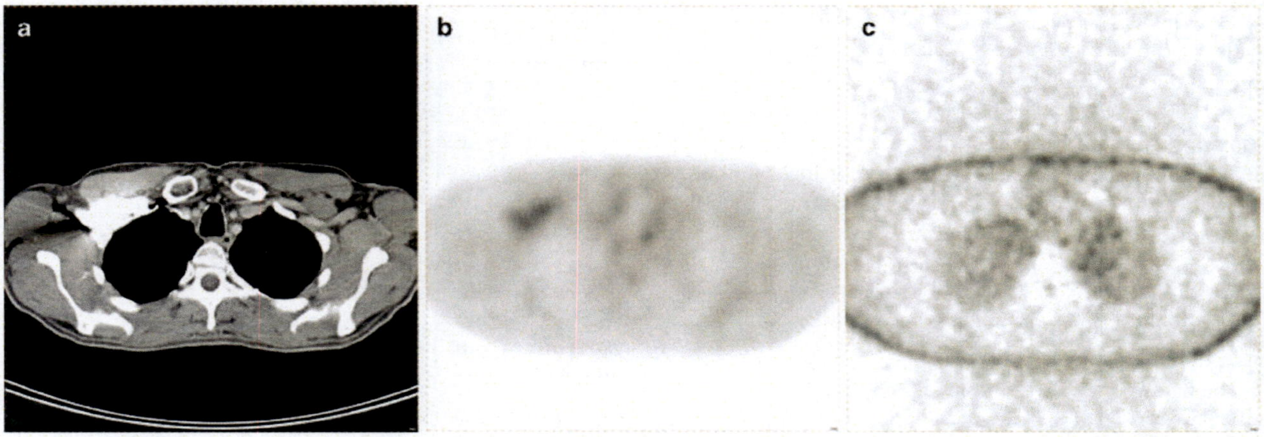

Fig. 10.7 Intravenous contrast related artifact on the attenuation corrected PET images. On the transaxial image (**a**) there is dense intravenous contrast material in the right axillary and subclavian veins. The density on the CT image results in ill-defined apparent increased tracer activity on the attenuation corrected FDG PET image (**b**), but this artifact is entirely absent on the non-attenuation-corrected FDG PET image (**c**). Note the level beam hardening artifact degrading the CT image; the artifact is actually more a problem for the CT images than the PET images

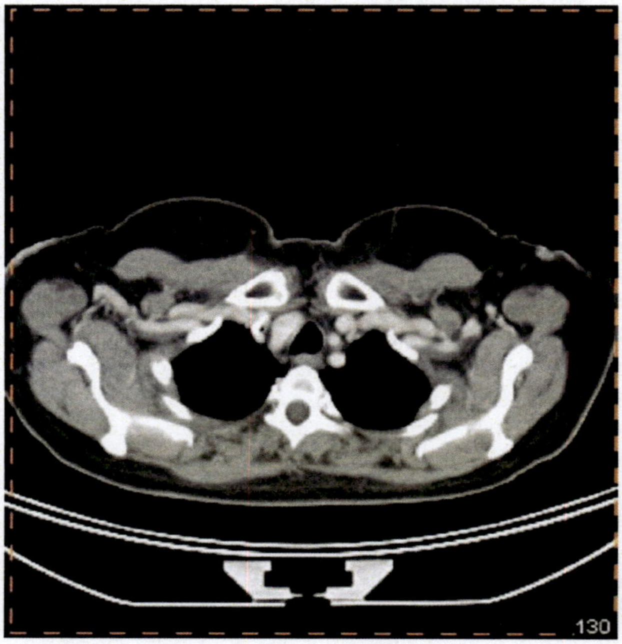

Fig. 10.8 Proper CT technique using intravenous contrast material. The transaxial contrast enhanced CT through the level of the shoulders shows no dense venous contrast material in the vein and the opacification of the arteries and veins is equal. Contrast was administered at the right arm peripheral vein, using a saline chase injection with the scan performed craniocaudad. Similar results can be obtained by scanning caudocraniad when using an arm injection

scanners with 16–64 slice CT capability, the breathing artifact at the lung bases when using quiet breathing and no breath hold is minimal in most patients, and acceptable for some indications, such as follow up scan for lymphoma, and generally causes few interpretive errors [14]. For optimal evaluation of the lung bases and organs at the upper abdomen, a breath hold during the CT scan acquisition is preferred, and this must be performed such that the position of the diaphragm on the breath-hold CT matches the average position of the diaphragm at quiet breathing, as depicted on the FDG PET images. This can be best achieved using near-end expiratory breath hold while scanning through the thorax and abdomen [4] Again, the advent of 16–64 slide CT PET-CT scanners has made such "on the fly" breath-hold single CT acquisition PET-CT protocols much easier, as patient breath hold of well under 10 s is easily accomplished with such fast-scanning CT capability. When there is a desire to optimally evaluate the lungs for small pulmonary nodules at the lung bases or other pulmonary details, a full inspiration breath hold while scanning through the lungs is required [15, 16]. In such settings including particularly lung cancer, initial assessment, and posttherapy assessment, a separate full-inspiration breath lung CT acquisition can be added to the whole torso acquisition easily [17], and this can be performed with relatively reduced beam current if desired to minimize additional patient dose.

The basic body oncology protocols for PET-CT are:

- Torso imaging from the base of the skull to the upper thighs ("skull base to thighs"), which accounts for the majority of examinations
- Whole body imaging from the cranial vertex to the feet, most often used for melanoma patients and certain cutaneous malignancies
- Head and neck imaging in which both PET and CT acquisition parameters are optimized for finer detail at the neck, and additional axial coverage may be limited

It should be noted that the skull base to thighs axial coverage is somewhat an arbitrary establishment of "one size fits all" axial coverage. While it may be appropriate to include the entire neck in a PET-CT performed for lymphoma, for example, it would not for ovarian cancer. Hence it has been suggested that axial coverage for PET-CT scans should be developed on an individual basis, rather than scanning from skull base to mid-thighs routinely [18].

Torso Imaging and Whole Body Imaging

PET-CT scan of the torso study typically extends from the skull base to the upper thighs, while a whole body extends from the skull vertex to feet. Arms above the head positioning is preferred if the patient can tolerate such for the total scan acquisition time. An initial scout image is taken to determine the table position for the desired axial coverage. If beam current modulation is employed to reduce patient dose, the patient's body must by centered in the scanner gantry to take full advantage of the beam current modulation. If intravenous contrast is employed, the contrast bolus is initiated and the CT scan acquisition commences after the bolus delay time (typically 60–65 s for adults). If a near-end expiration breath hold is to be performed, the patient is told to stop breathing as the scan passes through the thoracic inlet and then told to resume breathing as the scan passes through the pelvic inlet. If a separate breath-hold acquisition such as full inspiration acquisition of the lungs is desired, this can be acquired before or after the torso or whole body CT acquisition. When intravenous contrast is employed, this can easily be completed during the time of the contrast infusion and bolus delay (Fig. 10.9). If a full inspiration breath-hold CT of the thorax and full expiration breath-hold CT of the abdomen and pelvis are desired, a separate CT at quiet breathing for attenuation correction purposes would have to be acquired.

CT scanning parameters will vary between manufacturers. Applied tube voltage for adult patients ranges from 120 to 140 kVp, while for pediatric patients kVp will be reduces to as low as 80 kVp. Typical beam current for diagnostic CT of the body range from 40 to 160 mAs, although a higher range may be required for large and especially obese patients, and a lower range for very small children [7]. With beam current modulation an upper beam current limit is specified or a noise factor specified. Beam current will then be automatically modulated as the patient progresses axially through the scanner gantry, with reduced beam current while passing through the neck and lungs, and increased beam current while passing through the shoulders and abdomen and pelvis. Gantry rotation period is typically 0.5 s on contemporary PET-CT scanners, but table feed rate and gantry rotation

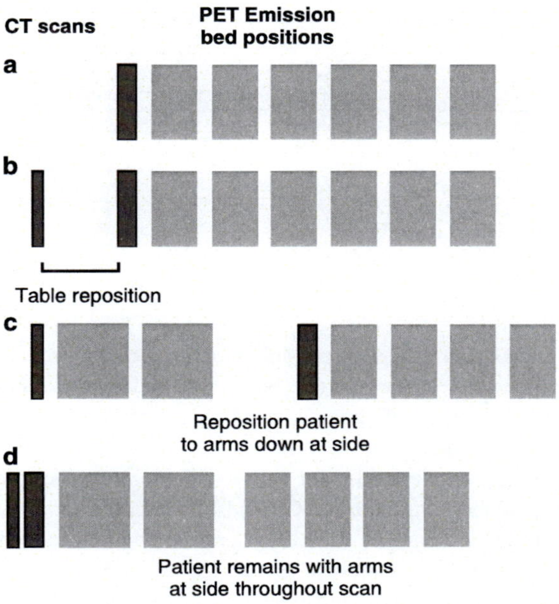

Fig. 10.9 PET-CT scan sequencing protocols. **a** Shows a typical torso exam with a single CT acquisition. **b** Shows an exam in which a full inspiration CT breath hold had been added for lung detail. The breath-hold portion of the exam can be performed before intravenous contrast is administered or during the arterial phase of contrast. **c** Shows a sequence for head and neck cancer with separate head and neck, and then the torso, PET-CT acquisitions with different (arms down vs arms up) patient positioning. **d** Shows a head and neck imaging sequence with no patient repositioning. In both (**c**) and (**d**) the acquisition parameters of both the CT and PET are specific for the head and neck acquisition, which differs from the acquisition parameters of the torso

period may be automatically determined based on desire noise factor setting and axial coverage of the scan.

The PET emission acquisition immediately follows the CT acquisition(s), commonly commencing caudocranial for torso exams and craniocaudad for whole body exams. The advantage of initiating the PET acquisition at the pelvis level is the configuration of the urinary bladder and position of the adjacent pelvic organs on the PET images will more closely match the CT image as this minimizes time for bladder distension due to normal urinary bladder filling. The emission acquisition time per table position varies among manufacturers, as well as the tradeoff between injected dose of FDG and desired image quality, but generally ranges from 2 to 4 min per bed position. Axial imaging field-of-view at each bed position varies with manufacturer and detector design options, typically 15–21.5 cm with varying degrees of bed position overlap such that an exam covering from skull base to thighs requires 5–7 bed positions. For whole body examinations, the CT and PET acquisition parameters for the head and neck are similar to the torso, but for the lower extremities emission acquisition parameters may be reduced to 1–2 min per bed position. Injected dose of FDG ranges from 225

Table 10.1 Comparison of radiation effective dose for FDG PET-CT scans

	Whole body	Red marrow	Breast	Gonads	Bladder
FDG PET (370 MBq)	7 mSv	4.6 mSv	3.5 mSv	5 mSv	59 mSv
CT torso (40 mAs)	5 mSv				
CT torso (120 mAs)	15 mSv				

to 555 MBq (6–15 mCi) for adult patients with dose reduced proportionally on a weight basis for pediatric patients. Reduced dose can be compensated by the increasing emission acquisition time.

The total patient dose for a PET-CT exam can be minimized by reducing both the CT and FDG contributions. CT dose reduction is most effectively achieved by first reducing redundant CT acquisitions as part of the PET-CT exam (eliminating so-called "localization CT" and using a single diagnostic CT acquisition or, if desired, using a true transmission scan (10 mAs) for attenuation correction purposes) and when at all possible, avoiding a CT of the chest, abdomen, and pelvis followed by a PET-CT exam a few days later in the evaluation of cancer patients. Dose-reducing features are now available on contemporary PET-CT scanners, including beam current modulation and fan beam collimator actuation, can be used routinely and the noise factor set to the lowest level that yields adequate diagnostic quality images. The FDG dosimetry is an important source of patient dose in a PET-CT examination (Table 10.1), and keeping the FDG administered dose low is an important aspect keeping overall patient exposure as low as reasonably achievable [18].

Head and Neck Imaging

PET-CT examinations performed for primary head and neck cancer can be specifically tailored for optimal image quality of both the PET and CT portions of the exam, recognizing the challenging anatomy and glucose metabolism physiology of this portion of the body. For these examinations arms should be down by the patient's sides to avoid beam-hardening degradation of the CT images and reconstruction artifacts due to arm movement between the CT and PET image acquisitions. To insure as little movement as possible of the neck between the CT and PET acquisitions, a dedicated head holder (see Fig. 10.3) should be utilized and the CT and PET acquisitions performed in close sequence. Mucosal (squamous cell carcinoma) cancer in the neck is typically a locoregional disease while nonmucosal cancers of the head and neck have a significant propensity for distant metastases. Since there are comorbid risk factors for mucosal head and neck cancer and lung cancer (tobacco abuse); there is a need on initial diagnosis and long-term follow-up exams to evaluate the chest for primary lung cancer as well, and consequently PET-CT exams for head and neck cancer will usually be performed with axial coverage including the thorax or remaining torso (Fig. 10.10).

With scanner there are two general options, a sequence of CT and PET acquisition of the neck optimized for the neck with arms down followed by a separate sequence of CT and PET of the chest or remaining torso with arms up optimized for this portion of the body, or a sequence of CT and PET acquisitions of the neck and chest/torso with arms down with a rapid switch of imaging parameters (see Fig. 10.9). The former protocol allows for optimization of CT and PET imaging for the neck and torso, but requires more overall scanner time as the patient spent be repositioning. The latter is efficient, but the chest/torso portion of the examination is compromised to some degree by having the arms down by the patient's side. The important aspect of either of these two options, or of a PET-CT scan limited to the neck, is the use of scanning acquisition parameters and image reconstruction parameters specifically optimal for the evaluation of the neck [19]. For the CT portion of the examination, the beam current employed while scanning through the neck will be higher (250 mAs or higher) than that used for scanning the torso in anticipation of the thinner slice thickness reconstruction (typically 1.25–2 mm) and narrower field-of-view reconstruction (and consequently smaller pixel size). For the PET portion of the examination the emission time per bed position (one or two bed positions are required depending on PET tomograph detector axial field-of-view) will be increased to 6–10 min in anticipation of use of a finer reconstruction matrix (256 instead of 125, for example), and a zoom factor that is greater than that used for torso imaging, to minimize pixel size. In either case, the dedicated neck portion of the study axial coverage is typically from the level of the internal auditory meatus to the thoracic inlet.

Oral Contrast

Oral contrast is valuable for the CT portion of the PET-CT when the abdomen and pelvis are included in the examination due to complex anatomy and variable appearance of the hollow viscera [9]. Both positive oral contrast containing dilute barium sulfate or water soluble contrast material and negative oral contrast consisting of water alone or sorbitol solutions having the same radiodensity as water can be used in the same manner as with body CT imaging alone. The dilute barium or water soluble positive contrast agents specifically used in CT will not cause hot spot artifacts on the

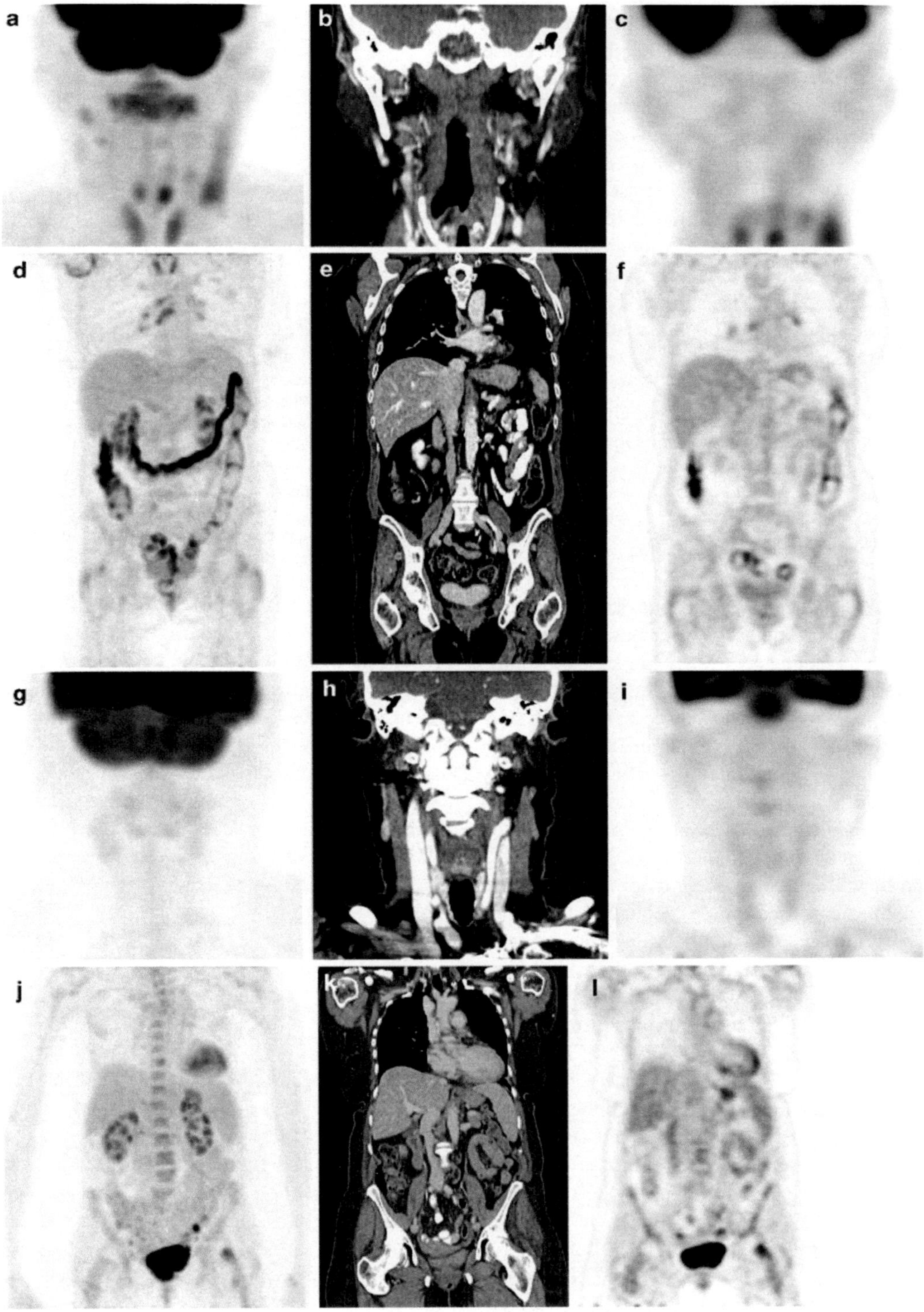

Fig. 10.10 Head and Neck cancer PET-CT scans. MIP (**a**) and coronal CT (**b**) and FDG PET (**c**) of the neck using fine matrix PET acquisition and CT beam current and field-of-view specifically for neck imaging, specifically for neck imaging (arms down) and PET and CT acquisition of the chest, abdomen and pelvis with repositioning (arms up). PET and CT acquisition of the chest and upper abdomen (**d**, **e**, **f**). Similar acquisition parameters but with no patient repositioning (arms remain down) is can be performed (**g**, **h**, **i**, **j**, **k**, **l**). The CTs of the neck and then chest or torso are performed in rapid succession, with respective optimized acquisition parameters using the same intravenous contrast bolus, and then the PET acquisitions, again with parameters tailored to the neck and then the chest/torso sequential CT and PET imaging acquisitions are performed

attenuation corrected PET images. Barium in bowel from a recent fluoroscopic GI study is of a density that will cause image degrading beam hardening artifacts on the CT images and spurious hot spot artifacts on the attenuation corrected PET images. Similar image degradation can be realized when dilute barium from a recent prior CT scan is concentrated in the colon. Generally, a positive oral contrast agent can be given at the time of the FDG dose administration and in the 1–2 h uptake time will have progressed through small bowel. For many centers this is sufficient; to achieve complete colon opacification typically requires ingestion of the oral contrast in stages prior to the appointment time. In adult patients with ample intraabdominal fat, particularly when intravenous contrast is used, some centers prefer negative oral contrast, as bowel wall features are well delineated. Optimal results, however, require rapid ingestion of volumes in excess of 1 L.

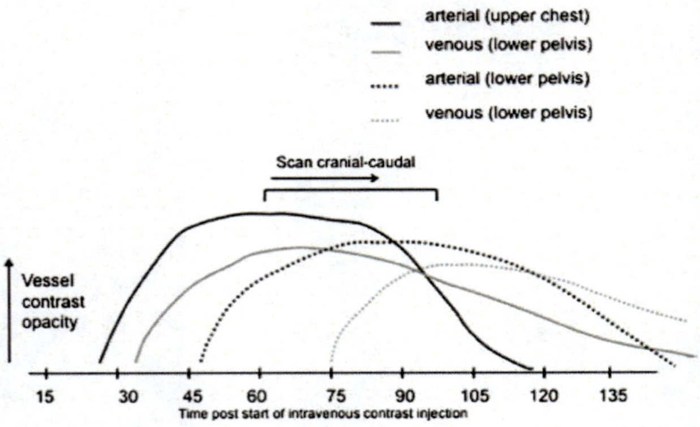

Fig. 10.11 Intravenous contrast bolus timing for whole torso single scan acquisition. When performing CT scans of extended axial coverage, the scan acquisition timing must follow the vascular circulation of the contrast material. The hypothetical curves show how, for craniocaudad scanning, with a typical 65-s bolus delay, opacification of the arteries and veins in the neck and shoulder level will be relatively equal, but the axial progression of the CT acquisition must allow for sufficient time for the contrast material to circulate to the lower torso and extremities and opacify the return venous system

Intravenous Contrast

Intravenous contrast can be employed in the same manner in PET-CT exams as in body and head and neck stand-alone CT scans. Preferred intravenous contrast is low or iso-osmolar iodinated contrast (75–150 cc) injected at typical rates of 2.5–3 cc/s. This can be followed by a 60 cc. saline flush (ideally with a dual injector) in order to eliminate any contrast retention in the subclavian and innominate veins, especially if the contrast enhanced CT is to be used for attenuation correction. As noted above, if the CT scans are performed with proper contrast technique, hot spot artifacts due to concentrated IV contrast will not occur when the intravenous contrast enhanced CT scan is used for the attenuation correction. More importantly, the CT scan will not be degraded by beam hardening artifact associated with the concentrated introduction route venous contrast (see Figs. 10.7 and 10.8).

Intravenous contrast is particularly valuable for PET-CT scans in the neck [19] and abdomen and pelvis [9]. To achieve optimal results, however, as with stand-alone CT, contrast bolus timing must be optimized. For most applications the goal is to have balanced opacification of the arterial and venous structures throughout the entire scan of the neck, chest, abdomen, and pelvis and scanning through the abdomen is at the portal venous phase (see Fig. 10.1). This can usually be accomplished by initiating the CT acquisition 60–65 s after initiation of the contrast injections. The rate of scanning in the axial direction, however, must be balanced to the rate and volume of contrast injected (Fig. 10.11), such that the bolus is not "outrun" resulting in arterial, but not venous opacification at the pelvis (when scanning craniocaudad) or upper chest and neck (when scanning caudocranial). For torso scanning the bolus delay many be lengthened in older patients or those with known compromised cardiac output, and shorted in younger patients and children, to account for the differences in blood transit time. Multiphase intravenous contrast enhancement, for example pulmonary arterial phase in the chest or late arterial phase in the abdomen, can be easily incorporated into the CT acquisition during the usual bolus delay time with repositioning of the patient (see Fig. 10.9) using the same contrast bolus [9, 17]. Similarly, when a dedicated head and neck acquisition is followed by a chest or torso acquisition without patient repositioning, the same contrast bolus can be used (see Fig. 10.10).

Image Reconstruction and Postprocessing

For PET-CT scans, there are two CT image reconstructions: one full field-of-view used for the attenuation correction of the PET emission images and one reduced field-of-view used for interpretation along with the PET images. The full field-of-view used for attenuation correction can be from a single diagnostic CT acquisition or separate CT scan acquisition performed only for attenuation correction purposes. For torso and whole body scans, the field-of-view will be limited to the maximum transverse dimension of the body, while for dedicated head and neck scans the field-of-view is reduced to the maximum dimension of the neck with resultant smaller pixel size. CT slice thickness reconstruction for torso and whole body scans is 2–3 mm while the slice thickness reconstruction dedicated head and neck scans is 1.25–2 mm. CT image reconstruction kernels for head and neck scans are also slightly finer detail than for body images. When a breath-hold CT scan of the lungs is performed, either dedicated full inspiration or on-the-fly, a lung kernel reconstruction of the projection data should also be performed to provide a lung detail image set of the chest.

PET image reconstruction is usually performed using iterative techniques, with inclusion of additional refinements to image spatial resolution and reduce image noise from scatter and random detection events. These reconstruction algorithms can take a matter of a few minutes per bed position, and exact method and total reconstruction time vary among manufacturers. With ordered subsets expectation maximization (OSEM) currently commonly used, the number of iterations and subsets employed in the reconstruction can be adjusted for desired reconstructed image properties and time of reconstruction. Increasing the effective iterations brings the image closer to depicting the true distribution of counts, but adds noise to the image. It should be noted that differences in the number of iterations can substantially alter Standardized Uptake Measurements (SUVs) for smaller lesions (cf. <2 cm) and is one of several factors that contribute to the non-standard nature of so-called "SUVs" [20, 21]. Filtered backprojection reconstruction is the same among different manufacturers and is very rapid, and does not demonstrate noise as focal small hot spots as do iterative image reconstruction methods. Since PET image reconstruction without attenuation correction will be free of any artifacts such as dense material depicted on the CT scan used for attenuation correction, it is advisable to have non-attenuation-corrected filtered backprojection image reconstruction as an additional PET image set for reference. The PET image reconstructed slice thickness in the transaxial plane is set to match the CT image reconstruction slice thickness. Likewise, sagittal and coronal reformats of the PET and CT images are set to matching slice thickness.

There are a variety of options for storage and distribution of reconstructed images [22]. Generally images set in PACs or local storage media should include the entire transaxial attenuation corrected PET iteratively reconstructed image set. As noted above, it is advisable to also have a non-attenuation-corrected PET image set available. Transaxial CT images sets are reconstructed using customary soft tissue kernels with the appropriate field-of-view. The full field-of-view CT images used for attenuation correction of the PET images are not needed in the diagnostic image archive. If CT images of the lungs were reconstructed with a lung kernel, this image set should be archived as well. It is optional to archive coronal and sagittal image reformats as these can be automatically generated on work stations from transaxial image sets. If CT transaxial image sets are to be used as source images for such reformats, there should be overlap of the reconstructed slices. It is likewise optional to archive fusion images, as these are generated automatically on work stations, and archived fusion images would have fixed fusion settings, limiting their usefulness.

PET-CT Performed for Radiation Therapy Planning

Increasingly PET-CT scan are performed for radiation therapy purposes, with the FDG PET information used to provide better initial staging and prognosis and improve locoregional staging to determine the optimal treatment fields. A high quality CT performed as part of the PET-CT can also be used in the simulation process. PET-CT scan performed for use in radiation therapy planning should be performed on a flat radiation therapy pallet (Fig. 10.12) available from all manufacturers, with the patient in the same restraint devices used to position the patient for treatment. Reference and fiducial markings placed with external reference lasers insure consistent positioning of the patient during treatment. The PET-CT protocol used for radiation therapy planning may be similar to a routine diagnostic PET-CT scan, although specific breath-hold positions of the CT acquisition or gated CT and even PET acquisitions may be required for thoracic malignancies. Image reconstruction may be slightly different in terms of slice thickness, overlap, and field-of-view, as specified for importation into radiation therapy planning software depending on the manufacturer.

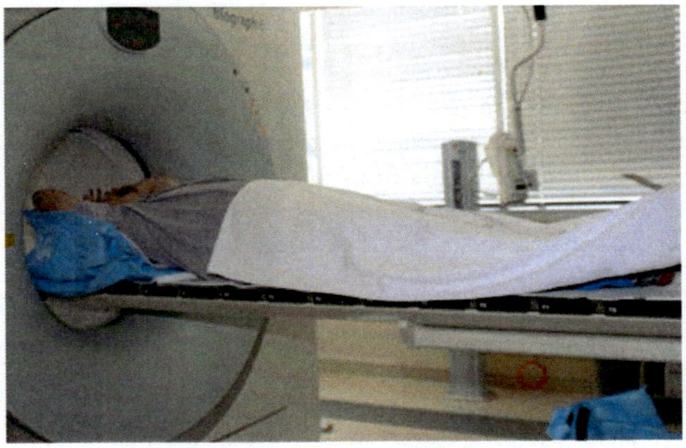

Fig. 10.12 Flat radiation therapy table. A radiation therapy pallet should be used when performing PET-CT for radiation therapy planning. This allows reproducible positioning of the patient on the treatment therapy table

Interpretation and Reporting of Body Oncology PET-CT Scans

PET-CT scans are of great value to oncologists, surgeons, and other medical specialists when the metabolic and anatomic information is properly integrated and the imaging findings put in the context of the patient's specific cancer and treatment history. These examinations, however, are among the most complex and time-consuming medical imaging studies to interpret and report. Patients typically undergoing PET-CT body oncology exams have complex histories related to their cancer and treatments and are additionally prone to related complications. Axial coverage of a majority of PET-CT scans for body oncology imaging is such that essentially the whole torso is imaged.

The tasks of interpretation of a PET-CT examination begin with full interpretation of the PET and CT images and integration of the findings. A fully capable workstation either of the scanner's manufacturer or PACs vendor with ample screen space is essential for the display of the transaxial PET and CT images and a coronal or sagittal image reformat of the PET and CT images, as well as the PET maximum intensity projection (MIP) rotating image display. Image display space must allow for CT images to be displayed of sufficient size such that they can be fully interpreted. This means, at least for whole-torso scan acquisitions, a coronal or sagittal image CT will usually need to fill an entire vertical aspect of the display screen. Fusion images require color-capable display screens, yet with sufficient resolution for CT interpretation, and such displays are now common. Having the PET and CT images registered and aligned allows for identification of the anatomic feature exhibiting a given focus of abnormal glucose metabolism and provides specificity in terms of whether the PET abnormality corresponds to a benign source of FDG tracer uptake or malignant neoplasm. There are additionally multiple clinically relevant CT findings both unrelated and related to the malignant disease only seen on the CT images.

Not all cancers and metastatic manifestations of malignancy are associated with increased glucose metabolism that will be detected on the FDG images. Such cancers often, however, are depicted on the CT images, whether fully optimized contrast-enhanced CT or reduced beam current noncontrast CT. For example, cancers that are not FDG avid or are not consistently highly FDG avid including renal cell carcinoma or bronchoalveolar lung cancer, hepatocellular carcinoma, carcinoid tumor, prostate cancer, as well as mucinous forms of colon, ovarian, and breast cancer can be only faintly positive, or even "cold", on FDG PET images (Table 10.2). Small (less than 5 mm) pulmonary nodules, are usually below the reliable detection threshold of FDG PET but are readily seen on a properly performed CT. Highly necrotic tumor masses can have little FDG tracer uptake due to the limited viable rim of malignant neoplasm. Certain manifestations of metastatic disease such as peritoneal carcinomatosis can be diagnosed more reliably on CT images than FDG PET images. The process of interpreting PET-CT examinations, then, requires the PET findings to be related to the corresponding CT findings, and CT images completely reviewed for clinically relevant abnormalities that may not be FDG avid.

Table 10.2 Cancers and manifestations of malignancy poorly detected on FDG PET

Highly necrotic primary or metastatic neoplasm's
Mucinous ovarian, breast, colon cancer
Cystic ovarian and pancreatic neoplasms
Peritoneal carcinomatosis
Small tumor mass (6 mm)
Brain metastases
Renal cell carcinoma, prostate cancer, carcinoid tumors, bronchoalveolar lung cancer, well differentiated adenocarcinomas, small lymphocyte subtype lymphoma, lobular breast cancer

Determining whether increased FDG tracer uptake reflects malignant neoplasm requires thorough knowledge of physiologic and normal variant sources of FDG tracer uptake [23]. Focal FDG tracer activity greater than mediastinal background or liver background tracer activity is suspicious for malignant neoplasm if not explained by normal physiologic or a benign pathologic process, as mild inflammatory and malignant neoplasm sources can give rise to the same level of FDG tracer accumulation. Qualitative assessment of abnormal FDG tracer uptake is readily determined on the MIP PET images, as this depiction of FDG tracer distribution allows comparison with all tissues and organs. Liver background tracer activity and mediastinal background activity, as well as cerebellum (a "hot" tissue reference) activity, have been shown to be reliable reference tissues in terms of intrasubject variation as well [24]

Standardized Uptake Values (SUVs) are subject to numerous factors that affect the SUV value obtained in a clinical setting, which if not properly accounted for will result in departures of SUV values from historic norms and renders comparison of values obtained amongst different institutions unreliable [20, 21] Consequently, SUV values should not be the sole criteria as to whether a focus of FDG tracer activity is deemed abnormal and hence suspicious for malignant neoplasm. Further, SUV values in the published literature are not necessarily comparable to values obtained at a given imaging center. SUV values can be useful for quantification of changes in tumor FDG tracer uptake in the setting of therapy response assessment, but this requires rigorous attenuation to consistency in terms of FDG uptake time, scanner and imaging parameters, image reconstruction method, type of region-of-interest analysis used, correction for lean body mass changes, and careful determination of the true activity of FDG administered intravenously. Whether SUVs are reported for diagnosis or staging, or for assessment of therapy response, it is recommended that an index SUV, such as of the liver, be reported as well for comparison with scans performed at other institutions [25].

There are three principal tasks in PET-CT interpretation in the setting of body oncology imaging (Table 10.3). Chief among these is integrating the PET abnormalities and corresponding morphologic abnormalities seen on the CT images as well as identifying any CT abnormalities that may reflect malignancy. Assessing the size and extent of local organ invasion by the primary tumor both in the setting of primary staging (T staging) and at recurrence is largely based on CT image interpretation. Similar morphologic assessment is important for certain staging criteria such as lymph node metastases, extracapsular spread, or necrosis in the setting of head and neck cancer or conglomeration of axillary nodal metastases in the setting of breast cancer. Incidental, but clinically relevant, CT findings not directly related to a patient's malignancy must also be assessed [26], requiring complete review of the CT images.

When interpreting PET-CT scans for body oncology applications, the FDG PET MIP images are particularly useful for overall assessment of the presence and extent of abnormal FDG tracer uptake. Foci of abnormal FDG tracer activity can then be further identified and morphologically characterized on the axial-, coronal-, or sagittal-registered and aligned PET and CT images. The entire set of CT images requires independent review to insure manifestations of malignancy negative on PET are not overlooked, and incidental clinically-relevant CT findings unrelated to malignancy are identified and reported. Some imaging physicians review the entire set of CT images before reviewing the FDG PET findings to insure relevant CT findings are not missed. Even when there has been a recently (within 4 weeks) performed CT scan of the corresponding body parts, the CT portion of the PET-CT exam still requires complete independent review, as a patient's condition can change in as little time or there can be interval procedures (for example, an interval port placement causing a pneumothorax), and important findings may have been overlooked or not reported on the recent CT interpretation. Further, findings mentioned on the prior CT report should be reinterpreted in light of the presence or absence of abnormal glucose metabolism depicted on the FDG PET images.

Table 10.3 Body oncology PET-CT interpretation

Identification and morphologic characterization of abnormal FDG tracer activity
T-staging and assessment of local invasion of primary and metastatic tumors
Unexpected and incidental findings on both CT and PET images

Note: The interpretative tasks and workload are the same for so-called "low dose" CT or "full diagnostic CT"

Table 10.4 Important incidental findings on PET-CT examinations

Focal abnormal FDG tracer activity in the colon, neck, or thyroid gland reflecting possible unsuspected primary cancer
Non-to minimally FDG avid malignancies
Pulmonary nodules too small to reliably assess on FDG PET
Deep venous thrombus and pulmonary thromboembolism
Large artery aneurysms
Improper positioning of central venous catheters
Pneumothorax following port placement or lung biopsy
Ascites, pleural effusions, pericardial effusions
Obstructive uropathy
Abscess including postoperative leaks
Active colitis, diverticulitis, cholecystitis

The report of a PET-CT exam should be treated as a consultation, with particular attention to a concise history and an impression that directly addresses the key clinical issues relevant to the patient's subsequent management [27]. PET-CT reports require an added level of depth due to the complex treatment history and number of prior imaging exams associated with patients typically undergoing these studies. In addition to the findings related to the known or suspected malignancy, unexpected [28] and incidental findings depicted on either the FDG PET images or the CT images must be recognized and reported (Table 10.4). When there are separate PET and CT reports, it is critically important the two reports are consistent. This is especially important when the PET and CT portions of the studies are interpreted by different physicians, in which case the readers must communicate and agree on the final impression.

The impression section of a PET-CT report should be just that, an impression, as opposed to a long list of abnormal findings. It should answer the question that the referring physician has posed. The impression component of the report should take into account all of the PET and CT findings as a whole, and be as definitive as possible. This is also best performed using a bulleted format.

References

1. Townsend DW. Combined positron emission tomography-computed tomography: the historical perspective. Semin Ultrasound CT MRI 2008;29:232–235.
2. Antoch G, Freudenberg LS, Statuss J, et al. Whole body positron emission tomography-CT: optimized CT using oral and IV contrast materials. Am J Roentgenol 2002;79:1555–1560.
3. Antoch G, Freudenberg LS, Beyer T, et al. To enhance or not to enhance? 18F-FDG and CT contrast agents in dual modality 18F-FDG PET/CT. J Nucl Med 2004;45:S56–S65.
4. Brechtel K, Klein M, Vogel M, et al. Optimized contrast-enhanced CT protocols for diagnostic whole-body 18F FDG PET/CT: technical

aspects of single-phase versus multiphase CT imaging. J Nucl Med 2006;47:470–476.
5. Kuehl H, Veit P, Rosenbaum SJ, et al. Can PET/CT replace separate diagnostic CT for cancer imaging? Optimizing CT protocols for imaging cancer of the chest and abdomen. J Nucl Med 2007;48: S45–S57.
6. Pfannenberg AC, Aschoff P, Brechtel K. Value of contrast-enhanced multiphase CT in combined PET/CT protocols for oncologic imaging. Br J Radiol 2007;80;437–445.
7. Nadel HR, Shulkin B. Pediatric positron emission tomography-computed tomography protocol considerations. Semin Ultrasound CT MRI 2008;29:271–276.
8. Soyka JD, Veit-Haibach P, Strobel K. Staging pathways in recurrent colorectal carcinoma: is contrast-enhanced 18F-FDG PET/CT the diagnostic tool of choice? J Nucl Med 2008;49:3354–3361.
9. Almusa O, Daly B, Shreve P. Protocol considerations for positron emission tomography-computed tomography of the abdomen and pelvis. Semin Ultrasound CT MRI 2008;29:251–262.
10. Antoch G, Freudenberg LS, Egelhop T, et al. Focal tracer uptake: a potential artifact in cotrast-enhanced dual-modality PET/CT scans. J Nucl Med 2002;43:1339–1342.
11. Yau YY, Chan WS, Tam YM, et al. Application of intravenous contrast in PET/CT: Does it really introduce significant attenuation correction error? J Nucl Med 2005;46:283–291.
12. Berthelsen AK, Holm S, Loft A, et al. PET/CT with intravenous contrast can be used for PET attenuation correction in cancer patients. Eur J Nucl Med Mol Imaging 2005;32:1167–1175.
13. Mawlawi I, Erasmus JJ, Munden RF, et al. Quantifying the effect of IV contrast media on integrated PET/CT: clinical evaluation. Am J Roentgenol 2006;186:308–319.
14. Osman, et al. Clinically Significant of Inaccurate Localization of Lesions with PET/CT: Frequency in 300 Patients. J Nucl Med 2003; 44:240–243.
15. Allen-Auerbach M, Yeom K, Park J, et al. Standard PET/CT of the chest during shallow breathing is inadequate for comprehensive staging of lung cancer. J Nucl Med 2006;47:298–301
16. Nehmeh SA, Erdi YE, Meirelles GSP, et al. Deep inspiration breath hold PET/CT of the thorax. J Nucl Med 2007;48:22–26.
17. Shyn PB. Protocol considerations for thoracic positron emission tomography-computed tomography. Semin Ultrasound CT MRI 2008;242–250.
18. Blodgett T. Best Practices in PET/CT: Consensus on performance of positron emission tomography-computed tomography. Semin Ultrasound, CT MRI 2008;29:236–241.
19. Escott EJ. Positron emission tomography-computed tomography considerations for head and neck cancer imaging. Semin Ultrasound CT MRI 2008;263–270.
20. Keyes JW. SUV: Standard uptake value or silly useless value? J Nucl Med 1995;36:1836–1839.
21. Boellaard R, Krak NC, Hoekstra OS, et al. Effects of noise, image resolution, and ROI definition on the accuracy of standardized uptake values: a simulation study. J Nucl Med 2004;45: 1519–1527.
22. Faasse T, Shreve P. Positron emission tomography-computed tomography patient management and workflow. Semin Ultrasound CT MRT 2008;29:277–282.
23. Shreve PD, Bui CDH. Normal variants in FDG PET imaging. In: Whal RL (ed.). Principals and practice of Positron Emission Tomography. Philadelphia, PA: Lippincott Williams & Williams, 2002:111–136.
24. Tann M, Miller M, Perry K, et al. Monitoring treatment response with FDG PET/CT: intrasubject variation of reference tissue SUV values with intercurrent therapy. J Nucl Med 2008; 49:326.
25. Wahl RL, Jacene H, Kasamon Y, Lodge MA. From RECIST to PERCIST: Evolving considerations for PET response criteria in solid tumors. J Nucl Med 2009;50:122S–150S.
26. Bruzzi JF, Truong MT, Marom EM. Incidental findings on integrated PET/CT that do not accumulate 18F-FDG. Am J Roentgenol 2006;187:1116–1123.
27. Agress H Jr, Wong TZ, Shreve P. Interpretation and reporting of positron emission tomography-computed tomography scans. Semin Ultrasound, CT MRI 2008;29:283–290.
28. Agress, H Jr, Cooper BZ. Detection of clinically unexpected malignant and premalignant tumors with whole-body FDG PET: histopathological comparison. Radiology 2004;23: 417–424.

Chapter 11
Pediatric Management and Preparation in PET-CT

Joseph J. Junewick and Paul Shreve

Preinjection Preparation

Protocol

A patient summary is requested from the referring clinician at the time the examination is scheduled. Pertinent information should include diagnosis, biopsy site and date, pathology report, treatment course (chemotherapy regimen, radiation therapy history, surgery history, bone marrow transplantation), and medications (especially glucose containing medicines, steroids and hematopoietic stimulants). Prior imaging examinations should also be made available. Protocols for the examinations are based on this information.

Glucose Status

Patients must be at basal glucose and insulin levels at the time of 18F-FDG injection. Glucose and 18F-FDG compete in tumor glycolysis, therefore high serum glucose will result in lower tumor uptake of 18F-FDG. Glucose restriction translates to fasting for most patients but also pertains to enteral feeding, TPN, glucose-containing intravenous fluids, certain medications, and syrups. In general, withholding glucose-containing food, drink, and medications for 6 h prior to administration of 18F-FDG is adequate; 4 h is probably adequate for preschool patients. If the patient is diabetic, insulin or oral hypoglycemic medication is given 4 h prior to injection. At our institution, all patients undergo serum blood glucose evaluation immediately before injection and 18F-FDG is only given to patients with levels <150 mg/dL. Hypoglycemia is rarely a problem. If the patient is not symptomatic, the injection is carried out in the routine fashion and glucose can be given intravenously or juice can be ingested after 30–90 min post-injection without significantly interfering with tumor uptake of 18F-FDG. If the patient is symptomatic before injection, hypoglycemia should be treated and the injection delayed or rescheduled.

Bowel Contrast

Intraperitoneal and retroperitoneal fat is significantly decreased in pediatric patients compared to adults and consequently unopacified bowel can simulate masses and inflammatory collections and may hinder evaluation of metastatic adenopathy and masses. Adequate bowel opacification will help mitigate these limitations. We use a 1–2% solution of iodixanol (Visipaque) diluted in a sugar-free beverage (Crystal Light). Patients are asked to rapidly drink a prescribed volume approximately 1 h prior to scanning and continually sip additional contrast until scanning is performed (Table 11.1).

Activity Restriction

It may be argued that only very vigorous physical activity that could deplete glycogen stores of muscle should be restricted before PET-CT. Children rarely achieve this level of exertion despite what most parents perceive. Also, the patient's disease status often restricts activity enough so this is not usually a concern. Some adolescents, particularly those able to compete in organized sports or with nondebilitating therapy, may exert themselves enough to result in excessive muscle uptake. Consequently, patients are asked to restrict such activity for the day prior to the examination.

J.J. Junewick (✉)
Department of Radiology, Spectrum Health Hospitals,
Helen de Vos Children's Hospital, Grand Rapids, MI, USA
and
Michigan State University College of Human Medicine,
Grand Rapids, MI, USA
e-mail: jjunewick@advancedrad.com

P. Shreve and D.W. Townsend (eds.), *Clinical PET-CT in Radiology: Integrated Imaging in Oncology*,
DOI 10.1007/978-0-387-48902-5_11, © Springer Science+Business Media, LLC 2011

Table 11.1 Bowel contrast protocol

Age	Volume 1 h prior	Additional sipping volume
<5 years	8 ounces (240 mL)	4 ounces (120 mL)
5–12 years	12 ounces (480 mL)	6 ounces (180 mL)
>12 years	16 ounces (480 mL)	8 ounces (240 mL)

Injection and Uptake

Vascular Access

Radiopharmaceutical dose is weight (lean body weight) adjusted based on 15 mCi standard. Vascular access is required for the radiopharmaceutical. Peripheral venous access with a 22-gauge catheter allows for optimum injections. Use of central venous catheters can be associated with several artifacts. Radiopharmaceutical can pool in a central catheter and adhere to the catheter or fibrin/thrombus associated with the catheter. Ample flushing of the catheter can compensate for the former but not the latter.

Hydration

Vascular access is maintained throughout the uptake and scanning periods. In the uptake period, the patient is hydrated with intravenous crystalloid 20 cc/kg. Hydration is critical in reducing background and minimizing exposure. The greatest patient dose is related to the urinary tract, and hydration and frequent urination significantly reduce dose.

Activity Restriction

After injection of the radiopharmaceutical, activity restriction is encouraged. Patients often watch television, read, do homework, rest, or other quiet activity (coloring, card games, board games, etc.). Activity restriction is most important in the early uptake phase when 18F-FDG availability is the highest. In some cases pharmacologic intervention may be necessary to minimize patient activity during the uptake phase and during scanning. Anxiolysis may be necessary in younger patients. Midazolam (Versed) can be used intravenously at the time of injection of the radiopharmaceutical or it may be administered orally or later as needed. Dosage is individualized and varies slightly, depending upon the patient's age and route of administration. We do not use versed in infants. Intravenously, 0.05 mg/kg up to 5 mg total is titrated slowly over 2 min to effect. Orally, a similar dose is used, although preschool age children may require 0.1 mg/kg. The effect is more predictable with the intravenous route, although the safety margin is higher with the oral route.

Scanning

Sedation

Sedation beyond anxiolysis may be needed to prevent misregistration between the CT and PET acquisitions. Physicians need to be knowledgeable of the sedative agents being used and be prepared to provide supportive care. Local sedation policy may require specific physician qualifications, patient preparation, and monitoring. Furthermore, sedations may require recovery and observation at the conclusion of the examination.

Pentobarbital sodium (Nembutal) is a fast-acting short-duration barbiturate sedative that is commonly employed in pediatric imaging (Table 11.2). It can be administered orally, rectally, or parenterally, but the intravenous route is most predictable. Because its onset of action is fast, it can be given with the patient on the table. Typically, a 2 mg/kg aliquot is administered by a slow intravenous push over 1 min. Additional aliquots can be given after a minute of observation up to 8 mg/kg total. Fentanyl (1 μg/kg) can be judiciously used as an adjunct if pentobarbital sedation is unsuccessful. (It is interesting that fentanyl premedication has been shown to reduce brown fat uptake of 18F-FDG.)

Deeper sedation or anesthesia may be necessary for some patients. Only professionals trained in advanced airway management and rescue and/or pediatric advanced life support should administer deep sedation or anesthesia. It should be noted that this level of sedation requires the need for close monitoring and will result in high radiation exposure to the attending medical personnel.

Iodinated Contrast

Iodinated vascular contrast is necessary to obtain diagnostic CT examinations in most oncologic settings. Vascular and visceral enhancement is optimal when iodinated contrast is administered with a power injector. If central lines are used,

Table 11.2 Anxiolysis and sedation protocol

	Drug	Dosage
Anxiolysis	Midazolam	0.05–0.1 mg/kg IV, PO (5 mg maximum)
Sedation	Pentobarbital	2 mg/kg IV, IM, PO, PR (up to 8 mg/kg)
	Fentanyl	0.1 μg/kg IV

iodinated contrast must be hand injected, although this can diminish the quality of the CT scans. Isoosmolar iodinated contrast (Visipaque, iodixanol) is administered with a power injector at 3 cc/s for a volume of 2 cc/kg (up to 150 cc) for neck and body imaging, and scanning begins approximately 60–70 s after the injection is completed. Dedicated imaging of the neck utilizes similar injection parameters, although scanning is initiated without delay. Dedicated brain imaging is often an isolated examination, with injection volume of 2 cc/kg (power or hand-injected) and scanning beginning approximately 2 min after the completion of the injection.

CT Scanning

Imaging parameters will vary between scanners. We obtain images at 3-mm intervals and reconstruct at 1.5-mm intervals. Images are reviewed utilizing standard, bone, and lung algorithms.

CT Radiation Dose Modulation

CT dose should be carefully monitored in pediatric patients. Both kV and mA can be significantly lowered compared to adult protocols and achieve diagnostic quality images. Our scanner employs CARE Solutions (Combined Applications to Reduce Exposure, Siemens) which prescribes dose based on patient age and weight. These preset parameters result in high-quality CT images but most pediatric radiologists will further reduce kV and mA to reduce patient exposure.

PET Scanning

PET scanning is performed after CT and approximately 2 h after the administration of 18F-FDG. Shorter uptake periods result in higher background activity and longer uptake periods result in lower background activity. While certain clinical situations may cause variation in the exact uptake time, we try to keep uptake time uniform to decrease variability between examinations.

The length of the PET portion of the examination is related to the number of bed positions and the emission time per bed position. Emission time varies but typically is 3 min for multiple bed position examinations and 5 min for dedicated single position examinations. While pediatric patients often require fewer bed positions to cover the pertinent anatomy compared to adults, the PET portion of the examination is considerably longer than the CT portion and as a result, the likelihood of motion increases. Often the region of greatest interest is imaged first. This will minimize the amount of misregistration related to motion.

Patient cooperation is crucial to a successful PET-CT examination. New situations are often a source of anxiety and can inhibit the child's ability to cooperate. Explanation of the procedure, practicing positioning, and touring the facility will help to curb the anxiety. Pediatric PET-CT examinations take a little bit longer to perform. Technologists must be patient and enjoy working with children. Parents can make or break the examination and their support will be instrumental for success. We have employed Child Life Specialists in our department to focus on the emotional, social, and developmental needs of our pediatric patients. The Child Life Specialist is knowledgeable of the requirements for obtaining diagnostic examinations and works with the patient, parents, and technologists to help complete. As a result, the patient gains control and anxiety is alleviated. We have found that examination quality has increased, the need for sedation has decreased, and overall patient satisfaction has improved.

Suggested Readings

Gelfand MJ, et al. Premedication to block [(18)F]FDG uptake in brown fat tissue of pediatric and adolescent patients. Pediatr Radiol 2005;35(10): 984–990.

Hahn K, Pfluger T. Has PET become an important clinical tool in paediatric imaging? Eur J Nucl Med Mol Imaging 2004;31(5):615–621.

Kaste SC. Issues specific to implementing PET/CT for pediatric oncology: what we learned along the way. Pediatr Radiol 2004;34(3):205–215.

Shulkin BL. PET Imaging in pediatric oncology. Pediatr Radiol 2004;34(3):199–204.

Chapter 12
PET-CT in Radiation Treatment Planning

Jacqueline Brunetti

Technologic advances in radiotherapy planning and delivery systems aimed at improving precision of target dosing and decreasing normal tissue exposure have significantly increased the importance medical imaging in radiation oncology. 3D conformal intensity-modulated radiation therapy (IMRT) techniques can now be coupled with further refinements in radiation therapy delivery systems that physically incorporate imaging capability. Such image-guided radiation therapy (IGRT) systems that have onboard fluoroscopy or cone-beam CT are now commercially available, allowing for dynamic adaptive radiation therapy (DART), a process that allows changes in field and dose during a treatment course to "adapt" to intrafraction changes to the tumor target. To achieve the full advantage of these sophisticated radiation therapy techniques, precise tumor targeting and accurate disease staging is critical. Positron emission tomography, and in particular PET-CT, has been shown to improve both tumor targeting as well as therapy decision making by virtue of the improved sensitivity and specificity of this imaging technique over other conventional imaging modalities.

Target Volumes

Better comprehension of the role of imaging in radiation oncology will be gained by understanding the approach a radiation oncologist employs in determination of the tumor target. Ideally, the target should receive a therapeutic dose sufficient to eradicate the tumor and nearby microscopic spread with adjacent, non-tumor-bearing tissue exposed to levels of radiation well within established tolerance levels. Initial delineation of a gross tumor volume (GTV) is defined as the extent of tumor as demonstrated at imaging. This encompasses not only the primary lesion, but also the extent of local metastatic disease. It is at this stage that benefits of functional imaging are most apparent both by delineating the local extent of the primary tumor mass and local metastases (Fig. 12.1). The clinical target volume (CTV) expands the GTV to account for the estimated microscopic tumor spread. The final treatment target is then further enlarged, typically an additional 1–2 cm, to compensate for motion and other inaccuracies and is defined as the planning target volume (PTV).

Clinical Applications

The earliest investigational report using PET in radiation treatment planning was published in 1987 by Schad et al., comparing combinations of data from CT, MRI, and PET for target definition of brain tumors [1]. With the increasing availability of PET, and now PET-CT scanners as well as improvements in image fusion software, application of these imaging modalities to radiation oncology has resulted in an increasing number of studies evaluating benefits in targeting, management change, and outcome. Collectively, these studies have shown that incorporating PET data significantly affects the planning, delivery, and surveillance of therapy patients by providing more accurate staging, tumor target delineation, and more accurate means of monitoring therapy response.

Non-small Cell Lung Cancer

The most extensive research on tumor targeting has been in patients with non-small cell lung cancer (NSCLC). Vanuytsel et al. reported in 2000 a theoretical retrospective study of 105 patients with non-small cell lung cancer (NSCLC) and known surgical pathology results [2]. GTV was defined based on conventionally using CT and for

J. Brunetti (✉)
Department of Radiology, Holy Name Medical Center, 718 Teaneck Rd, Teaneck, NJ, 07666, USA
e-mail: brunetti@mail.holyname.org; jcb1@columbia.edu

P. Shreve and D.W. Townsend (eds.), *Clinical PET-CT in Radiology: Integrated Imaging in Oncology*,
DOI 10.1007/978-0-387-48902-5_12,

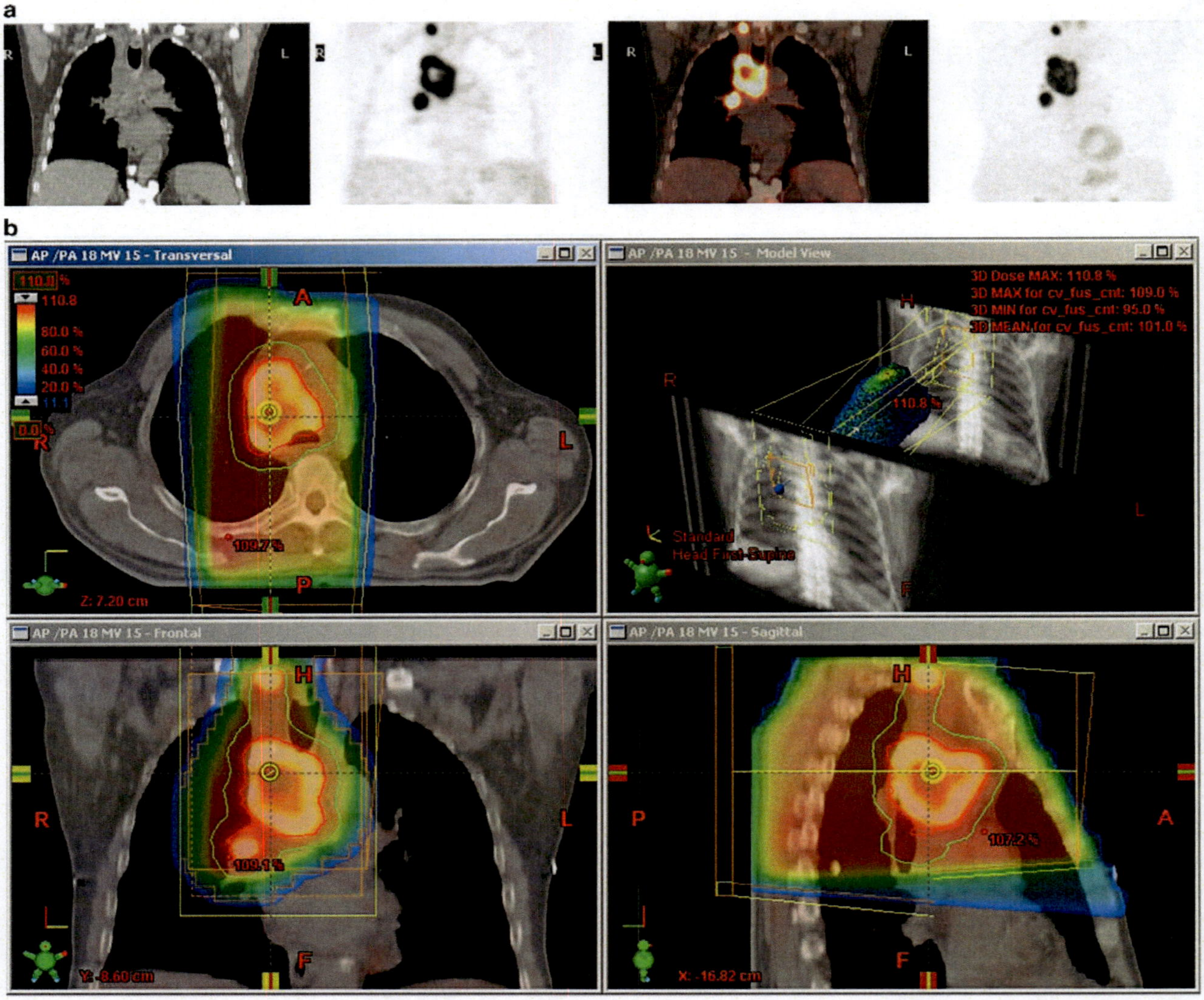

Fig. 12.1 (**a**) Coronal images obtained at radiation therapy simulation PET-CT demonstrate a large right paratracheal mass and metastatic right hilar adenopathy. A right supraclavicular metastatic lymph node had not been identified on a prior chest CT. (**b**) The patient's radiation field was extended to include the right supraclavicular node. (**c**) Coronal images from a PET-CT scan obtained 20 months after completion of radiation therapy demonstrate right apical activity at a site of postradiation pneumonitis, but no evidence of residual or recurrent disease

comparison based on computer fusion images using FDG PET and CT data. Accuracy of nodal detection and inclusion in the GTV increased from 75% with CT-defined volumes to 89% with PET-CT-defined GTV. Overall treatment volume changes occurred in 62%, with the GTV reduced in ten patients. The authors concluded that in the subgroup of patients considered for curative radiotherapy, inclusion of FDG PET data improves accuracy of tumor coverage, and when volumes may be reduced, these patients may become candidates for treatment intensification. Bradley et al. came to similar conclusions in a report of 26 patients with NSCLC evaluating the impact of PET imaging on target volumes and toxicity profiles [3]. In these studies patients were immobilized in the treatment planning position and underwent separate FDG-PET and CT imaging on the same day. Contouring was performed for both CT and computer-fused PET-CT images. The authors report that PET data resulted in alteration of TNM stage in 31% of patients, with radiation plan changed from curative to palliative in two patients as a result of detection of unexpected metastatic disease. PET altered radiation volumes in 58%, and where target volumes were decreased, this resulted in decrease in normal-tissue toxicity. More recently, van Der Wel et al. describe a modeling study to estimate the potential gain from incorporating FDG PET in radiation therapy planning [4]. CT-based PTV was compared with a PET-CT-defined PTV for 21 patients with NSCLC. For this group, toxicity data was calculated for esophagus, spinal

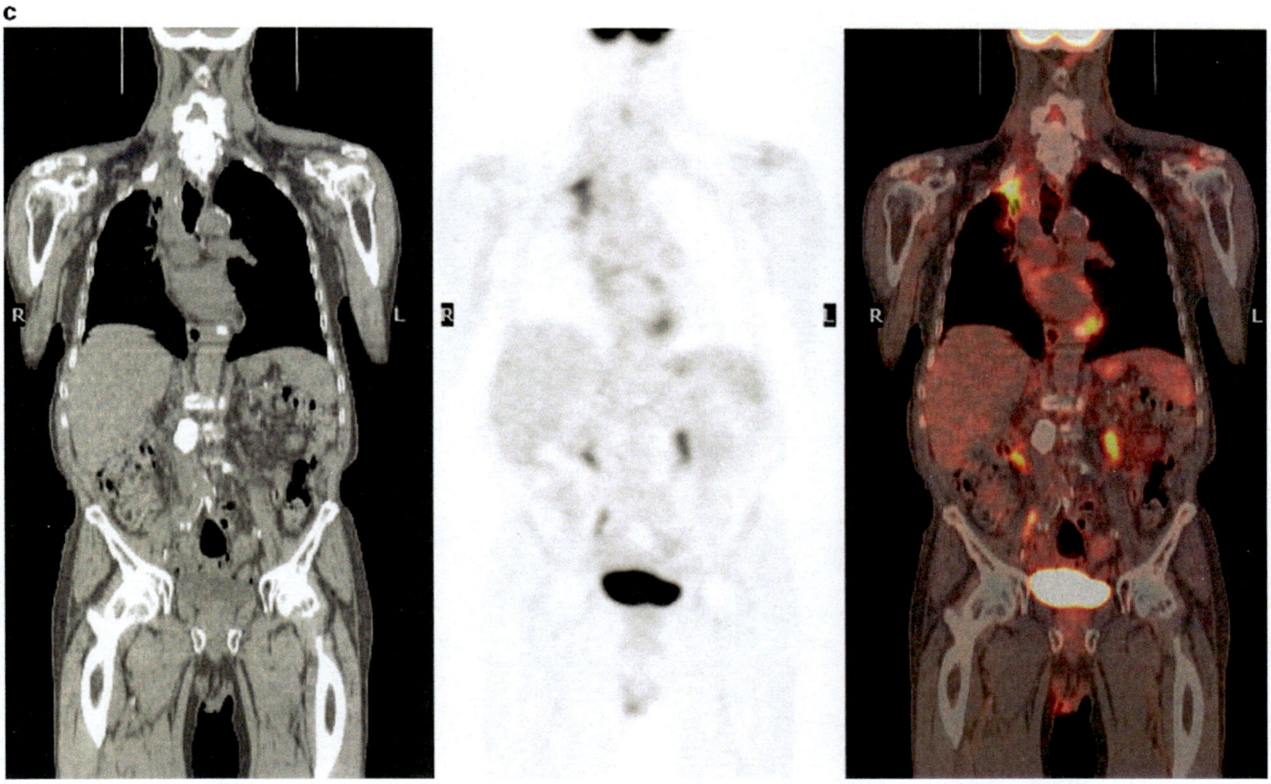

Fig. 12.1 (continued)

cord, and lung and tumor control probability (TCP) was estimated based on radiation dose. PET-CT-defined PTV resulted in less radiation exposure to the esophagus and normal lung. The authors state that by using PET-CT GTV, the radiation dose could be increased from 56 to 71 Gy with no change in the toxicity levels for lung, esophagus, and spinal cord, and as a result, estimated TCP increased from 12.5% to 18.3%.

Accuracy in detection of locoregional lymph node metastases in lung cancer is critical in diminishing the possibility of geographic miss in the course of radiation therapy treatment, and here the improved diagnostic performance of PET-CT is particularly important. Cerfolio et al. compared the accuracy of PET-CT compared with dedicated PET alone for staging of patients with NSCLC [5]. In a prospective study of 129 candidates for lung surgery, PET and PET-CT images were reviewed separately and TNM status assigned by the interpreting radiologist. All patients underwent biopsy and histologic analysis. The authors find that integrated PET-CT is a better predictor for all stages of NSCLC. PET-CT was shown to be more accurate than PET alone in determination of T status (70% vs. 47%), and N status (90% vs. 56%). To date, there is little published data evaluating patterns of disease recurrence in NSCLC in patients treated with radiation therapy planned using the addition of PET data. De Ruysscher et al. performed a prospective study of 44 patients with NSCLC without detectable distant metastases treated with radiation therapy planned with PET and CT [6]. Patients received a dose of either 61.2 Gy delivered in 34 fractions or 64.8 Gy delivered in 36 fractions to the primary tumor and to only the PET-positive mediastinal nodes. Isolated nodal failure was defined by the authors as recurrence in the regional nodes outside the CTV in the absence of in-field failure. After a median follow-up time of 16 months, 11 patients developed local recurrence, but only one patient developed an isolated nodal failure, reflecting the value of FDG PET images for the detection of lymph node metastases. Outcome data of 35 patients with non-small cell lung cancer treated with radiotherapy treatment volumes derived from PET-CT simulation are reported by Klopp et al. [7]. Patients received radiation dosed of 60–70 Gy to a treatment volume restricted to lymph nodes that were determined positive by a diagnostic radiologist on PET-CT and CT. The criterion for positivity was FDG uptake greater than mediastinal background, with uptake in nodes less than 1.5 cm in diameter deemed an unreliable indicator of metastasis. Patients underwent follow-up CT or PET-CT for 2 years. Distant metastatic disease developed in 20% of patients. Concurrent in-field and out-of field failure rate was 14.3%. Recurrence rates correlated with high SUV and

a

b

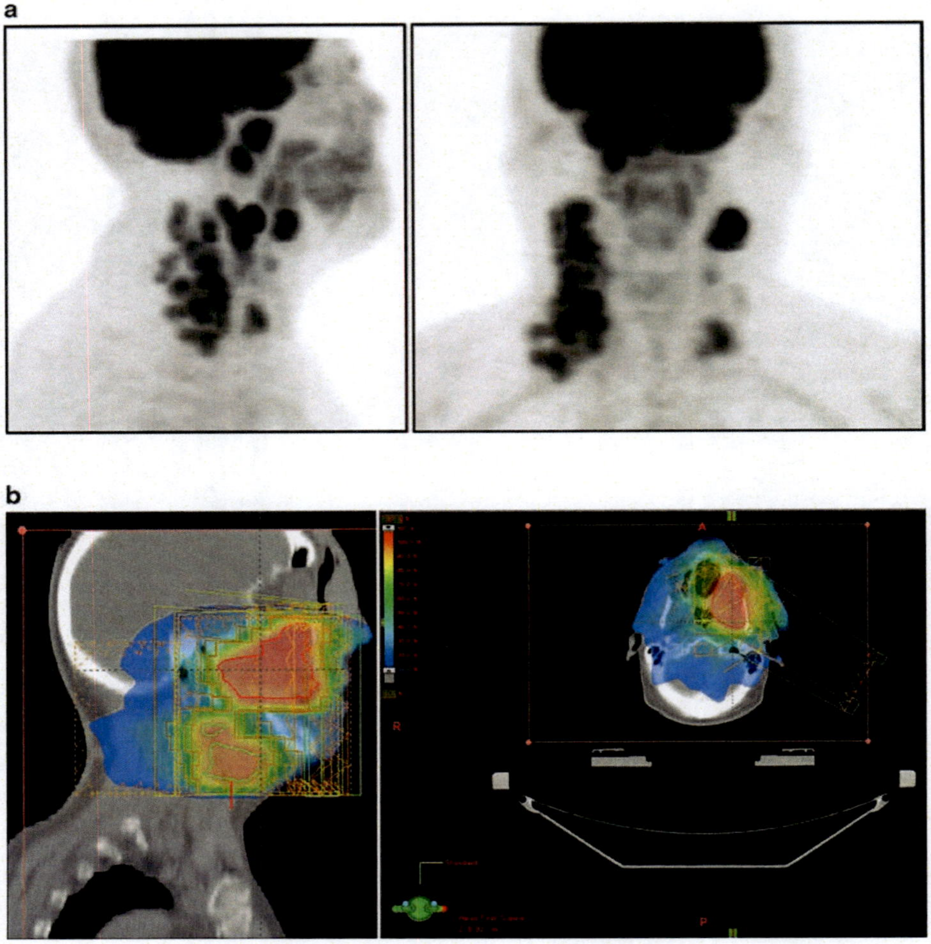

c

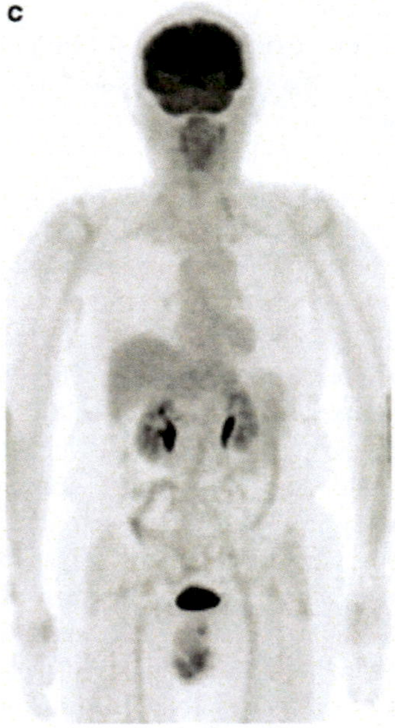

Fig. 12.2 (**a**) Coronal and saggital radiation simulation PET-CT images of patient with nasopharyngeal carcinoma reveal intense hypermetabolic activity at the primary tumor site as well as in bilateral cervical nodes. (**b**) 3D IMRT radiotherapy plan demonstrates low dose to the spinal cord and high exposure to the primary tumor. (**c**) Post-radiation PET-CT obtained *8* months after completion of radiation reveals no evidence of residual disease

increasing volume, with rates highest in regions with SUVs greater than ten and volumes greater than 11.3 cm^3. No recurrence was found in nodes less than 1 cm. A low isolated out-of field recurrence rate of 5.7% as reported in this series was similar to recurrence rates found in CT-based planning and supports limiting radiation treatment to PET-positive disease.

Head and Neck Cancer

Highly focused radiotherapy techniques are standard in treating patients with head and neck (H&N) cancer; moreover, treatment choices currently strive to preserve form and function, permitting improved quality of life for patients with this disease. The high diagnostic accuracy in staging in H&N cancer and in delineating the primary target provided by PET and PET-CT has resulted in a significant impact in radiation therapy planning (Fig. 12.2).

Accurate staging in H&N cancer is critical to the increasing precision in radiotherapy delivery. In early stage disease with a clinically negative neck (N0) the accuracy of FDG PET in identifying disease is poor, as 20% of nodal metastasis will be less than 3 mm in size [8]. In spite of this limitation, FDG-PET imaging is a marked improvement over the clinical exam (sensitivity 35% and specificity 35%), ultrasound fine needle aspiration (sensitivity 42%), and CT (sensitivity 77% and specificity 95%). In a retrospective study of 56 patients comparing FDG PET with biopsy results or patient outcome, Sigg et al. reported sensitivity for PET of 94%, specificity of 97%, and accuracy of 96% in identification of cervical nodal disease and a sensitivity of 93%, specificity of 100%, and accuracy of 94% for identification of the primary tumor [9]. PET-CT has been shown to be more accurate than PET alone in patients with H&N cancer. Schoder et al., in a review of 68 patients found that PET-CT reduced equivocal findings on FDG PET alone by 53% and increased accuracy from 90% to 96% [10]. The value of PET-CT over CT alone in preradiotherapy staging of patients with H&N cancer is supported by a pilot study reported by Schwartz et al. comparing CT and PET-CT staging with surgical pathology obtained at neck dissection [11]. Preoperative FDG-PET and contrast-enhanced CT were performed on 63 patients with squamous cell carcinoma of oral cavity, oropharynx, larynx, and hypopharynx. Primary and nodal volumes were generated for the CT and fused PET-CT data on radiation treatment planning software and compared to neck dissection specimens. The PET-CT resulted in a nodal level staging sensitivity of 96% and specificity of 98.5%. Agreement between PET-CT and pathology was greater than for contrast CT alone. This same group reported results of a theoretical study in which IMRT plans were developed based on PET-CT image findings and compared to surgical pathology results with the purpose of investigating the feasibility of dose escalation [12]. In this series no PET-CT generated IMRT plan missed pathologically verified disease and, moreover, it was theoretically possible to escalate the dose to 95% of the PTV.

Posttherapeutic surveillance with FDG PET has been shown to be more accurate than conventional imaging in H&N cancer [13, 14]. There is some controversy as to the timing of FDG-PET scans after radiotherapy, as postradiation inflammation may confound interpretation. Early investigations recommended performing these scans more than 3 months after treatment to eliminate false-positive results from inflammation [15]. In addition, Greven et al. reported false-negative results on FDG PET when scans were obtained 1 month after therapy [16]. In this series of 45 patients imaged at 1, 4, and 24 months after radiation therapy for head and neck cancer, 28% of patients with 1 month post-therapy negative FDG-PET scans developed local recurrence within 1 year after radiation. The authors found in their series that the FDG PET scans obtained at 4 months after therapy were more accurate for identification of residual tumor.

Other Malignancies

PET and PET-CT imaging has also been utilized for radiation therapy planning in other malignancies that are FDG-avid. PET and PET-CT improves pretherapy staging as well as targeting cervical cancer, as it is more accurate that CT or MRI in identification of metastatic paraortic lymph nodes and distant metastatic disease [17, 18]. There is increasing data that support the use of PET-CT in target definition of other cancers such as esophageal cancer and lymphoma [19–23].

Technical Issues in PET-CT Treatment Planning

Of prime concern in radiation therapy is establishing certainty of, and consistency with, the target location throughout the course of therapy. It is particularly crucial in the delivery of curative radiation that these prescribed high doses of radiation accurately conform to the tumor target and spare the adjacent normal tissues or organs at risk. To achieve this goal, imaging performed with a patient immobilized on a flat table in the treatment position is routine in radiation planning. With the exception of brain cancer, for which both CT and MRI are utilized, imaging for radiation planning is typically performed on a CT scanner with a flat table insert and in a room equipped with positioning lasers. Patients are positioned by radiation therapy technologists according to localization markers predetermined in the radiation simulation session. CT images provide exquisite anatomic data for development of 3D treatment plans, critical for sculpting out organs at risk from the radiation field, and also provide raw tissue density data for dose calculations.

The addition of FDG-PET to the radiation therapy planning process can be performed at a variety of levels of sophistication from simple visual fusion of PET with CT simulation images, fusion of images from separate PET and CT scanners with third party image fusion software, and optimally, to imaging of the immobilized patient on a PET-CT scanner. PET-CT is advantageous, as both anatomic and functional images are obtained sequentially on the same device, diminishing the possibility of image alignment and registration error. Newer generation PET-CT scanners with wide-bore gantries allow easier adaptation, as patient positioning while in immobilization cradles or other devices is less challenging. Although only a limited PET-CT of the area of interest is required for radiation therapy planning, it is prudent with cancers such as lung cancer to obtain a whole body scan for each patient to insure accurate staging prior to therapy (i.e., detection of unsuspected distant metastases or second primary cancer). As there is not yet a digital imaging and communication in medicine (DICOM) standard for fused PET-CT images, the separate sets of PET and CT images obtained during the simulation session are exported to the radiation therapy work station for generation of treatment planning contours. DICOM compatibility must exist between scanner and radiation therapy planning computer to allow exportation of these images.

As with most programs that involve coordinating the efforts of separate departments, attention must to paid to additional logistical issues such as patient and staff scheduling as well as monitoring radiation dose to the radiation oncology staff.

Defining the Target

The introduction of FDG-PET and PET-CT images into a planning protocol requires multidisciplinary cooperation by Radiation Oncologist, Radiologist, or Nuclear Physician, and department physicists. This collaborative approach is necessary for the members of each discipline to understand the clinical issues and challenges associated with interpretation of functional images and accepted contouring techniques. It is critical that the imaging physician interprets the PET-CT simulation images with the radiation oncologist to foster an understanding not only of how to optimize image display for the most accurate lesion detection but also demonstrate the differences between sites of benign physiologic uptake and malignant hypermetabolic FDG concentration. Owing to the nature of this functional imaging technique, lesion size and extent can vary greatly simply by the choice of display intensity chosen (Fig. 12.3). Various approaches to this problem have been suggested. Some centers simply set the intensity to the level considered by the interpreting Radiologist or Nuclear physician that best displays the pathology for each specific patient. There are commercially available segmentation programs that will allow automated edge-detection based on an

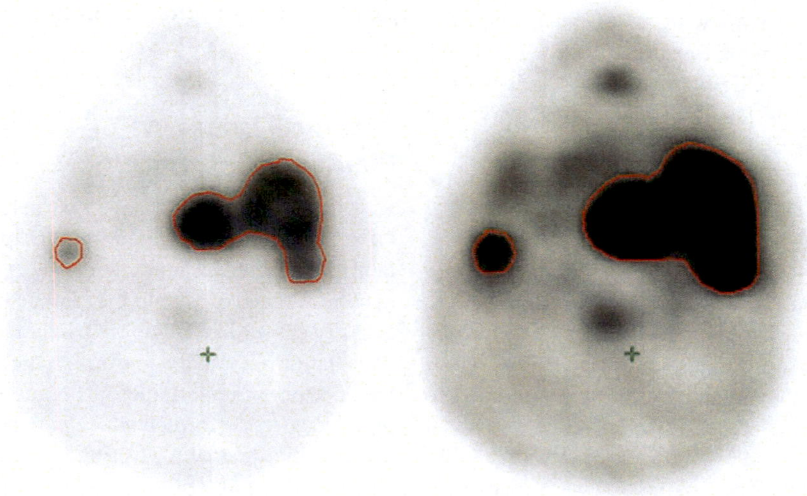

Fig. 12.3 GTV contours generated on the same axial slice set with two different PET intensities. PET intensity is set too high on the image on the right and the PET contour overestimates the CT boundaries of this right hilar lesion

assigned SUV value. Erdi et al. describe a method of scaling the PET image by identifying the highest activity pixel in the lesion region of interest and then setting the upper window of the intensity display to this value and the lower window to 42% of the maximum level [24, 25]. This approach has recently been shown to have limitations in a recent article by Nestle et al., comparing GTV's obtained using simple visual analysis, a threshold of 40% SUVmax, an isocontour of 2.5 SUV, and an additional in-house algorithm [26]. The authors report differences in GTV of up to 41% depending on the method employed and found that these differences correlated with lesion size, SUVmax level and tumor inhomogeneity. The authors suggest that more accurate PET-defined contour delineation might be forthcoming with system-specific contrast-oriented algorithms for FDG-PET edge detection.

In spite of these challenges PET and PET-CT defined targeting has been demonstrated to reduce observer variation in target delineation as well as decreasing the number of corrections and overall contouring time [27, 28]. Of additional interest is a comparison of CT, MRI, and FDG PET-defined GTV with macroscopic surgical specimen in nine patients with pharyngolaryngeal squamous cell carcinoma [29]. In this series, the authors found the PET-defined GTV (derived by an automated segmentation algorithm) to be smaller than both CT and MRI derived volumes but was most equivalent to the size of the surgical specimen.

Future Directions for Radiation Therapy Planning

Biologic Target Volume

Local therapeutic failure in radiation therapy is due to cellular mechanisms of radioresistance and repair as well as the limitations of maximal dose restricted by the radiation tolerance of surrounding normal tissue. By predefining each particular neoplasm's biologic phenotype, it may be possible to predict therapy response and allow modification of treatment in order to optimize the radiation response. For example, for tumors with a high hypoxia fraction, radiosensitizers might be administered in conjunction with radiotherapy. Tumors may be imaged during the course of radiotherapy treatment to assess behaviors such as reoxygenation, or changes in proliferation fraction, which may have an impact on choice of further adjuvant treatment.

It is possible, with currently available radiotherapy systems to deliver different radiation doses to specific regions of a 3D target volume, allowing higher doses to regions of more aggressive or possibly more resistant tissue. New positron tracers currently under development may provide a method to image critical cellular processes facilitating the prescription of tumor specific therapies based on the biologic phenotype. FDG provides information of tumor viability as a reflection of tumor glycolysis and overexpression of glucose transporters. Other investigational PET tracers can image hypoxia (18F-fluoromisonidazole -FMISO), blood flow (oxygen15 labeled water), apoptosis (annexin V), angiogenesis and metastases (18F-Galacto-RGD), and cellular proliferation (18F-labeled 3′-fluorothymidine -FL T) [30]. An interesting application of hypoxia imaging is reported by Hicks et al. [31]. Fifteen patients with advanced head and neck cancer were imaged with serial FMISO and FDG-PET scans and treated with hypoxia-targeted therapy, chemoradiation and tirapazamine, a cytotoxin for hypoxic cells. All sites initially positive at baseline demonstrated marked reduction in activity at 4 weeks. Only four patients developed locoregional failure. The authors conclude that the high prevalence of FMISO uptake in this patient group is consistent with the advanced disease state, but that the early resolution of FMISO during treatment is associated with excellent locoregional control and these early findings would support further investigation in tumor hypoxia imaging.

Tumor Motion

Respiratory-gated radiation therapy synchronizes the delivery of the beam with the patient's respiratory cycle with potential for decreasing the size of the radiation field and potentially increasing target dose [32, 33]. With these so-called 4D imaging techniques, both respiratory gated CT and PET allow visualization of the tumor target location throughout the respiratory cycle, thereby replacing estimates of motion by actual determination of target location at the point in the breathing cycle where motion is minimized [34–36]. Preliminary data indicate that there is an increase in recovered tracer activity in lesions as measured by SUV on respiratory gated FDG PET images [37, 38]. Although the exact role of respiratory-gated PET-CT in radiation therapy planning has yet to be determined, [39] noted that treatment margins in respiratory-gated radiation therapy can only be reduced if combined with respiratory correlated image guidance. This supports a role of 4-D CT imaging with the value of 4D-PET to be determined.

Conclusions

There is an increasing volume of evidence to support the inclusion of PET-CT imaging in radiation therapy planning.

In spite of possible inaccuracies in edge detection relating to the resolution of PET, the overall gain in improvement in target delineation as well as the contribution to more accurate staging is a clear step toward individualized cancer therapy. The anticipated development of additional positron tracers that will allow pretherapeutic identification of tumor biologic phenotype, coupled with continuing advances in delivery techniques, may ultimately result in further refinement in target definition with the potential to increase tumoricidal dose to the tumor target without increasing toxicity to normal tissues. Further studies are essential to determine whether changes in therapy resulting from biologic targeting as defined on FDG-PET images result in improvement in patient outcome.

References

1. Schad LR, Boesecke R, Schlegel W, Hartmann GH, Sturm V, Strauss LG, Lorenz WJ. Three dimensional image correlation of CT, MR, and PET studies in radiotherapy treatment planning of brain tumors. J Comput Assist Tomogr 1987;11(6):948–954.
2. Vanuytsel LJ, Vansteenkiste JF, Stroobants SG, De Leyn PR, De Wever W, Verbeken EK, Gatti GG, Huyskens DP, Kutcher GJ. The impact of 18F-fluoro-2-deoxy-D- glucose positron emission tomography (FDG-PET) lymph nodes staging on radiation treatment volumes in patients with non-small cell lung cancer. Radiother Oncol 2000;55:317–324.
3. Bradley JB, Thorstad WL, Mutic S, Miller TR, Dehdashti F, Siegel BA, Bosch W, Bertrand RJ. Impact of FDG-PET on radiation therapy volume delineation in non-small cell lung cancer. Int J Radiat Oncol Biol Phys 2004;59(1):78–86.
4. van Der Wel A, Nijsten S, Hochstenbag M, Lamers R, Boersma L, Wanders R, Lutgens L, Zimny M, Bentzen SM, Wouters B, Lamblin P, De Ruysscher D. Increased therapeutic ratio by 18FDG-PET CT planning in patients with clinical CT stage N2-N3M0 non-small cell lung cancer: a modeling study. Int J Radiat Oncol Biol Phys 2005;61(3):649–655.
5. Cerfolio RJ, Ojha B, Bryant AS, Raghuveer V, Mountz JM, Bartolucci AA. The accuracy of integrated PET-CT compared with dedicated PET alone for the staging of patients with non-small cell lung cancer. Ann Thorac Surg 2004;78(3):1017–1023.
6. De Ruysscher D, Wanders S, van Haren E, Hochstenbag M, Geeraedts W, Utama I, Simons J, Dohmen J, Rhami A, Buell U, Thimister P, Snoep G, Boersma L, Verschueren T, van Baardwijk A, Minken A, Bentzen SM, Lambin P. Selective mediastinal node irradiation based on FDG-PET scan data in patients with non-small-cell lung cancer: a prospective clinical study. Int J Radiat Oncol Biol Phys 2005;62(4):988–994.
7. Klopp AH, Chang JY, Tucker SL, Sulman EP, Balter PA, Liu HHL, Bucci MK, Macapinlac HA, Komaki R, Cox JD. Intrathoracic patterns of failure for non-small-cell lung cancer with positron-emission tomography/computed tomography defined target delineation. Int J Radiat Oncol Biol Phys 2007;69(5):1409–1416.
8. Brouwer J, de Bree R, Comans EF, Castelijns JA, Hoekstra OS, Leemans CR. Positron emission tomography using [(18)F]fluordeoxyglucose (FDG-PET) in the clinically negative neck: is it likely to be superior? Eur Arch Otorhinolaryngol 2004;261(9):479–483.
9. Sigg MB, Steinert H, Gratz K, Hugenin P, Stoeckli S, Eyrich GK. Staging of head and neck tumors: [18F]fluordeoxyglucose positron emission tomography compared with physical examination and conventional imaging modalities. J Oral Maxillofac Surg 2003; 61(9):1002–1029.
10. Schoder H, Yeung HW, Gonen M, Kraus D, Larson SM. Head and neck cancer: clinical usefulness and accuracy of PET/CT image fusion. Radiology 2004;231(1):65–72.
11. Schwartz DL, Ford E, Rajendran J, Yueh B, Coltrera MD, Virgin J, Anzai Y, Haynor D, Lewellyn B, Mattes D, Meyer J, Phillips M, Leblanc M, Kinahan P, Krohn K, Eary J, Laramore GE. FDG-PET/CT imaging for preradiotherapy staging of head-and-neck squamous cell carcinoma. Int J Radiat Oncol Biol Phys 2005;61(1):129–136.
12. Schwartz DL, Ford E, Rajendran J, Yueh B, Coltrera MD, Virgin J, Anzai Y, Haynor D, Lewellyn B, Mattes D, Kinahan P, Meyer J, Phillips M, Leblanc M, Krohn K, Eary J, Laramore GE. FDG-PET/CT guided intensity modulated head and neck radiotherapy: a pilot investigation. Head Neck 2005;27(6):478–487.
13. Ryan WR, Fee WE, Le QT, Pinto HA. Positron-emission tomography for surveillance of head and neck cancer. Laryngoscope 2005;115(4):645–650.
14. McCollum AD, Burrell SC, Haddad RI, Norris CM, Tishler RB, Case MA, Posner MR, Van den Abbeele AD. Postron emission tomography with 18F-fluorodeoxyglucose to predict pathologic response after induction of chemotherapy and definitive chemoradiotherapy in head and neck cancer. Head and neck 2004;26(10): 890–896.
15. Greven KM, Williams DW, Keyes JW, McGuirt WF, Harkness BA, Watson NE, Raben M, Frazier LC, Geisinger KR, Cappellari JO. Distinguishing tumor recurrence from irradiation sequelae with positron emission tomography in patients treated for larynx cancer. Int J Radiat Oncol Biol Phys 1994;29(4):841–845.
16. Greven KM, Williams DW, Mcguirt WF, Harkness BA, D'Agostino RB, Keyes JW, Watson NE. Serial positron emission tomography scans following radiation therapy of patients with head and neck cancer. Head Neck 2001;23(11):942–946.
17. Yildrim Y, Sehirali S, Avci ME, Yilamz C, Ertopcu K, Timar S, Duman Y, Sayhan S. Integrated PET/CT for the evaluation of para-aortic nodal metastasis in locally advanced cervical cancer patients with negative conventional CT findings. Gynecol Oncol 2008;108(1):154–159.
18. Loft A, Berthelsen AK, Roed H, Ottosen C, Lundvall L, Knudsen J, Nedergaard L, Hojgaard L, Engelholm SA. The diagnostic value of PET/CT in patients with cervical cancer: a prospective study. Gynecol Oncol 2007;106(1):29–34.
19. Gondi V, Bradley K, Mehta M, Howard A, Khuntia D, Ritter M, Tome W. Impact of hybrid fluorodeoxyglucose positron-emission tomography/computed tomography on radiotherapy planning in esophageal and non-small cell lung cancer. Int J Radiat Oncol Biol Phys 2007;67(1):187–195.
20. Leong T, Everitt C, Yuen K, Condron S, Hui A, Ngan SY, Pitman A, Lau EW, MacManus M, Binns D, Ackerly T, Hicks RJ. A prospective study to evaluate the impact of FDG-PET on CT-based radiotherapy for oesophageal cancer. Radiother Oncol 2006;78(3): 254–261.
21. Specht L. 2-[18F]fluro-2-deoxyglucose positron-emission tomography in staging, response evaluation and treatment planning of lymphomas. Semin Radiat Oncol 2007;17(3):190–197.
22. Hutchings M, Loft A, Hansen M, Berthelsen AK, Specht L. Clinical impact of FDG-PET/CT in the planning of radiotherapy for early stage Hodgkin lymphoma. Eur J Haematol 2007;78(3):206–212.
23. Baardwijk A, Baumert BG, Bosmans G, van Kroonenburgh M, Stroobants S, Gregoire V, Lambin P, De Ruysscher D. The current status of FDG-PET in tumour volume definition in radiotherapy treatment planning. Cancer Treatment Rev 2006;32(4): 245–260.
24. Erdi Y, Mawlawi O, Larson SM, Imbriaco M, Yeung H, Finn R, Humm JL. Segmentation of lung lesion volume by adaptive positron

emission tomography image thresholding. Cancer 1997;80:(12 Suppl):2505–2509.
25. Erdi Y, Rosenzweig K, Erdi A, Macapinlac H, Hu Y, Braban LE, Humm JL, Squire OD, Chiu C, Larson SM, Yorke ED. Radiotherapy planning for patients with non-small cell lung cancer using positron emission tomography (PET). Radiother Oncol 2002;62: 51–60.
26. Nestle U, Kremp S, Schaefer-Schuler A, Sebastian-Welsch C, Hellwig D, Rube C, Kirsch CM. Comparison of different methods for delineation of 18F-FDG PET-positive tissue for target volume definition in radiotherapy of patients with non-small cell lung cancer. J Nucl Med 2005;48(8):1342–1348.
27. Caldwell CB, Mah K, Ung YC, Danjoux CE, Balogh JM, Ganguli SN, Ehrlich LE. Observer variation in contouring gross tumour volume in patients with poorly defined non-small-cell lung cancer on CT: the impact of 18FDG-hybrid PET fusion. Int J Radiat Oncol Biol Phys 2001;51(4):923–931.
28. Steenbakkers RJ, Duppen JC, Fitton I, Deurloo KE, Zijp LJ, Comans EF, Uitterhoeve AL, Rodrigus PT, Kramer GW, Bussink J, De Jaeger K, Belderbos JS, Nowak PJ, van Herk M, Rasch CR. Reduction in observer variation using matched CT-PET for lung cancer delineation: a three-dimensional analysis. Int J Radiat Oncol Biol Phys 2006;64(2):435–448.
29. Daisne JF, Duprez T, Weynand B, Lonneux M, Hamoir M, Reychler H, Gregoire V. Tumor volume in pharyngolaryngeal squamous cell carcinoma: comparison at CT, MR imaging and FDG PET and validation with surgical specimen. Radiology 2004;233(1): 93–100.
30. Zanzonico P. PET-based biologic imaging for radiation therapy treatment planning. Criti Rev Eukaryot Gene Expr 2006;16(1): 61–101.
31. Hicks RJ, Rischin D, Fisher R, Binns D, Scott AM, Peters LJ. Utility of FMISO PET in advanced head and neck cancer treated with chemoradiation incorporating a hypoxia-targeting chemotherapy agent. Eur J Nucl Med Mol Imaging 2005;32(12):1384–1391.
32. Berson AM, Emery R, Rodriguez L, et al. Clinical experience using respiratory gated radiation therapy: comparison of free-breathing and breath-hold techniques. Int J Radiat Oncol Biol Phys 2004; 60(2):419–426.
33. Butler LE, Forster KM, Stevens CW, et al. Dosimetric benefits of respiratory gating: a preliminary study. J Appl Phys 2004;5(1):1–9.
34. Keall P. 4-Dimensional computed tomography imaging in treatment planning. Semin Radiat Oncol 2004;14(1):81–90.
35. Nehmeh SA, Erdi YE, Pan T, Yorke E, Mageras GS, Rosenzweig KE, Schoder H, Mostafavi H, Squire O, Pevsner A, Larson SM, Humm JL. Quantitation of respiratory motion during 4D-PET/CT acquisition. Med Phys 2004;31(6):1333–1338.
36. Brunetti J, Caggiano A, Rosenbluth B, Vialotti C. Technical aspects of positron emission tomography/computed tomography fusion planning. Semin Nucl Med 2008;38(2):129–136.
37. Erdui Y, Nehmeh SA, Pan T, Pevsner A, Rosenzweig KE, Mageras G, Yorke ED, Scoder H, Hsiai W, Squire OD, Vernon P, Ashman JB, Mostafavi H, Larson, S, Humm JL. The CT motion quantitation of lung lesions and its impact on PET-measured SUVs. J Nucl Med 2004;45(8):1287–1292.
38. Brunetti JC, Caggiano A, Greenstein E. Respiratory-gated (4D) FDG-PET: effect on SUV measurements. Eur J Med Mol Imaging 2004;31(S2):S286(abstr).
39. Korreman SS, Juhler-Nottrup T, Fredberg Persson G, Navrsted Pedersen A, Enmark M, Nystrom H, Specht L. The role of image guidance in respiratory gated radiotherapy. Acta Oncol. 2008; 47(7):1390–6.

Chapter 13
Probability and the Principles of Diagnostic Certainty in Medical Imaging

Steven Kymes and James W. Fletcher

At its most basic level, diagnosis is the process of translating quantitative or qualitative data into a form that allows a clinician to make a yes or no decision. The yes/no question may take a number of forms: Does the patient have X condition? Should I order an additional test? Is the patient's condition progressing? Has the patient developed a functional impairment? Regardless of the question, the answer has a dichotomous form, which mathematically can be represented with 0 or 1.

Most data available to clinicians is not in a 0/1 form. It is typically continuous (e.g., uptake values, blood pressure) or qualitative (e.g., evidence of the presence of adenopathy). Such information does not easily translate into yes/no decisions. Instead, the clinician is required to construct in his or her mind a model that allows him or her to convert clinical information into an estimate of the probability of disease. The process requires that four questions be answered:

- How valid is the source of the information linking the clinical information (e.g., diagnostic test result, physical finding) to the patient's condition?
- What does the clinical information infer concerning the presence of disease?
- Given the clinical information provided and what we know about the patient, what is the probability that the patient has the condition in question?
- Given this information, what should be done?

Validity of Clinical Information Provided

In performing a diagnostic test, the clinician and patient engage in a game of chance. Like any form of gaming, this is a probabilistic exercise. The patient and physician seek to learn the patient's true disease status so they can make decisions regarding treatment. They know there is a procedure that can provide them with near perfect information (i.e., commonly referred to as the *Gold Standard test,* but here we will use the more precise term *reference test*). However, the procedure that will yield them the perfect information is often fraught with increased risk and expense, so a safer and less costly option is sought. Of course, in doing this, they must accept that the safer and less costly option (which we refer to as the *index test*) will not provide perfect information. Thus, they are left to gamble that the index test will ultimately yield enough information that a decision congruent with the patient's goals can be made.

Consider the following example. We could determine with nearly absolute certainty whether a man has lung cancer by subjecting him to an exploratory thoracotomy. This of course would expose him to countless risks including infection and post- and intraoperative complications. It would also require weeks of rehabilitation and tens of thousands of dollars in expense for each procedure. The upside would be that once the procedure was over, we would know whether the patient had lung cancer, and assuming he survived the procedure and did not suffer a permanent disability he might find some satisfaction in that knowledge (of course, his contentment would be somewhat reduced when he is told he will need to undergo the same procedure in 2 years to ascertain whether the cancer remained or returned in the interim). The downside, of course, is that he might not survive the procedure.

Thankfully, this is not the typical method for diagnosis of lung cancer. Patients and their physicians do not feel that perfect precision in the diagnosis of lung cancer in asymptomatic patients is necessary. Our hypothetical patient and his physician have the benefit of plain film chest x-rays, thoracic CT, and PET to provide clinical information regarding the presence of lung cancer, and less invasive ways to obtain tissue samples. None of these modalities subject the patient to the risks and inconvenience of thoracotomy, but neither are any of them completely accurate in determining whether the patient has lung cancer.

S. Kymes (✉)
Department of Ophthalmology and Visual Sciences,
Washington University School of Medicine, 660 South Euclid,
St. Louis, MO 63110, USA
e-mail: kymes@vrcc.wustl.edu

P. Shreve and D.W. Townsend (eds.), *Clinical PET-CT in Radiology: Integrated Imaging in Oncology*,
DOI 10.1007/978-0-387-48902-5_13,

The acceptance of this lack of accuracy is what the patient selects in return for a safer, less expensive procedure. But in order to "hedge" his bets, the patient (and the physician) seek a concurrent understanding of the degree of inaccuracy that can be characterized as a probability. There are a number of statistical methods for expressing this probability, and they will be described in the next section of this chapter. Here we will discuss the sources of data, and potential bias that underlie these statistics.

It is well established that the efficacy of therapeutic interventions is best established through randomized clinical trials (RCT) [1]. This is due to three features of the RCT that improve the investigator's ability to infer causality between the intervention and outcome of interest: the prospective design, the concurrent control arm, and randomization [2]. However, while the RCT is considered to be the penultimate option for evaluation of therapeutic interventions, the RCT is not considered to be optimal for evaluation of diagnostic tests [3]. The reason for this lies in the nature of the research question being asked. In a diagnostic trial the concern is not with causality, but correlation between the index test and reference standard (Fig. 13.1). Therefore, the issue of temporal sequencing that is essential in the RCT is not important in a diagnostic trial. At the same time, factors that may confound the association between the index and reference test take on additional importance.

In the diagnostic trial, each study participant acts as her or his own control (Fig. 13.2). This allows for control over factors that may confound the correlation between the index and reference test due to temporal or biological factors to an extent that is superior to the RCT for this purpose. However, the diagnostic trial has potential for bias as well.

Spectrum (Selection) Bias

As with any clinical trial, the external validity (generalizability) of a diagnostic trial is limited by the characteristics of the study sample selected. In the case of therapeutic trial; this bias is referred to as *selection bias*. In diagnostic trial, this bias is referred to as *spectrum bias*, as it refers to the spectrum of clinical characteristics represented by the patients in the diagnostic trial [4]. Ideally, the trial to establish efficacy or effectiveness should be conducted in a sample that is randomly chosen from the population in which the test will be used. This is, however, rarely the case. The accuracy of diagnostic tests is commonly set in diagnostic trials that are conducted in academic settings where there is a high prevalence of disease, but used in community settings where there is a relatively low prevalence of disease. This bias can have significant impact on the interpretation of results of early diagnostic trials. For instance, a study concerning diagnosis of urinary tract infection found that in patients with severe disease there was a sensitivity of 92%, while patients with a lower pretest probability of disease had a sensitivity of 56% [5]. Thus, a community physician relying on estimates of sensitivity set in an academic setting would vastly overestimate the significance of negative finding on the test. Similarly, early trials of SPECT imaging for diagnosis of coronary artery disease found a much higher result for specificity than was found in later trials and common clinical practice [6].

It is often impractical to conduct diagnostic trials in community settings due to the paucity of participants at a single site. As an alternative, if investigators have a comprehensive knowledge of the risk factors associated with the disease, as well as the prevalence of those risk factors, a stratified

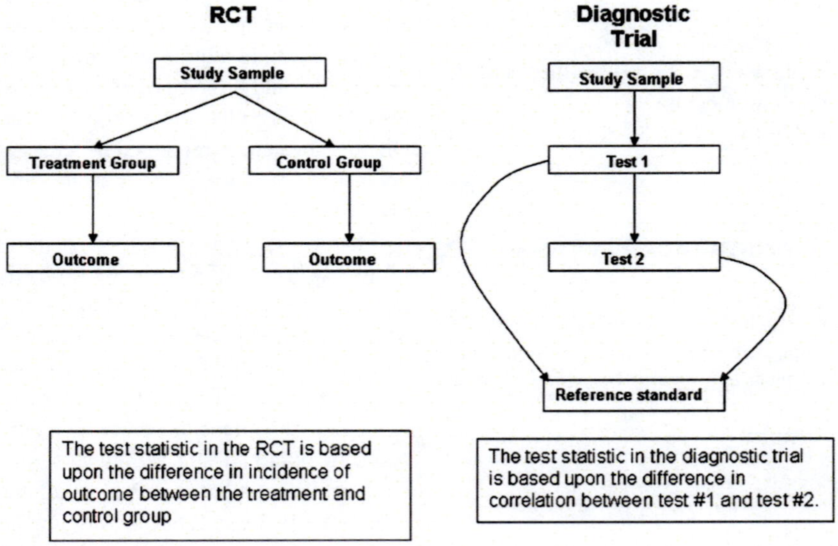

Fig. 13.1 Comparison of randomized clinical trial and diagnostic trial

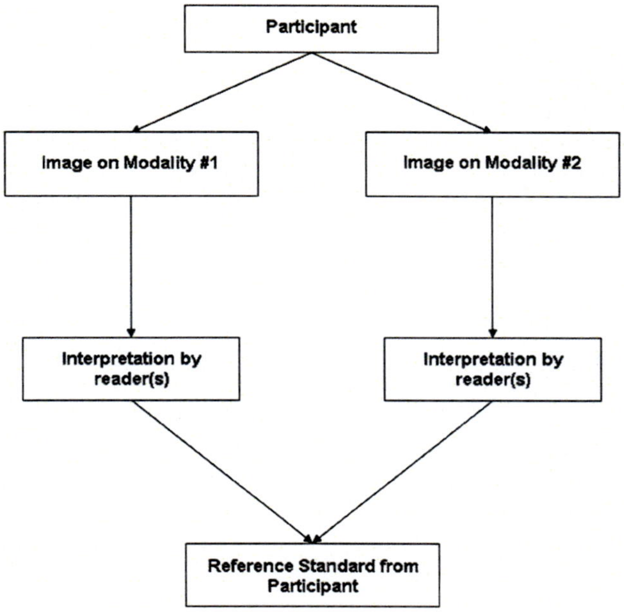

Fig. 13.2 Schematic of diagnostic trial

analysis can be conducted to adjust the crude findings to reflect that which might be found in a community setting [7]. Alternatively (or concurrently) the study can be designed so that spectrum bias is reduced. Studies of the accuracy of PET in the diagnosis of lung cancer have traditionally relied on participants with positive or indeterminate results referred from CT. In such studies, the generalizability of PET accuracy would be limited to patients with a higher risk of lung cancer following CT (i.e., PET accuracy would be conditional on a positive or indeterminate CT result). In such a case, spectrum bias would exist if the results were applied to cases referred directly from screening with chest x-ray, or from CT where the patient had a benign finding. Investigators in a recent study of PET addressed this by recruiting participants from a sample of those with a qualifying pulmonary nodule identified on chest x-ray [8]. The consequence of this study design was to increase the proportion of participants in the sample with a benign finding on the reference standard, and to extend the external generalizability of findings to settings where patients have a lower risk of disease.

Diagnostic and Test Review Bias

Diagnostic review bias and test review are two separate types of bias that are a function of study design. They occur when the interpretation of the reference test and index test are not independent of each other [9–11]. In the design of therapeutic trials, measurement of the intervention and the outcome must be independent. Typically, this is accomplished through use of the double blind study design and an independent assessment of outcome. If such independence does not exist, there is a threat to internal validity due to the potential for correlation between the intervention and outcome that has an unknown influence on the estimate of effect.

Consider the following diagnostic trial as an example. An investigator conducts a retrospective review of the records of 100 people to estimate the accuracy of echocardiography in the diagnosis of coronary artery disease (CAD). She uses coronary angiography as the reference standard. She is a cardiologist who directs an echocardiography lab and (after undergoing the proper review by a Human Studies Committee), selects the records of consecutive patients who meet the inclusion criteria and underwent angiography after having echocardiography in her lab. In order to avoid bias that may result from her knowledge of pretest clinical data, she chooses only those patients whose echo was read by her colleagues. She intends to reread these tests using standardized clinical records prepared by her research assistant.

So far, she has done well. Yes, we can nit-pick her for having only one reader, and the requirement that the patient undergo angiography is, as we will discuss in the following section, problematic. But she has done better in designing her study than most that we see in the literature. So, now let us assume that she begins her investigation by reviewing the angiography reports of the patients in the assembled sample. Her primary concern, as it would be for any investigator, is that the test was done correctly and the result was recorded correctly in the study records. Having done this, she then turns to reviewing the echocardiography data to assess the index test result.

Would this be a bias? Indeed it is, this is referred to as *test review bias* and is the result of interpreting the results of the index test with knowledge of the reference test. Diagnostic review bias would occur if the investigator has knowledge of the index test result when reviewing the reference test. To many, it may seem obvious that such forms of bias should be avoided, but various rationalizations can be offered for the approach:

- There is sufficient temporal separation between review of the two tests so it is not reasonable to assume that the investigator can remember the result from one test to the other.
- Identifying headers for the index and reference test were removed so the investigator cannot easily link the results of the index and reference tests.
- The investigator attempts to consider only the data presented by the index (or reference) test, when interpreting that test, blocking out any knowledge of the other test to insure an unbiased result.

These justifications fail to recognize that the clinician reading a report on the study is not concerned with whether the investigator interpreting the index (or reference) test maintained an unbiased mindset in interpreting the test result. The clinician is concerned with the fact that there was an element of the study design that was potentially biased, and therefore the clinician must consider the result of the study as biased. This problem is compounded because the reader cannot know in what direction the bias influenced the result. A recent systematic review of sources of bias identified seven studies that assessed the influence of diagnostic and test review bias and found that sometimes it resulted in increased accuracy, other times decreased accuracy, and yet other times it affected sensitivity and specificity differently [12].

The defense against these biases is to incorporate features into the study design that insure independence between the assessment of the index and reference tests. At minimum, the assessment of the index and reference test should be conducted by two individuals blinded to each other's findings. Larger studies routinely take more extreme measures. For a recent multisite study of PET in the diagnosis of lung cancer, the PET reading was performed by a panel of readers who were not involved in care of the study participant, at a time and place remote from the patient recruitment and testing. An independent reading such as this virtually eliminates the risk of test review bias [8]. Efforts to eliminate diagnostic review bias were not as rigorous. The reference standard was assessed by a local pathologist who was asked to remain blinded to imaging results and patient history as the interpretation was made. A superior approach would be to contract with an independent pathology lab employed in order to insure an unblinded assessment of the reference standard.

Verification Bias

Verification bias is common in nearly all diagnostic trials [13]. It is a form of bias that can be reduced by study design, or adjusted for statistically, but realistically cannot be eliminated from imaging studies because of the nature of the reference standard test.

Discussion of verification bias is complicated by a lack of consensus on what it is. Some have referred to verification bias as work-up bias or sequential-ordering bias, [4] while others have suggested that it is a particular variety of workup bias [14]. Recently others have sought to distinguish between ignorable and nonignorable verification bias [15]. We will not attempt to fuel this discussion of the finer points of study design theory, but we can present the definition on which we will base our further discussion:

> [*Verification bias*]...occurs when patients with positive (or negative) test results are preferentially referred for the gold standard procedure after which the sensitivity and specificity are calculated only based on those cases who underwent the gold [reference] standard procedure [14].

Let us return to our hypothetical cardiologist. In an effort to insure that her reference standard is "squeaky clean" she selected only those patients for whom she had a well-defined angiography result. Intuitively, this may seem obvious; however, such precautions limit the generalizability of findings. Echocardiography is performed on patients with a wide range of risk of disease – those referred to angiography for further diagnosis and those who are not. In excluding from the study those who are not referred for the reference standard test, we create a threat to external validity. The consequence of this exclusion is to overestimate sensitivity and underestimate specificity. Shaw and Pryor [16] showed that this bias can be rather severe, resulting in an estimate of sensitivity or specificity that varies from the "true" population based estimate by as much as 20% points.

Verification bias can be addressed through a number of statistical methods [14, 17]. In these methods the assumption is made that the estimates of sensitivity and specificity are biased due to missing data, and that most missing data are from patients who had a negative result on the index test. Thus, the patient's status of "missing" or "not-missing" is conditioned on their test result. The statistical adjustment uses maximum likelihood methods to describe the most likely distribution from which the missing data were drawn.

It is this link between test result and missing data that leads to the often confusing description of verification bias as being present when referral to the reference test is dependent upon the index test result [18]. This would certainly be the case in most retrospective diagnostic trials (hence, verification bias is a greater risk in retrospective trials). However, this is a very limited definition of verification bias. Prospective trials can easily be designed in which referral to the reference standard is not dependent upon the index test result, but the trial may still may suffer from verification bias. For instance, assume we are conducting a trial to estimate the diagnostic accuracy of CT imaging. Our reference standard will be definitive diagnosis based upon tissue biopsy, either surgical of percutaneous. We require that all patients upon enrollment agree to undergo both CT and biopsy, and all those who enroll do. By the definition above, we have eliminated verification bias, but that is not the case. It is likely that patients with a lower risk of disease will either not be asked to join the study (as the investigator seeks to avoid exposing them to risk of an invasive procedure with no clinical benefit) or the patient declines to participate in a study that will expose him or her to risk and discomfort.

Simply unlinking eligibility for the reference test from the index test result is not sufficient to avoid verification bias. Use of statistical methods is one approach to address this problem, but there is no current method to validate such estimates in a specific sample, so investigators may view them with suspicion, particularly when the adjusted estimate varies substantially from the unadjusted. In this case, a superior method to reduce verification bias is through study design. Verification bias is an issue when the disease status of patients with a low risk of disease cannot be verified because they are not enrolled in the study or decline to undergo the reference test (i.e., are "lost to follow-up"). If an acceptable alternative reference standard can be established for patients with a lower risk of disease, they might be included in the study, and verification bias reduced. In many studies, a long-term follow-up with the patient to evaluate changes in disease status has been used. In a study of pulmonary embolism (PIOPED), patients who did not have angiography were followed at regular intervals for a year to assess relevant events [19]. A study of breast cancer followed participants who did not have biopsy for a year to determine if there was any change in breast characteristics [20]. In a study of the accuracy of PET in the diagnosis of lung cancer, participants who did not have biopsy were followed for 2 years, with those who did not have a change in the size of the solitary pulmonary nodule of interest being considered to have benign disease [8].

Other Sources of Bias in Diagnostic Studies

There are a number of other sources of bias in diagnostic trials that have not been studied as thoroughly as those considered here [12, 20–22]. In general, these are variations of those considered above; therefore we refer interested readers to the above citations.

Clinical Information and the Presence of Disease

Sensitivity and Specificity

Estimation of the accuracy of a diagnostic test begins with a 2×2 table to classify the results according to the index test result and the patient's disease status (as determined by the reference standard (Table 13.1)).

Note that in the above example, we do not consider indeterminate results from the index test. This is not an unrealistic manner in which to consider such a finding. Depending on the consequences associated with misdiagnosis, a clinician will consider an indeterminate result as evidence of disease (and continue the disease workup or move to treatment) or benign (and move to watchful waiting).

In the 2×2 table, TP, FP, FN, and FP refer to true positive, false positive, false negative, and false positive results, respectively. From these data, we calculate the primary indices of diagnostic accuracy: sensitivity and specificity [1].

Table 13.1 2×2 table of test results

		Reference test	
		+	–
Index test result	+	TP	FP
	–	FN	TN

$$\text{Sensitivity} = \text{TP} / (\text{TP} + \text{FN})$$

$$\text{Specificity} = \text{FP} / (\text{TN} + \text{FP})$$

Sensitivity represents the probability that a person with the disease will have a positive test result. Specificity represents the probability that a person without the disease will have a negative test result. These are attractive measures to those involved in evaluation of diagnostic tests, as they are not sensitive to the prevalence of disease in the population in which the test was conducted (as opposed to positive and Negative Predictive Value, which are discussed in the next section). However, these statistics are of little use to clinicians. Sensitivity and specificity begin by assuming that the patient's disease status is known. (In the language of Bayesian mathematics, sensitivity and specificity are the accuracy of the test, conditional on the patent's disease status.) If the clinician knows the patient's disease status, he or she would not order the test (at least for the purpose of diagnosis).

The Receiver Operating Characteristic (ROC) Curve

Sensitivity and specificity have another important limitation that needs to be addressed at length. Consider Fig. 13.3 in which we graph the distribution of a hypothetical disease marker. Let us assume for the purposes of this discussion that the value on the *x*-axis is the standardized uptake value (SUV) associated with a pulmonary nodule as measured by PET and the *y*-axis is the number of people with a nodule having recorded that particular SUV. The two distributions (1 and 2) were constructed by biopsying the nodule identified and having a qualified pathologist determine whether the tissue was benign ("Well") or malignant ("Diseased"). On average, people with a malignant nodule (Distribution 2) have a higher tumor SUV value than those with benign nodules (Distribution 1). Also, while this relationship exists, there are a substantial number of people with a benign nodule who have SUVs higher than some with malignant tumors.

If we want to know how good SUV is at classifying tumors as benign or malignant, we want to construct a 2×2 table similar to Table 13.1 to calculate sensitivity and specificity. To do this, we need to determine at what level of SUV

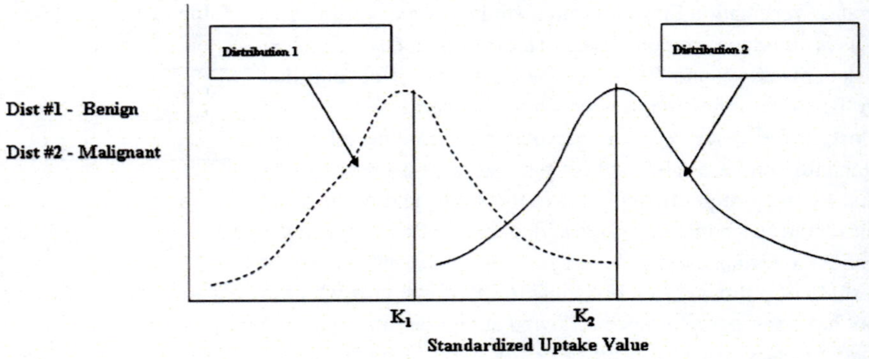

Fig. 13.3 Distribution of disease markers in a population

we will declare a tumor to be malignant. One option would be to use the value at K_1 (which we refer to as our *decision threshold*). We would choose this value because we would achieve 100% sensitivity, correctly characterizing all malignant tumors. But note that at this decision threshold we would also characterize at least half of benign tumors as malignant as well (achieving 50% specificity). If this is unacceptable, perhaps we would shift the threshold to K_2 so that we achieve 100% specificity, but now we incorrectly characterize half of malignant tumors as benign (i.e., 50% sensitivity).

This tension (and inverse correlation) between sensitivity and specificity is a characteristic of all diagnostic tests. The degree to which tradeoff occurs between sensitivity and specificity occurs is a function of several factors, including technical characteristics of test itself (such as reliability), but it is primarily a function of the variance within the underlying distributions and difference in mean between them. If one were to vary "*K*" across a range of decision thresholds, the corresponding sensitivity and specificity values could be calculated. We may then wish to examine the relationship between these pairs graphically, so we would graph them in a two dimensional plane creating a graph similar to Fig. 13.4. By convention, the points are plotted in a plane with sensitivity on the *y*-axis and 1-specificity on the *x*-axis. The resulting plane, bounded by 1.0 on both the *x*- and *y*-axis is referred to as the ROC space.

If we fit a smooth curve between the points, the result is the receiver operating characteristic curve, or more commonly the ROC curve (Fig. 13.5). It is a graphic representation of the expected accuracy of the test in a population similar to the sample in which the test was studied [23]. Alternatively, one might consider the ROC curve as representing the possible combinations of sensitivity and specificity that might be achieved with the testing modality.

The area bounded by the ROC curve (i.e., the area under the curve or AUC) provides an index for comparing the accuracy of diagnostic tests that is superior to comparisons of point estimates [24]. When applied to diagnostic imaging, the AUC represents the probability that a clinician choosing a particular image from a pool will correctly classify the image as either diseased or not diseased [23]. For example, suppose that in our example of using PET SUV values to characterize malignancy we found that PET had an AUC of 0.91. This would indicate that if one were to use the SUV of a randomly selected nodule to determine malignancy, there would be a 91% probability of correctly characterizing the nodule.

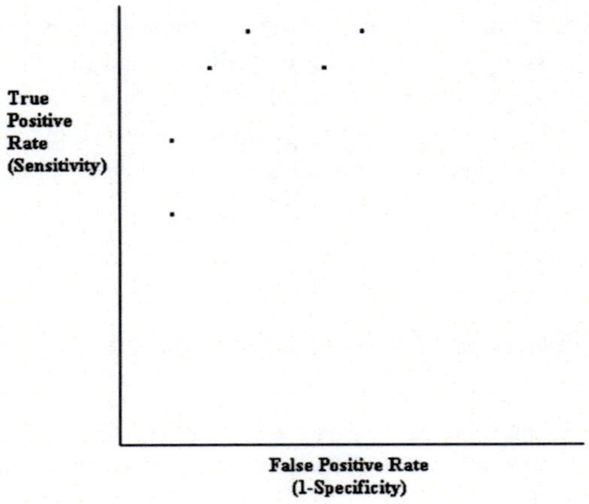

Fig. 13.4 Sensitivity/specificity pairs

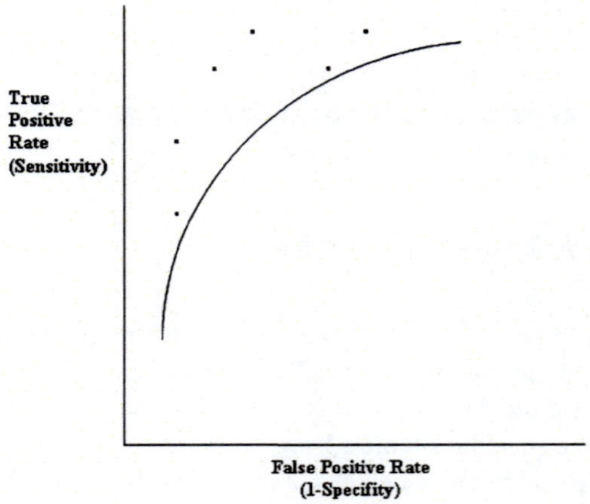

Fig. 13.5 Receiver operating characteristic (ROC) curve

Table 13.2 Sensitivity/specificity at varied decision thresholds

"Malignant" defined as "worse"	PET		CT	
than (but not including)	Sensitivity	Specificity	Sensitivity	Specificity
Definitively benign	98%	56%	99%	13%
Probably benign	94%	81%	94%	50%
Indeterminate	88%	87%	73%	79%
Probably malignant	39%	96%	4%	99%

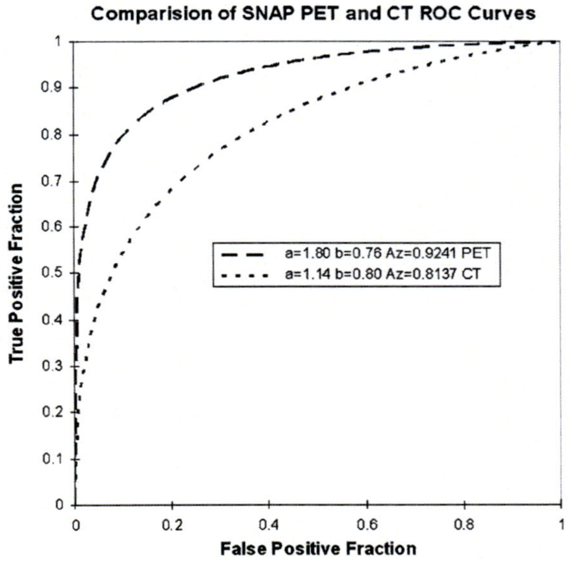

Fig. 13.6 Using receiver operating characteristic (ROC) curves to compare two diagnostic tests

Let us consider a hypothetical example. We will compare the accuracy of PET and CT in diagnosis of lung cancer. Both modalities were used on each patient, and the reference standard was established with minimal verification bias. Readers of both imaging methods rated diagnosis on a five point ordinal scale ranging from "Definitely Benign" to "Definitely Malignant." Our decision threshold problem then becomes at what point on this ordinal scale we declare the nodule as malignant. We consider each option and calculate the sensitivity and specificity at each threshold (Table 13.2).

It may seem obvious that the best option is to define malignant as a rating of Worse Than Probably Benign, or possibly Indeterminate, but as we discuss in the following sections, in setting the ideal cutpoint, we must consider a number of factors in addition to accuracy, particularly the benefit associated with treatment of disease, as well as the cost of a false positive result [11].

In Fig. 13.6 we present two ROC curves that result from this data. The curves were constructed using ROCKIT, one of the most commonly used ROC software packages (for further information see http://xray.bsd.uchicago.edu/krl/KRL_ROC/software_index.htm). ROCKIT uses a parametric method developed by Dorfman and Alf [25] and later refined by Metz [26] to draw the curve and compare the AUCs to establish statistical significance. The parameters on which the curves are based ("a" and "b") are given for each curve, as well as the AUC (parameter Az). The difference between these two curves is statistically significant ($p<0.001$), indicating that in this hypothetical sample PET had superior overall accuracy when compared to CT. In addition, note that the two curves do not cross at any point. This indicates that there is no decision threshold that could be chosen at which CT would have superior accuracy to PET.

Clinical Information, Patient Characteristics, and the Probability of Disease

Sensitivity/specificity and ROC curves do not provide clinicians direct evidence that an individual patient has disease. Instead, these methods inform clinicians of the probability, given a patient's disease status, that the index test will yield the "correct" result [11]. The ROC curve has the additional property that it describes the range of performance of a test (in terms of combinations of sensitivity and specificity), with the AUC providing an estimate of the probability that a clinician will "correctly" classify a random patient selected from a defined population. However, as we have defined the ROC curve thus far, it does not provide information regarding the decision threshold that should be applied to a specific patient.

What the clinician caring for a real patient wants to know is, "If this test gives me a normal (abnormal) result, what is the probability that the patient does not (or does) have disease?" Note that this is precisely the inverse of the information offered by sensitivity and specificity. It should be readily apparent that this information is contained in the rows of the table (as opposed to the columns on which we based sensitivity and specificity). If we take the row for positive (abnormal) test result (Table 13.3), we can calculate the probability of a person having disease by dividing the number of true positives by the total number of positive test results. This is referred to as the Positive Predictive Value or PPV of the test:

$$PPV = TP / (TP + FP)$$

Conversely, the probability of a patient with a negative (normal) test result not having disease is calculated by dividing the number of true negatives by the total number of negative

Table 13.3 2×2 table of test results

		Reference test	
		+	–
Index test	+	TP	FP
result	–	FN	TN

test results. This is called the "Negative Predictive Value" or NPV of the test:

$$NPV = TN / (FN + TN).$$

PPV and NPV are often criticized as being sensitive to the prevalence of disease found in the study on which the measure was based. This is not dissimilar to the problems related to spectrum bias that we discussed above, but here the problem is that instead of being an artifact of reader performance, it is inherent in the design of the statistic itself [18]. Consider the following table comparing the PPV and NPV that was found in two separate studies, both evaluating the diagnostic accuracy of PET in identifying patients with lung cancer. In the first study, patients who were found to have a suspicious nodule on chest radiograph were recruited to the study, and in the second, the patients selected were those who had indeterminate nodules on thoracic CT [27]. For purposes of this example, we have set the sensitivity and specificity of the two tests at the same level. However, we have not "fixed" the prevalence of disease. In the first study, the prevalence of malignancy was found to be 55% (200/365) and in the second study it was 67% (60/89). In Table 13.4 we see that even this scant 12-point swing in prevalence resulted in a flip of the relationship between PPV and NPV. If the prevalence in the second study were 75%, a level frequently seen in such studies, the result would be a ten-point difference in PPV and NPV between the two studies.

While these differences may seem small, and might even be clinically inconsequential, recall that these differences are seen even though sensitivity and specificity have not changed between the studies. It is strictly a function of the prevalence of disease in the population in which the study is tested. Given that it is nearly inevitable that the test will be used in a setting where the prevalence of disease is different (most likely less) than the tested setting, PPV and NPV have come to be viewed with considerable concern by most clinical epidemiologists, who advise that they should not be used [11].

Sensitivity and specificity are measures of diagnostic accuracy that are not sensitive to prevalence. Therefore, a method that relies only on sensitivity and specificity (that is, a measure that is calculated using the column values of the 2×2 table) for estimating the patient's probability of disease conditional on the test result would address the limitations of PPV and NPV. Every patient who comes to a physician carries with him or her a certain risk of disease. The physician considers the patient's complaints and determines the pretest probability of disease based on the prevalence of disease among people with similar complaints. For instance, for patients similar to those in Study #1 mentioned previously, the prevalence of malignancy is 55%. Therefore if our patient is similar to those in the study, we could say that his or her pretest probability of disease is 55%. The purpose of a diagnostic test is to change the pretest probability of disease to such a point that a clinician might make a treat/no treat decision based upon the posttest probability of disease [10]. Let us assume that our patient had a positive (abnormal) test result. We know based on the results given in Table 13.2 that the sensitivity of the test is 88% (assuming we define our decision threshold as "indeterminate"). So, if our patient is diseased, there is an 88% chance that the test would give a positive result. But what is the probability of getting a positive test result if he (or she) does not have disease? That would be the complement to specificity, or 1/0.87, or 13%. Now, we can ask ourselves, given these probabilities and a positive test result, what would be the odds, that the patient is diseased? That would be the ratio of the probability of getting the positive result if the patient has the disease (sensitivity) divided by the probability of getting the positive test result if the patient does not have disease (1 – specificity). In the Bayesian world, this ratio is called the likelihood ratio (positive):

$$LR+ = \frac{\text{Sensitivity of test}}{1 - \text{Specificity of test}} \qquad (13.1)$$

Let us apply this ratio to our patient. First we need to estimate the likelihood ratio (positive) for a thoracic PET scan in diagnosing lung cancer:

$$LR+ = 0.88 / (1 - 0.87) = 0.88 / 0.13 = 6.77$$

In English, this means that for every person who has a positive test result and does not end up having lung cancer, there are 6.77 who do have lung cancer (alternatively, you could say that people who have an abnormal PET scan are 6.77 times more likely to have lung cancer than those who do not). As this is an odds ratio, we need to estimate our patient's posttest probability of disease in terms of odds so we are doing and "apples to apples" comparison. The pretest odds are given by the ratio:

$$\text{Odds of disease} = \text{Probability of disease} / \text{Probability of no disease}$$

Given that we have estimated the probability of disease already as 55%, we can estimate the odds that our patient has disease as:

$$\text{Odds of disease} = 0.55 / 0.45 = 1.22$$

Meaning that for every person with a suspicious lung nodule seen on chest x-ray who does not have disease, there are 1.22 who had an abnormal CXR who do have lung cancer.

Table 13.4 Positive/negative predictive value in two studies with different prevalence of disease

	Study #1						Study #2					
	Reference test						Reference test					
Index test result	+	–	SN	SP	PPV	NPV	+	–	SN	SP	PPV	NPV
Positive	188	31	94%	81%	86%	92%	56	6	94%	81%	90%	85%
Negative	12	134					4	23				
Total	200	165					60	29				

Now, we can bring together these two pieces of information by multiplying the pretest odds of disease by the LR+ to get the posttest odds of disease:

$$1.22 \times 6.77 = 8.27$$

As it is easier to understand, we should consider converting this back to a probability which we do with a simple formula:

$$\text{Probability of disease} = \text{Odds of disease} / \left(1 + \text{Odds of disease}\right)$$

In the case of the patient before us this would be:

$$\text{Probability of disease} = 8.27 / \left(1 + 8.27\right) = 0.893$$

Or, following a positive PET scan, our patient's probability of having lung cancer is 89.3%.

What if our patient had a negative test result? Our concern is still with the probability of disease, but now our question is: What are the odds of finding a negative test result in someone who has disease? This would be given by dividing the probability of finding a negative test result in someone without the disease (or, 1 − sensitivity), by the probability of finding a negative test result in someone without the disease, which is specificity. So, the likelihood ratio (negative) would be as shown in 13.2.

$$\text{LR}- = \frac{1 - \text{Sensitivity of test}}{\text{Specificity}} \qquad (13.2)$$

Based on our hypothetical results, for PET in diagnosis of lung cancer, this would be:

$$\text{LR}- = \left(1 - 0.88\right) / 0.87 = 0.12 / 0.87 = 0.138$$

When applied to our hypothetical patient the result is:

$$1.22 \times 0.138 = 0.168$$

Using our conversion formula, we convert this back to probability:

$$\text{Probability of disease} = 0.168 / \left(1 + 0.168\right) = 0.144$$

indicating that after a negative test result, our patient has a 14.4% chance of having lung cancer.

A Few Notes of Caution Regarding Uncertainty

In this entire discussion, we have, for the sake of simplicity made the assumption that our estimates are extremely precise. But it must be acknowledged that this is a completely unrealistic assumption. First, we must recognize that the entire Bayesian process described above begins with the assumption that the physician can properly estimate the patient's pre-test probability of disease. For the sake of our discussion here we based our pretest probability on a single hypothetical study. In practice the clinician should carefully consider the evidence that is presented concerning the patient's risk factors and associated risk of disease. Seeking systematic reviews or the most current population based studies of prevalence of disease is preferable to relying on expert opinion or poorly designed case series [2, 28]. However, in the absence of a valid estimate of the patient's pretest probability of disease, it should be noted that the methods described above are robust in estimating the importance of a positive or negative test result if the lack of precision in the base estimate is recognized.

More importantly, our statistical estimates (i.e., sensitivity, specificity, AUC, PPV, NPV, LR+ and LR–) are just that, estimates. By definition, the science of statistics is an effort to characterize uncertainty, and as such it must be recognized that each of these estimates is bracketed by an interval describing the range of values it might take. This bracket is referred to as the *confidence interval* and the best known version of this is the 95% confidence interval (CI) [29]. The purpose of the CI is to inform the reader of the range of values within which the "true" mean associated with the estimate may lie [30]. For instance, in the example above, we found that the sensitivity of PET in diagnosis of lung cancer is 88.5%. The 95% CI about this estimate is 83.2% to 92.6%, meaning that we can say with 95% confidence that the true sensitivity of PET in the population from which the sample was drawn would be no less than 83.2% and no better than 92.6%. The width of the CI is inversely related to the sample size of the study that provided the data used to construct the 2×2 table. With a few notable exceptions, most imaging studies are relatively small, and therefore tend to have considerable uncertainty.

We will not address the methods to calculate CIs, other than to give this caution – the confidence intervals about proportions such as sensitivity and specificity are not typically symmetric [29]. Proportions are bounded by 0 and 1, and as one approaches the boundary (as one would in most estimates of diagnostic accuracy) the CI becomes more and more asymmetric. Failure to adjust for this asymmetry in reporting the CI will result in an overestimation of the precision of the estimate, and most importantly, will underestimate the length of the tail which represents the lower bound.

Confidence intervals should also be calculated and reported for likelihood ratios [31]. It should be noted that while the LR is not a proportion, it is similarly bound (by zero and infinity) and when properly calculated, the interval will often be asymmetric, particularly for the LR–, which will often approach zero.

Meta-Analysis and Evidence in Diagnostic Trials

The purpose of a meta-analysis is to create a precise and definitive answer when the results of individual studies disagree or are inconclusive [32]. It does this using a systematic method to acquire and analyze data, and creating a summary statistic using rigorous statistical methods [33]. Meta-analysis begins by reviewing the relevant literature and identifying all studies that have been conducted to address the clinical question at hand. It is essential at this point in the analysis to cast a net that is too wide rather than too narrow [34]. Following this, the data is graded to assess its quality. The purpose of grading is to determine which biases might differentially affect the summary estimates [34]. For example, if a third of reports used in the meta-analysis that come from a foreign source, and there is a substantially different method of medical referral from that system, this would threaten the validity of a pooled estimate. Consequently, grading must be done prior to pooling of data.

Heterogeneity has been defined as a factor that causes a change in the effect size from one patient series to another, such that the resulting meta-estimate (when the series are combined) is meaningless [35]. Thompson has distinguished two types of heterogeneity: statistical and clinical [36]. Clinical heterogeneity is defined as those clinically important differences that exist between the trials that constitute the meta-analysis. Sources of clinical heterogeneity would include the process of patient selection, baseline disease severity, and differences in study design or clinical procedures. Statistical heterogeneity exists when quantitative results in a meta-analysis are incompatible. This is often the result of clinical heterogeneity or methodological differences in study design (as in the case of combining a randomized controlled trial with a retrospective study). Where clinical heterogeneity is present the data reported must be stratified in order to provide meaningful information to clinical decision-makers.

The two primary methods for combining meta-analytic data are the fixed-effects model, and the random-effects model. Both of these create summary point estimates of accuracy (i.e., sensitivity = 95%) and differ only in the way they treat heterogeneity in the component studies. The fixed-effects model assumes that all potential sources of bias have been identified and the data stratified prior to combination, so it assumes that all sources of heterogeneity have been controlled. The random-effects model assumes that there is unidentified or uncontrolled heterogeneity and in estimating confidence intervals allows for more variation. Thus the random effects model yields wider confidence intervals than the fixed effects model [33]. While some have argued that use of the random effects model corrects for heterogeneity, this is not the case. If there is a source of clinical heterogeneity that is unaddressed by stratifying the sample of studies, the result can be a meaningless estimate of accuracy regardless of the method used to create summary estimates [36]. For example, a recent meta-analysis compared SPECT and echo imaging in diagnosis of CAD [37]. In constructing their estimates the authors combined SPECT studies that were scored using a visual approach with developmental studies of quantitative scoring software. In essence the authors were creating a weighted average of the two methods, but this does not reflect clinical practice. Clinicians use one approach or the other in interpreting SPECT images, not both. A subsequent critique of this report demonstrated that had the investigators stratified their analysis to take this heterogeneity into account, the previous claim of superiority of echo in diagnosis of CAD would not be supported [38].

As we noted previously, in evaluating diagnostic tests, the usefulness of point estimates of accuracy is severely limited, and thus ROC curves have an important role in describing accuracy of tests. This is similar in meta-analysis. The information contained in several studies can be summarized in ROC curves, described in this context, not surprisingly, as summary ROC (SROC) curves [39]. The curves thus created are interpreted in a manner similar to single study curves. The structure of ROC (and SROC) curves allow for changes in the patient characteristics (by recognizing that clinicians change the decision threshold based upon the patient's pretest likelihood of disease), thus the SROC curve is not sensitive to most sources of statistical heterogeneity. However, the SROC curve cannot correct for sources of clinical heterogeneity related to instrumentation or study design; these must be addressed (as demonstrated in the example above) by stratification of the sample.

Given This Information, What Should Be Done?

Now that the clinician has evaluated the quality of the data describing the accuracy of the diagnostic test, calculated the accuracy and likelihood ratios associated with the test, estimated pre- and post-test probability of disease, and considered the degree of uncertainty about the estimates – what should she or he do? After all, what we have is a number – one that ranges from 0 to 1. It tells us the probability of disease, it does not tell us whether to treat, or test, or watch, or send the patient home happy that they are well. The contribution by the diagnostic test to the clinical algorithm is a function of the accuracy of the test, but this is only the beginning of the manner in which the efficacy of the test is judged. Fryback and Thornbury addressed this in a hierarchy of efficacy associated with diagnostic imaging (Table 13.5) [40]. Thus far, the statistics we have considered address only the first two types of efficacy described in this hierarchy. Addressing higher levels of efficacy requires that we consider the influence of clinical information on clinical decision making or the degree to which the information assisted the patient and society to meet their goals.

Table 13.5 Fryback/Thornbury hierarchy for efficacy for diagnostic imaging

Level/name	Suggested measures
Level 1	Resolution of line pairs
Technical efficacy	Gray-scale range
	Sharpness
Level 2	Predictive value (positive/negative)
Diagnostic accuracy efficacy	Sensitivity/specificity
	Measures of ROC curve ("area under the curve")
Level 3	Number of cases judged "helpful" in making diagnosis
Diagnostic thinking accuracy	Entropy change in diagnosis probability distribution
	Difference in subjective pre- and posttest probability
Level 4	Percentage of times judged helpful in planning treatment
Therapeutic efficacy	Percentage of times avoided unnecessary treatment
	Percentage of times therapy changed
Level 5	Percentage of patients whose outcome improved with test
Patient outcome efficacy	Change in quality adjusted life expectancy
	Cost per QALY saved with new information
Level 6	Cost/benefit analysis for society
Societal efficacy	Cost/effectiveness analysis for society

Clinical trials evaluating the influence of imaging devices on diagnostic and therapeutic thinking (Levels 3 and 4) are quite rare. A search of the literature in 2005 found only one that had been conducted [41], and one that was planned but for which the findings had not been reported [8]. However, such studies have great social import. It is rare that the adoption of a new technology leads to obsolescence of an old one [42], and one can speculate that a major reason for this is the failure on the part of investigators to determine if the proposed test provides incremental information, or simply provides clinicians a "new toy." The failure to consider the impact of new technology has two important consequences: (1) It results in wasteful use of scarce social resources; and (2) it can result in iatrogenic harm to the patient as he/she is subjected to unnecessary testing and delay in treatment.

Economic Evaluation: Diagnostic Efficacy at Levels 5 and 6

Efficacy as measured at levels 5 and 6 concerns whether the patient, and ultimately society, benefit from the test. Economic evaluation of diagnostic tests is a process that seeks to measure the relationship between the resources expended on an intervention and the benefit gained [43]. The basic principles of economic evaluation are well established [33, 43, 44]. The economic investigator must determine if the information provided by the test to clinicians and their patients justifies the cost of the test, measured in terms of monetary expenditures and those things that are given up in order to perform the test (the latter referred to as *opportunity cost* by economists) [45]. Frequently, the adoption of a new test represents a tradeoff between the increase in cost for the new test and an increase in the quality of information gained (or conversely, a decrease in cost weighed against lower quality of information). These principles are demonstrated graphically (Table 13.6). Where a test saves resources and provides greater or similar benefit (northeast quadrant of the table), it is said to dominate the current test and should be adopted [43]. Similarly, a test that costs more but does not deliver additional benefit (falling in the southwest quadrant) is said to be dominated by the current test, and should be rejected. Tests that fall on the diagonal from northwest to southeast are ambiguous. These represent tests that are either

Table 13.6 Evaluating the cost-effectiveness of tests

	Benefit of test	
Cost of test	Lower than previous	Higher than previous
Lower than previous	Ambiguous	Accept new intervention
Higher than previous	Reject new intervention	Ambiguous

cost saving with fewer benefits, or have higher benefits at a higher cost.

Tests considered to be ambiguous in their initial evaluation are evaluated using the incremental cost-effectiveness ratio (ICER) [44]:

$$\frac{\text{Incremental Costs of Intervention}}{\text{Incremental Effectiveness of Intervention}} \tag{13.3}$$

In its broadest sense, cost-effectiveness analysis estimates the amount of resources necessary to "purchase" a unit of effectiveness (e.g., years of life saved, number of lives saved, number of screening cases identified) [44]. However, the use of different measures of effectiveness limits the ability of policy makers to compare interventions. For instance, consider a CMS policymaker considering whether to authorize coverage for use of PET in diagnosis of Alzheimer's. He is presented information that use of PET costs $150,000 per year of life saved. Should such use be authorized? Suppose the decision to authorize payment for PET scans in Alzheimer's patients is being weighed against screening for glaucoma that costs $75,000 per year of vision saved? Which represents a better option?

One could argue that one way to measure effectiveness would be by assessing health-related quality of life (HRQoL) through function status measures such as the widely used SF-36 or similar instruments [46]. These instruments examine distinct domains of living (i.e., physical function, mental health, role function, etc.) by asking questions about ability to perform tasks (e.g., walking a mile) or to function (e.g., "feeling blue," "having pep") [47]. However, the limitation of such methods is that they evaluate quality of life by inquiring concerning physical or mental function, but the instrument does not concern itself with the importance of that function to the person. This can on occasion lead to contradictory results when examining the impact of functional measures in dissimilar populations. A recent report compared vision-related quality of life in people with keratoconus and macular degeneration [48]. Keratoconus is a corneal disease that affects the young, while macular degeneration is a retinal disease affecting the elderly. Keratoconus has minimal impact on visual acuity, and people with advanced macular degeneration are often nearly blind. Examining the overall score on vision-related quality of life, the people with keratoconus have higher scores (reflecting the better visual acuity); yet, on the mental health, role difficulties, and ocular pain scales the people with keratoconus had scores that were equal to or lower than those with macular degeneration. This may be indicative of the difference in perception between young adults and older people of the importance of visual disability and related morbidity.

Economists address this by measuring quality of life using the person's preference for health and health states. The metric used for this purpose is described as the *utility* and is measured on a scale of 0 to 1 (with zero typically being death, and one, perfect health). Maximum utility for a community is achieved when the aggregate utility cannot be increased through a change to any individual in the community [43]. In estimating the ICER using utilities (referred to as cost-utility analysis), effectiveness is defined as the expected remaining life span weighted by the expected utility over that life span. The resulting measure is the quality-adjusted life year (QALY), with the result being the cost/QALY (or the resources required to purchase a quality adjusted life year) [49].

There are three primary methods for measuring utility: the visual analog scale (VAS), the standard gamble (SG), and the time trade-off (TTO). In the VAS, the person is asked to rate their perception of health state on a line, with one end being death and the other perfect health [44]. In the latter two methods the person is asked to consider what they would trade to gain perfect health (in SG, the risk of immediate death; in TTO a portion of their remaining life span) [50]. The latter two methods are considered to be more consistent with economic theory [51].

The results of cost-utility analysis have important consequences in the context of the hierarchy of efficacy. Since utility represents a persons preference for a health state, analysis based upon this metric can be translated into a person's preference for an intervention. Consider for instance the use of PET in the diagnosis of lung cancer. The decision to undergo a test represents a complex calculus weighing costs (the charge for the test, the time spent having the test performed, radiation exposure, pain of the needle stick, the need to remain motionless over a period of time, etc.) and benefits, all weighted by probabilities associated with misdiagnosis, treatment, and progression. Using preference measures, the investigator can model the decision that a patient would make if they had full understanding of the costs, benefits, and probabilities associated with their condition.

The unit of effectiveness being "purchased" when cost-utility analysis is conducted is the QALY. So, to determine the patient's decision when they have weighed the costs, benefits, and probabilities, one must know what the patient is willing to pay for a QALY. At this point the science associated with this work remains unsettled, largely because in most Western countries, people do not perceive that they pay for their health care. It is paid for by governmental entities or the patient's employer. Therefore, the question of how much a QALY is worth becomes a social policymaking question (i.e., efficacy level 6). Many have suggested a limit of $50,000/QALY [52], but more recently many health economists have recognized $100,000/QALY as the upper limit [53], and some have argued for a threshold in excess of $200,000 [54].

Use of the ROC Curve to Compare Cost-Effectiveness of Tests

As we discussed previously, in comparing diagnostic tests, the test with the greatest area under the ROC curve has the greatest accuracy in a population [23]. However, it has been pointed out that this method has important limitations [55]. Assume that in Fig. 13.7, the curve representing Test A clearly has the greater area under the curve due to its superior specificity at lower levels of sensitivity. This would imply that Test A would be the preferred technology to be used when diagnosing the condition of interest. However, note that on the right side of the graph, the ROC curve for Test B is clearly above that of the curve for Test A. This would indicate that in a setting where sensitivity would be valued (i.e., a setting where the pretest probability of disease is relatively high) Test B might be the preferred technology.

A second limitation of the AUC is that it ignores the costs of the test. Each point on the curve has associated with it an ICER associated with the sensitivity/specificity found at that point. Summing these up would provide a summary CUR for the test. This being the case, the weighted difference in AUC would represent the value society would place on the more accurate test. If this value were less than the difference in cost between the two technologies, then the gain in diagnostic accuracy represented by the larger area under the curve would not translate into improved cost-effectiveness. It should be noted, however, that methods to do this have not been developed beyond some very preliminary efforts [56, 57].

It has been suggested that the lack of information regarding patient costs and preferences limit the usefulness of ROC curve data [55]. However, some have suggested that the ideal use of ROC curves would be to identify the ideal combination of sensitivity/specificity to use for a specific patient with known clinical characteristics. This point would balance the cost and benefit of diagnosis and treatment. Consider the expected cost associated with diagnosis and treatment in 13.4 [24]:

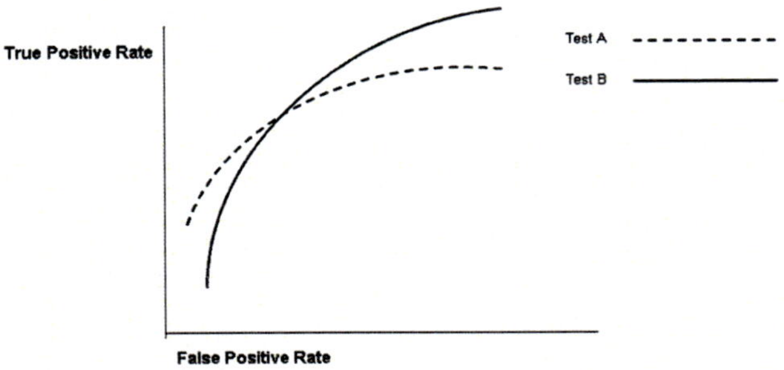

Fig. 13.7 Comparison of two competing technologies using receiver operating characteristic (ROC) curves

$$\begin{aligned}\mathrm{EC} = C_0 &+ \{C_{\mathrm{TP}} \times P(\mathrm{D+}) \times P(\mathrm{T+}\mid\mathrm{D+})\} \\ &+ \{C_{\mathrm{TN}} \times P(\mathrm{D-}) \times [1 - P(\mathrm{T+}\mid\mathrm{D-})]\} \\ &+ \{C_{\mathrm{FP}} \times P(\mathrm{D-}) \times P(\mathrm{T+}\mid\mathrm{D-})\} \\ &+ \{C_{\mathrm{FN}} \times P(\mathrm{D+}) \times [1 - P(\mathrm{T+}\mid\mathrm{D+})]\} \qquad (13.4)\end{aligned}$$

where:

EC = Expected cost

C_0 = Overhead cost of test (i.e., the resource consumption associated with the test itself)

C_{xx} = Specific cost associated with the clinical pathway for that test result

T+ (or −) = Test result ("+" diseased, "−" not diseased)

D+ (or −) = Disease status ("+" disease, "−" not diseased)

P = Probability of test result

From this equation the slope associated with the ideal operating point on the ROC curve might be derived [24]:

$$\text{Optimal operating point} = \frac{P(\mathrm{D-})}{P(\mathrm{D+})} \times \frac{[C_{\mathrm{FP}} - C_{\mathrm{TN}}]}{[C_{\mathrm{FN}} - C_{\mathrm{TP}}]} \qquad (13.4.1)$$

Note that this is structured as a cost-effectiveness problem, without utility being considered. Thus, the patient's preference for treatment would not be considered unless it can be quantified (one alternative would be to use a net health benefit approach to characterizing the benefit of treatment [58], but this approach has not been previously considered in identifying the optimal point on the ROC curve). The consequence of this is that the "ideal" point thus identified is addressing a Level 4 efficacy question by improving the clinician's therapeutic thinking, and thus may not be meeting the goals of the patient or society addressed in Levels 5 and 6.

Summary

In addressing probability and the principles of diagnostic certainty associated with medical imaging in this chapter, we have in essence described the science of clinical decision making, of which medical imaging is only one component. In recent years this has come under the rubric of Evidence-Based Clinical Practice (EBCP). EBCP is an approach to health care practice that explicitly acknowledges the evidence that bears on each patient management decision, the strength of that evidence, the benefits and risk of alternative management strategies, and the role of patients' values and preferences in trading off those benefits and risks. Having the evidence assists the clinician, the health policymaker, and patients to know what to do, to do what is known, and to understand what is done.

For the clinician, the best sources of evidence will be found in the published literature under such titles as *systematic reviews*, *meta-analysis*, and practice and procedure guidelines published and promulgated by professional medical organizations. An excellent example of a publication that addresses standardization on reporting of studies of diagnostic accuracy, the STARD Initiative [59], provides a comprehensive summary of those facets of reporting that will allow readers to assess the potential for bias in the study and evaluate its generalizability. The article developed by a multinational group of experts provides a foundation of reporting in medical journals on studies of diagnostic accuracy that should prove to be highly advantageous to the clinician, the researcher, reviewers, journals, and the patient.

References

1. Sackett DL, Haynes RB, Guyatt GH, Tugwell PX. Clinical Epidemiology: A Basic Science for Clinical Medicine, 2nd edn. Boston: Little, Brown, 1991.
2. Guyatt GH, Haynes RB, Jaeschke R, et al. Users' guide to the medical literature – XXV. Evidence-based medicine: principles for applying the users' guide to patient care. JAMA 2000;284(10):1290–1296.
3. Valk PE. Randomized controlled trials are not appropriate for imaging technology evaluation. J Nucl Med 2000;41(7):1125–1126.
4. Ransohoff DF, Feinstein AR. Problems of spectrum and bias in evaluating the efficacy of diagnostic tests. NEJM 1978;299(17):926–930.
5. Lachs MS, Nachamkin I, Edelstein PH, Goldman J, Feinstein AR, Schwartz JS. Spectrum bias in the evaluation of diagnostic tests: lessons from the rapid dipstick test for urinary tract infection. Ann Intern Med 1992;117(2):135–140.
6. Diamond GA. How accurate is SPECT thallium scintigraphy? J Am Coll Cardiol 1990;16(4):1017–1021.
7. Mulherin SA, Miller WC. Spectrum bias of spectrum effect? Subgroup variation in diagnostic test evaluation. Ann Intern Med 2002;137(7):598–602.
8. Kymes SM, Lee K, Fletcher JW. Improving studies of diagnostic tests: a case study from Department of Veterans Affairs Cooperative Study #027 (SNAP) – a study of positron emission tomography (FDG-PET) imaging in patients with solitary pulmonary nodules. Clin Trials 2005; Under Review.
9. Babu AN, Kymes SM, Carpenter-Fryer SM. Eponyms and the diagnosis of aortic regurgitation: what says the evidence? Ann Intern Med 2003;138(9):736–742.
10. Jaeschke RZ, Guyatt GH, Sackett DL. Users' guides to the medical literature: III. How to use an article about a diagnostic test: A. Are the results of the study valid? JAMA 1994;271(5):389–391.
11. Sox HC, Blatt MA, Higgins MC, Marton KI. Medical Decision Making. Boston: Butterworth-Heinemann, 1988.
12. Whiting P, Rutjes AWS, Reitsma JB, Glas AS, Bossuyt PM, Kleijnen J. Sources of variation and bias in studies of diagnostic accuracy: a systematic review. Ann Intern Med 2004;140(1):189–202.
13. Reid MC, Lachs MS, Feinstein AR. Use of methodological standards in diagnostic test research: getting better, but still not good. JAMA 1995;274(8):645–651.
14. Zhou X-H, Obuchowski NA, McClish DK. Statistical Methods in Diagnostic Medicine. New York: Wiley, 2002.
15. Kosinski AS, Barnhart HX. Accounting for nonignorable verification bias in assessment of diagnostic tests. Biometrics 2003;59:163–171.
16. Shaw LK, Pryor DB. Sensitivity and specificity of the history and physical examination for coronary artery disease (letter, comment). Ann Intern Med 1994;120(4):344–345.
17. Begg CB, Greenes RA. Assessment of diagnostic tests when disease verification is subject to selection bias. Biometrics 1983;39:207–215.
18. Kent DL, Haynor DR, Larson EB, Deyo RA. Diagnosis of lumbar spinal stenosis in adults: a metaanalysis of the accuracy of CT, MR, and Myelography. AJR 1992;158:1135–1144.
19. Investigators P. Value of the ventilation perfusion scan in acute pulmonary embolism: results of the prospective investigation of pulmonary embolism diagnosis (PIOPED). JAMA 1990;263:2753–2759.
20. Kent DL, Haynor DR, Longstreth WT, Larson EB. The clinical efficacy of magnetic resonance imaging in neuroimaging. Ann Intern Med 1994;120(10):856–871.
21. Kent DL, Larson EB. Magnetic resonance imaging of the brain and spine: is clinical efficacy established after the first decade? Ann Intern Med 1988;108(3):402–424.
22. Lijmer JG, Mol BW, Heisterkamp S, et al. Empirical evidence of design related bias in studies of diagnostic tests. JAMA 1999;282(11):1061–1066.
23. Hanley JA, McNeil BJ. The Meaning and use of the area under a receiver operating characteristic (ROC) curve. Radiology 1982;143:29–36.
24. Metz CE. Basic principles of ROC analysis. Sem Nuc Med 1978;8(4):283–298.
25. Dorfman DD, Alf E. Maximum likelihood estimations of parameters of signal detection theory and determination of confidence intervals. Rating method data. J Math Psychol 1969;6:487–496.
26. Metz CE, Herman BA, Roe CA. Statistical comparison of two roc-curve estimates obtained from partially-paired datasets. Med Decis Making 1998;18(1):110–121.
27. Lowe VJ, Fletcher JW, Gobar L, et al. Prospective investigation of postiron emission tomography in lung nodules. J Clin Oncol 1998;16(3):1075–1084.
28. Cook DJ, Mulrow CD, Haynes RB. Systematic reviews: synthesis of best evidence for clincal decisions. Ann Intern Med 1997;126(5):376–380.
29. Newcombe RG. Two-sided confidence intervals for the single proportion: comparison of seven methods. Stat Med 1998;17:857–872.
30. Fleiss JL. Statistical Methods for Rates and Proportions. New York: Wiley, 1973.
31. Simel DL, Samsa GP, Matchar DB. Likelihood ratios with confidence: sample size estimation for diagnostic test studies. J Clin Epidemiol 1991;44(8):763–770.
32. Egger M, Schneider M, Smith GD. Meta-analysis: spurious precision? Meta-analysis of observational studies. BMJ 1998;316:140–144.
33. Pettiti DB. Meta-Analysis, Decision Analysis, and Cost-Effectiveness Analysis: Methods for Quantitative Synthesis in Medicine, vol 24. New York: Oxford University Press, 1994.
34. Lau J, Ioannidis JPA, Schmid CH. Quantitative synthesis in systematic reviews. Ann Intern Med 1997;127(9):820–826.
35. Bailer JC. Passive smoking, coronary heart disease, and meta-analysis (editorial). NEJM 1999;340(12):958–959.
36. Thompson SG. Why sources of heterogeniety in meta-analysis should be investigated. BMJ 1994;309:1351–1355.
37. Fleischmann KE, Hunink MGM, Kuntz KM, Douglas PS. Exercise echocardiography or exercise SPECT imaging? A meta-analysis of diagnostic test performance. JAMA 1998;280(10):913–920.
38. Kymes SM, Fletcher JW, Shaw L, Bruns D, Gillespie KN. Anatomy of a meta-analysis: a critical review of "Exercise echocardiography or exercise SPECT imaging? A meta-analysis of diagnostic test performance." (Letter, comment). J Nuc Cardiol 2002;9(1):133–134.
39. Littenberg B, Moses LE. Estimating diagnostic accuracy from multiple conflicting reports: a new meta-analytic method. Med Decis Making. 1993;13(4):313–321.

40. Fryback DG, Thornbury JR. The efficacy of diagnostic imaging. Med Decis Making. 1991;11(2):88–94.
41. Tsushima Y, Aoki J, Endo K. Contribution of the diagnostic test to the physician's diagnostic thinking: new method to evaluate the effect. Acad Radiol 2003;10(7):751–755.
42. Eisenberg JM. Ten lessons for evidence-based technology assessment. JAMA 1999;282(19):1865–1869.
43. Gold MR, Siegel JE, Russell LB, Weinstein MC. Cost-Effectiveness in Health and Medicine. New York: Oxford University Press, 1996.
44. Drummond MF, O'Brien B, Stoddart GL, Torrance GW. Methods for the Economic Evaluation of Health Care Programmes, 2nd edn. Oxford: Oxford University Press, 1997.
45. Drummond MF, Richardson WS, O'Brien B, Levine M, Heyland DK. Users' guides to the medical literature: XIII. How to use an article on economic analysis of clinical practice A. Are the results of the study valid? JAMA 1997;277(19):1552–1556.
46. McHorney CA, Ware JE, Lu JFR, Sherbourne CD. The MOS 36-item short-form health survey (SF-36): III. Tests of data quality, scaling assumptions, and reliability across diverse patient groups. Med Care 1994;32(1):40–66.
47. Bergner M. Quality of life, health status, and clinical research. Med Care 1989;27 (3 Suppl):S148–156.
48. Kymes SM, Walline JJ, Zadnik K, Gordon MO. Quality of life in keratoconus: baseline findings from the Collaborative Longitudinal Evaluation of Keratoconus (CLEK) Study. Am J Ophthalmol 2004;138(4):527–535.
49. Torrance GW, Feeny DH. Utilities and quality adjusted life years. Int J Technol Assess Health Care 1989;5:559–575.
50. Torrance GW. Social preferences for health states: an empirical evaluation of three measurement techniques. Soc Sci Med 1976;10:129–136.
51. Kymes SM, Frick KD. Value based medicine: let's get it right (letter). Br J Ophthalmol 2005;89(5):643–644.
52. Laupacis A, Feeny D, Detsky AS, Tugwell P. Tentative guidelines for using clinical and economic evaluations revisited. CMAJ 1993;148(6):927–929.
53. Gillick MR. Medicare coverage for technological innovations – time for new criteria? NEJM 2004;350(21):2199–2203.
54. Ubel PA, Hirth RA, Chernew ME, Fendrick AM. What is the price of life and why doesn't it increase with the rate of inflation? Arch Intern Med 2003;163:1637–1641.
55. Metz CE, Goodenough DJ, Rossmann K. Evaluation of receiver operating characteristic curve data in terms of information theory, and applications in radiography. Radiology 1973;109:297–303.
56. Phelps CE, Mushlin AI. Focusing technology assessment using medical decision theory. Med Decis Making 1988;8(4):279–289.
57. Hunink MGM, Kuntz KM, Fleischmann KE, Brady TJ. Noninvasive imaging for the diagnosis of coronary artery disease: focusing the development of new diagnostic technology. Ann Intern Med 1999;131(9):673–680.
58. Stinnett AA, Mullahy J. Net health benefits: a new framework for the analysis of uncertainty in cost-effectiveness analysis. Med Decis Making 1998;18(2 Suppl):S68–S80.
59. Bossuyt PM, Reitsma JB, Bruns DE, Gatsonis CA, et al. Towards complete and accurate reporting of studies of diagnosstici accuracy: the STARD Initiative. Ann Intern Med 2003;138:40–44

Chapter 14
Principles of Medical Imaging in the Diagnosis and Staging of the Cancer Patient

Anthony F. Shields

Staging of cancer involves determining the extent of tumor spread; this provides predictive information that is critical in assessing prognosis independent of treatment effects and choosing the best therapy. This information is obtained with a combination of physical exam, laboratory studies, imaging, and pathology. One of the first regular uses of staging was in the assessment and treatment of breast cancer. It was noted that the progression and spread of breast cancer was initially manifest as local involvement, followed by appearance in the axillary lymph nodes, and subsequently to other organs. Halstead used this information to develop his surgical approach including the primary tumor and draining nodes within the then standard radical mastectomy. More recent studies have demonstrated that the removal of axillary lymph nodes is more important for predicting survival, rather than of direct therapeutic importance. This surgical approach has been applied to many, but not all, tumor types and over time has led to the standardization of the staging with international agreement on the elements of staging and study of its implications. As indicated above, it was understood early on that the extent of the local tumor, its spread to lymph nodes, and evidence of metastases all were important considerations in staging. Around 1940, the efforts of Denoix led to the formal incorporation of these elements into the TNM (tumor-nodes-metastases) staging system [1]. For example, depending on the cancer being studied, each of these elements is graded from one to four. These elements are then combined to determine an overall stage, varying between I and IV; designating local involvement up to distant spread [2]. While the exact staging criteria varies from tumor to tumor and undergoes occasional revision, as will be discussed, general principals make communication and understanding between physicians more rapid and succinct.

A.F. Shields (✉)
Department of Internal Medicine, Karmanos Cancer Institute, Wayne State University, 4100 John R St., HWCRC, Detroit, MI, 48201-2013, USA
e-mail: ShieldsA@Karmanos.org

TNM Staging

T stage describes the local tumor and includes elements describing the local extent of invasion and tumor size. Lesions that show histologic changes typical of cancer without evidence of invasion into surrounding tissues are generally described as Tis (carcinoma in situ). In this situation, if there is no spread to nodes or elsewhere in the body, the stage would be TisN0M0. For tumors of epithelial origin, such lesions are usually curable with simple surgical removal. T1 lesions have begun to invade the surrounding normal tissue, with the depth of invasion and size of the lesion differentiating T1, T2, and T3 lesions (Tables 14.1, 14.2, and 14.3). For example, in breast cancer an invasive lesion of less than 2 cm in diameter is termed T1, a T2 lesion is from 2 cm up to 5 cm, and a lesion of greater than 5 cm is T3. If the lesion extends to the skin or chest wall it is termed T4. Invasion into adjacent normal organs that are continuous with the primary tumor are generally defined as T4, even if the lesion is smaller in size. For breast cancer this includes involvement of the skin or chest wall. It should be noted that the pattern of invasion and spread needs to be carefully considered for each tumor type and it depends on the tissue of origin and the normal structures. In the case of colon cancer, which arises in the superficial epithelium of the bowel, the depth of penetration of the tumor through the normal histologic layers of the intestine determines T stage. For example, T1 lesions invade through the muscularis mucosa, but not into the muscularis propria, while T2 lesions invade into the muscularis propria. T3 lesions in the colon invade through the complete bowel wall into the surrounding adipose tissue. Size is not included in the staging criteria for colon cancer, although depth of invasion correlates with size. From this example one can see that while T stage is based on tumor anatomy, it is not always determined by a CT or MR procedure. One usually needs pathology to accurately judge the depth of invasion for colon cancer. At times, an estimate of tumor depth can be obtained in rectal cancer using endoscopic ultrasound (EUS). Such information is often used in deciding if a patient should receive pre-operative treatment.

P. Shreve and D.W. Townsend (eds.), *Clinical PET-CT in Radiology: Integrated Imaging in Oncology*,
DOI 10.1007/978-0-387-48902-5_14,

Table 14.1 American Joint Committee on Cancer TNM staging of breast cancer (From Ref. [2]. With permission)

TX	Primary tumor cannot be assessed
T0	No evidence of primary tumor
Tis	Carcinoma in situ
Tis (DCIS)	Ductal carcinoma in situ
Tis (LCIS)	Lobular carcinoma in situ
Tis (Paget's)	Paget's disease of the nipple NOT associated with invasive carcinoma and/or carcinoma in situ (DCIS and/or LCIS) in the underlying breast parenchyma. Carcinomas in the breast parenchyma associated with Paget's disease are categorized based on the size and characteristics of the parenchymal disease, although the presence of Paget's disease should still be noted.
T1	Tumor ≤ 20 mm in greatest dimension
	T1mi Tumor ≤ 1 mm in greatest dimension
	T1a Tumor >1 mm but ≤ 5 mm in greatest dimension
	T1b Tumor >5 mm but ≤ 10 mm in greatest dimension
	T1c Tumor >10 mm but ≤ 20 mm in greatest dimension
T2	Tumor >20 mm but ≤ 50 mm in greatest dimension
T3	Tumor >50 mm in greatest dimension
T4	Tumor of any size with direct extension to the chest wall and/or to the skin (ulceration or skin nodules). Note: Invasion of the dermis alone does not qualify as T4.
	T4a Extension to the chest wall, not including only pectoralis muscle adherence/invasion
	T4b Ulceration and/or ipsilateral satellite nodules and/or edema (including peau d'orange) of the skin which do not meet the criteria for inflammatory carcinoma
	T4c Both T4a and T4b
	T4d Inflammatory carcinoma (see Rules for Classification)
Regional lymph nodes (N)	
Clinical	
NX	Regional lymph nodes cannot be assessed (e.g., previously removed)
N0	No regional lymph node metastases
N1	Metastases to movable ipsilateral level I, II axillary lymph node(s)
N2	Metastases in ipsilateral level I, II axillary lymph nodes that are clinically fixed or matted; or in clinically detected[a] ipsilateral internal mammary nodes in the *absence* of clinically evident axillary lymph node metastases
	N2a Metastases in ipsilateral axillary lymph nodes fixed to one another (matted) or to other structures
	N2b Metastases only in clinically detected[a] ipsilateral internal mammary nodes and in the *absence* of clinically evident axillary lymph node metastases
N3	Metastases in ipsilateral infraclavicular (level III axillary) lymph node(s) with or without level I, II axillary lymph node involvement; or in clinically detected[a] ipsilateral internal mammary lymph node(s) with clinically evident level I, II axillary lymph node metastases; or metastases in ipsilateral supraclavicular lymph node(s) with or without axillary or internal mammary lymph node involvement
	N3a Metastases in ipsilateral infraclavicular lymph node(s)
	N3b Metastases in ipsilateral internal mammary lymph node(s) and axillary lymph node(s)
	N3c Metastases in ipsilateral supraclavicular lymph node(s)
Pathologic (pN)[b]	
pNX	Regional lymph nodes cannot be assessed (e.g., previously removed, or not removed for pathologic study)
pN0	No regional lymph node metastasis identified histologically
	Note: Isolated tumor cell clusters (ITC) are defined as small clusters of cells not greater than 0.2 mm, or single tumor cells, or a cluster of fewer than 200 cells in a single histologic cross-section. ITCs may be detected by routine histology or by immunohistochemical (IHC) methods. Nodes containing only ITCs are excluded from the total positive node count for purposes of N classification but should be included in the total number of nodes evaluated.
	pN0(i−) No regional lymph node metastases histologically, negative IHC
	pN0(i+) Malignant cells in regional lymph node(s) no greater than 0.2 mm (detected by H&E or IHC including ITC)
	pN0(mol−) No regional lymph node metastases histologically, negative molecular findings (RT-PCR)
	pN0(mol+) Positive molecular findings (RT-PCR),[c] but no regional lymph node metastases detected by histology or IHC
pN1	Micrometastases; or metastases in 1–3 axillary lymph nodes; and/or in internal mammary nodes with metastases detected by sentinel lymph node biopsy but not clinically detected[d]
	pN1mi Micrometastases (greater than 0.2 mm and/or more than 200 cells, but none greater than 2.0 mm)
	pN1a Metastases in 1–3 axillary lymph nodes, at least one metastasis greater than 2.0 mm
	pN1b Metastases in internal mammary nodes with micrometastases or macrometastases detected by sentinel lymph node biopsy but not clinically detected[d]
	pN1c Metastases in 1–3 axillary lymph nodes and in internal mammary lymph nodes with micrometastases or macrometastases detected by sentinel lymph node biopsy but not clinically detected

(continued)

Table 14.1 (continued)

pN2	Metastases in 4–9 axillary lymph nodes; or in clinically detected[e] internal mammary lymph nodes in the *absence* of axillary lymph node metastases
	pN2a Metastases in 4–9 axillary lymph nodes (at least one tumor deposit greater than 2.0 mm)
	pN2b Metastases in clinically detected[e] internal mammary lymph nodes in the *absence* of axillary lymph node metastases
pN3	Metastases in 10 or more axillary lymph nodes; or in infraclavicular (level III axillary) lymph nodes; or in clinically detected[e] ipsilateral internal mammary lymph nodes in the *presence* of 1 or more positive level I, II axillary lymph nodes; or in more than 3 axillary lymph nodes and in internal mammary lymph nodes with micrometastases or macrometastases detected by sentinel lymph node biopsy but not clinically detected[d]; or in ipsilateral supraclavicular lymph nodes
	pN3a Metastases in 10 or more axillary lymph nodes (at least one tumor deposit greater than 2.0 mm); or metastases to the infraclavicular (level III axillary lymph) nodes
	pN3b Metastases in clinically detected[e] ipsilateral internal mammary lymph nodes in the *presence* of 1 or more positive axillary lymph nodes; or in more than 3 axillary lymph nodes and in internal mammary lymph nodes with micrometastases or macrometastases detected by sentinel lymph node biopsy but not clinically detected[d]
	pN3c Metastases in ipsilateral supraclavicular lymph nodes
Distant metastases (M)	
M0	No clinical or radiographic evidence of distant metastases
	cM0(i+) No clinical or radiographic evidence of distant metastases, but deposits of molecularly or microscopically detected tumor cells in circulating blood, bone marrow or other non-regional nodal tissue that are no larger than 0.2 mm in a patient without symptoms or signs of metastases
M1	Distant detectable metastases as determined by classic clinical and radiographic means and/or histologically proven larger than 0.2 mm

Anatomic stage • Prognostic groups			
Stage IA	T1[f]	N0	M0
Stage IB	T0	N1mi	M0
	T1[f]	N1mi	M0
Stage IIA	T0	N1[g]	M0
	T1[f]	N1[g]	M0
	T2	N0	M0
Stage IIB	T2	N1	M0
	T3	N0	M0
Stage IIIA	T0	N2	M0
	T1[f]	N2	M0
	T2	N2	M0
	T3	N1	M0
	T3	N2	M0
Stage IIIB	T4	N0	M0
	T4	N1	M0
	T4	N2	M0
Stage IIIC	Any T	N3	M0
Stage IV	Any T	Any N	M1

See further categorization in the American Joint Committee on Cancer staging guidelines [2]

[a] *Clinically detected* is defined as detected by imaging studies (excluding lymphoscintigraphy) or by clinical examination and having characteristics highly suspicious for malignancy or a presumed pathologic macrometastasis based on fine needle aspiration biopsy with cytologic examination. Confirmation of clinically detected metastatic disease by fine needle aspiration without excision biopsy is designated with an (f) suffix, e.g., cN3a(f). Excisional biopsy of a lymph node or biopsy of a sentinel node, in the absence of assignment of a pT, is classified as a clinical N, e.g., cN1. Information regarding the confirmation of the nodal status will be designated in site-specific factors as clinical, fine needle aspiration, core biopsy, or sentinel lymph node biopsy. Pathologic classification (pN) is used for excision or sentinel lymph node biopsy only in conjunction with a pathologic T assignment

[b] Classification is based on axillary lymph node dissection with or without sentinel lymph node biopsy. Classification based solely on sentinel lymph node biopsy without subsequent axillary lymph node dissection is designated (sn) for "sentinel node," e.g., pN0(sn)

[c] RT-PCR: reverse transcriptase/polymerase chain reaction

[d] *Not clinically detected* is defined as not detected by imaging studies (excluding lymphoscintigraphy) or not detected by clinical examination

[e] *Clinically detected* is defined as detected by imaging studies (excluding lymphoscintigraphy) or by clinical examination and having characteristics highly suspicious for malignancy or a presumed pathologic macrometastasis based on fine needle aspiration biopsy with cytologic examination

(continued)

Table 14.1 (continued)

[f] T1 includes T1mi.

[g] T0 and T1 tumors with nodal micrometastases only are excluded from Stage IIA and are classified Stage IB.

• M0 includes M0(i+)

• The designation pM0 is not valid; any M0 should be clinical

• If a patient presents with M1 prior to neoadjuvant systemic therapy, the stage is considered stage IV, and remains stage IV regardless of response to neoadjuvant therapy

• Stage designation may be changed if postsurgical imaging studies reveal the presence of distant metastases, provided that the studies are carried out within 4 months of diagnosis in the absence of disease progression and provided that the patient has not received neoadjuvant therapy

• Postneoadjuvant therapy is designated with "yc" or "yp" prefix. Of note, no stage group is assigned if there is a complete response (CR) to neoadjuvant therapy, e.g., ypT0ypN0cM0

Table 14.2 American Joint Committee on Cancer TNM staging of colon cancer (From Ref. [2]. With permission)

TNM classification	Description
Tis	Carcinoma in situ
T1	Tumor invades submucosa
T2	Tumor invades muscularis propria
T3	Tumor invades through the muscularis propria into the subserosa, or into nonperitonealized pericolic or perirectal tissues
T4	Tumor perforates the visceral peritoneum or directly invades other organs or structures
N1	Metastasis in 1–3 regional lymph nodes
N2	Metastasis in ≥ 4 regional lymph nodes
M0	No distant metastasis
M1	Distant metastasis present

Stage grouping of colon cancer

	Primary tumor (T)	Regional lymph nodes (N)	Distant metastases (M)
0	Tis	N0	M0
I	T1	N0	M0
	T2	N0	M0
IIA	T3	N0	M0
IIB	T4	N0	M0
IIIA	T1–T2	N1	M0
IIIB	T3–T4	N1	M0
IIIC	Any T	N2	M0
IV	Any T	Any N	M1

See further categorization in the American Joint Committee on Cancer staging guidelines [2]

Definitions of TNM

The same classification is used for both clinical and pathologic staging.

Primary tumor (T)

TX	Primary tumor cannot be assessed
T0	No evidence of primary tumor
Tis	Carcinoma in situ: intraepithelial or invasionof lamina propria[a]
T1	Tumor invades submucosa
T2	Tumor invades muscularis propria
T3	Tumor invades pericolorectal tissues
T4a	Tumor penetrates the visceral peritoneum[b]
T4b	Tumor directly invades or is adherent to other organs or structures[b,c]

(continued)

Table 14.2 (continued)

Regional lymph nodes (N)	
NX	Regional lymph nodes cannot be assed
N0	Regional lymph node metastasis
N1	Metastasis in 1 ro 3 regional lymph nodes
N1a	Metastasis in 1 regional lymph node
N1b	Metastasis in 2–3 regional lymph nodes
N1c	Tumor deposit(s) in the subserosa, or nonperitonealized pericolic or perirectal tissues without regional nodal metastasis
N2	Metastasis in 4 or more regional lymph nodes
N2a	Metastasis in 4–6 regional lymph nodes
N2b	Metastasis in 7 or more regional lymph nodes

Note: A satellite peritumoral nodule in the pericolorectal adipose tissue of a primary carcinoma without histologic evidence of residual lymph node in the nodule may represent discontinuous spread, venous invasion with extravascular spread (V1/2) or a totally replaced lymph node (N1/2). Replaced nodes should be counted separately as positive nodes in the N category, whereas discontinuous spread or venous invasion should be classified and counted in the Site-Specific Factor category Tumor Deposits (TD).

Distant metastasis (M)	
M0	No distant Metastasis
M1	Distant Metastasis
M1a	Metastasis confined to one organ or site (e.g., liver, lung, ovary, nonregional node)
M1b	Metastases in more than one organ/site or the peritoneum

Anatomic stage • Prognostic groups

Stage	T	N	M	Dukes[d]	MAC[d]
0	Tis	N0	M0	–	–
I	T1	N0	M0	A	A
T2	N0	M0	A	B1	
IIA	T3	N0	M0	B	B2
IIB	T4a	N0	M0	B	B2
IIC	T4b	N0	M0	B	B3
IIIA	T1–T2	N1	M0	C	C1
	T1	N2a	M0	C	C1
IIIB	T3–T4a	N1	M0	C	C2
	T2–T3	N2a	M0	C	C1/C2
	T1–T2	N2b	M0	C	C1
IIIC	T4a	N2a	M0	C	C2
	T3–T4a	N2b	M0	C	C2
	T4b	N1-N2	M0	C	C3
IVA	Any T	Any N	M1a	–	–
IVB	Any T	Any N	M1b	–	–

cTNM is the clinical classification, pTNM is the pathologic classification. The y prefix is used for those cancers that are classified after neoadjuvant pretreatment (e.g., ypTNM). Patients who have a complete pathologic response are ypT0N0cM0 that may be similar to Stage Group 0 or I. The r prefix is to be used for those cancers that have recurred after a disease-free interval (rTNM)

[a]Tis includes cancer cells confined within the glandular basement membrane (intraepithelial) or mucosal lamina propria (intramucosal) with no extension through the muscularis mucosae into the submucosa

[b]Direct invasion in T4 includes invasion of other organs or other segments of the colorectum as a result of direct extension through the serosa, as confirmed on microscopic examination (for example, invasion of the sigmoid colon by a carcinoma of the cecum) or, for cancers in a retroperitoneal or subperitoneal location, direct invasion of other organs or structures by virtue of extension beyond the muscularis propria (i.e., respectively, a tumor on the posterior wall of the descending colon invading the left kidney or lateral abdominal wall; or a mid or distal rectal cancer with invasion of prostate, seminal vesicles, cervix, or vagina)

[c]Tumor that is adherent to other organs or structures, grossly, is classified cT4b. However, if no tumor is present in the adhesion, microscopically, the classification should be pT1-3 depending on the anatomical depth of wall invasion. The V and L classifications should be used to identify the presence or absence of vascular or lymphatic invasion whereas the PN site-specific factor should be used for perineural invasion

[d]Dukes B is a composite of better (T3 N0 M0) and worse (T4 N0 M0) prognostic groups, as is Dukes C (any TN1 M0 and Any T N2 M0). MAC is the modified Astler-Coller classification

Table 14.3 American Joint Committee on Cancer TNM Staging of Lung Cancer[a] (From Ref. [2]. With permission)

Primary tumor	
Tis	Carcinoma in situ
T1	Tumor 3 cm or less in greatest dimension surrounded by lung or visceral pleura without bronchoscopic evidence of invasion more proximal than the lobar bronchus (i.e., not in the main bronchus)
T2	Tumor with any of the following features of size or extent: More than 3 cm in greatest dimension Involves main bronchus 2 cm or more distal to the carina Invades the visceral pleura Associated with atelectasis or obstructive pneumonitis that extends to the hilar region but does not involve the entire lung
T3	Tumor of any size that directly invades any of the following: Chest wall (including superior sulcus tumors), diaphragm, mediastinal pleura, parietal pericardium Tumor in the main bronchus less than 2 cm distal to the carina, but without involvement of the carina Associated atelectasis or obstructive pneumonitis of the entire lung
T4	Tumor of any size that invades any of the following: mediastinum, heart, great vessels, trachea, esophagus, vertebral body, carina; or separate tumor nodules in the same lobe; or tumor with malignant pleural effusion
Regional lymph nodes	
N1	Metastasis to ipsilateral peribronchial and/or ipsilateral hilar lymph nodes, and intrapulmonary nodes including involvement by direct extension of the primary tumor
N2	Metastasis to ipsilateral mediastinal and/or subcarinal lymph nodes
N3	Metastasis to contralateral mediastinal, contralateral hilar, ipsilateral or contralateral scalene, or supraclavicular lymph nodes
Distant metastasis	
M1	Distant metastasis present

Stage grouping			
Occult Carcinoma	TX	N0	M0
Stage 0	Tis	N0	M0
Stage IA	T1	N0	M0
Stage IB	T2	N0	M0
Stage IIA	T1	N1	M0
Stage IIB	T2	N1	M0
	T3	N0	M0
Stage IIIA	T1	N2	M0
	T2	N2	M0
	T3	N1	M0
	T3	N2	M0
Stage IIIB	Any T	N3	M0
	T4	Any N	M0
Stage IV	Any T	Any N	M1

[a] See further categorization in the American Joint Committee on Cancer staging guidelines

On the other end of the spectrum is Hodgkin's lymphoma, which is often limited to the lymph nodes with less likelihood of local invasion. In this tumor the TNM staging system is not used; rather the separate Ann Arbor system has been developed, which takes into account the pattern of lymph node involvement along with other organ spread.

Nodal or N stage denotes the involvement and extent of tumor bearing lymph nodes. The definition varies with tumor type and takes into account the usual pattern or spread and often includes information about the size and number of involved nodes. For example, in breast cancer N1 includes ipsilateral nodes that are movable, while if the nodes are fixed to each other or nearby structures they are N2. N3 is reserved for spread to ipsilateral internal mammary nodes. Staging of lung cancer is similar in that the location of involved nodes is crucial in assessing N stage and size is not directly included. On the other hand, the staging system for colon cancer now simply denotes those with three or fewer involved regional nodes as being N1, while four or more nodes are described as N2. Location of the nodes is not considered since all mesenteric nodes within the specimen are judged similarly. Clearly one limitation of such a system is that the number of lymph nodes recovered for analysis may vary with the aggressiveness of the clinical and pathologic examination.

It should be noted that for each of these solid tumors, lymph nodes outside of the region defined by the specific staging system are judged as having widespread metastatic involvement, as if they had distant organ spread. Spread to certain local nodes is called metastatic according to the standard definition of the term, as the noncontiguous tumor growth arises from the primary tumor. Such patients are not considered to have distant metastases and are defined as M0 within the TNM system. Metastatic spread to more distant lymph nodes and other organs is defined as present (M1). Physicians often speak of a cancer as being locoregional in nature. While this term is not strictly defined in common usage, it generally means that the tumor does not have distant metastases. It does not necessarily mean that the tumor is resectable. For example, pancreatic cancer invading the mesenteric artery would be clinically considered locoregional, staged as M0, but the tumor can't be surgically removed.

Clinical and Pathologic Staging

The information on tumor extent, nodal spread, and metastases (TNM) are combined to describe the overall stage. Stage I generally includes small tumors with limited local invasion, while stage II tumors are larger or have a greater extent of local invasions. Stage III disease generally includes spread to regional lymph nodes while distant spread is categorized as stage IV.

The TNM staging system takes into account the level of evidence of spread of the tumor differentiating the extent of disease as determined by physical exam and imaging studies from that determined by pathologic examination of the tumor, nodes, and distant sites. While the diagnosis of cancer clearly requires pathologic confirmation, the extent of tumor spread may be based on pathologic or imaging evidence of tumor spread. Over the last decades cross-sectional imaging with CT and MR has clearly added to our evaluation of patient stage. More recently, PET and PET-CT have been found to bring new information that is valuable in assessing patient stage. The integration of such techniques into routine clinical care continues as more information is gained [3]. The primary treating physician, taking into account all the clinical, imaging, and pathologic information, generally determines the actual determination of tumor stage. At most cancer centers a form that details the TNM staging information is filled out for each new patient. While imaging clearly contributes to the overall stage, the actual stage determination may take into account follow up findings needed to verify the results. Even the pathology report alone may not provide a complete picture of the patient's stage. For example, resection of the primary tumor in a patient with colon cancer may indicate that a patient has local lymph node involvement (stage III), but the pathologist may not be aware of image results showing evidence of distant metastases.

When a patient has evidence of recurrent disease they are restaged. Once again all available evidence from the clinical exam, laboratory studies, imaging results, and pathology are combined to determine the extent of disease. The same forms are used for staging as done for the initial diagnosis, but there is a place to indicate that the staging is being done after initial treatment. Unfortunately, the recurrence is often to a distant site and the patient will be stage IV. The TNM staging is frequently indicated as TxNxM1 in such a situation, since no information is available (or needed) about the local tumor and lymph nodes.

Limitations of TNM Staging

The overall goal of TNM staging is to assist in providing prognostic information that is useful in making therapeutic decisions. As treatment advances, the therapeutic options can change altering prognosis and resulting in suggestions that eventually lead to changes in the staging criteria. For example, the present TNM staging for proximal cholangiocarcinoma of the extrahepatic biliary ducts describes patients with tumors invading adjacent organs, such as the liver, as having T3 lesions, which are classified as stage IVa. This becomes stage IVb if distant metastases are present. These staging criteria made sense before the surgical resection of part of the liver was routinely done. Today, such a staging system makes less sense when involvement of either the right or left hepatic duct can be surgically treated with curative intent by partial hepatectomy, while bilateral liver involvement would preclude surgery short of transplantation. New staging schemes that take such differences into account have been proposed for cholangiocarcinoma [4]. While PET/CT may assist in appropriately identifying such situations, clearly the greater problem is the appearance of unexpected metastases in patients with cholangiocarcinomas, as it is in other tumor types [5, 6].

Staging Issues with New Technology

"When the Okies left Oklahoma and moved to California they raised the average intelligence level in both states." This statement, attributed to Will Rogers, is of importance in its implications for staging and can prove to significantly change treatment results [7]. Stage migration and new diagnostic techniques are sources of misleading statistics for survival in cancer. The role of staging is to group patients with similar types of tumors and risk factors together to assist in better understanding prognosis, limit ambiguity and help treatment selection. The problem pointed out by Will Rogers arises by what has been termed stage migration. If one now divides up a stage grouping using a new approach and thus removes those with the worst prognosis from a given stage, then patients left behind in the previous staging category will overall have a better prognosis (Table 14.4). The more surprising effect is that if such patients are moved into a higher stage, one may also find that the higher-risk patients are also now doing better, since they may have less bulky or aggressive disease than those initially included in the higher category. Simply reformulating the staging criteria too quickly can result in the effect of shifting statistical data that may lead to an inappropriate prognostic conclusion. This was recently demonstrated as a result of changes in the staging system for breast cancer over the last decade [8]. The new 2002 AJCC staging system was compared with the 1988 system by analyzing a group of 1,350 patients, which resulted in moving 54% of the patients with stage IIb disease to stage III. Previously those with any number of positive moveable ipsilateral nodes were classified as N1, while the newer stages changed those with four to nine positive nodes into N2 and hence increased those patients from stage II to stage III [8]. Overall, such changes resulted in increasing the 10 year survival rates for stages II and III from 65% to 76% and from 45% to 50%, respectively.

The use of PET in restaging patients with colon cancer can also produce "improved" results of treatment. Patients with a limited number of liver metastases can have the tumor surgically removed and about 30% survive at 5 years. A recent study has shown that those undergoing surgery after re-staging with PET have about a 58% 5-year survival [9]. This can be attributed to the detection of additional foci of metastatic disease, which preclude surgery. The removal of those with more widespread disease, through the use of PET, produces a surgical group with a better survival rate, thus demonstrating the Will Rogers phenomenon. In this situation, all the patients were stage IV, but PET has been able to further sub-divide these patients into groups of different prognosis.

Improvements in pathologic, molecular biology, and imaging techniques will also result in stage migration. For example, in the assessment of breast cancer, evaluation of axillary lymph nodes with fine sectioning and immunohistochemical staining will find small foci of tumor cells. How to best handle this new type of information is still under study. The staging criteria for breast cancer now categorize nodes that have foci of tumor cells that are less than 0.2 mm as being node negative, but the full implications of such results requires further study. Molecular techniques such as the polymerase chain reaction (PCR) evaluation of tissues have also been done to look for evidence of tumor spread. Notably, this has been done on bone marrow samples in patients with prostate cancer. While one would expect that such an approach would be more sensitive than either routine imaging or even histology, the predictive value of positive marrow findings was surprisingly low; the 2-year disease-free survival was 77.5 % in one series of patients with PCR positive marrow samples. This demonstrates that while a limited number of tumor cells may be present in other locations in the body, this does not prove that such cells are capable of surviving. While new molecular approaches will undoubtedly gain more widespread use because of their sensitivity, knowledge of the presence of macroscopic lesions as detected by PET/CT will also be important. Larger lesions will likely become of greater clinical significance and more predictive of disease progression, but more study is needed to integrate all of these approaches into the routine clinical care of patients with cancer. The optimal utility of staging techniques will vary from tumor to tumor and require sophisticated Bayesian analysis of the available data at each step in the patient's initial staging.

PET-CT Imaging and Staging

Staging with CT, and more recently PET, has become standard in the evaluation of a number of tumor types. PET is now routinely used in the initial evaluation of many patients with lung, esophageal, and head and neck cancers. It is regularly employed with other tumor types in particular clinical situations, such as restaging after initial therapy and suspected recurrence. The more recent advent of combined

Table 14.4 The Will Rogers' effect in action: a theoretic example of how changing stage can affect stage-specific survival[a]

Staging	Initial			Revise staging results	
	Survival	%Survival		Survival	%Survival
II	70/100	70	40% survival	50/60	83
III	30/100	30	50% survival	50/140	36
Overall	100/200	50		100/200	50

[a] This example demonstrates the effect of reclassifying patients who were initially judged as stage II, but using new approaches classified as stage III.

PET/CT scanners has further improved the evaluation of lesions, by combining the images of activity seen with PET with much improved anatomic localization.

The description of data for the utility of PET for staging of each type of cancer is further discussed in the individual chapters, but a couple of examples are worth presenting. PET has gained regular use in the staging of esophageal cancer because the undetected but frequent metastases produced by this tumor led to unnecessary surgery. A recent meta-analysis of 12 studies examining the staging of esophageal cancer with PET found that the sensitivity and specificity for the detection of regional metastases was 0.51 and 0.84, respectively [10]. The limitation of PET in this situation may in part be ascribed to activity in the primary tumor masking the nearby lymph nodes. Lack of specificity may be the result of inflammation in the area of the tumor and the surrounding nodes, leading to FDG uptake. Overall, endoscopic ultrasound (EUS) has been the preferred technique in this situation, since it can assess the penetration of the tumor and enlargement of the local nodes. PET has superior clinical benefit in the assessment of tumor metastases where it has a sensitivity and specificity 0.67 and 0.97, respectively [10]. This includes spread to more distant nodes, including the celiac and cervical areas, as well as other organs. As one would expect, microscopic involvement is often missed with PET, but detected at the time of surgery. The benefit of PET is the detection of tumor that increases the patient stage and provides information for treatment selection more appropriate to the stage. The present staging classification, however, may not take full advantage of all the information now available with PET. For example, in esophageal cancer staged with PET, additional independent prognostic information was obtained when considering the number of PET-positive lymph nodes and length of the tumor as determined by PET [11]. This was most evident in patients with stage III disease, where those with greater than three positive nodes had a particularly poor outcome. The present esophageal staging classification does not take into account the number of involved nodes, but inclusion of this criterion has been proposed [12].

A recent study has retrospectively evaluated the use of PET-CT in the staging of a variety of cancers [13]; mainly lung, head, and neck, and gastrointestinal in origin. Staging was compared using CT alone, PET alone, both modalities read side by side (PET+CT), and using fused images (PET-CT) in 260 patients who were staged using the TNM system. Combined PET-CT was found to be superior, with 84% of patients correctly staged compared with 63% and 64% with CT alone and PET alone, respectively. Fused PET-CT was statistically superior to the two approaches when read side by side (76% accuracy). As one might predict all four approaches did not provide any significant improvement in assessingT stage. N stage was best assessed by PET-CT, even when compared to PET and CT read together. M stage was determined with equal accuracy with both PET-CT and PET + CT. Overall, PET-CT changed patient management 6% of the time compared with PET + CT, and 15% and 17% with either modality alone.

In summary, staging is a critical issue in the evaluation, prognosis, and treatment planning for patients with cancer. Newer imaging techniques play an important role in determining the extent of cancer and the optimal treatment regimen. The recent introduction of PET and PET-CT has been shown to increase the stage of many patients, leading to changes in the treatment plan. Stage migration will lead to improved treatment results, which must be kept in mind when viewing historical data.

References

1. Doll R. The Pierre Denoix Memorial Lecture: nature and nurture in the control of cancer. Eur J Cancer 1999;35(1):16–23.
2. Cancer AJCC. AJCC Cancer Staging Manual, 6th edn. New York: Springer-Verlag, 2002.
3. Gospodarowicz MK, Miller D, Groome PA, Greene FL, Logan PA, Sobin LH. The process for continuous improvement of the TNM classification. Cancer 2004;100(1):1–5.
4. Fong Y, Kemeney N, Lawrence T. Cancer of the liver and biliary tree. In: DeVita Jr VT, Hellman S, Rosenberg SA (eds.). Cancer Principles & Practice of Oncology, 6th edn. Philadelphia: Lippincott Williams & Wilkins, 2001:1182
5. Kluge R, Schmidt F, Caca K, et al. Positron emission tomography with [(18)F]fluoro-2-deoxy-D-glucose for diagnosis and staging of bile duct cancer. Hepatology 2001;33(5):1029–1035.
6. Kim YJ, Yun M, Lee WJ, Kim KS, Lee JD. Usefulness of 18F-FDG PET in intrahepatic cholangiocarcinoma. Eur J Nucl Med Mol Imaging 2003;30(11):1467–1472.
7. Feinstein AR, Sosin DM, Wells CK. The Will Rogers phenomenon. Stage migration and new diagnostic techniques as a source of misleading statistics for survival in cancer. N Engl J Med 1985;312(25): 1604–1608.
8. Woodward WA, Strom EA, Tucker SL, et al. Changes in the 2003 American Joint Committee on Cancer staging for breast cancer dramatically affect stage-specific survival. J Clin Oncol 2003;21(17): 3244–3248.
9. Fernandez FG, Drebin JA, Linehan DC, Dehdashti F, Siegel BA, Strasberg SM. Five-year survival after resection of hepatic metastases from colorectal cancer in patients screened by positron emission tomography with F-18 fluorodeoxyglucose (FDG-PET). Ann Surg 2004;240(3):438–447; discussion 447–450
10. van Westreenen HL, Westerterp M, Bossuyt PM, et al. Systematic review of the staging performance of 18F-fluorodeoxyglucose positron emission tomography in esophageal cancer. J Clin Oncol 2004;22(18):3805–3812.
11. Choi JY, Jang HJ, Shim YM, et al. 18F-FDG PET in patients with esophageal squamous cell carcinoma undergoing curative surgery: prognostic implications. J Nucl Med 2004;45(11):1843–1850.
12. Eloubeidi MA, Desmond R, Arguedas MR, Reed CE, Wilcox CM. Prognostic factors for the survival of patients with esophageal carcinoma in the U.S.: the importance of tumor length and lymph node status. Cancer 2002;95(7):1434–1443
13. Antoch G, Saoudi N, Kuehl H, et al. Accuracy of whole-body dual-modality fluorine-18-2-fluoro-2-deoxy-D-glucose positron emission tomography and computed tomography (FDG-PET/CT) for tumor staging in solid tumors: comparison with CT and PET. J Clin Oncol 2004;22(21):4357–4368.
14. Gao CL, Dean RC, Pinto A, et al. Detection of circulating prostate specific antigen expressing prostatic cells in the bone marrow of radical prostatectomy patients by sensitive reverse transcriptase polymerase chain reaction. J Urol. Apr 1999; 161(4); 1070–1076.

Chapter 15
Principles of PET in Cancer Treatment for the Assessment of Chemotherapy and Radiotherapy Response and for Radiotherapy Treatment Planning

Natalie Charnley, Terry Jones, and Pat Price

PET and Response Assessment

Changes in FDG signal following treatment can give a reflection of cell kill, so making PET more sensitive than MRI or CT. It may also detect an earlier response to treatment. In a study of patients with relapsed high grade glioma, glucose metabolic rate (MRGlu) was assessed following one cycle of chemotherapy. All patients who had a reduction in MRGlu greater than 25% had a subsequent radiologic/clinical response at 8 weeks [1] (Fig. 15.1). ^{11}C-methionine PET has been used to assess response of patients with locally advanced hypopharyngeal cancer following a cycle of Cisplatin/5-FU chemotherapy. The PET response defined by SUV max after 1 cycle of chemotherapy correlated well with the MRI response at the end of three courses of neoadjuvant chemotherapy [2]. The implication of this is that patients who are identified as an early nonresponder may be changed to an alternative treatment.

A particular benefit of PET in response assessment is where standard imaging is confounded by the mode of action of the anticancer therapy. Biologic therapies are often cytostatic rather than cytotoxic, so tumor shrinkage may not be apparent so soon after treatment. As PET can reflect cell kill, this would be a more useful imaging tool than CT or MRI. The rare gastrointestinal stromal tumors (GIST) respond to the biologic therapy imatinib by becoming more cystic, and with a reduction in Hounslow units on CT, rather than shrinking. True responders are often mistaken for nonresponders. The value of PET, CT, and PET-CT has been compared for assessing response of these tumors to imatinib. PET-CT accurately diagnosed tumor response in 95% of patients at 1 month and 100% at 3 months; for PET alone, these figures were 85% and 100%, and for CT, 44% and 60%, respectively [3]. The additional benefit of PET-CT over PET alone observed in this study may partially be due to reproducibility of positioning of the region of interest.

N. Charnley (✉)
Wolfson Molecular Imaging Centre, University of Manchester, 15 Grosvenor Place, Ashton Preston, Lancs, PR2 1ED, United Kingdom
e-mail: natalie.charnley@manchester.ac.uk

PET has the potential to detect response or disease progression after neoadjuvant chemotherapy prior to surgery. Chen's group assessed response of patients with locally advanced breast cancer following neoadjuvant chemotherapy. Radiologic response measured with PET and MRI was compared to pathologic response. PET correctly predicted lack of response in five of six patients, whereas MRI did not correctly identify response in any patient [4]. PET has been used to assess response of patients with locally advanced adenocarcinoma of the esophagogastric junction, receiving a 3-month course of neoadjuvant chemotherapy prior to surgery. A PET scan was performed before treatment, and 2 weeks after initiation of treatment. Histologic responders had a larger decrease in SUV compared to non-responders at 2 weeks. [5]. This study was followed by a phase II trial, where after 2 weeks of chemotherapy, metabolic nonresponders had treatment terminated and proceeded to surgery [6]. This rationale should be extended to other tumor sites.

Functional imaging with PET improves detection of residual disease following therapy. However, following treatment, the biologic phenotype of the tumor may be altered. The sensitivity and specificity of PET to detect tumor following treatment are not the same as the values for diagnosis of treatment naïve tumor. A recent study has shown that a PET scan 1 month following chemoradiation for rectal cancer, correctly identified 79% of patients with a pathologic response, but sensitivity to response was only 45% [7]. Thus negative predictive value for response is better than the positive predictive value. This relationship has also been confirmed in testicular tumors [8].

Detection of residual masses can guide decisions on further treatment. For example, PET scanning is used in patients with Hodgkin's lymphoma following partial or complete response to induction chemotherapy, to identify residual tumor masses, in order to avoid unnecessary consolidation radiotherapy if there is no active residual disease. An economic model predicts a reduction in unnecessary consolidation. Radiotherapy from 36% using CT to 4% using PET; however, this practice of PET assessment for residual disease has not actually been verified [9]. In patients with non-small cell lung cancer (NSCLC) residual and recurrent disease

P. Shreve and D.W. Townsend (eds.), *Clinical PET-CT in Radiology: Integrated Imaging in Oncology*,
DOI 10.1007/978-0-387-48902-5_15, © Springer Science+Business Media, LLC 2011

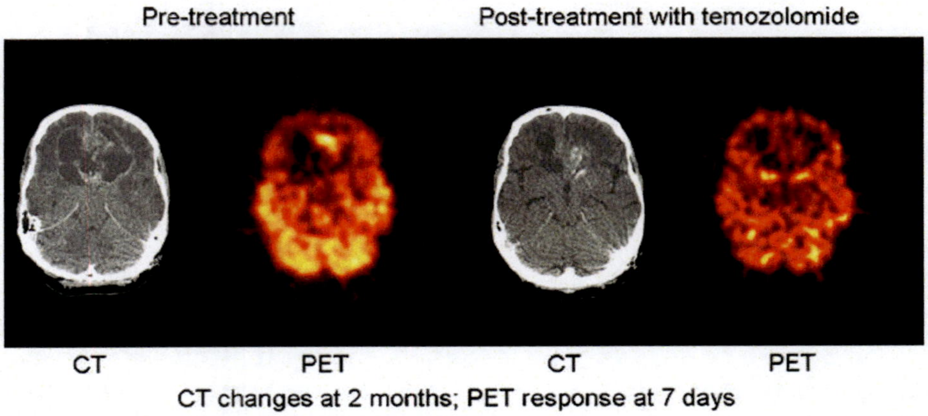

Fig. 15.1 Response to temozolomide in patients with high-grade glioma. Early PET response at 7 days, compared to CT response at 2 months (From Ref. [47]. With permission)

may be detected by PET following pneumonectomy, and indicate a need for irradiation [10]. With new radiotherapy technologies, i.e., intensity modulated radiotherapy (IMRT), small residual PET-positive masses following the end of a course of radiotherapy may potentially be boosted, with minimum toxicity to normal surrounding tissues. However, a positive PET scan suggests rather than confirms the presence of residual disease, and a negative PET scan does not exclude microscopic residual disease.

Timing of the PET scan following treatment is critically important. Anticancer therapy may lead to increased FDG uptake, due to glycolytic inflammatory processes, so causing a false positive signal. This has been observed 24 h following chemotherapy for glioma [11] and after 7–10 days after administration of hormones for breast cancer [12]. Timing is especially important following radiotherapy, as radiotherapy can induce an inflammatory response. Increased FDG uptake has been observed following radiotherapy for glioma [13], and rectal cancer [14]. In a study of PET for response assessment in head and neck cancer following radiotherapy, scans performed greater than 1 month after the completion of radiation had a significantly higher sensitivity than those performed within 1 month [15]. In view of this, many advocate a 3-month interval before assessing tumor response following radiotherapy.

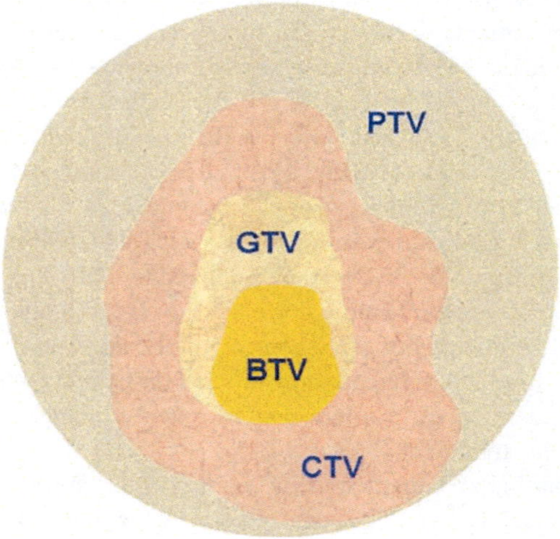

Fig. 15.2 Definition of radiotherapy planning target volumes. *BTV* Biologic target volume. Defined by molecular imaging. *GTV* Gross tumor volume. Image defined; uses high spatial resolution imaging, CT, or MRI. *CTV* Clinical target volume. Clinician defined; accounts for microscopic tumor spread. *PTV* Planning target volume. Physics defined; incorporates margins for tumor motion and setup errors

PET and Radiotherapy Planning

The aim of radiotherapy planning is to treat all the tumor, encompassing areas of potential microscopic spread, with enough margins to account for tumor movement and inaccuracies in setup, but to minimize dose to uninvolved organs at risk. Traditionally, high spatial resolution imaging is used to define the gross tumor volume (GTV) (Fig. 15.2).

Delineation of the ideal GTV is not always achieved. There is a potential for this process to be improved with incorporation of functional images, which show metabolically active areas of tumor.

Technicalities of Planning

Conventional radiotherapy treatment planning uses diagnostic imaging (simple x-ray or CT) to locate the tumor. Additional information may be provided by clinical examination. Attention is paid to reproducibility of patient positioning so that the planning episode simulates the radiotherapy treatment position.

Treatment planning with PET has mostly been done by visual analysis of CT and PET images. PET-CT scanners such as PET-CT GE Discovery LS are however becoming increasingly available. There are several important issues. Patient positioning needs to be reproducible for PET and for treatment. This may include the use of a flat bed insert for the PET scanner, careful attention to patient immobilization, treatment angle, and the use of lasers. Jarrit reports the use of a "cold session" to set up patient position and defining region of interest for the "hot session" where PET-CT images are obtained [16]. Radiographers involved in patient setup, may be exposed to huge and impractical absorbed doses during this hot session. This risk can be minimized if CT Simulator images are coregistered with PET-CT data taken on a different occasion [17]. The PET-CT dataset is created, transferred to the treatment planning system, and manually registered to the CT simulator dataset procured during a "cold session."

Challenges of Clinical Applications

Significance of Clinical Evidence

In recent years there has been an explosion of studies of PET and treatment planning in a range of sites. Most of these studies use PET-CT image coregistration, but more recent studies employ PET-CT. The most common sites published are in non-small cell lung cancer (NSCLC) [18, 19], head and neck cancer [20], and brain [21], but include lymphoma [22] and esophagus [23].

The majority of these studies show that incorporating PET data effects a change in staging and thus strategy of treatment due to metastatic or nodal disease, and a change in shape and size of PTV, with modification of treatment portals. Modeling can establish potential gain due to decreased dose to organs at risk and subsequent dose escalation [24]. In lung cancer, PET enhances characterization of abnormal lung parenchyma. PET can define lung nodules, and has been shown to lead to a reduction of the size of radiotherapy portals for patients with tumor-associated atelectasis [25]. Several planning studies extend CT-based volumes to include PET defined nodal disease. However, false-positive findings are common, and increased FDG uptake can occur in many benign processes, for example inflammation. In one lung cancer study, the positive predictive value was as low as 49.3% [26]. For nodal disease in head and neck cancer, sensitivity and specificity range from 50% to 96% and 88% to 100% respectively, which are not superior to CT [27]. It would be inadvisable to change clinical practice based on these figures.

Sensitivity of PET to define primary tumor is equally important. In rectal cancer, automated segmentation of the PET signal can allow definition of a PTV which does correlate with the CT derived PTV, though correlation with pathologic PTV is not ideal ($r^2=0.77$) [28]. In a study of patients with pharyngolaryngeal cancer, PET, CT, and MRI based volumes were compared against the histologic "gold standard." The GTVs defined by CT, MRI, and the pathologic specimen were all different sizes, and several false-positive results were seen [29]. Thus for PET to affect clinical practice, PET defined volumes need to be validated against histology.

Though many studies have confirmed modification of treatment with PET imaging, there is little evidence that this translates into an actual clinical benefit. There is only one published study to date to demonstrate a survival benefit with PET. In this study, patients received radiotherapy for recurrent high grade glioma. GTV was defined using ^{11}C- Met PET or SPECT with CT/MRI fusion or CT/MR fusion alone. Methionine is of use in delineating brain tumor GTVs, as normal brain has a high uptake of FDG but not amino acids, and so this gives better distinction from normal brain. Defining GTV with PET(SPECT)/CT/MRI imaging compared to CT/MRI led to improved survival with median survival times of 9 months versus 5 months [21].

Jankowska's group investigated use of PET in patients with occult primary head and neck cancers [30]. Early analysis of this retrospective data suggest that where PET suggested a primary and management was altered, survival and local control were increased. Before PET can be routinely incorporated into treatment planning, there needs to be more studies confirming outcome benefit.

Planning Inaccuracies

Incorporating PET-CT in treatment planning leads to several inaccuracies, which need to be accounted for. There may be inaccuracies in coregistration of PET and CT images. A study using Automatic Mutual Information-based Registration suggested that co-registration accuracy in patients was less than 4 mm, but that this may increase as the distance from the image centre increases [31].

Current PET-CT whole body scanners have, at best, a resolution of 4 mm, which is far inferior to CT and MRI. Therefore microscopic disease cannot be visualized. PET imaging gives no indication of anatomy, and so offers no advantage when determining invasion of surrounding structures by the tumor. The GTV edge is usually clearly defined by standard imaging. The edge of a PET image, however, is smeared. The CTV size can vary significantly depending on the SUV threshold chosen for determination of the CTV edge [32]. It has yet to be determined which SUV threshold matches most closely the actual tumor limits. In addition, the threshold itself can vary according to tumor size and background intensity [33].

Interpretation of CT images may sometimes be met with clinicians' inaccuracies, but PET image interpretation is even more challenging. It is likely that multidisciplinary involvement by clinical oncologist, radiologist, and nuclear medicine physicist, will lead to optimal definition of target volumes. This having been said, a more consistent definition of NSCLC CTV by clinicians has been demonstrated when PET images are used [34].

Consideration must be given to respiratory gating. PET data acquisition time is over several minutes, whereas CT is a few seconds, and with breath hold. PET imaging inherently shows the tumor's complete trajectory, which may give useful information about margins needed for tumor motion [34]. This does, however, reduce the quality of the data. Respiratory gating techniques can reduce smearing of the PET image and improve quantitation of SUVs [35]. For treatment planning with PET/CT, however, integrated respiration correlation would be necessary to limit respiratory inaccuracies.

All the above factors can impair the usefulness of PET in radiotherapy planning. Each center will need to define its own margins for PTV definition, depending on the precision of its own systems. The relative contribution of these inaccuracies will be established only when outcome data are available.

The Future of PET in Treatment Planning: Imaging Biologic Phenotype In Vivo

There has been a growth in development of new tracers for molecular imaging and with this, an expansion in the potential to image biologic phenotypes in vivo. There is a range of processes we can now image, including glucose metabolism (FDG), hypoxia (FMISO) [36], and blood flow (oxygen-15 labeled water) [37], Apoptosis (annexin V) [38], and angiogenesis and metastases [(18)F]Galacto-RGD) [39]. Proliferation may be imaged using the thymidine analogue FLT [40] (Fig. 15.3). Many of these tracers have already been validated against histopathology.

Biologic phenotypes may predict for response and allow intensification of treatment accordingly. Proliferation as measured by FLT has the potential to be exploited in radiotherapy by using different fractionation schedules. Tumors may be imaged throughout radiotherapy to assess behaviors such as reoxygenation, reduction in proliferation, or accelerated repopulation, which may have an impact on choice of further adjuvant treatment.

In the future, PET technology may result in reduction of normal tissue damage. In the radical treatment of lung cancer, PET has the potential to guide radiation beams through areas

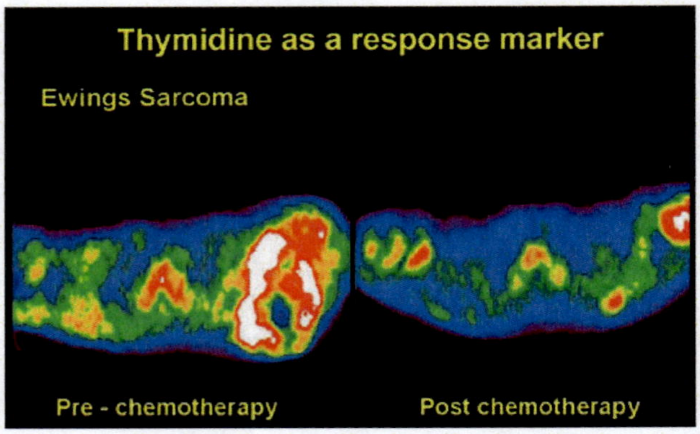

Fig. 15.3 Thymidine as a response marker following chemotherapy in a patient with Ewing's sarcoma

of damaged lung in preference to healthy tissue, by assessing lung perfusion with ^{15}O-water, or ventilation with ^{15}O-oxygen. Assessment of functional heterogeneity of lung has been shown to be feasible, using SPECT to assess perfusion [41]. In an animal model it is possible to image pulmonary fibrosis [42]. If we had validated PET markers for tissue repair and radiotherapy fibrosis, it would be possible to predict which survivors of radiotherapy would have late tissue damage.

Dose Painting and Biologic Target Volume

Intensity modulated radiotherapy (IMRT) delivers radiation more conformally to a tumor, and provides the opportunity for dose painting. There is thus a potential to boost more aggressive areas of tumor, such as areas which are hypoxic or highly proliferative. A pilot dose escalation study has been performed in patients with head and neck cancer in which FDG avid areas with a high glucose metabolism were boosted by IMRT [43]. IMRT feasibility studies have also been performed where hypoxic areas [44] were boosted.

There are problems associated with boosting a BTV apart from the limitations in resolution. In dose painting of hypoxic areas, hypoxia is dynamic, so the question is, when to image and which volume to boost? IMRT itself does have its limitations, and it would not be feasible to dose paint multiple miniscule BTVs. In addition, a murine model suggests that uptake of FMISO can be impaired if the hypoxic areas are scattered rather than confluent [45]. We know that hypoxic tumors are more resistant to radiation, and a model has been derived to predict the potential increased gain with a hypoxic boost [46]. However, there is no direct evidence that outcome is improved when an increased dose is given to a hypoxic area, or indeed to an area with increased FDG uptake. Much work has yet to be done in this area before boosting biologic target volumes becomes a clinical reality.

Conclusions

Inclusion of PET images to guide radiotherapy planning has advantages. Definition of target volumes of areas equivocal for malignancy can be done with greater certainty, but depends on sensitivity and specificity at that site. There is a huge potential for biologic dose planning using IMRT, which will expand with the development of new tracers.

However, only one published study demonstrates a survival benefit from incorporating PET into treatment planning [21]. Further clinical studies and outcome analysis are required to evaluate cost effectiveness and overall utility before a change in practice can be recommended. For current radiotherapy treatment planning, PET images are best used as a guide alongside CT images and should be done so with caution.

References

1. Brock CS, Young H, O'Reilly SM, et al. Early evaluation of tumor metabolic response using [18F]fluorodeoxyglucose and positron emission tomography: a pilot study following the phase II chemotherapy schedule for temozolomide in recurrent high-grade gliomas. Br J Cancer 2000;82:608–615.
2. Chesnay E, Babin E, Constans JM, et al. Early response to chemotherapy in hypopharyngeal cancer: assessment with (11) C-methionine PET, correlation with morphological response, and clinical outcome. J Nucl Med 2003;44:526–532.
3. Antoch G, Kanja J, Bauer S. Comparison of PET, CT, and dual-modality PET/CT imaging for monitoring of imatinib (STI571) therapy in patients with gastrointestinal stromal tumors. J Nucl Med 2004;45:357–365.
4. Chen X, Moore MO, Lehman CD. Combined use of MRIU and PET to monitor response and assess residual disease for locally advanced breast cancer treated with neoadjuvant chemotherapy. Acad Radiol 2004;11:1115–1124.
5. Weber WA, Ott K, Becker K, et al. Prediction of response to preoperative chemotherapy in adenocarcinomas of the esophagogastric junction by metabolic imaging. J Clin Oncol 2001;19:3058–3065.
6. Lordick F, Ott K, Krause BJ, et al. PET to assess early metabolic response and to guide treatment of adenocarcinoma of the oesophagogastric junction: the MUNICON phase II trial. Lancet Oncol 2007;8:797–805.
7. Capirci C, Rubello D, Chierichetti F, et al. Restaging after neoadjuvant chemoradiotherapy for rectal adenocarcinoma: role of F18-FDG PET. Biomed Pharmacother 2004;58:451–457.
8. Putra LJ, Lawrentschuk N, Ballok Z et al. 18F-fluorodeoxyglucose positron emission tomography in evaluation of germ cell tumor after chemotherapy. Urology 2004;64:1202–1207.
9. Facey K, Bradbury I, Laking G, Payne E. Ultra rapid review positron emission tomography. PET imaging in cancer management. Health Technology Assessment NHS R&D HTA Programme 2004.
10. Roberts KB, Manus MP, Hicks RJ, et al. Lung cancer. PET imaging for suspected residual tumor or thoracic recurrence of non-small cell lung cancer after pneumonectomy. Lung Cancer 2005;47:49–57
11. De Witte O, Hildebrand J, Luxen A, et al. Acute effect of carmustine on glucose metabolism in brain and glioblastoma. Cancer 1994;74:2836–2842.
12. Dehdashti F, Flanagan FL, Mortimer JE, et al. Positron emission tomographic assessment of metabolic flare to predict response of metastatic breast cancer to antioestrogen therapy. Eur J Nucl Med 1999;26:51–56.
13. Spence AM. [18F]Fluoro-2-deoxyglucose and glucose uptake in malignant gliomas before and after radiotherapy: correlation with outcome. Clin Cancer Res 2002;8:971–979.
14. Haberkorn U, Strauss LG, Dimitrakopolou A, et al: PET studies of fluorodeoxyglucose metabolism in patients with recurrent colorectal tumors receiving radiotherapy. J Nucl Med 1991;32:1485–1490.
15. Ryan WR, Fee WE Jr, Le QT, Pinto HA. Positron-emission tomography for surveillance of head and neck cancer. Laryngoscope 2005;15:645–650.
16. Carson KJ, Young VA, Cosgrove VP et al. Personnel radiation dose considerations in the use of an integrated PET-CT scanner for radiotherapy treatment planning. Br J Radiol 2009; 82(983):946–9.
17. Hall L, Severn O, Rosenberg I et al. The UCLH experience in registration of PET/CT fused images with radiotherapy planning CT studies. BJR S. 2005 BIR Meeting.
18. Caldwell CB, Mah K, Ung YC, et al. Observer variation in contouring gross tumor volume in patients with poorly defined non-small-cell lung tumors on CT: the impact of 18FDG-hybrid PET fusion. Int J Radiat Oncol Biol Phys 2001;51:923–931.
19. Mah K, Caldwell CB, Ung YC, et al. The impact of (18)FDG-PET on target and critical organs in CT-based treatment planning of patients with poorly defined non-small-cell lung carcinoma: a prospective study. Int J Radiat Oncol Biol Phys 2002;52:339–350.
20. Schwartz DL, Ford E, Rajendran J, et al. FDG-PET/CT imaging for preradiotherapy staging of head-and-neck squamous cell carcinoma. Int J Radiat Oncol Biol Phys 2005;61:129–136.
21. Grosu AL, Weber WA, Franz M, et al. Reirradiation of recurrent high-grade gliomas using amino acid PET (SPECT)/CT/MRI image fusion to determine gross tumor volume for stereotactic fractionated radiotherapy. Int J Radiat Oncol Biol Phys 2005;63:511–519.
22. Lee YK, Cook G, Flower MA, et al. Addition of 18F-FDG-PET scans to radiotherapy planning of thoracic lymphoma. Radiother Oncol 2004;73:277–283.
23. Konski A, Doss M, Milestone B, et al. The integration of 18-fluoro-deoxy-glucose positron emission tomography and endoscopic ultrasound in the treatment-planning process for esophageal carcinoma. Int J Radiat Oncol Biol Phys 2005;61:1123–1128.
24. van Der Wel A, Nijsten S, Hochstenbag M, et al. Increased therapeutic ratio by 18FDG-PET CT planning in patients with clinical CT stage N2-N3M0 non-small-cell lung cancer: a modeling study. Int J Radiat Oncol Biol Phys 2005;61:649–655.
25. Nestle U, Walter K, Schmidt S, et al. 18F-deoxyglucose positron emission tomography (FDG-PET) for the planning of radiotherapy in lung cancer: high impact in patients with atelectasis. Int J Radiat Oncol Biol Phys 1999;44:593–597.
26. Graeter TP, Hellwig D, Hoffmann K, et al. Mediastinal lymph node staging in suspected lung cancer: comparison of positron emission tomography with F-18-fluorodeoxyglucose and mediastinoscopy. Ann Thorac Surg 2003;75:231–235.
27. Gregoire V. Is there any future in radiotherapy planning without the use of PET: unraveling the myth. Radiother Oncol 2004;73:261–263.
28. Ciernik IF, Huser M, Burger C, et al. Automated functional image guided radiation treatment planning for rectal cancer. Int J Radiat Oncol Biol Phys 2005;62:893–900.
29. Daisne JF, Duprez T, Weynand B, et al. Tumor volume in pharyngolaryngeal squamous cell carcinoma: comparison at CT, MR imaging, and FDG PET and validation with surgical specimen. Radiology 2004;233:93–100.
30. Jankowska P, Goodchild K, Lemon C, et al. The impact of FDG PET on local control and survival in patients with occult primary head and neck cancers. BJR S 2005 BIR meeting.

31. Lavely WC, Scarfone C, Cevikalp H, et al. Phantom validation of coregistration of PET and CT for image-guided radiotherapy. Med Phys 2004;31:1083–1092.
32. Bradley J, Thorstad WL, Mutic S, et al. Impact of FDG-PET on radiation therapy volume delineation in non-small-cell lung cancer. Int J Radiat Oncol Biol Phys 2004;59:78–86.
33. Yaremko B, Riauka T, Robinson D, et al. Threshold modification for tumor imaging in non-small-cell lung cancer using positron emission tomography. Nucl Med Commun 2005;26:433–440.
34. Caldwell CB, Mah K, Skinner M, Danjoux CE. Can PET provide the 3D extent of tumor motion for individualized internal target volumes? A phantom study of the limitations of CT and the promise of PET. Int J Radiat Oncol Biol Phys 2003;55:1381–1393.
35. Nehmeh SA, Erdi YE, Ling CC, et al. Effect of respiratory gating on quantifying PET images of lung cancer. J Nucl Med 2002;43:876–881.
36. Lehtio K, Eskola O, Viljanen T, et al. Imaging perfusion and hypoxia with PET to predict radiotherapy response in head and neck cancer. Int J Radiat Oncol Biol Phys 2004;59:971–982.
37. Anderson H, Yap JT, Wells P, et al. Measurement of renal tumor and normal tissue perfusion using positron emission tomography in a phase II clinical trial of razoxane. Br J Cancer 2003;89:262–267.
38. Collingridge DR, Glaser M, Osman S, et al. In vitro selectivity, in vivo biodistribution and tumor uptake of annexin V radiolabelled with a positron emitting radioisotope. Br J Cancer 2003;89: 1327–1333.
39. Haubner R, Weber WA, Beer AJ, et al. Noninvasive visualization of the activated alphavbeta3 integrin in cancer patients by positron emission tomography and [(18)F]Galacto-RGD. PLoS Med 2005;2:e70.
40. Barthel H, Cleij MC, Collingridge DR, et al. 3′-deoxy-3′-[18F]fluorothymidine as a new marker for monitoring tumor response to antiproliferative therapy in vivo with positron emission tomography. Cancer Res 2003;63:3791–3798.
41. Nioutsikou E, Partridge M, Bedford JL, Webb S. Prediction of radiation induced normal tissue complications in radiotherapy using functional image data. Phys Med Biol 2005;50:1035–1046.
42. Wallace WE, Gupta NC, Hubbs AF, et al. Cis-4-[(18)F]fluoro-L-proline PET imaging of pulmonary fibrosis in a rabbit model. J Nucl Med 2002;43:413–420.
43. Schwartz DL, Ford EC, Rajendran J, et al. FDG-PET/CT-guided intensity modulated head and neck radiotherapy: A pilot investigation. Head Neck 2005;27:478–487.
44. Lee NY, Mechalakos JG, Nehmeh S, et al. Fluorine-18-labeled fluoromisonidazole positron emission and computed tomography-guided intensity-modulated radiotherapy for head and neck cancer: a feasibility study. Int J Radiat Oncol Biol Phys 2008;70:2–13
45. Sorensen M, Horsman MR, Cumming P, et al. Effect of intratumor heterogeneity in oxygenation status on FMISO PET, autoradiography, and electrode Po2 measurements in murine tumors. Int J Radiat Oncol Biol Phys 2005;62:854–861.
46. Nahum AE, Chapman J. Boosting the dose to hypoxic regions-what does a TCP model tell us about the increase in local control? Radiotherapy Oncology 2004;73(Suppl):S188.
47. Aboagye E, Saleem A, Price P. Tumor imaging applications in the testing of new drugs. In Baguley B, Kerr D (eds), Anticancer Drug Development. San Diego: Academic, 2002.

Chapter 16
PET-CT Imaging of Lung Cancer

Vikram Krishnasetty and Suzanne L. Aquino

Over 170,000 patients will be diagnosed with lung cancer in the USA in a year [1]. The majority of lung cancers, 80%, will be non-small cell (NSCLC) [1]. The treatment plan and prognosis of NSCLC depend greatly on the staging of disease at diagnosis. Early stage disease, with an absence of local lymph node involvement, is treated by surgical resection. Tumors of more advanced stages are more likely to be treated with a combination of chemotherapy and radiation therapy. On the other hand, surgery usually plays no role in the treatment of small cell lung cancer (SCLC). Therefore, chemotherapy is the mainstay of treatment for both limited and extensive stage SCLC.

Traditionally, CT has been the primary imaging technique for the diagnosis and staging of patients with lung cancer. The basis of oncologic imaging by CT is based on its superior anatomic resolution. However, the interpretation of CT primarily depends on a change in morphology. With the advent of PET technology, the addition of physiologic data has supplemented the radiologic staging and diagnosis of malignant disease [2]. Research has shown that the added metabolic information regarding abnormal glucose metabolism within malignant cells in FDG PET imaging has significantly improved radiologic staging of patients with lung cancer. The use of FDG PET imaging has been shown to significantly and appropriately change the management in the majority of patients with lung cancer. In a study by Hicks et al. [3], the addition of PET to conventional staging techniques identified patients with metastases to be converted to palliative therapy, sparing patients unnecessary surgery. An additional 10% of the patients in their study were downstaged based on PET results converting their therapy regimen from palliative to curative.

Recent advances in combined PET-CT imaging systems [4] as well as software generated PET-CT image registration [5, 6] has further improved lung cancer staging and management by combining the anatomically specific information of CT with the more sensitive metabolic findings of FDG PET. In this chapter, we will review the role of PET-CT imaging in the initial diagnosis, staging, and re-staging of lung cancer.

Primary Diagnosis of Lung Cancer

The detection and diagnosis of lung cancer is a foremost subject in thoracic imaging. Detection of lung cancer in its earliest stage as a solitary pulmonary nodule (Stage 1), when it is potentially curable, is an important goal of thoracic imaging. Lesions evaluated by CT are categorized into nodules or masses by size criteria. Lesions less than 3 cm maximum diameter are termed nodules, and those greater than 3 cm maximum diameter are termed masses. The likelihood of malignancy increases with the increasing size of a nodule/mass.

Traditionally, invasive techniques such as transthoracic needle aspiration/biopsy and thoracoscopic resection are used to differentiate malignant from benign solitary pulmonary nodules. In addition to the risks associated with invasive techniques to evaluate a pulmonary nodule, negative results from these techniques cannot always be accepted as true negatives. For example, in a study by Larscheid et al. in which CT-guided transthoracic needle aspiration (TTNA) of discrete pulmonary lesions was evaluated in 130 patients, the overall diagnostic accuracy of TTNA was only 76% [7]. Although transthoracic core biopsy has been shown to have an increased diagnostic accuracy over needle aspiration, it is also associated with an increased incidence of pneumothorax [8]. Generally, pulmonary nodules less than 1 cm in diameter are too small for transthoracic needle aspiration/biopsy. Because over 50% of radiographically indeterminate pulmonary nodules resected by thoracoscopy were benign [9], the noninvasive differentiation between malignant and benign nodules is important, especially in avoiding unnecessary surgery and therapy.

The management of the solitary pulmonary nodule detected radiographically is challenging. Roughly one third to nearly half of pulmonary nodules are malignant depending on the risk factors of the patient population. Because of the risk of complications resulting from invasive sampling

V. Krishnasetty (✉)
Columbus Radiology Corp., 471 East Broad St., Suite 1500, Columbus, OH 43215, USA
e-mail: vkrishnasetty@gmail.com

P. Shreve and D.W. Townsend (eds.), *Clinical PET-CT in Radiology: Integrated Imaging in Oncology*, DOI 10.1007/978-0-387-48902-5_16, © Springer Science+Business Media, LLC 2011

procedures, noninvasive imaging techniques are often sought in the initial workup of an indeterminate pulmonary nodule. Although chest CT is useful for assessing the size and stability of a nodule over time, it lacks sufficient specificity to provide a definitive diagnosis. A uniformly densely calcified pulmonary nodule is reliably classified as a benign granuloma. The detection of calcifications by CT densitometry or visible detection of central/coarse calcification, such as in a granuloma or hamartoma, favors a benign pulmonary nodule [10]. It is generally accepted that a nodule, regardless of calcifications or lack of calcifications, can be considered benign if stability on radiologic imaging is established for at least a 2-year period [11]. Most nodules are noncalcified and therefore are indeterminate on the basis of CT alone.

FDG PET has been shown to be both highly sensitive and specific in the diagnosis of malignancy in a solitary pulmonary nodule relative to morphologic imaging alone. Sensitivity for FDG PET alone has been greater than 90%, while specificity has typically been in the range of 85–90% [12–15]. Specificity varies with geographic region of the patient population due to differences in the prevalence of granulomatous infection. High prevalence contributes to false-positive pulmonary lesions, resulting in a specificity of FDG PET as low as 80% in some series [13]. The absence of FDG tracer uptake within a pulmonary nodule identifies it as more likely benign. As demonstrated in a study by Lowe et al. [15], when FDG uptake within nodules was analyzed, a highly statistically significant difference was found between the PET SUV value of malignant and benign lesions. A patient with no FDG uptake within a nodule could potentially avoid resection or invasive histologic sampling and be followed by serial CT scans instead. Because there is overlap in the amount of FDG tracer uptake due to malignancy with the amount of tracer uptake due to inflammatory processes, there is no clean cutoff for malignancy based on semiquantitative (or truly quantitative, for that matter) measures. The reported SUV of 2.3, as the line between benign versus malignant, for example, only specifies a certain relationship of sensitivity and specificity [16]. A lower value selected would result in higher sensitivity at the expense of specificity, and a higher value conversely.

The decision to resect, biopsy, or follow a pulmonary nodule depends on the likelihood of malignancy and the patient's clinical condition. PET-CT evaluation of a pulmonary nodule includes both a qualitative or semiquantitative assessment of FDG tracer uptake in the pulmonary nodule and assessment of morphologic features of the nodule as depicted by CT. The relative likelihood ratios for malignancy of a nodule's morphologic features, the presence or absence of abnormal FDG tracer uptake, clinical signs, and predisposing risk factors have been estimated [14]. The likelihood of malignancy increases for any nodule with increased glucose metabolism, CT morphologic features such as spiculation, lobulation, or mixed ground glass/solid [17], or increasing size on serial CT imaging.

Thus, in reporting the findings of a pulmonary nodule on a PET-CT scan, it is important to include morphologic features including size; nature of any calcifications; density, e.g., solid, fat-containing, ground glass, or mixed solid/ground glass; and margins, e.g., lobulation, spiculation, as well as the presence or absence of abnormal FDG tracer uptake (Fig. 16.1).

FDG PET is limited for the evaluation of pulmonary nodules less than 8 mm since the limiting reconstruction resolution of most commercially available PET scanners is 7–8 mm [14]. Studies have also revealed that certain malignancies in the thorax, e.g., bronchioloalveolar cell carcinoma [18, 19] and carcinoid tumor [20, 21], demonstrate low FDG uptake. In these instances, CT characteristics of a lung nodule may need to be factored into the analysis of a nodule evaluated by PET-CT. Nodules that have ground glass or mixed ground glass appearance on CT may need to be more aggressively approached, even in the absence of abnormal FDG tracer uptake, since these patterns are more likely to be associated with bronchoalveolar carcinoma (BAC) [22]. Carcinoid tumors are less distinct radiographically but may manifest as a discrete nodule associated with a bronchus (Fig. 16.2) [23]. On the other hand, pulmonary diseases other than malignancy may create false-positive interpretations resulting from increased FDG activity that has been observed in a variety of benign conditions such as granulomatous diseases and infections such as focal or organizing pneumonias. These will be discussed in more detail below.

It is important at this juncture to briefly discuss the interpretation of FDG tracer uptake on FDG PET scans before continuing any further. FDG tracer uptake in clinical practice is assessed by either qualitative means on visual interpretation or semiquantitative means as standardized uptake values (see Chap. 6). In our clinical practice, we employ the qualitative assessment of FDG uptake. SUVs are subject to variations dependent on FDG uptake time, non-lean body mass, method of PET image reconstruction and attenuation correction, method of region-of-interest analysis, and circulating serum glucose levels [24]. In addition, studies demonstrate a wide overlap of individual SUVs between malignant and benign lesions, even though overall SUVs are higher in malignant lesions than benign lesions [25]. Lapela et al. found it preferable to identify the presence of tumor recurrence in patients with head and neck cancers using qualitative methods rather than SUV determinations. In the thorax, FDG uptake can be qualitatively assessed using visual comparison to mediastinal uptake as the baseline [26]. FDG tracer above mediastinal background activity is considered abnormal. In practice, it is useful to evaluate FDG tracer uptake in pulmonary nodules based on the presence of abnormal FDG tracer uptake (greater than mediastinal background and thus suspicious for malignancy), equivocally abnormal (same or less than mediastinal background activity but still readily perceptible on

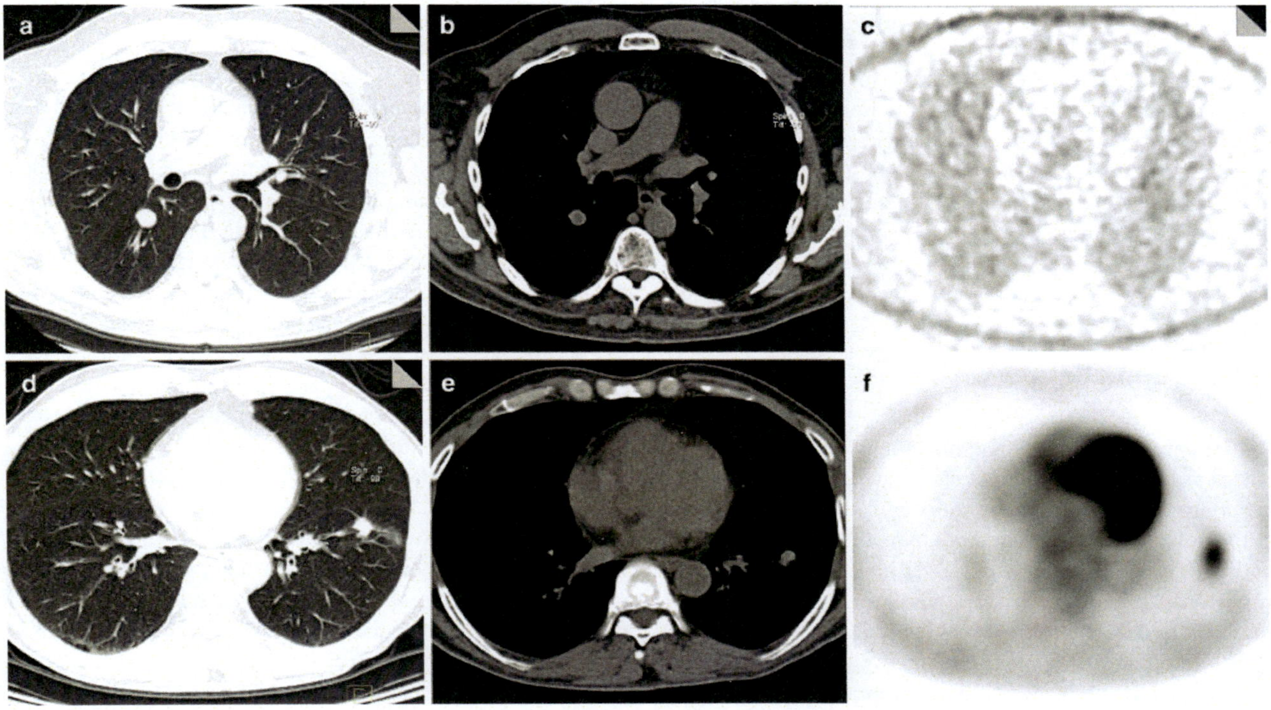

Fig. 16.1 Benign versus malignant solitary pulmonary nodule. A solitary pulmonary nodule in the superior segment of the right lower lobe is smoothly marginated on the lung window CT image (**a**) and noncalcified on the soft tissue window CT image (**b**), and without any discernable FDG uptake on even nonattenuation corrected FDG PET image (**c**) indicating the nodule FDG tracer activity is as low as lung background tracer activity. This would be considered a benign nodule such as a noncalcified granuloma. In a different patient a solitary pulmonary nodule in the superior segment of the left lower lobe is shown to be spiculated on CT lung window images (**d**) and noncalcified on soft tissue CT images (**e**), and is associated with increased FDG tracer uptake well above mediastinal background on the FDG PET images (**f**). This nodule was considered highly suspicious for malignancy and proved to be adenocarcinoma on biopsy

Fig. 16.2 Carcinoid tumor manifest as solitary pulmonary nodule. (**a**) Combined PET-CT imaging demonstrates low level FDG tracer uptake within a right lower lobe lung nodule proven to be carcinoid tumor by histologic sampling. (**b**) Although the level of FDG uptake within the nodule is equivalent to mediastinal background tracer uptake, the close association with a bronchus seen on the CT image suggests a carcinoid tumor

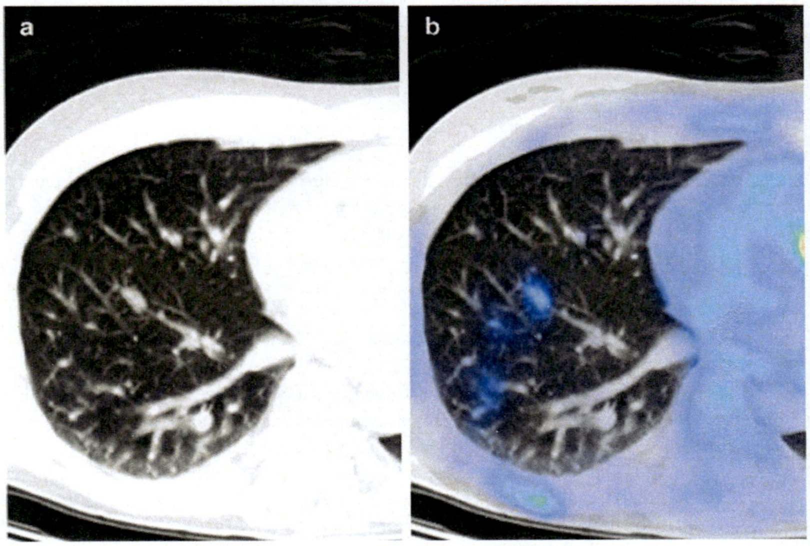

attenuation corrected images, considered low to moderate suspicion for malignancy), and no appreciable FDG tracer uptake in the nodule (minimal, if any, uptake above lung background activity – best assessed on the nonattenuation corrected images, and considered very low suspicion for malignancy). As noted previously, close attenuation to the morphologic features of the nodule is essential for interpretation of the FDG PET findings in proper context.

For larger nodules and masses, which are clearly suspicious for malignancy based on abnormal FDG tracer uptake and additional morphologic features, the fused images of PET and CT datasets can be helpful in determining the preferred biopsy site when transthoracic needle biopsy is planned. Areas of low FDG uptake due to adjacent scar or necrosis can be avoided in favor of areas of increased FDG uptake that are more likely to have viable tumor, and therefore raise the diagnostic yield.

Staging Lung Cancer with PET-CT

The primary role of radiologic imaging in patients with lung cancer is initial staging. Accurate staging is particularly important for management of non-small cell lung cancer due to the roles of surgery and radiation therapy [1]. Recent studies evaluating combined PET-CT have shown significant improvement in the accuracy of lung cancer staging over both PET and CT performed separately [4, 6].

The International System for Staging Lung Cancer published by Mountain in 1997 [27] incorporates the TNM classification. Stage I tumors are essentially confined to the lung and are subdivided into stage IA (T1N0M0) and stage IB (T2N0M0). The division between T1 and T2 tumors is important because of the prognostic implications. In patients with no evidence of lymph node disease or other metastases, T1 lung cancer carries a 61% 5-year survival rate compared to T2 lung cancer, which carries a 38% 5-year survival rate [27]. The *AJCC Cancer Staging Manual,* seventh edition, TNM description for lung cancer is presented in Table 16.1.

Patients with stage II lung cancer have local lymph node involvement in the lung or hila. As in stage I lung cancer, stage II tumors are subdivided into stage IIA (T1N1M0) and stage IIB (T2N1M0 and T3N0M0). Although clinical stage IIA cancers occur infrequently, the higher 5-year survival rate of 34% distinguish it from stage IIB cancers that have a 5-year survival rate of 24% for T2 malignancies and 22% for T3 malignancies [27]. Stage I and stage II patients are considered candidates for lobectomy or pneumonectomy as the primary means of treatment.

Stage III lung cancers have a significant decline in 5-year survival to 9–13% [27]. Stage IIIA lung cancer includes the four subsets: T3N1M0, T1N2M0, T2N2M0, and T3N2M0. Stage IIIA lung cancers reflect the involvement of lymph nodes in the ipsilateral mediastinum or mediastinal nodal involvement. Although these lesions are considered surgically resectable, patient survival is relatively poor, ranging from 9% to 23% 5-year survival. Patients who fall into this group generally will receive neoadjuvant therapy prior to surgical resection [27]. In this group, patients with T3N1M0 tumors have the poorest cumulative survival rate of 9% at 5 years [27]. Stage IIIB cancers include T4 tumors and/or

Table 16.1 AJCC definitions of TNM for lung cancer (Used with the permission of the American Joint Committee on Cancer (AJCC), Chicago, IL. The original source for this material is the *AJCC Cancer Staging Manual*, seventh edition (2010) published by Springer Science and Business Media LLC. www.springer.com)

Primary tumor (T)	
TX	Primary tumor cannot be assessed, or tumor proven by the presence of malignant cells in sputum or bronchial washings but not visualized by imaging or bronchoscopy
T0	No evidence of primary tumor
Tis	Carcinoma in situ
T1	Tumor 3 cm or less in greatest dimension, surrounded by lung or visceral pleura, without bronchoscopic evidence of invasion more proximal than the lobar bronchus (i.e., not in the main bronchus)[a]
T1a	Tumor 2 cm or less in greatest dimension
T1b	Tumor more than 2 cm but 3 cm or less in greatest dimension
T2	Tumor more than 3 cm but 7 cm or less or tumor with any of the following features (T2 tumors with these features are classified T2a if 5 cm or less)
	Involves main bronchus, 2 cm or more distal to the carina
	Invades visceral pleura (PL1 or PL2)
	Associated with atelectasis or obstructive pneumonitis that extends to the hilar region but does not involve the entire lung
T2a	Tumor more than 3 cm but 5 cm or less in greatest dimension
T2b	Tumor more than 5 cm but 7 cm or less in greatest dimension
T3	Tumor more than 7 cm or one that directly invades any of the following: parietal pleural (PL3) chest wall (including superior sulcus tumors), diaphragm, phrenic nerve, mediastinal pleura, parietal pericardium; or tumor in the main bronchus (less than 2 cm distal to the carina,[a] but without involvement of the carina; or associated atelectasis or obstructive pneumonitis of the entire lung or separate tumor nodule(s) in the same lobe
T4	Tumor of any size that invades any of the following: mediastinum, heart, great vessels, trachea, recurrent laryngeal nerve, esophagus, vertebral body, carina, separate tumor nodule(s) in a different ipsilateral lobe
Regional lymph nodes (N)	
NX	Regional lymph nodes cannot be assessed
N0	No regional lymph node metastases

(continued)

Table 16.1 (continued)

N1	Metastasis in ipsilateral peribronchial and/or ipsilateral hilar lymph nodes and intrapulmonary nodes, including involvement by direct extension		
N2	Metastasis in ipsilateral mediastinal and/or subcarinal lymph node(s)		
N3	Metastasis in contralateral mediastinal, contralateral hilar, ipsilateral or contralateral scalene, or supraclavicular lymph node(s)		
Distant metastasis (M)			
M0	No distant metastasis		
M1	Distant metastasis		
M1a	Separate tumor nodule(s) in a contralateral lobe; tumor with pleural nodules or malignant pleural (or pericardial) effusion[b]		
M1b	Distant metastasis		
Anatomic Stage • Prognostic Groups			
IA:	T1[a]	N0	M0
	T1[b]	N0	M0
IB:	T2[a]	N0	M0
IIA:	T2[b]	N0	M0
	T1[a]	N1	M0
	T1[b]	N1	M0
	T2[a]	N1	M0
IIB:	T2[b]	N1	M0
	T3	N0	M0
IIIA:	T1[a]	N2	M0
	T1[b]	N2	M0
	T2[a]	N2	M0
	T2[b]	N2	M0
	T3	N1	M0
	T3	N2	M0
	T4	N0	M0
	T4	N1	M0
IIIB:	T1[a]	N3	M0
	T1[b]	N3	M0
	T2[a]	N3	M0
	T2[b]	N3	M0
	T3	N3	M0
	T4	N2	M0
	T4	N3	M0
IV:	Any T	Any N	M1a
	Any T	Any N	M1b

[a]The uncommon superficial spreading tumor of any size with its invasive component limited to the bronchial wall, which may extend proximally to the main bronchus, is also classified as T1a

[b]Most pleural (and pericardial) effusions with lung cancer are due to tumor. In a few patients, however, multiple cytopathologic examinations of pleural (pericardial) fluid are negative for tumor, and the fluid is nonbloody and is not an exudate. Where these elements and clinical judgment dictate that the effusion is not related to the tumor, the effusion should be excluded as a staging element and the patient should be classified as M0

involvement of contralateral lymph nodes. Nodules within the same lobe as the primary tumor are considered T4 disease and nodules within other lobes or the contralateral lung are considered distant metastases (M1). Patients with stage IIB disease have a poor prognosis (3–7% 5-year survival) and are usually treated with chemotherapy or radiation therapy without surgery [27].

Stage IV disease involves the presence of distant metastases and carries a 1% 5-year survival rate [27]. Distant metastases of non-small cell lung cancer are usually to liver, bone, bone, brain, lung, and pleura, and adrenal glands and kidneys. Osseous metastases tend to be widespread in potential location, and soft tissue metastases are not rare. Patients with stage IV lung cancers are not considered surgical candidates and are treated with chemotherapy and radiation therapy.

T Staging

In the standard TNM staging system, the diameter of the tumor is used to distinguish T1 from T2 tumors. Neoplasms less than 3 cm in greatest dimension are considered T1, while those greater than 3 cm are classified as T2. However, a small tumor that involves a bronchus (but >2 cm distance from the tracheal carina) will be classified as T2. Any tumor that demonstrates involvement of the visceral pleura/hilum or any tumor associated with obstructive pneumonitis is classified as T2. A tumor is categorized as T3 if it directly invades the chest wall, diaphragm, mediastinal pleura, or parietal pericardium. A tumor is also considered T3 if it is located within 2 cm of the carina but does not involve the trachea or cause obstructive pneumonitis of an entire lung. Tumors that invade the mediastinum, heart, or spine are classified as T4. Tumors are also classified as T4 if there is an ipsilateral malignant pleural effusion or metastatic pulmonary nodules within the same lobe as the primary tumor. In general, involvement of a site is characterized by increased FDG uptake on PET or combination of soft tissue thickening or direct extension of tumor seen on CT.

Although the high spatial resolution of multidetector CT makes it an excellent modality for assessing the size and extent of the primary tumor (T), combined PET-CT can improve the accuracy of primary tumor evaluation further [4]. For example, Lardinois et al. [4] found that combined PET-CT more accurately demonstrates chest wall, diaphragm, and mediastinal invasion as compared to PET alone, CT alone, or visually correlated PET and CT (Fig. 16.3). According to Goerres et al. [28], images from PET-CT more precisely delineated the primary tumor because of the exact anatomic correlation of the extent of FDG-uptake. This in turn helped improve the detection of any involvement of the chest wall or pleura. An example of this is seen in Fig. 16.4, in which there is distinct thickening of the pleura adjacent to a primary lung cancer. On the combined PET-CT, the thickened pleura clearly demonstrates intense FDG uptake, which upstages the tumor from T1 to a T2 lesion. According to Nestle et al. [29], the fusion of registered and aligned PET and CT images also improved the delineation between an obstructing tumor and adjacent postobstructive atelectasis (Fig. 16.5). This improved anatomic localization improves the accuracy of tumor measurement (T staging) and allows for better targeting of radiation therapy. Nestle et al. demonstrated that 35% of radiation portals were changed (primarily reduced) after more accurate T staging was achieved with combined PET and CT imaging.

The combination of PET and CT imaging may also help distinguish benign from malignant pleural effusions. The presence of a malignant effusion will define a tumor as T4. Malignant pleural effusions have been shown to demonstrate more intense uptake than the usual background FDG uptake seen in benign pleural effusions [30].

Lymph Node Staging

Non-small cell lung cancer generally metastasizes first by lymphatic spread. The pattern of spread and lymph nodes most likely to be involved depends to some degree on the

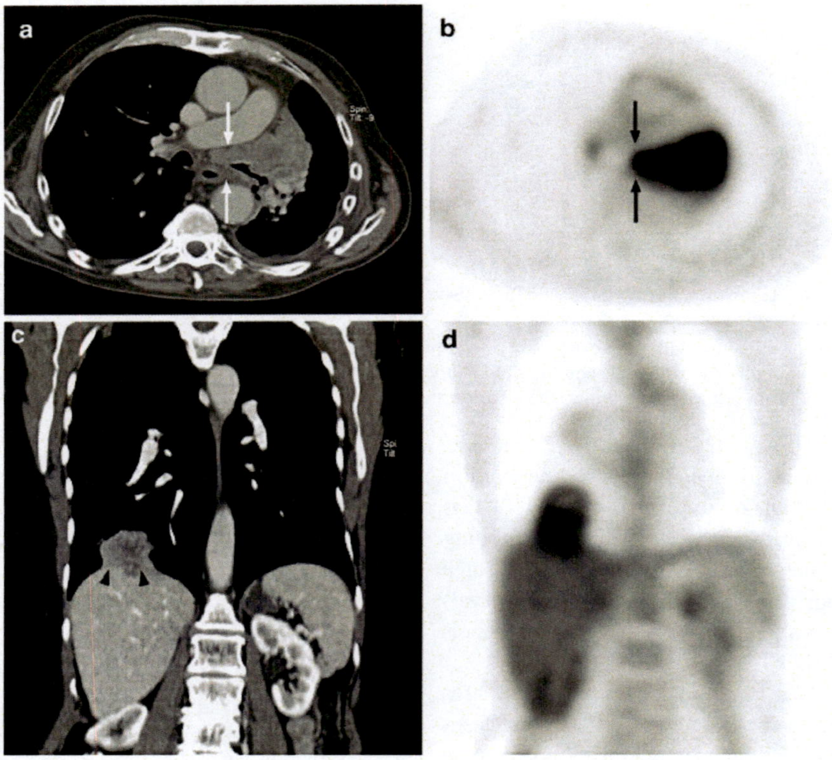

Fig. 16.3 T4 primary lung tumor. Transaxial contrast enhanced CT (**a**) and FDG-PET (**b**) images of a left upper lobe bronchogenic carcinoma contiguously involving the left hilum and extending into the mediastinum posterior to the pulmonary artery. The enhancing soft tissue is FDG avid and extends to the mediastinal midline (*arrows*). Coronal contrast enhanced CT (**c**) and FDG PET (**d**) images of a mass at the base of the right lower lobe demonstrates intense abnormal FDG tracer uptake extending below the margin of the diaphragm into the hepatic dome. The portal venous phase contrast enhanced CT images reveals abnormal soft tissue extending into the hepatic parenchyma (*arrowheads*) at the dome of the liver. T4 status renders these patients at least stage IIIB

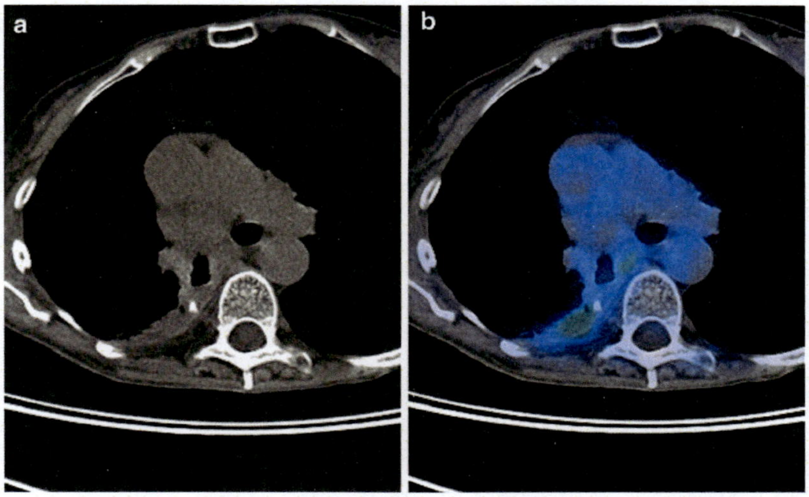

Fig. 16.4 Contiguous pleural involvement of primary lung cancer. Transaxial CT image (**a**) demonstrates thickened pleura adjacent to a known malignant right lower lobe pulmonary nodule. On the CT images alone, it is uncertain whether the thickened pleura are related to the primary tumor or of benign etiology. On the PET-CT fusion image (**b**) the thickened pleura clearly demonstrate abnormal FDG tracer uptake most consistent with pleural extension, rendering the nodule a T2 rather than a T1 tumor

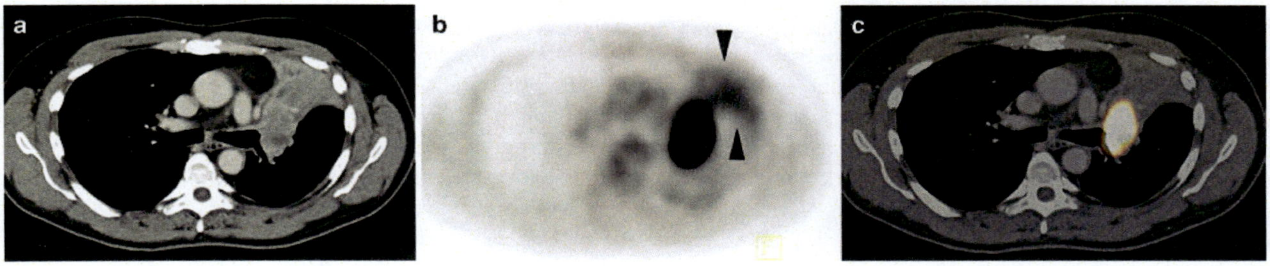

Fig. 16.5 Bronchogenic carcinoma with associated post-obstructive atelectasis extending to the hilum (T3 primary lung tumor). Transaxial contrast enhanced CT (**a**) and FDG-PET (**b**) images reveal a mass abutting the superior left hilum obstructing the left upper lobe bronchus. Atelectatic lung extends to the anterior chest wall, and on the CT images the underlying mass is not completely delineated from postobstructive lung. Intense abnormal FDG tracer uptake delineates the primary tumor, and there is low level FDG tracer uptake in the postobstructive atelectatic lung is seen on the FDG PET image (*arrowheads*). FDG PET-CT fusion image (**c**) depicts the relationship of the underlying primary tumor and associated adjacent postobstructive atelectatic lung

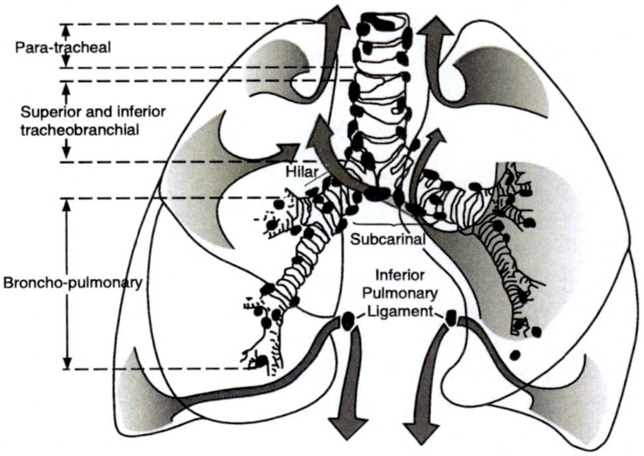

Fig. 16.6 Patterns of lymphatic drainage in the thorax. See text (From [31]. With permission)

location of the primary tumor (Fig. 16.6). Tumors located in the upper lobes tend to spread to the paratracheal lymph nodes. The middle lobe, lingular segment, and lateral aspects of the lower lobes tend to spread to ipsilateral hilar and to the tracheobronchial nodes between the middle and lower lobe bronchus or the right and the upper and lower lobe bronchus on the left. The middle lobe and anterolateral right lower lobe also tend to spread to right lower tracheobronchial lymph nodes. Lower lobe tumors tend to spread to the lower tracheobronchial lymph nodes including subcarinal lymph nodes, and paraesophageal nodes. Basilar lower lobe tumors can further spread via the pulmonary ligament to subdiaphragmatic lymph nodes.

It should be noted that definitions for lymph node locations used in staging have been based on anatomic landmarks relevant to mediastinoscopy and thoracotomy [32]. In an effort to produce a reproducible classification of lymph node location, the American Joint Committee on Cancer (AJCC) adopted a 14-numbered station schema for lymph node classification. However, since the AJCC classification of regional lymph node stations is based on surgical landmarks, it is not intended to be used for the description of imaging findings alone. By convention in thoracic imaging, lymph node locations are described by locations referenced to anatomic landmarks depicted on cross-sectional imaging. Hence, for PET-CT, as with CT, lymph node stations are denoted by terms such as hilar, peribronchial, tracheobronchial, paratracheal, aortopulmonary window, subcarinal, precarinal, azygoesophageal recess, prevascular, retrosternal, and paraesophageal.

In the TNM staging classification, the absence of nodal disease is defined as N0. N1 is defined as local metastases to intrapulmonary, ipsilateral hilar, or peribronchial lymph nodes. N2 disease is defined as the presence of ipsilateral mediastinal and/or subcarinal involvement; and N3 disease is defined as contralateral mediastinal/hilar or involvement of any scalene or supraclavicular lymph nodes. Other lymph node involvement, such as axillary, cervical, or retroperitoneal nodes constitute distant metastatic (M1) disease.

In patients with lung cancer, CT has been the imaging modality used to evaluate lymph nodes for metastatic involvement and to detect distant metastatic disease. The standard method used with CT to evaluate lymph nodes for metastatic involvement has been by measurement of a lymph node's short-axis diameter, since long-axis measurements are variable depending on the cross-sectional plane in which the lymph node is seen. A mediastinal or hilar lymph node greater than 1 cm short-axis measurement is defined as pathologically enlarged. It has been well known, however, that the use of morphologic criteria is limited in detecting metastatic nodal disease. In a study by McLoud et al. [33], 33% of enlarged lymph nodes on CT in patients with lung cancers were benign. Further, nonenlarged lymph nodes can be entirely replaced by metastatic neoplasm, yet would be considered uninvolved by CT criteria based on the normal short-axis diameter. Pieterman et al. demonstrated that small metastatic lymph nodes that were missed on CT were better detected by FDG PET [34]. In their study, PET was 91% sensitive and 86% specific compared to CT, which was 75% sensitive and 66% specific for the detection of mediastinal nodal metastases in patients with non-small cell lung cancer on preoperative evaluation.

The combination of both FDG PET and CT registered and aligned images further improves this sensitivity and specificity. Antoch et al. [35] reported sensitivity of 89% and specificity of 94% in regional nodal staging with combined PET-CT scan as compared to 89% sensitivity and 89% specificity with PET alone. Shim and co-workers reported somewhat lower sensitivity and specificity of 85% and 84%, respectively, for PET-CT as compared to sensitivity and specificity of 70% and 69%, respectively, for CT alone [36]. Aquino et al. [37] reported improved sensitivities and specificities in detecting nodal metastases and overall staging among their readers when they compared staging of CT and PET images interpreted side-by-side with CT-PET datasets fused with registration software.

PET-CT thus provides more accurate lymph node staging for lung cancer and is the preferred modality for this purpose. It is important to identify lymph nodes by both abnormal FDG tracer uptake as well as abnormal enlargement when interpreting PET-CT examinations. The sensitivity and specificity of FDG PET findings are not independent from lymph node size. Enlarged mediastinal lymph nodes have a lower false-positive rate on FDG PET, while the sensitivity of FDG PET for malignancy decreases with lymph node size. When assessing the locoregional spread of lung cancer it is important to distinguish whether isolated hilar disease is caused by contiguous involvement from a perihilar mass, or by distinctly separate lymph node metastases, as the latter is associated with a poorer prognosis. The presence of ipsilateral mediastinal lymph node metastases, as noted above, is significant as the N2 status renders a patient stage III (Fig. 16.7). Contralateral mediastinal involvement and supraclavicular/scalene lymph node metastases are similarly very important findings, rendering a patient at least stage IIIB, and consequently not a surgical candidate (Fig. 16.8). While FDG PET and, as a result, PET-CT have significantly improved locoregional lymph node staging of lung cancer, it is vitally important to understand that false-positive FDG PET findings occur in mediastinal and hilar lymph nodes at a relatively high rate, as high as 15–20%, accounting for the limited observed sensitivity. This reflects inflammatory processes which are a relatively common occurrence in these lymph nodes due to constant exposure of the aeorepithelium to the outside environment. As is the case with pulmonary nodules, the false-positive rate varies with patient population and region. In regions with high prevalence of histoplasmosis activity; for example, false-positive rates are elevated. For this reason, abnormal mediastinal lymph nodes on PET-CT that would render a patient a nonsurgical candidate should, when at all possible, be histologically proven as positive for malignancy by transbronchial or mediastinoscopy biopsy.

Detection of Metastases

Non-small cell lung cancer can metastasize to a variety of sites throughout the body. Stenbygaard et al. found that the common metastatic sites documented at autopsy in decreasing order of occurrence were mediastinal lymph nodes, pleura, liver, bone, brain, adrenals and pericardium [38]. Studies have found that whole-body FDG PET has an 11–12% incidence of detecting metastases that were missed by conventional staging methods [34, 39]. A study by Bury et al. demonstrated the usefulness of whole body FDG PET in the detection of bone metastases in patients with NSCLC [40]. The exception is the use of FDG PET in the evaluation of brain metastases. Rohren et al. demonstrated only a 61% sensitivity of FDG PET in the detection of cerebral metastases from non-central nervous system malignancies [41]. Rohren et al. theorized that the insensitivity of FDG PET in the detection of cerebral

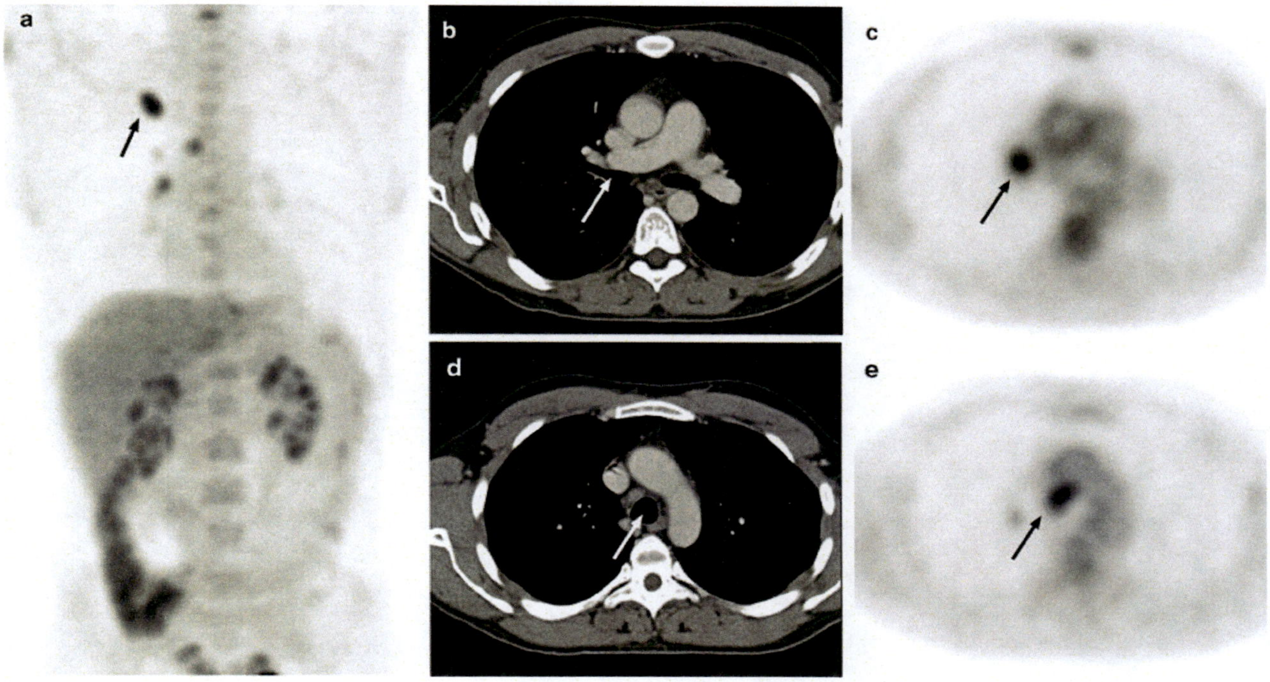

Fig. 16.7 Ipsilateral mediastinal lymph node metastasis. Anterior FDG PET MIP image (**a**) shows primary right upper lobe lung cancer (*arrow*) as well as small focus of FDG tracer uptake in the right hilum and right mediastinum. Transaxial contrast-enhanced CT (**b**) and FDG PET (**c**) images demonstrate a nonenlarged (7-mm) right superior hilar lymph node (*arrow*) associated with abnormal FDG tracer uptake. At a higher transaxial level, the contrast enhanced CT (**d**) and FDG PET (**e**) images demonstrate a nonenlarged (9-mm) right paratracheal lymph node (*arrow*) that is also FDG avid. Ipsilateral mediastinal lymph node metastases confer N2 status and renders the patient stage III

metastases may be secondary to the small size of the metastases as well as the inherent FDG-uptake of the gray matter. For these reasons, contrast enhanced CT and MRI remains the standard for the assessment of cerebral metastases.

The detection of distant metastatic disease is further improved by PET-CT. Metastatic lesions that are not clearly evident or are missed on CT may be more easily identified with the addition of registered and aligned FDG PET images of PET-CT. Prabhakar et al. [42] found that 17.6% of cancer patients who received combined PET-CT scans had findings on combined image interpretation that were missed on CT alone. For the overall staging of non-small cell lung cancer, Lardinois found accuracy improved to 88% with combined PET-CT from 65% for visual correlation of PET and CT images [4].

Due to the propensity of lung cancer to metastasize visceral organs, distant lymph nodes and in a generally unpredictable fashion in the skeleton, whole body coverage that includes at least from the base of the neck to below the hips should be used when staging lung cancer. Small extrathoracic lung cancer metastases may be undetectable or subtle on even fully optimized contrast-enhanced CT images, however, are more likely to be detected on FDG PET scans [34, 43]. Because urinary FDG tracer and normal renal parenchymal activity can obscure renal metastases, special attention to the kidneys on CT is required (Fig. 16.9). Although osseous metastases of non-small cell lung cancer tend to be lytic and may be subtle or indiscernible on CT, it is not unusual to have fairly extensive corresponding FDG PET abnormalities. Additionally, careful attention to technique and interpretation of the lung CT images is required to ensure that small pulmonary nodules, which may be below the detection threshold of FDG PET, are not missed. As with locoregional lymph node staging, PET-CT is the preferred modality for staging distant metastatic disease of non-small cell lung cancer, with the exception of cerebral metastases [35, 41].

Bronchioloalveolar Carcinoma

Bronchioloalveolar carcinoma (BAC) accounts for 2–10% of all lung cancers but has increased in incidence over the past few years [44]. This tumor is a well-differentiated adenocarcinoma, which frequently exhibits very slow growth. The revised 1999 WHO classification divides BAC into three smaller subtypes: (1) nonmucinous; (2) mucinous; and (3) mixed or indeterminate. Studies prior to the reclassification of BAC suggested poor reliability of detection of BAC by FDG PET [18, 19]. Kim et al. [19] theorize that the unique lepidic growth of BAC accounts for the lower peak SUV

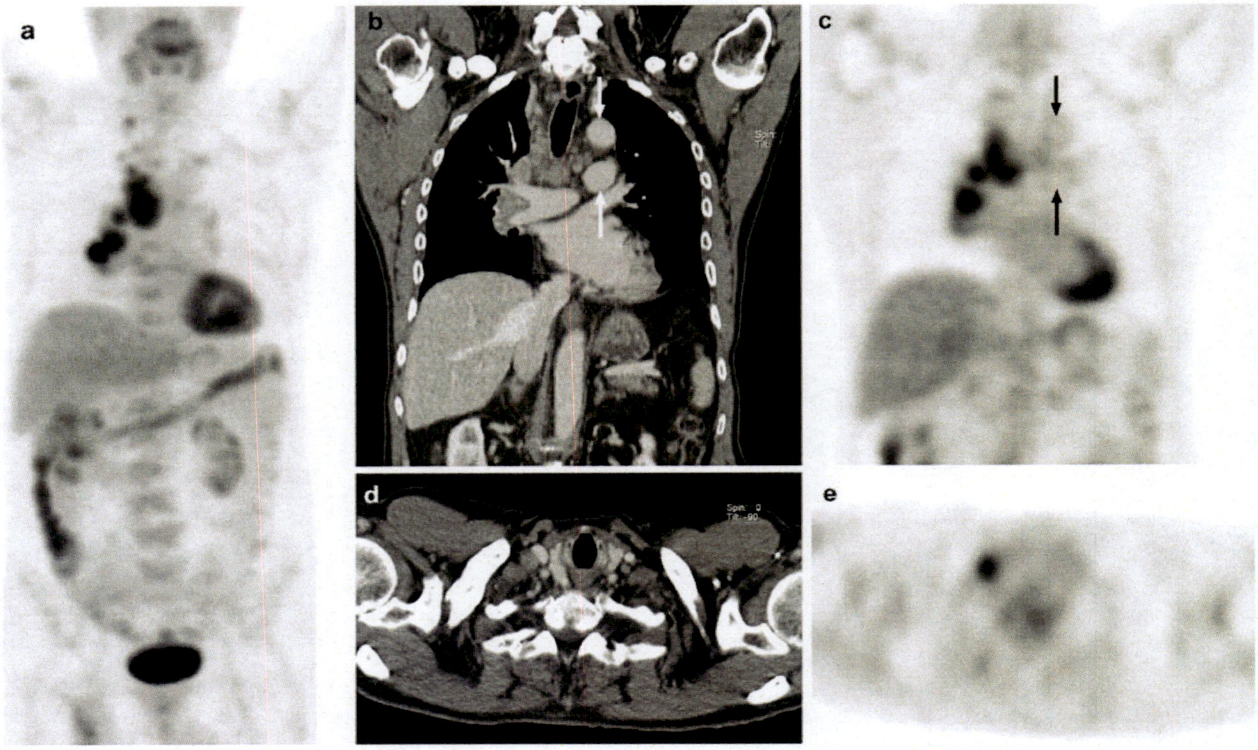

Fig. 16.8 Supraclavicular lymph node metastasis. Anterior FDG PET MIP image (**a**) shows intense FDG tracer uptake in the right hilum and mediastinum, as well as a subtle focus of tracer uptake in the right supraclavicular region. Coronal contrast-enhanced CT (**b**) and FDG PET (**c**) images reveal enlarged right hilar and right paratracheal lymph nodes associated with intense abnormal FDG tracer uptake, and borderline enlarged AP window lymph nodes that are not FDG avid (*small arrows*). Transaxial contrast enhanced CT (**d**) and FDG PET (**e**) images demonstrate a borderline enlarged (10-mm) right supraclavicular lymph node, partially effacing the right jugular vein, which is associated with abnormal FDG tracer uptake. Supraclavicular lymph node metastasis confers N3 status and renders the patient stage IIIB

values, thus decreasing the reliability of PET for the detection of BAC. However, a recent study by Yap et al. [44] demonstrated an 87% sensitivity for the detection of BAC by PET. In all of these studies, however, FDG PET had the lowest sensitivity and specificity in the detection of pure BAC (100% BAC component) [19, 44].

Although no study has yet examined combined PET-CT in the diagnosis of BAC, the addition of CT morphologic features and improved lesion localization likely will improve accuracy over FDG PET alone. Even though the peak SUV of pure BAC lesions may not be as high as other types of bronchogenic carcinoma, the combination of a ground glass or mixed solid/ground glass CT appearance with slightly higher levels of uptake on FDG PET may allow for better BAC detection by combined PET-CT. Fig. 16.10 demonstrates a case of histologically proven BAC. Although the level of FDG uptake within the nodules is equivalent to mediastinal uptake and not as intense as seen in other types of NSCLC, the slightly elevated level of FDG uptake above lung background in combination with the morphologic CT features sufficient to consider these lesions as not benign and is suspicious for BAC.

Small Cell Lung Cancer

Unlike non-small cell lung cancer, small cell lung cancer (SCLC) is rarely treated surgically. Currently, most patients with SCLC are treated with chemotherapy and/or radiation therapy. Although the staging criteria used for NSCLC can be applied to SCLC staging, the most important prognostic factor for patients with SCLC is clinical stage, which is divided into limited disease and extensive disease [45]. Limited disease is defined as disease confined to one hemithorax, mediastinum, and regional lymph nodes. In other words, disease that can be targeted with one radiation portal field is considered limited disease [46]. A malignant pleural effusion or disease extent outside the thorax is considered extensive disease. At initial presentation, two thirds of the patients present with extensive disease [45].

The primary role of diagnostic imaging is to accurately distinguish limited disease from extensive disease for initial staging and radiation planning. Patients with limited disease SCLC are treated with a combination of chemotherapy and chest irradiation. Those patients with extensive disease are treated primarily with chemotherapy alone. Traditionally, CT,

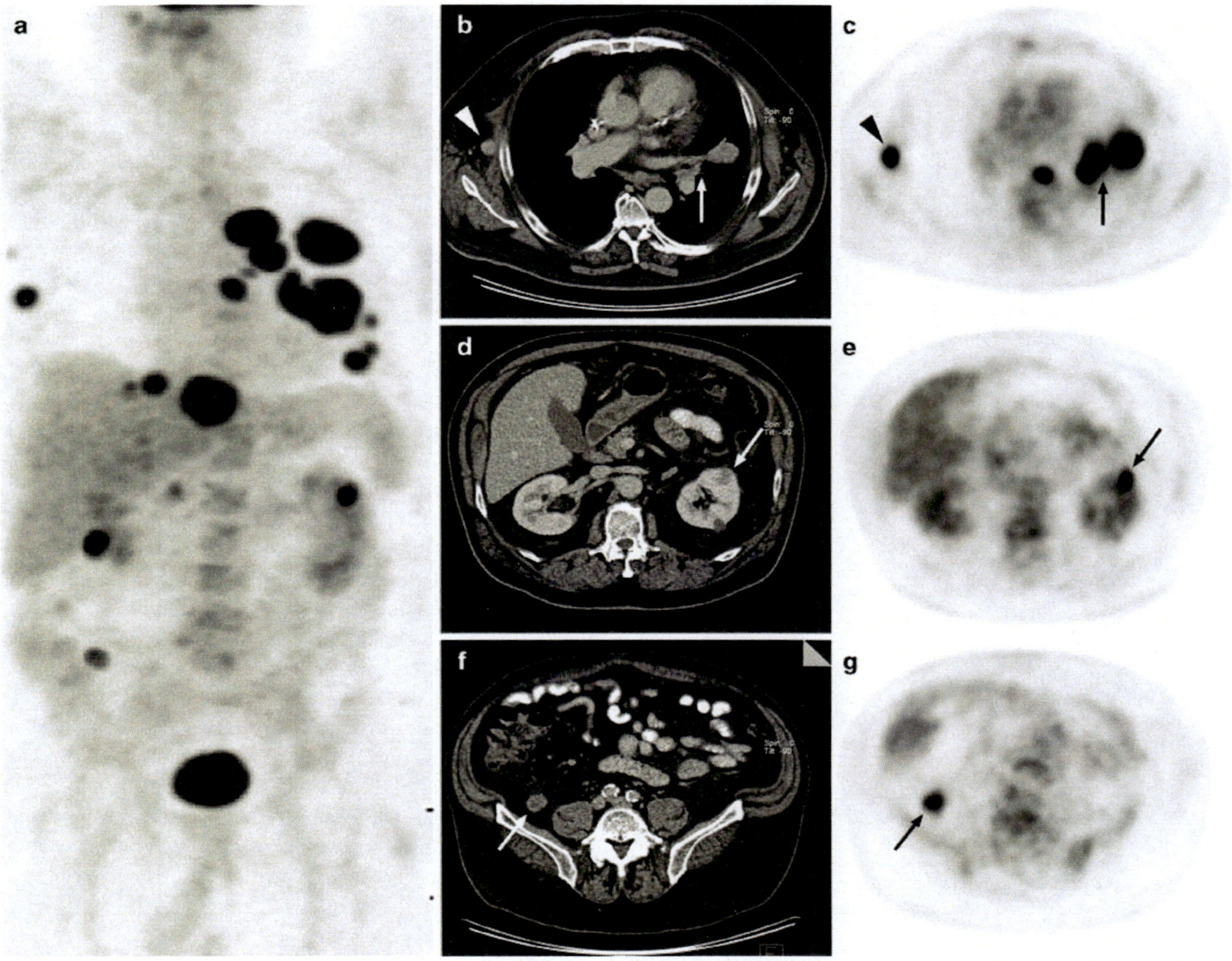

Fig. 16.9 Lung cancer with distant metastatic disease (stage IV). Anterior FDG-PET-MIP image (**a**) demonstrates multiple intrathoracic and extrathoracic foci of intense FDG tracer uptake. Transaxial contrast enhanced CT (**b**) and FDG PET (**c**) images demonstrate the primary lingular mass (3 cm maximum dimension), and a 1.2-cm left hilar lymph node (*arrow*) and 1-cm subcarinal lymph node (*small arrow*), all of which are intensely FDG avid, consistent with N2 nodal disease. The additional 1.5 cm soft tissue nodule in the subcutaneous fat at the right chest wall (*arrowhead*), also associated with intense FDG tracer uptake, is classified as a distant metastasis. Transaxial contrast-enhanced CT (**d**) and FDG PET (**e**) images at the mid-abdomen reveals a 1.6-cm soft tissue attenuation mass in the anterior mid left kidney (*arrow*) associated with intense FDG tracer uptake, consistent with a renal metastasis. There is a simple cyst in the posterior mid-left kidney. Transaxial contrast enhanced CT (**f**) and FDG-PET (**g**) images at the level of the pelvis reveals a 1.6-cm intensely FDG avid soft nodule in the intrapelvic fat (*arrow*), reflecting an additional soft tissue metastasis. Non-small cell lung cancer commonly metastasized to bone, liver, adrenal glands, and brain; however, renal and soft tissue metastases also occur

MRI, and bone scan are the mainstay of the diagnostic modalities used for the staging of SCLC. However, recent studies have demonstrated that the addition of FDG PET imaging affected staging and management in 29% of the 42 patients with SCLC in their study [46]. Kamel et al. showed that FDG PET was able to demonstrate otherwise occult metastatic sites that changed patients from a limited disease to extensive disease category. In addition, Kamel et al. demonstrated that FDG PET excluded metastases in 12% of patients with suspicious lesions found on CT and MRI. Hence, PET-CT is likely to become the standard modality for staging of SCLC as it has become for NSCLC.

Restaging Lung Cancer with PET-CT

Treatment of bronchogenic carcinoma varies with a number of factors including stage at presentation (as discussed above) and cell type. The therapeutic response and potential for recurrence are continually reassessed with imaging studies given that approximately 50% of patients with resected NSCLC will have recurrence [47]. Until the advent of FDG PET, imaging studies relied on changes in anatomy to distinguish post-therapy changes from residual or recurrent tumor. However, this is extremely difficult to assess in the background of architectural distortion from surgery or radiation therapy.

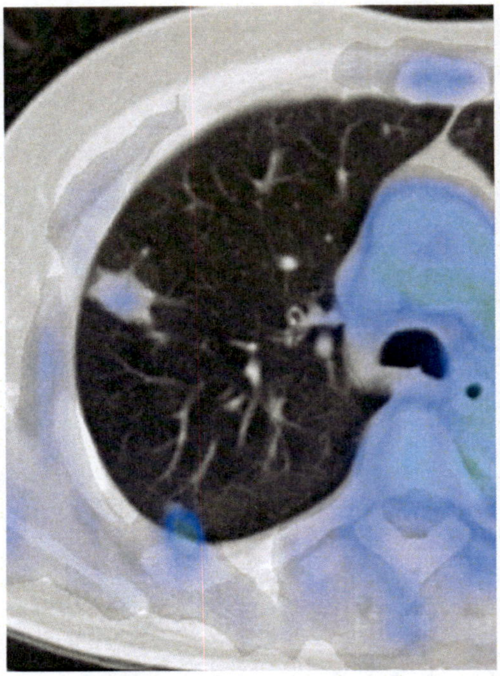

Fig. 16.10 Combined PET-CT imaging demonstrates low level FDG tracer uptake within two nodules with ground glass appearance in the right lung, proven to be bronchoalveolar adenocarcinoma (BAC) by histologic sampling. The level of FDG tracer uptake within the nodules is equivalent to mediastinal tracer uptake, which is considered borderline abnormal for malignancy. FDG tracer uptake associated with BAC is typically not as intense as seen in other types of non-small cell lung cancer. The ground glass morphologic appearance on the CT images can be helpful in raising suspicion of BAC; however, BAC can also present as solid noncalcified pulmonary nodules

Regional Recurrence of Lung Cancer Following Surgical Treatment

Patients in the immediate postoperative period may show increased FDG uptake at the surgical site. Many patients after a pneumonectomy will have a postoperative inflammatory response. Early postsurgical changes may be difficult to distinguish from recurrent disease. However, late postsurgical changes should demonstrate background low-level FDG uptake. Recurrence should be suspected if there is intense FDG uptake or if the abnormal areas of FDG uptake extend to locations that should not have been affected by the surgery (Fig. 16.11). Recurrence is also manifest in distant metastatic disease, including nodal, visceral, osseous, cerebral, and soft tissue metastases.

Recurrence at the bronchial stump after pneumonectomy has traditionally been difficult to diagnose before disease progression beyond the bronchial stump [48]. In a study by Verleden, 3.4% of patients followed after radical resection for NSCLC developed bronchial stump recurrence [49]. They found a significant relationship between the time of recurrence and the distance of the primary tumor from the bronchial stump. Although studies have suggested that the appearance of soft tissue at the bronchial stump or change in the sharp appearance of the bronchial stump on CT can be used as signs of recurrence [50], the addition of FDG PET images can be useful in the evaluation of such recurrence (see Fig. 16.11). Keidar et al. reported a case where PET-CT was useful in excluding bronchial stump recurrence in a patient where CT findings were equivocal [51].

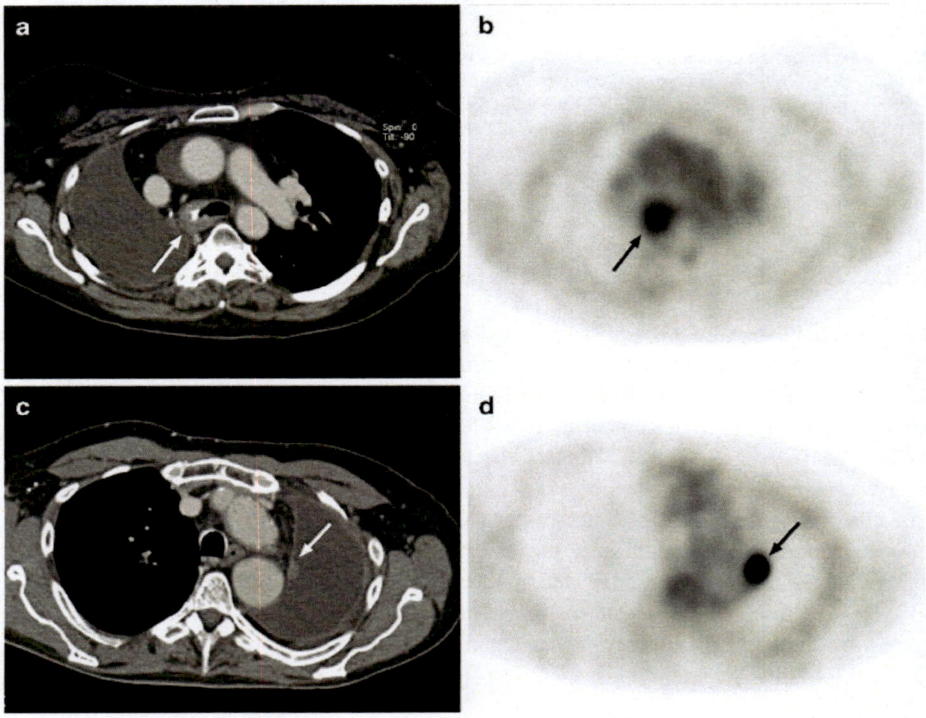

Fig. 16.11 Local recurrence following pneumonectomy. Transaxial contrast enhanced CT (**a**) and FDG PET (**b**) images of a patient 10 months following right pneumonectomy demonstrates prominent soft tissue at the right bronchial stump which is associated with intense abnormal FDG tracer uptake (*arrow*), consistent with local recurrence of lung cancer. Postoperative changes can be difficult to distinguish from recurrent neoplasm on CT images alone. FDG tracer uptake at the bronchial stump due to normal inflammation related to healing postoperatively is generally low level and resolved within a few weeks. Transaxial contrast enhanced CT (**c**) and FDG PET (**d**) images of a patient 4 months post left pneumonectomy reveal a 4-mm soft tissue pleural based nodule at the medial left hemithorax (*arrow*) which is intensely FDG avid, consistent with recurrence in the pneumonectomy space

Recurrence of Lung Cancer Following Radiation Therapy

Virtually all patients who receive therapeutic doses of radiation will have some type of lung parenchymal reaction [52]. Early radiation damage (1–4 months) results in radiation pneumonitis. Exposure of the lung parenchyma to radiation leads to cellular damage and subsequent repair [52]. Some of the biochemical pathways involved in cellular repair depend on ATP as a source of energy [53], which may help explain the association of increased FDG uptake and radiation induced pneumonitis. The typical CT findings of acute radiation include indistinct pulmonary vasculature, air space disease, and dense consolidation. On FDG PET these areas show moderate FDG uptake within the boundaries of the radiation port [52, 54]. Late radiation changes manifest as fibrosis on CT [52]. The typical CT findings of radiation fibrosis include well-defined areas of architectural distortion, fibrosis, traction bronchiectasis, and volume loss. On FDG PET these areas of fibrosis will show relatively very low levels of FDG uptake similar to background soft tissue uptake [52, 54].

The differentiation between posttreatment changes in the lungs from residual/recurrent tumor can be difficult during the period in which FDG uptake has not normalized. Studies have demonstrated that FDG PET imaging is useful in the differentiation between late posttreatment changes from recurrent or residual tumor in the lungs. In a study by Patz et al. [55], persistent FDG uptake 2 months posttreatment was considered suspicious for malignancy since FDG uptake from posttreatment changes should have normalized in that time period. More recent studies, such as that by Keidar et al. suggest that persistent FDG uptake can be seen up to 6 months posttreatment [51]. Although standalone FDG PET is sensitive for the detection of recurrence, it lacks the anatomic detail to localize suspicious findings, or differentiate benign inflammatory processes from malignancy (Fig. 16.12). Treatment related distorted anatomy along with posttherapeutic inflammation may hinder the diagnosis of recurrence. Keidar et al. [51] demonstrated that combined PET-CT scans

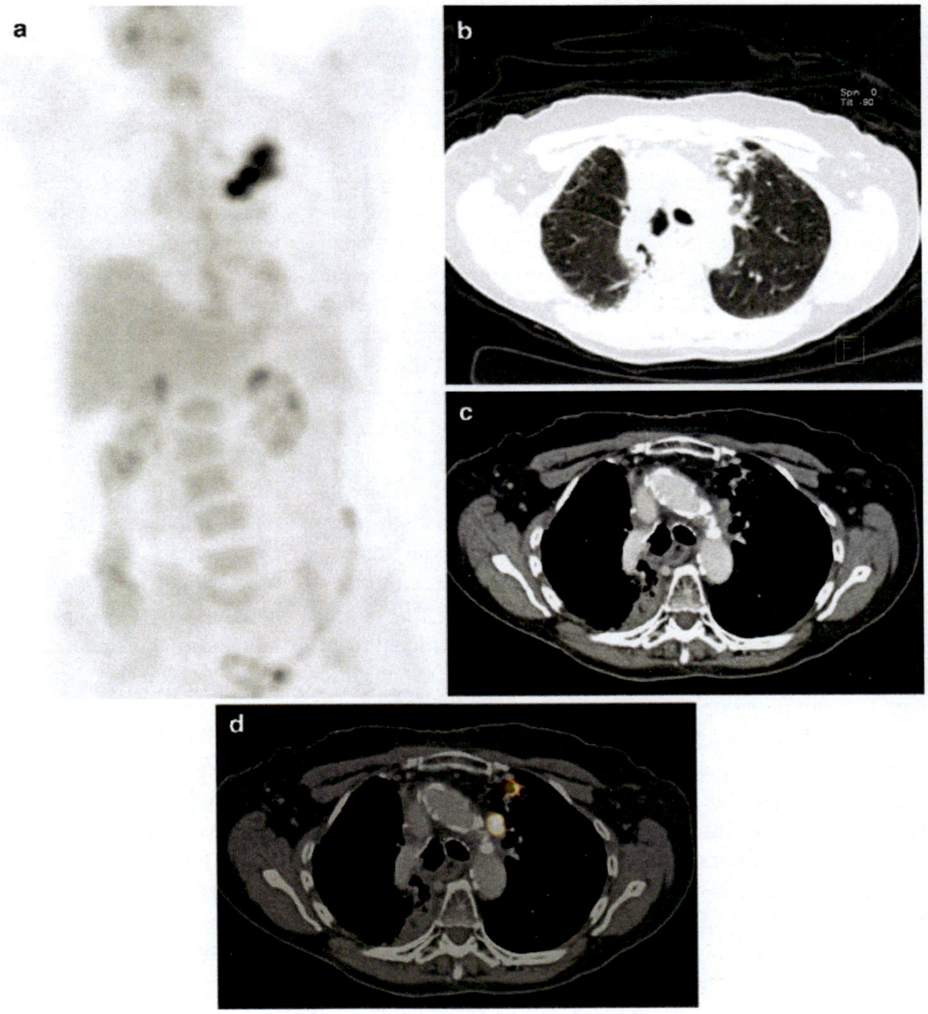

Fig. 16.12 Radiation pneumonitis. Anterior FDG PET MIP (**a**) image demonstrates a region of increased FDG tracer uptake in lung in the upper left hemithorax. Transaxial CT lung window images (**b**) and CT soft tissue window images (**c**) and FDG PET-CT fusion images (**d**) show bilateral paramediastinal fibrotic changes typical of postradiation therapy lung parenchymal reaction. In the anteromedial left upper lung there are areas of diffuse and focal increased FDG tracer activity corresponding to pleural parenchymal thickening related to active postradiation therapy pneumonitis. Paramediastinal fibrotic changes in the right lung are without any active inflammatory reaction

improved the anatomic localization of suspicious lesions compared to PET or CT alone in patients with suspected NSCLC recurrence. Aquino et al. [37] found that fusion of registered and aligned PET and CT images of patients treated for lung cancer and other thoracic neoplasms improved the detection of recurrent or metastatic tumor.

The administration of talc into the pleural space during thoracotomy may create false-positive findings on FDG PET. Talc causes a chronic granulomatous reaction in the pleural space which can mimic pleural tumor. The registered and aligned images of PET-CT will show correlation of the dense talc deposits in the pleura with these foci of increased FDG uptake. According to Kwek et al. pleural talc deposits will be abnormal on FDG PET for an indefinite period of time [56]. Therefore, patient history may be essential for proper interpretation. In any case, it is important to carefully identify regions of abnormal FDG tracer uptake along the pleural surface and correlate with pleural morphology, pleural density, and evidence of prior thoracotomy on CT to avoid false interpretation.

Therapy Monitoring with PET-CT

FDG PET imaging may be a valuable addition to CT and MRI in the monitoring of therapy in patients with lung cancer. Because PET imaging evaluates the metabolic rate of tumor cells, this technique has been shown to evaluate effectiveness of various treatments earlier than anatomic imaging modalities in certain cancers, particularly lymphoma. Initial studies with stand-alone FDG PET have described the usefulness of FDG PET for monitoring response to chemotherapy or radiation therapy and determining prognosis after therapy for lung cancer [57–59]. Mac Manus and coworkers [60] reported significantly longer survival of patients with non-small cell lung cancer that had complete resolution of abnormal findings on FDG PET in response to chemoradiation therapy. Hoekstra and coworkers [61] found that the residual mediastinal lymph node FDG uptake on FDG PET imaging after induction chemotherapy predicted survival in patients treated with induction chemotherapy for stage IIIA non-small cell lung cancer. Pottgen and coworkers [62] found PET-CT predicted histopathologic response and survival of patients after neoadjuvant therapy based on the degree of decrease of FDG tracer uptake in the primary tumor and mediastinal lymph node metastases following three cycles of chemotherapy. Currently the role of PET-CT in monitoring response to chemotherapy or radiation therapy has not been fully established. Generally, a complete normalization of FDG tracer uptake in a lung mass or metastases is most predictive of a favorable response and improved survival, even when there is little or no change in size of the tumor or metastases [57] (Fig. 16.13).

PET-CT in Radiation Therapy Planning

Because radiation therapy plays an important role in the treatment of non-small cell lung cancer stages IIB, IIIA, and IIIB, as well as recurrent disease, the application of PET-CT in radiation therapy planning for lung cancer is currently among the most developed applications. A discussion of current experience specific to non-small cell lung cancer can be found in Chap. 12.

Pitfalls of Combined PET-CT Imaging of Pulmonary Malignancies

Both neoplasm and inflammation exhibit increased FDG uptake and, therefore, acute inflammatory lesions may be erroneously interpreted as malignant. For example, active granulomatous disease such as histoplasmosis, mycobacterial infection, or sarcoidosis will show intense FDG uptake. False-positive uptake has been reported in diseases such as Wegener's granulomatosis, acute and organizing pneumonias, and lipoid pneumonia [63]. Lowe et al. also found that acute infections, particularly infections such as tuberculosis, coccidiomycosis, aspergillosis, and histoplasmosis were sources of false-positive findings on FDG PET. The authors also reported that some nongranulomatous pneumonias and viral infections displayed relatively lower levels of FDG uptake than malignancies [16]. Further complication of the issue arises when both an acute inflammatory process and malignancy coexist such as in a postobstructive pneumonia. Although Nestle et al. [29] found PET useful in distinguishing primary tumor from post obstructive atelectasis, Strauss et al. [53] found inconclusive results in attempting to differentiate tumor from inflammation based on the intensity of FDG uptake. They found that visual interpretation and calculation of SUVs were not helpful in the differentiation of tumor when acute inflammation had to be excluded. As noted above, there is an unavoidable false-positive rate in hilar and mediastinal lymph nodes on FDG PET, and in general, patients with positive mediastinal lymph nodes on PET images should undergo bronchoscopic or mediastinoscopic biopsy of the abnormal lymph nodes to prove malignant involvement (Fig. 16.14).

While lung cancer is generally highly FDG avid, mucinous dominant adenocarcinoma can be associated with very low levels of FDG tracer uptake, both in the primary lung mass as well as metastases. As has been mentioned previously, bronchoalveolar carcinoma frequently is associated with only mild FDG uptake.

Healing fractures are typically associated with FDG tracer uptake. Hence focal tracer uptake in ribs or at vertebral

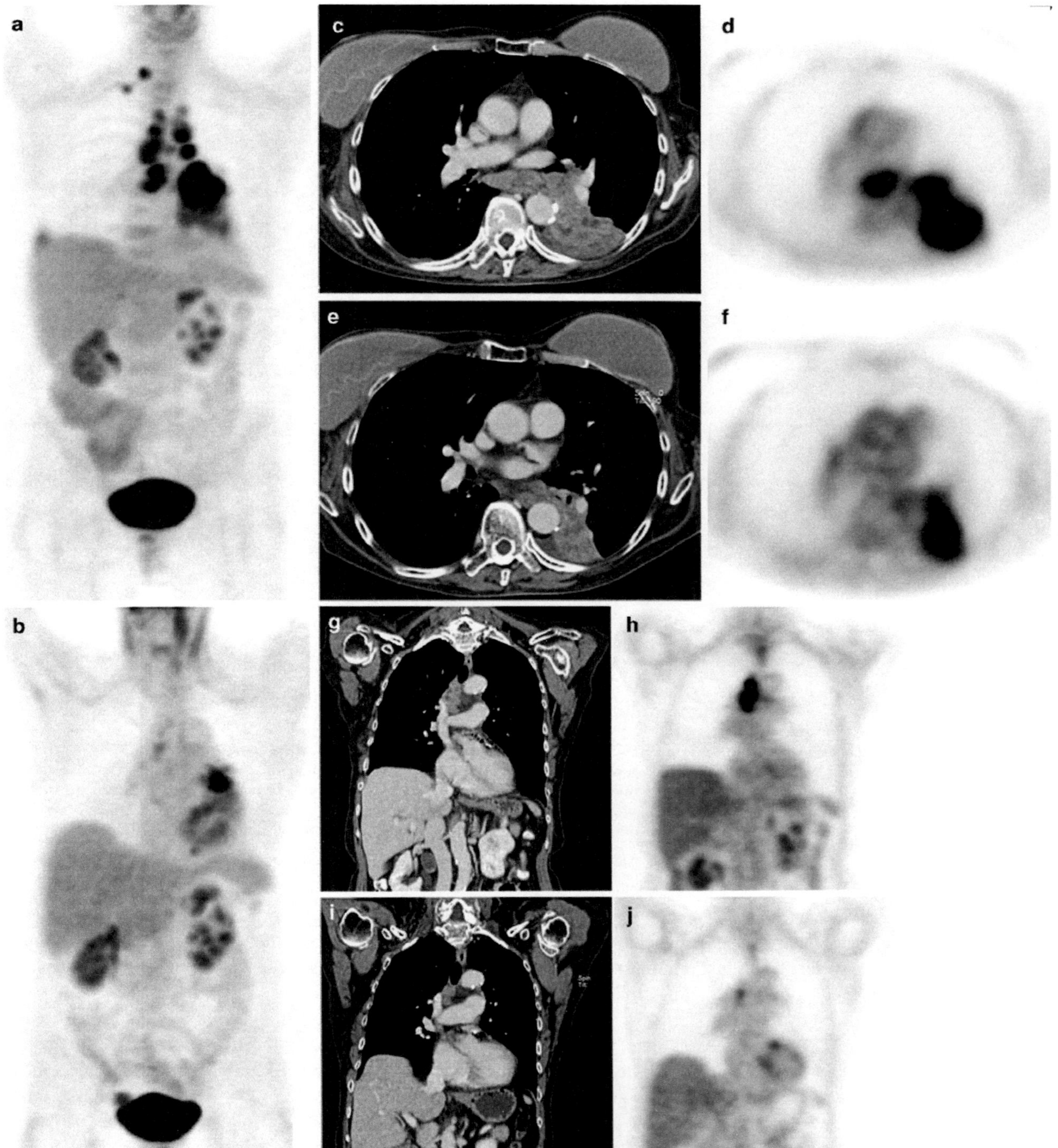

Fig. 16.13 PET-CT assessment of therapy response. Stage IIIB squamous cell carcinoma treated with six cycles of chemotherapy. Anterior FDG PET MIP images (**a**) prior to chemotherapy and (**b**) following completion of six cycles of chemotherapy demonstrate nearly complete resolution of the abnormal FDG tracer uptake associated with the mediastinal and right supraclavicular lymph node metastases, and substantial reduction in the abnormal FDG tracer activity associated with the left lower lobe mass. Transaxial contrast enhanced CT (**c**) and FDG PET (**d**) images at the level of the primary lung neoplasm prior to chemotherapy and after completion of chemotherapy (**e, f**) demonstrate resolution of the subcarinal mass and left infrahilar soft tissue and reduction in size of the medial left lower lobe mass; however, persistent intense abnormal FDG tracer uptake in the residual pulmonary soft tissue mass indicates substantial residual viable neoplasm. Coronal contrast enhanced CT (**g**) and FDG PET (**h**) images prior to chemotherapy and after completion of chemotherapy (**i, j**) reveal substantial reduction in the size of the right paratracheal lymphadenopathy; however, there is persistent mildly abnormal FDG tracer uptake in the remaining 1.2-cm low right paratracheal lymph node, indicating some residual viable neoplasm in the mediastinal lymph node metastasis

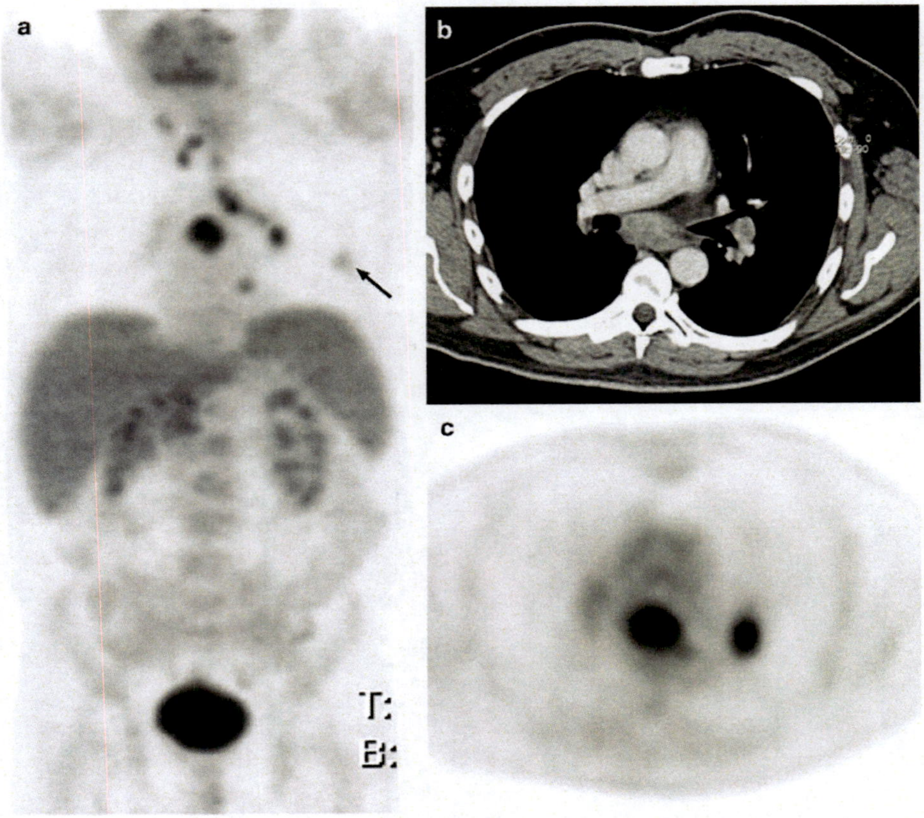

Fig. 16.14 False-positive mediastinal lymph nodes on PET-CT evaluation of lung nodule. Anterior FDG PET MIP (**a**) image shows intense focal abnormal FDG tracer activity in the mediastinum involving upper paratracheal, left tracheobronchial, subcarinal, and left hilar lymph nodes. A peripheral small left lung nodule is associated with only modest FDG tracer uptake (*arrow*). Transaxial contrast enhanced CT (**b**) and FDG PET (**c**) images show intense abnormal FDG tracer uptake in the enhancing subcarinal and left hilar lymphadenopathy. On mediastinoscopy, the upper mediastinal lymph nodes were negative for malignancy, but contained extensive caseating granulomatous inflammatory changes

end plates should be correlated with CT evidence of fracture, including assessment of benign versus pathologic fracture. Sacral fractures can be associated with fusiform or focal FDG tracer uptake and often only subtle CT findings for fracture [64].

Brown adipose tissue (BAT) can accumulate FDG to levels well within the range of lung cancer or other malignant neoplasms. The first description of BAT is generally attributed to Konrad Gessner, who detected BAT in hibernating marmots more than 450 years ago [65]. Only recently has it become evident that BAT is a highly specialized thermogenic tissue that plays an important role in body temperature regulation [65]. In addition to the typical distribution at the base of the neck, supraclavicular fossa and high axillary fat regions, and paraspinous fat, brown adipose tissue FDG tracer uptake can occur within the mediastinal and upper abdominal fat (Fig. 16.15). Generally, with PET-CT the distribution of the FDG tracer uptake on the FDG PET images and localization this tracer activity to fat attenuation on the CT images allows for ready identification of brown adipose tissue source. The presence of brown adipose FDG uptake, however, does not preclude coexisting lymph node metastases such as those to supraclavicular nodes or mediastinal nodes.

Brown fat is a known component of lipomatous hypertrophy of the interatrial septum (LHIS). This focus of increased fat deposit in the heart between the right and left atria may show very intense uptake on FDG PET, which may mimic tumor spread as a mediastinal lymph node metastases in a patient with lung cancer. According to Fan et al. [66], registered and aligned PET and CT images correctly localizes the area of intense uptake to the interatrial septum, correctly identifying the LHIS source.

Similar to uptake in metabolically active fat, FDG uptake in muscle may be problematic. Focal uptake at the origin or insertion of muscles, such the scalene muscles of the neck, may be falsely attributed to abnormal uptake within supraclavicular lymph nodes. With accurate image registration on combined PET-CT, these areas of increased uptake can be localized to these specific muscle groups.

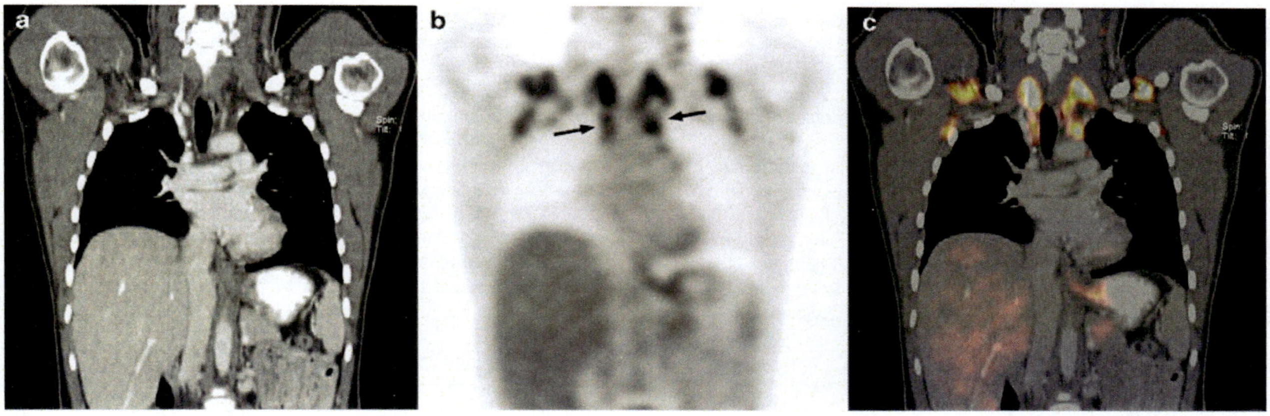

Fig. 16.15 Physiologic brown fat FDG tracer uptake. Coronal contrast enhanced CT (**a**), FDG PET (**b**), and FDG PET-CT fusion (**c**) images demonstrate intense abnormal FDG tracer uptake in fat at the base of the neck, deep axilla, and supraclavicular fossa regions, a common distribution. Note additionally the physiologic brown fat FDG uptake in paratracheal fat in the upper mediastinum (*arrows*). Physiologic brown fat FDG uptake can occur in deeper in the mediastinal fat as well as the interatrial septum, and subdiaphragmatic fat in the upper abdomen

In summary, combined PET-CT imaging has made a significant improvement on the radiologic diagnosis, staging, and restaging of lung cancer. Integrated PET-CTs more accurate anatomic localization of FDG tracer uptake and associated CT morphologic characterization of FDG PET findings allows for improved specificity in staging of lymph nodal disease and for more accurate identification of physiologic uptake that would otherwise be potential causes for false-positive interpretation. PET-CT is rapidly coming into routine use for radiation therapy treatment planning for lung cancer, and there is growing experience with treatment monitoring. With a solid understanding of the normal physiologic distribution of FDG, radiologists and nuclear medicine physicians have the ability to significantly contribute to the management of lung cancer patients with combined PET-CT imaging.

References

1. Vesselle H, et al. The impact of fluorodeoxyglucose F 18 positron-emission tomography on the surgical staging of non-small cell lung cancer. J Thorac Cardiovasc Surg 2002;124(3):511–519.
2. Eubank WB, et al. Imaging of oncologic patients: benefit of combined CT and FDG PET in the diagnosis of malignancy. Am J Roentgenol 1998;171(4):1103–1110.
3. Hicks RJ, et al. (18)F-FDG PET provides high-impact and powerful prognostic stratification in staging newly diagnosed non-small cell lung cancer. J Nucl Med 2001;42(11):1596–1604.
4. Lardinois D, et al. Staging of non-small-cell lung cancer with integrated positron-emission tomography and computed tomography. NEJM 2003;348(25):2500–2507.
5. Krishnasetty V, et al. Comparison of alignment of computer-registered data sets: combined PET-CT versus independent PET and CT of the thorax. Radiology 2005;237(2):635–639.
6. Aquino SL, et al. Improved radiologic staging of lung cancer with 2-[18F]-fluoro-2-deoxy-D-glucose-positron emission tomography and computed tomography registration. J Comput Assist Tomogr 2003;27(4):479–484.
7. Larscheid RC, Thorpe PE, Scott WJ. Percutaneous transthoracic needle aspiration biopsy: a comprehensive review of its current role in the diagnosis and treatment of lung tumors. Chest 1998;114(3): 704–709.
8. Klein JS, Salomon G, Stewart A. Transthoracic needle biopsy with a coaxially placed 20-gauge automated cutting needle: results in 122 patients. Radiology 1996;198(3):715–720.
9. Mack MJ, et al. Thoracoscopy for the diagnosis of the indeterminate solitary pulmonary nodule. Ann Thorac Surg 1993;56(4): 825–830; discussion 830–832.
10. Dewan NA, et al. Likelihood of malignancy in a solitary pulmonary nodule: comparison of Bayesian analysis and results of FDG PET scan. Chest 1997;112(2):416–422.
11. Yankelevitz DF, Henschke CI. Does 2-year stability imply that pulmonary nodules are benign? Am J Roentgenol 1997;168(2):325–328.
12. Patz EF Jr, et al. Focal pulmonary abnormalities: evaluation with F-18 fluorodeoxyglucose PET scanning. Radiology 1993;188(2): 487–490.
13. Lowe VJ, et al. Prospective investigation of positron emission tomography in lung nodules. J Clin Oncol 1998;16(3):1075–1084.
14. Gould MK, et al. Accuracy of positron emission tomography for diagnosis of pulmonary nodules and mass lesions: a meta-analysis. JAMA 2001;285(7):914–924.
15. Lowe VJ, Naunheim KS. Current role of positron emission tomography in thoracic oncology. Thorax 1998;53(8):703–712.
16. Lowe VJ, et al. Semiquantitative and visual analysis of FDG PET images in pulmonary abnormalities. J Nucl Med 1994;35(11): 1771–1776.
17. Henschke CI, et al. CT screening for lung cancer: frequency and significance of part-solid and nonsolid nodules. Am J Roentgenol 2002;178(5):1053–1057.
18. Higashi K, et al. Fluorine-18-FDG PET imaging is negative in bronchioloalveolar lung carcinoma. J Nucl Med 1998;39(6): 1016–1020.
19. Kim BT, et al. Localized form of bronchioloalveolar carcinoma: FDG PET findings. Am J Roentgenol 1998;170(4):935–939.
20. Jadvar H, Segall GM. False-negative fluorine-18-FDG PET in metastatic carcinoid. J Nucl Med 1997;38(9):1382–1383.
21. Erasmus JJ, et al. Evaluation of primary pulmonary carcinoid tumors using FDG PET. Am J Roentgenol 1998;170(5):1369–1373.
22. Henschke CI, et al. Computerized tomography screening for lung cancer: new findings and diagnostic work-up. Semin Thorac Cardiovasc Surg 2003;15(4):397–404.

23. Fink G, et al. Pulmonary carcinoid: presentation, diagnosis, and outcome in 142 cases in Israel and review of 640 cases from the literature. Chest 2001;119(6):1647–1651.
24. Sugawara Y, et al. Reevaluation of the standardized uptake value for FDG: variations with body weight and methods for correction. Radiology 1999;213(2):521–525.
25. Lapela M, et al. Experience in qualitative and quantitative FDG PET in follow-up of patients with suspected recurrence from head and neck cancer. Eur J Cancer 2000;36(7):858–867.
26. Gupta N, et al. Dynamic positron emission tomography with F-18 fluorodeoxyglucose imaging in differentiation of benign from malignant lung/mediastinal lesions. Chest 1998;114(4):1105–1111.
27. Mountain CF. Revisions in the International System for Staging Lung Cancer. Chest 1997;111(6):1710–1717.
28. Goerres GW, von Schulthess GK, Steinert HC. Why most PET of lung and head-and-neck cancer will be PET-CT. J Nucl Med 2004;45(Suppl 1):66S–71S.
29. Nestle U, et al. 18F-deoxyglucose positron emission tomography (FDG PET) for the planning of radiotherapy in lung cancer: high impact in patients with atelectasis. Int J Radiat Oncol Biol Phys 1999;44(3):593–597.
30. Gupta NC, et al. Clinical role of F-18 fluorodeoxyglucose positron emission tomography imaging in patients with lung cancer and suspected malignant pleural effusion. Chest 2002;122(6): 1918–1924.
31. Richter E, Feyerabend T, Bondorf W (eds.). *Normal Lymph Node Topography: CT Atlas*. New York: Springer, 2004.
32. Mountain CF, Dresler CM. Regional lymph node classification for lung cancer staging. Chest 1997;111(6):1718–1723.
33. McLoud TC, et al. Bronchogenic carcinoma: analysis of staging in the mediastinum with CT by correlative lymph node mapping and sampling. Radiology 1992;182(2):319–323.
34. Pieterman RM, et al. Preoperative staging of non-small-cell lung cancer with positron-emission tomography. NEJM 2000;343(4): 254–261.
35. Antoch G, et al. Non-small cell lung cancer: dual-modality PET-CT in preoperative staging. Radiology 2003;229(2):526–533.
36. Shim SS, et al. Non-small cell lung cancer: prospective comparison of integrated FDG PET-CT and CT alone for preoperative staging. Radiology 2005;236(3):1011–1019.
37. Aquino SL, et al. Improved image interpretation with registered thoracic CT and positron emission tomography data sets. Am J Roentgenol 2002;178(4):939–944.
38. Stenbygaard LE, et al. Metastatic pattern in non-resectable non-small cell lung cancer. Acta Oncol 1999;38(8):993–998.
39. Reske SN, Kotzerke J. FDG PET for clinical use. Results of the 3rd German Interdisciplinary Consensus Conference, "Onko-PET III", 21 July and 19 September 2000. Eur J Nucl Med 2001;28(11): 1707–1723.
40. Bury T, et al. Fluorine-18 deoxyglucose positron emission tomography for the detection of bone metastases in patients with non-small cell lung cancer. Eur J Nucl Med 1998;25(9):1244–1247.
41. Rohren EM, et al. Screening for cerebral metastases with FDG PET in patients undergoing whole-body staging of non-central nervous system malignancy. Radiology 2003;226(1):181–187.
42. Prabhakar H, et al. Impact of dual PET-CT findings on the interpretation of thoracic CT in patients with malignancy. Chicago: RSNA Abstract, 2004.
43. Weder W, et al. Detection of extrathoracic metastases by positron emission tomography in lung cancer. Ann Thorac Surg 1998;66(3): 886–892; discussion 892–893.
44. Yap CS, et al. FDG PET imaging in lung cancer: how sensitive is it for bronchioloalveolar carcinoma? Eur J Nucl Med Mol Imaging 2002;29(9):1166–1173.
45. Tas F, et al. Factors influencing the distribution of metastases and survival in extensive disease small cell lung cancer. Acta Oncol 1999;38(8):1011–1015.
46. Kamel EM, et al. Whole-body (18)F-FDG PET improves the management of patients with small cell lung cancer. J Nucl Med 2003;44(12):1911–1917.
47. Martini N, et al. Incidence of local recurrence and second primary tumors in resected stage I lung cancer. J Thorac Cardiovasc Surg 1995;109(1):120–129.
48. Miura H, et al. Recurrence at the bronchial stump after resection of lung cancer. Ann Surg 1994;219(3):306–309.
49. Verleden G, Deneffe G, Demedts M. Bronchial stump recurrence after surgery for bronchial carcinoma. Eur Respir J 1990;3(1): 97–100.
50. Gruden JF, Campagna G, McGuinness G. The normal CT appearances of the second carina and bronchial stump after left upper lobectomy. J Thorac Imaging 2000;15(2):138–143.
51. Keidar Z, et al. PET-CT using 18F-FDG in suspected lung cancer recurrence: diagnostic value and impact on patient management. J Nucl Med 2004;45(10):1640–1646.
52. Logan PM. Thoracic manifestations of external beam radiotherapy. Am J Roentgenol 1998;171(3):569–577.
53. Strauss LG. Fluorine-18 deoxyglucose and false-positive results: a major problem in the diagnostics of oncological patients. Eur J Nucl Med 1996;23(10):1409–1415.
54. Lin P, et al. Fluorine-18 FDG dual-head gamma camera coincidence imaging of radiation pneumonitis. Clin Nucl Med 2000;25(11): 866–869.
55. Patz EF Jr, et al. Persistent or recurrent bronchogenic carcinoma: detection with PET and 2-[F-18]-2-deoxy-D-glucose. Radiology 1994;191(2):379–382.
56. Kwek BH, Aquino SL, Fischman AJ. Fluorodeoxyglucose positron emission tomography and CT after talc pleurodesis. Chest 2004;125(6):2356–2360.
57. Patz EF Jr, Connolly J, Herndon J. Prognostic value of thoracic FDG PET imaging after treatment for non-small cell lung cancer. Am J Roentgenol 2000;174(3):769–774.
58. Erdi YE, et al. Use of PET to monitor the response of lung cancer to radiation treatment. Eur J Nucl Med 2000;27(7):861–866.
59. Kostakoglu L, Goldsmith SJ. PET in the assessment of therapy response in patients with carcinoma of the head and neck and of the esophagus. J Nucl Med 2004;45(1):56–68.
60. Mac Manus MP, et al. Metabolic (FDG PET) response after radical radiotherapy/chemoradiotherapy for non-small cell lung cancer correlates with patterns of failure. Lung Cancer 2005;49(1):95–108.
61. Hoekstra CJ, et al. Prognostic relevance of response evaluation using [18F]-2-fluoro-2-deoxy-D-glucose positron emission tomography in patients with locally advanced non-small-cell lung cancer. J Clin Oncol 2005;23(33):8362–8370.
62. Pottgen, C., et al. Value of 18F-fluoro-2-deoxy-D-glucose-positron emission tomography/computed tomography in non-small-cell lung cancer for prediction of pathologic response and times to relapse after neoadjuvant chemoradiotherapy. Clin Cancer Res, 2006;12(1): 97–106.
63. Asad S, et al. False-positive FDG positron emission tomography uptake in nonmalignant chest abnormalities. Am J Roentgenol 2004;182(4):983–989.
64. Fayad LM, et al. Sacral fractures: a potential pitfall of FDG positron emission tomography. Am J Roentgenol 2003;181(5):1239–1243.
65. Weber WA. Brown adipose tissue and nuclear medicine imaging. J Nucl Med 2004;45(7):1101–1103.
66. Fan CM, et al. Lipomatous hypertrophy of the interatrial septum: increased uptake on FDG PET. Am J Roentgenol 2005;184(1): 339–342.

Chapter 17
PET-CT of Esophageal Cancer

Gary J.R. Cook

Esophageal carcinoma is more frequent in later life, being relatively uncommon under the age of 45 years. It is twice as common in men and has been increasing in frequency over the last 30 years. Associated causative risk factors include tobacco and alcohol use. There may be a relation to diet as this cancer is more common in the Far East. Medical conditions associated with an increased risk of esophageal cancer include Barrett's esophagus and gastroesophageal reflux (adenocarcinoma) and achalasia (squamous cell carcinoma).

Squamous cell carcinoma accounts for approximately half of new cases and tends to occur in the upper third and middle esophagus. Adenocarcinoma is increasing in incidence and most commonly occurs in the lower third of the esophagus.

Approximately 20% of patients presenting with carcinoma of the esophagus will be eligible for attempted curative surgical resection (usually stage IIB or less). The overall 5-year survival is approximately 5–10%, increasing to 10–25% of patients who have surgery. This ranges from above 50% in stage I to almost zero in stage IV. Surgery alone may be offered to patients with stage I but neoadjuvant chemotherapy may be used in stages II and III prior to surgery. In high squamous cell carcinomas radical combined chemotherapy and radiotherapy may be offered with curative intent. Chemotherapy and/or radiotherapy may be used as adjuvant treatment in those considered at high risk of recurrence following attempted curative surgery. Palliative options in advanced disease include chemotherapy and radiotherapy, either alone or in combination, palliative surgery and stenting of esophageal strictures, as well as newer techniques, including lasers and photodynamic therapy.

G.J.R. Cook (✉)
Department of Nuclear Medicine and PET,
Royal Marsden Hospital,
Downs Rd, Sutton, Surrey SM2 5PT, UK
e-mail: gcook@icr.ac.uk

Diagnosis

There is no established role for the use of 18FDG PET in the screening or initial diagnosis of esophageal carcinoma. The diagnosis remains essentially the province of endoscopic biopsy. Endoscopic biopsy of an esophageal stricture can be negative, and in such cases when suspicion of an esophageal cancer is high, PET-CT can offer diagnostic and staging information (Fig. 17.1). Incidental note may occasionally be made of abnormal uptake of 18FDG in the esophagus in a segmental pattern when using PET for the management of another cancer [1]. Such FDG uptake most commonly caused by esophagitis is relatively frequent. Esophageal cancer, however, can present as long segmental FDG uptake as well due to the relative ease of spread of esophageal cancer along the lymphatic network of the esophagus (Fig. 17.2). In such instances the esophageal wall may not be detectably thickened on the CT images, and hence PET-CT cannot distinguish between esophagitis and esophageal cancer. Endoscopic examination is required for definitive diagnosis.

Staging

Management decisions in esophageal carcinoma are dependent on accurate staging (Table 17.1) with stage being closely related to survival (Table 17.2) [2]. Once the diagnosis has been made histologically, then T staging is best made by a combination of CT and endoscopic ultrasound (EUS). Although the vast majority of esophageal cancers show enhanced uptake of 18FDG, the resolution of PET is insufficient to determine the depth of invasion, although T4 tumors may be diagnosed with PET-CT. The criteria for T4 disease on the CT component of the study includes the obliteration of fat planes between esophageal tumors and adjacent mediastinal structures, extension into the trachea or bronchi with displacement, compression, or bulging of the posterior wall of the carina or left main bronchus and obliteration of a

P. Shreve and D.W. Townsend (eds.), *Clinical PET-CT in Radiology: Integrated Imaging in Oncology*,
DOI 10.1007/978-0-387-48902-5_17, © Springer Science+Business Media, LLC 2011

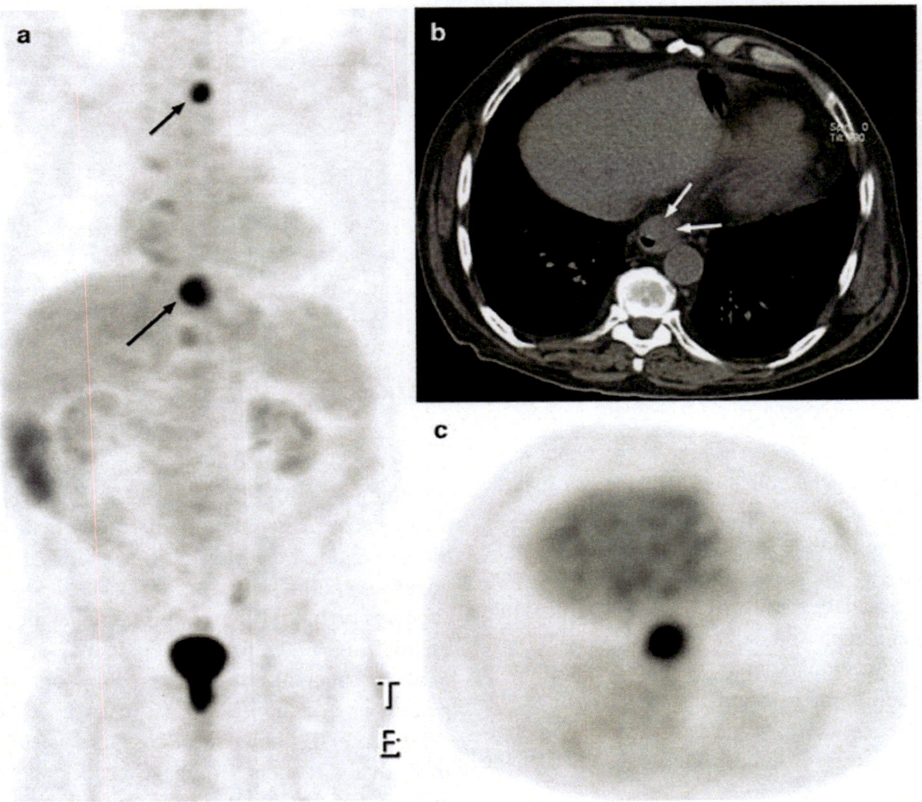

Fig. 17.1 Stenosis at the gastroesophageal junction on endoscopy with negative biopsy in an 80-year-old patient with dysphagia and weight loss. On the FDG PET anterior MIP image (**a**) intense focal FDG uptake is present at gastroesophageal junction (*arrow*) as well as in a high left paraesophageal mediastinal lymph node (*small arrow*). Transaxial CT (**b**) and FDG PET (**c**) at the level of the gastroesophageal junction shows eccentric thickening of the esophageal wall (*arrowheads*), which is associated with intense abnormal FDG tracer uptake

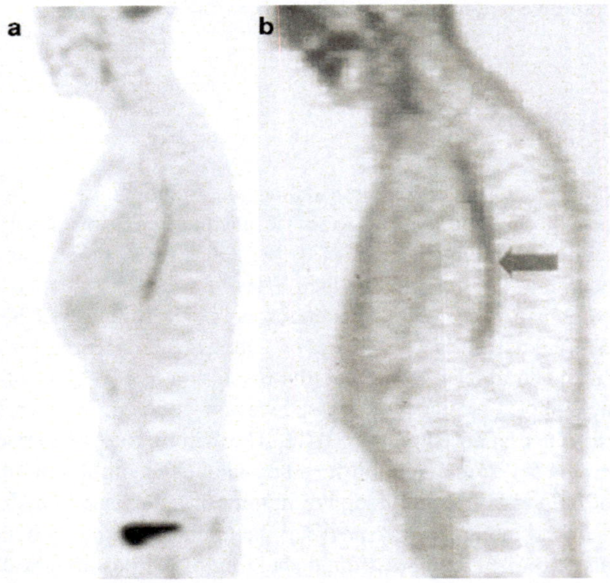

Fig. 17.2 Sagittal 18FDG images of esophageal carcinoma (**a**) and esophagitis (**b**), demonstrating how similar the different pathologies can appear on FDG PET

greater than 90° arc of the fat plane between the esophagus and aorta (Fig. 17.3). The few primary tumors that are not visible with PET are usually small T1 tumors [3].

The pattern of spread of lymph node metastases depends on the site of the primary tumor (Fig. 17.4). Upper esophageal tumors metastasize predominantly to cervical and mediastinal nodes, although more than 10% are associated with abdominal nodes. Lower esophageal tumors are more commonly associated with abdominal and mediastinal nodes, although almost 30% may also have nodes in the cervical region, commonly in supraclavicular nodes [5]. Distant metastases are most frequently found in lung, liver, and bone [6].

Lymph node staging is crucially important and one of the most important prognostic factors. Clinical N staging has previously relied on size criteria of detecting nodes of greater than 10 mm in short axis, but it is recognized that this has limitations and that normal nodes vary in size depending on anatomic site, for example, some use a criteria of greater than 5 mm for retrocrural nodes and greater than 8 mm for celiac and left gastric nodes for positivity. Lymph node staging can be divided into N stage concerning periesophageal nodes extending from cervical to celiac nodes (Fig. 17.5) or more

Table 17.1 AJCC staging for esophageal cancer (Used with the permission of the American Joint Committee on Cancer (AJCC), Chicago, IL. The original source for this material is the *AJCC Cancer Staging Manual,* Seventh Edition (2010) published by Springer Science and Business Media LLC. www.springer.com)

Definitions of TNM

Primary tumor (T)[a]

TX	Primary tumor cannot be assessed
T0	No evidence of primary tumor
Tis	High-grade dysplasia[b]
T1	Tumor invades lamina propria, muscularis mucosae, or submucosa
T1a	Tumor invades lamina propria or muscularis mucosae
T1b	Tumor invades submucosa
T2	Tumor invades muscularis propria
T3	Tumor invades adventitia
T4	Tumor invades adjacent structures
T4a	Resectable tumor invading pleura, pericardium, or diaphragm
T4b	Unresectable tumor invading other adjacent structures, such as aorta, vertebral body, trachea, etc.

Regional lymph nodes (N)[c]

NX	Regional lymph nodes cannot be assessed
N0	No regional lymph node metastasis
N1	Metastasis in 1–2 regional lymph nodes
N2	Metastasis in 3–6 regional lymph nodes
N3	Metastasis in 7 or more regional lymph nodes

Distant metastasis (M)

M0	No distant metastasis
M1	Distant metastasis

[a](1) At least maximal dimension of the tumor must be recorded, and (2) multiple tumors require the Tm suffix

[b]High-grade dysplasia includes all noninvasive neoplastic epithelia that was formerly called carcinoma in situ, a diagnosis that is no longer used for columnar mucosae anywhere in the gastrointestinal tract

[c]The number must be recorded for total number of regional nodes sampled and total number of reported nodes with metastases

Table 17.2 Anatomic stage, prognostic group, and 5-year survival in esophageal cancer

Stage	Prognostic Group	Five-year survival (%)
Stage I	T1, N0 M0	66%
Stage IIa	T2 or T3, N0, M0	40%
Stage IIb	T1 N1 M0, T2 N1 M0	19%
Stage III	T3 N1, M0, T4, any N, M0	16%
Stage IV	Any T, any N, M1	2%

distant nodal involvement considered MI disease, (Fig. 17.6). Regional lymph nodes have recently been redefined to include any paraesophageal node from cervical to celiac groups (Table 17.1). A number of studies have confirmed the inferiority of FDG PET in detecting periesophageal nodes compared to CT and EUS [7–9], although when detected, PET shows good specificity. The reason for the inferior sensitivity of PET alone is likely to be due to the inability to separately resolve small focal areas of uptake within nodes that are in close proximity to the high activity demonstrated in an adjacent primary tumor (see Fig. 17.5). It is likely that combination PET-CT may be more accurate in this regard than PET alone [10]. PET may enable detection of disease in subcentimeter nodes, although enlarged nodes on CT in the expected distribution of metastases that are PET negative may be regarded as indeterminate, requiring further evaluation with EUS. EUS has been reported to be more sensitive in detecting periesophageal and celiac nodes than PET and CT [11], and also has the advantage of the ability to guide endoscopic biopsy for histologic confirmation and should be regarded as complementary to PET-CT in the full TNM staging of patients with esophageal cancer.

It is in the detection of distant metastatic lymph nodes and other organ metastases that FDG PET is more accurate than EUS and CT combined [11–16]. Distant nodal metastases are usually located in the supraclavicular fossae or retroperitoneum (Fig. 17.7), while distant visceral metastases are most frequently in the liver, lung, or skeleton [6]. Skeletal metastases are usually lytic in nature and not infrequently can be invisible on the CT component of PET-CT, while being strongly positive on the PET images (Fig. 17.8). It is rarer for there to be distant metastases on the CT component that are not seen on PET except in the lung where the sensitivity for the PET component at less than 1 cm is inferior. It is largely due to the detection of distant metastatic nodal and visceral disease in approximately 15–25% of patients that PET frequently alters management from a surgical to palliative approach, saving patients from futile major surgery and saving healthcare costs. As PET and PET-CT cannot give all the information that is required for optimal staging, particularly with regard to T staging, they should be considered as complementary to EUS and diagnostic CT in the initial staging of esophageal cancer being considered for radical therapy. A recent large prospective US study of 189 patients showed that although 22% of eligible patients did not undergo esophagectomy, FDG-PET after standard clinical staging for esophageal carcinoma identified M1b disease in 5% of patients, which was subsequently confirmed. Unconfirmed PET evidence of M1 disease and regional adenopathy resulted in definitive nonsurgical or induction therapy in additional patients [17]. Other than the pitfalls that can occur in imaging any cancer with 18FDG PET, false-positive uptake in hilar nodes has been described as being the most common in esophageal cancer [18]. As the positive predictive value of PET is not 100%, it is important to confirm PET-positive abnormalities histologically if a patient is to be denied a curative procedure as a result of the PET findings alone. CT is likely to remain more sensitive than PET alone is detecting small (e.g., <5 mm) lung metastases, although PET is more specific, but this deficiency is overcome with combined PET-CT. Similarly, PET alone is insensitive for detecting brain metastases, an area where contrast CT or MRI remain the most accurate.

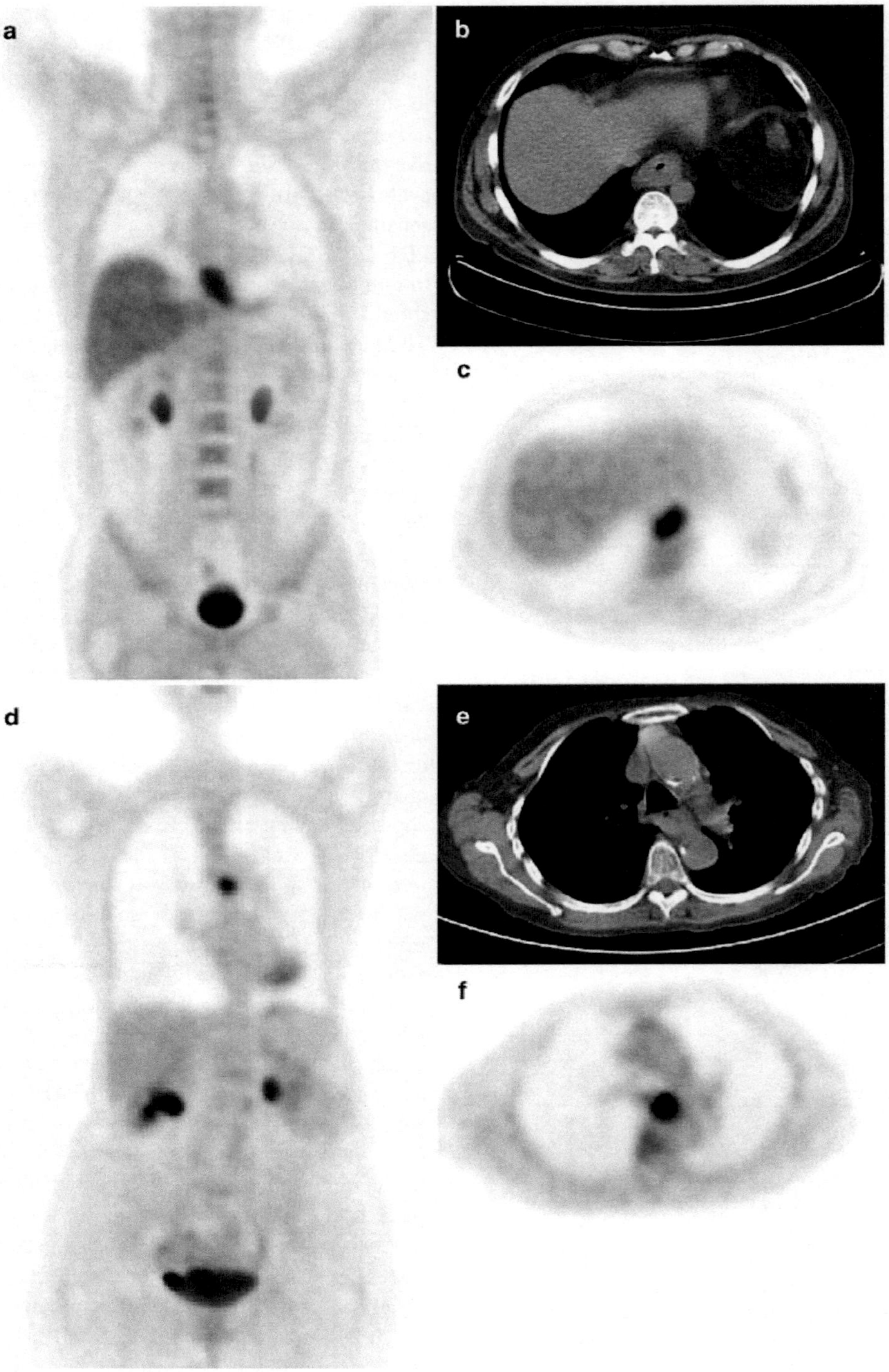

Fig. 17.3 Primary esophageal tumor local extension. On coronal FDG PET (**a**) intense FDG tracer activity is seen in the distal esophagus. Transaxial CT (**b**) and FDG PET (**c**) images show a large concentric distal esophageal mass which is intensely FDG avid, but a very thin fat plane is maintained between the mass and the descending thoracic aorta. In another patient, coronal FDG PET image (**d**) demonstrates a focus of intense abnormal FDG tracer activity in the mid-esophagus. On transaxial CT (**e**) and FDG PET (**f**) a posterior mid-esophageal mass with luminal narrowing is seen which is intensely FDG avid, and the fat plane between the esophagus and left superior pulmonary vein is entirely lost on the CT image, indicating T4 disease. This was confirmed on endoscopic ultrasound

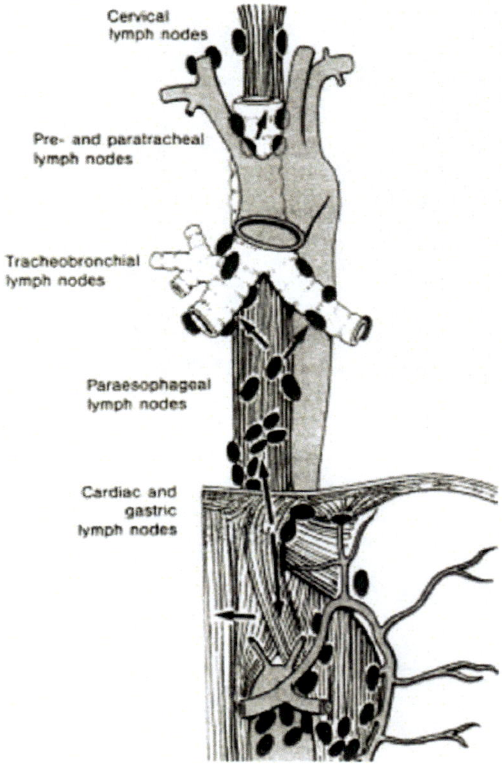

Fig. 17.4 Directions of lymphatic flow and regional lymph nodes of the esophagus. Above the level of the aortic arch, lymphatic flow is to cervical and pretracheal and paratracheal upper mediastinal lymph nodes. At the mid-level of the esophagus, lymphatic flow is bidirectional and includes tracheobronchial lymph nodes. Below the level of the pulmonary veins, lymphatic drainage is primarily directed toward subdiaphragmatic lymph nodes (From [4]. With permission)

Restaging

Recurrent esophageal carcinoma is common, reflecting the relative insensitivity of conventional staging techniques in selecting patients for radical therapy and due to the aggressive nature of this type of cancer. Recurrence can occur close to the surgical margins at anastomoses or in regional lymph nodes or distant organs. Locoregional recurrence (Fig. 17.9) predominates in upper and middle third carcinomas (largely squamous cell carcinoma), while in carcinomas of the lower third of the esophagus (largely adenocarcinomas) distant recurrence (Fig. 17.10) is more common [6].

Despite PET showing high sensitivity for detecting perianastomotic recurrences, this is at the expense of a number of false-positives primarily due to inflammatory changes at the anastomotic site (specificity 57%) [12] (Table 17.3). It remains unknown whether PET-CT may improve this specificity owing to the additional morphologic information. It should be noted, however, that in this situation EUS has proven remarkably accurate (sensitivity 100%, specificity 93%) [18].

For regional metastases, similar overall accuracy has been reported for FDG PET versus anatomic imaging (PET 88%, conventional imaging 83%), but FDG PET has been shown to be superior in detecting distant metastases [18] (see Fig. 17.7). It would appear, likely, therefore, that a combination of EUS and PET-CT are required to optimally stage recurrent esophageal cancer. Additional information from PET has been reported in 27% of patients with suspected recurrence confirming the value of the FDG PET component of PET-CT in this situation. Additionally, the combination of PET-CT is likely to improve specificity by reducing false-positives due to uptake in benign variants and reduce the number of equivocal interpretations, as has been shown in other PET-CT studies [10]. False-positive findings have been particularly reported following dilatation of esophageal strictures or following surgery with false-positive uptake being reported several months after dilatation or surgery [18].

Therapy Monitoring

Outcomes in the treatment of locally advanced esophageal cancer are improved in patients who respond to neoadjuvant chemoradiation therapy. Response of esophageal cancer to chemoradiation adjuvant therapy includes resolution of abnormal glucose metabolism as depicted on FDG PET, and reduction in size of the tumor, as depicted on CT (Fig. 17.11). Compared to conventional criteria for measuring response to neoadjuvant chemotherapy in adenocarcinomas of the gastroesophageal junction (e.g., reduction of tumor length and wall thickness by >50% at 3 months), change in SUV from baseline FDG PET to FDG PET performed at 14 days is significantly different in responding tumors (–54% ± 17%) compared to nonresponding tumors (–15% ± 21%) [19]. An optimal cutoff of 35% reduction in SUV at 14 days predicted a clinical response with a sensitivity and specificity of 93% and 95%, respectively. The metabolic changes as depicted on FDG PET in response to neoadjuvant therapy for adenocarcinoma of the gastroesophageal junction were shown to precede tumor wall thickness changes and were of twice the magnitude in responding patients [20]. FDG PET-CT response has been used to guide subsequent treatment [21]. Patients showing a greater than 35% reduction in SUV completed chemotherapy before surgery, but those deemed not to respond went straight to surgery. Prognosis was better in responders than nonresponders, and this trial showed the feasibility of tailoring treatment according to individual tumor biology.

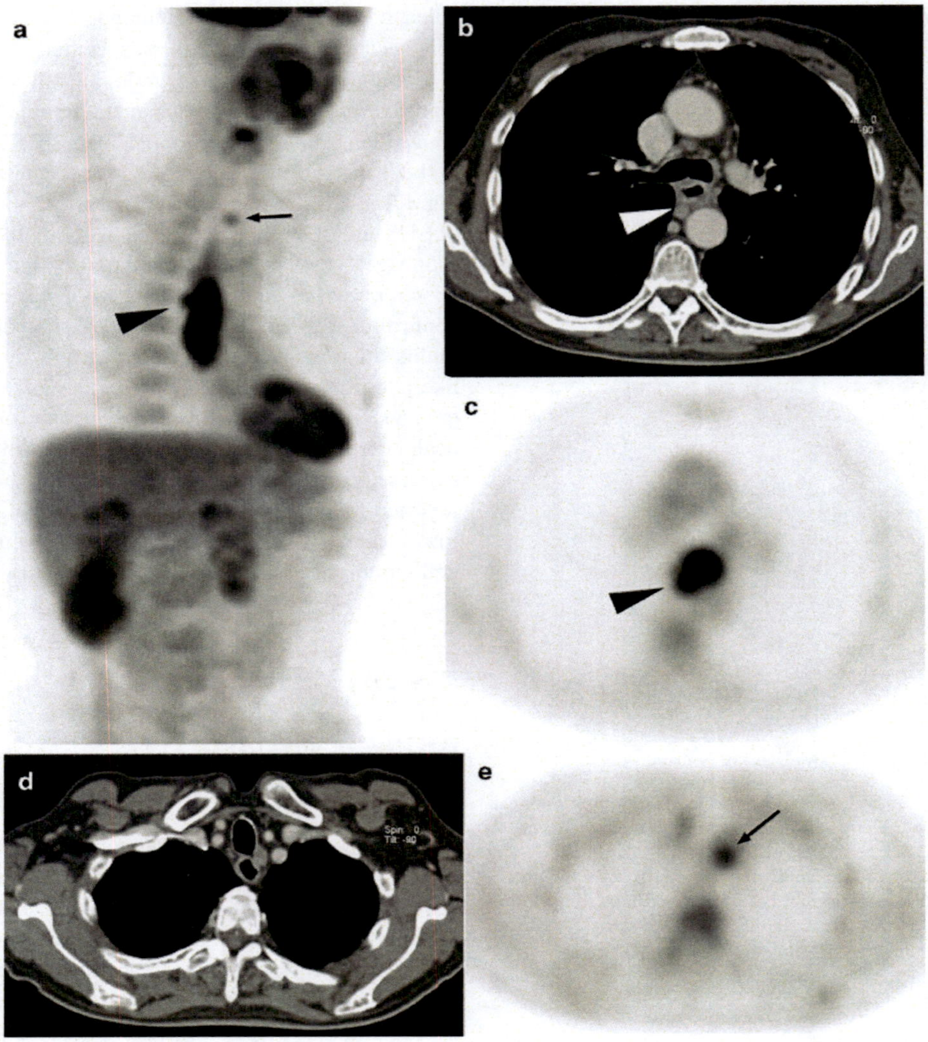

Fig. 17.5 Squamous cell carcinoma of the mid-esophagus on endoscopy. Left anterior oblique FDG PET MIP image (**a**) shows intense fusiform increased 18FDG uptake at the mid esophagus with an associated adjacent focus of tracer activity (*arrowhead*) partially obscured by the intensity of the esophageal mass, and an additional high left mediastinal focus (*arrow*) of abnormal tracer uptake. Transaxial (*arrowhead*) CT (**b**) (*arrow*) and FDG PET (**c**) images reveal an 8-mm paraesophageal lymph node at the level of the primary esophageal mass (*arrowhead*) and an additional paraesophageal FDG avid 11-mm lymph node (*arrow*) in the upper mediastinum (**d**, **e**), consistent with regional (N1) lymph node metastases

Serial FDG PET has also been used to predict response to neoadjuvant combined radiotherapy and chemotherapy with a sensitivity of 71% and specificity of 82% [22]. The presence of lymph node or distant metastases on the baseline PET study was much more likely to be associated with a poor response than those without evidence of metastatic disease. However, a poor PET response is a better predictor of overall survival than lymph node involvement on a baseline PET scan.

A similar study comparing baseline and 3 week 18FDG PET scans in neoadjuvant chemoradiotherapy for squamous cell carcinomas of the esophagus predicted clinical response with a sensitivity of 100% and specificity of 55% when using a cutoff of 52% decrease [23]. High pretreatment FDG uptake in locally advanced esophageal cancer or a large decrease in tumor FDG uptake after chemoradiation therapy were correlated with histopathologic response with an overall accuracy of 88% [24]. Another study failed to find a correlation between reduction in SUV and histopathologic response, possibly due to increased uptake in therapy induced esophagitis [25]. When assessing the response to radiotherapy

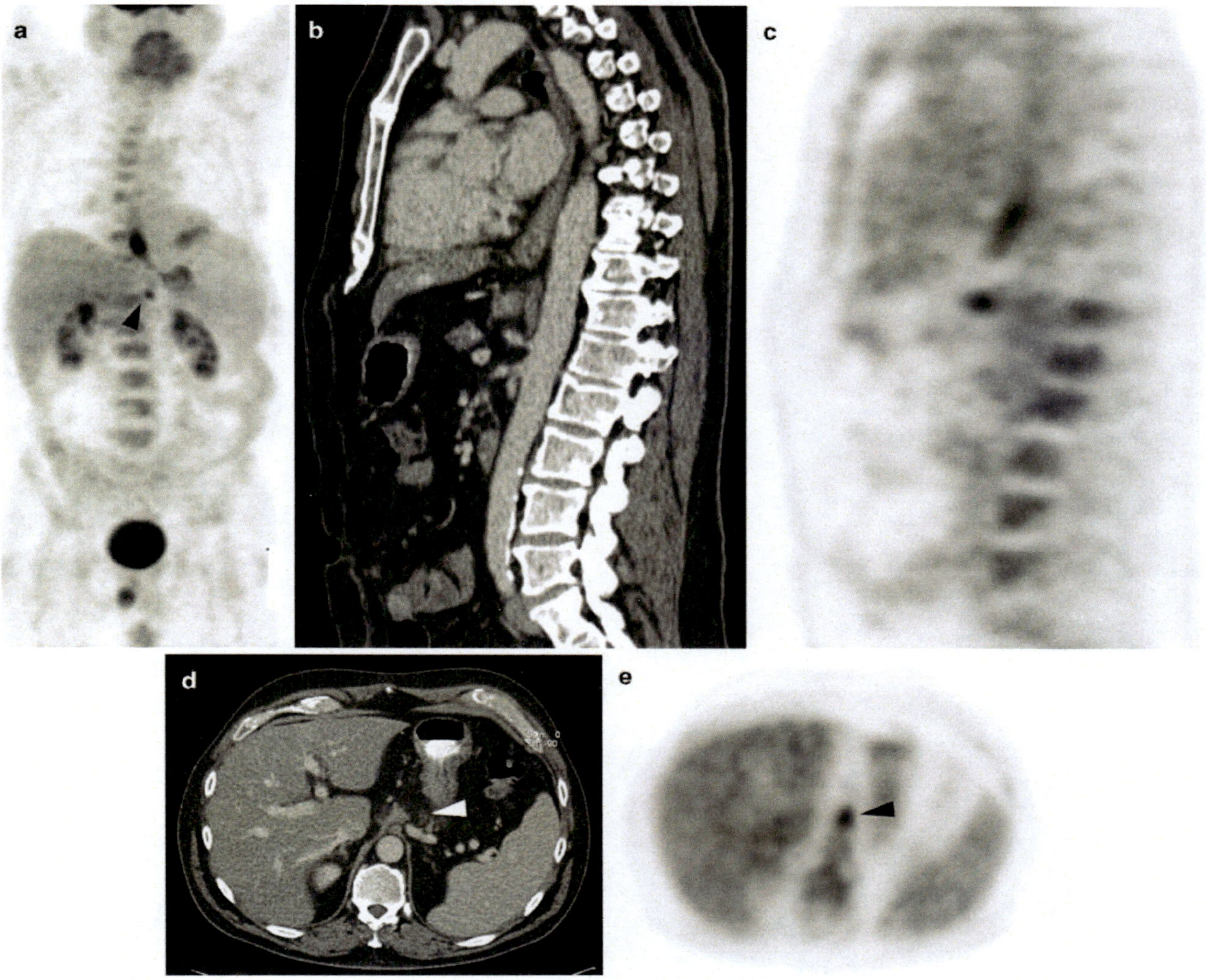

Fig. 17.6 Adenocarcinoma of the distal esophagus on endoscopic biopsy. The anterior FDG PET MIP image (**a**) shows focal abnormal FDG tracer uptake at the distal esophagus and a small focus of FDG tracer uptake near midline in the upper abdomen (*arrowhead*). Sagittal CT (**b**) (*arrowhead*) and FDG PET (**c**) (*arrowhead*) images demonstrate slightly fusiform FDG avid thickening of the distal esophagus (*arrowhead*) corresponding to the primary tumor and a FDG avid lymph node just superior to the celiac axis (*arrowhead*), which measures 7 × 9 mm on transaxial CT (**d**) and FDG (*arrowhead*) PET (**e**).

alone in squamous cell carcinoma, 18FDG PET may predict tumor response but may not be able to sufficiently differentiate residual disease from complete response [26]. It would appear that using 18FDG PET to evaluate response in primary esophageal tumors may be more reliable with chemotherapy alone (Fig. 17.12) than with regimens including radiotherapy, possibly due to the benign inflammatory uptake of 18FDG that may be associated with this form of therapy.

Although the use of 18FDG PET-CT would appear promising as a tool to noninvasively monitor neoadjuvant therapy, further work is required before practical guidelines can be issued on how this should be used in routine practice at the current time. However, an unequivocal progression of T stage by PET-CT or EUS or the appearance of new metastases on PET-CT would likely preclude surgery after neoadjuvant therapy.

RT Planning

Radiotherapy planning of primary esophageal tumors relies mostly on morphologic techniques, including CT and EUS. 18FDG PET-CT has the potential to more accurately delineate

Fig. 17.7 Newly diagnosed adenocarcinoma of the gastroesophageal junction. Anterior FDG PET MIP image (**a**) shows intense focal FDG tracer uptake at the gastroesophageal junction (*arrow*) and less intense foci of abnormal FDG tracer uptake in the mid-abdomen just superior to the physiologic tracer uptake in the gastric antrum (*arrowheads*). There is also modest focal FDG activity in the right upper thorax reflecting a subcentimeter pulmonary metastasis (*arrowheads*). The mid-abdominal tracer uptake corresponds to retroperitoneal metastases including a FDG avid 1.1 × 2.8 cm portocaval lymph node (*arrowhead*) and a FDG avid 1.2-cm aortocaval lymph node (*arrowhead*), seen on the transaxial CT (**b**) and FDG PET (**c**) images

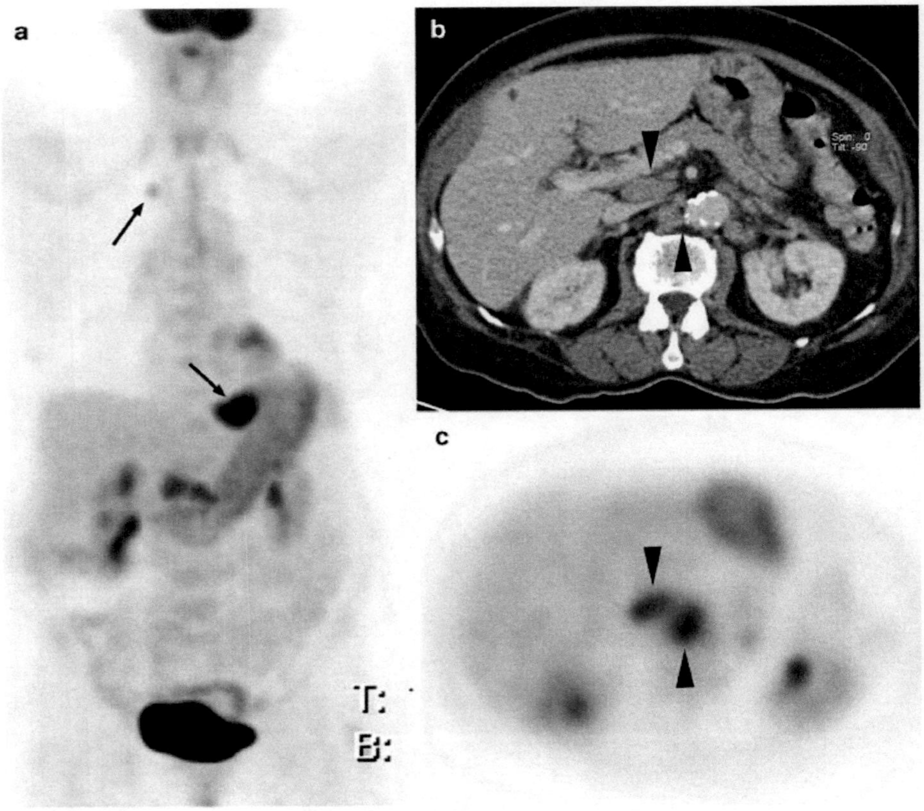

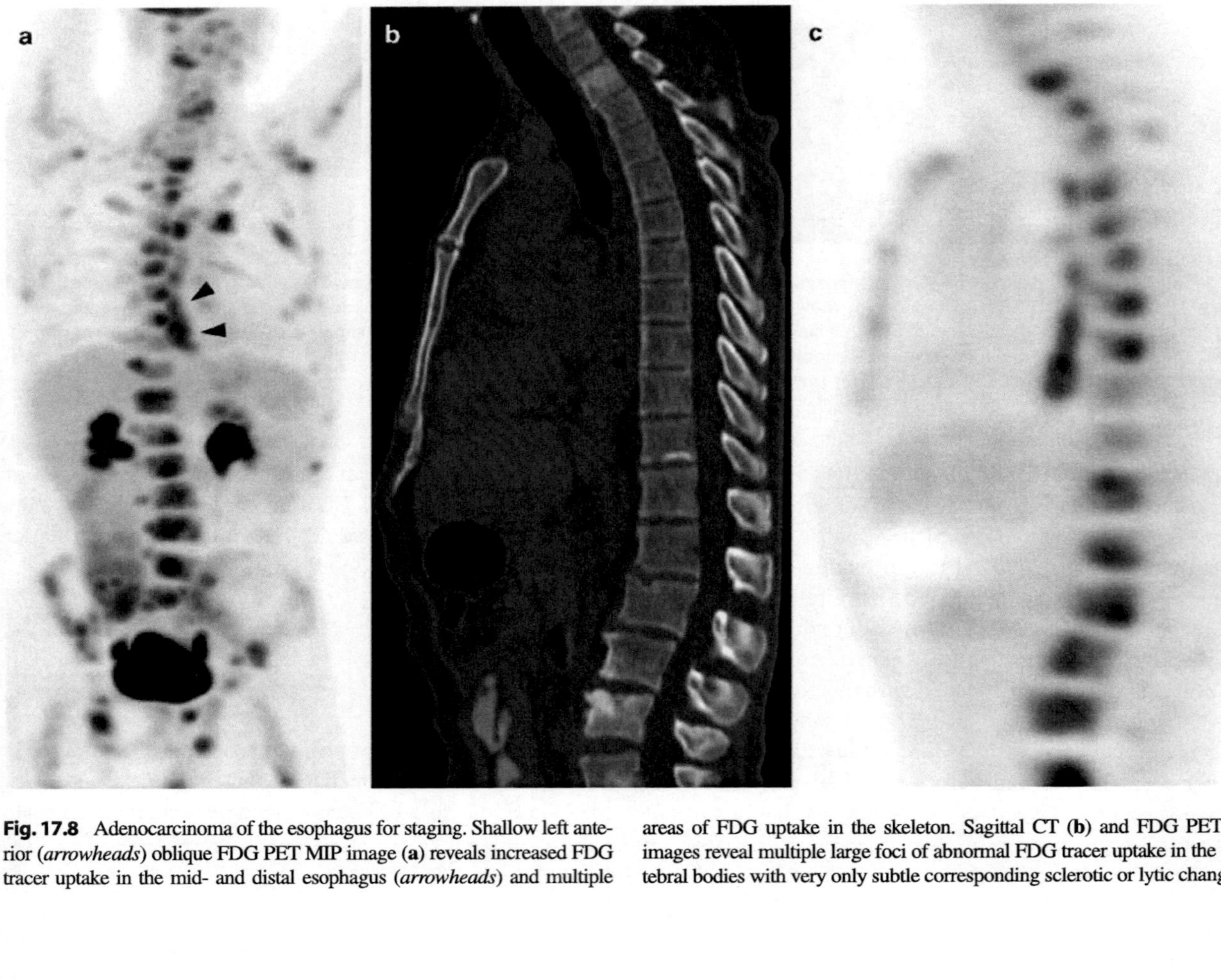

Fig. 17.8 Adenocarcinoma of the esophagus for staging. Shallow left anterior (*arrowheads*) oblique FDG PET MIP image (**a**) reveals increased FDG tracer uptake in the mid- and distal esophagus (*arrowheads*) and multiple areas of FDG uptake in the skeleton. Sagittal CT (**b**) and FDG PET (**c**) images reveal multiple large foci of abnormal FDG tracer uptake in the vertebral bodies with very only subtle corresponding sclerotic or lytic changes

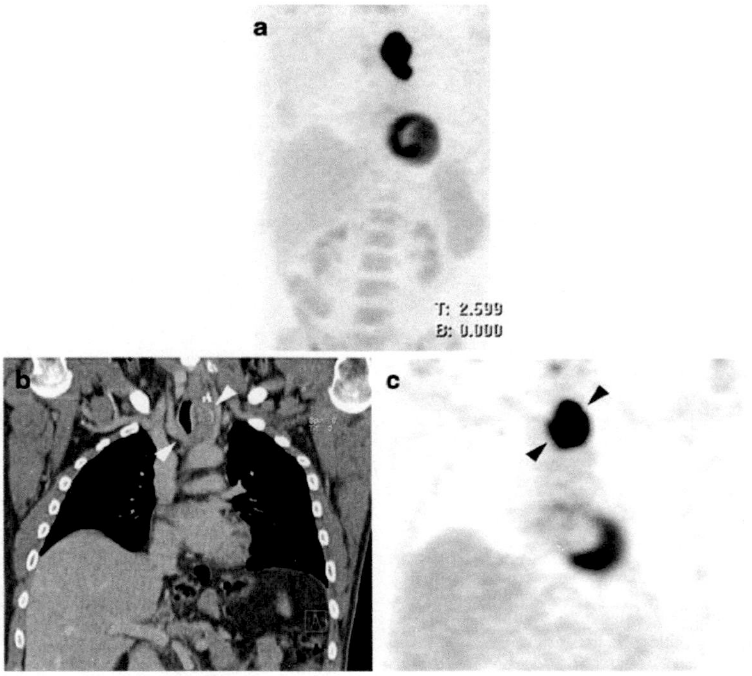

Fig. 17.9 Recurrent esophageal cancer (squamous cell carcinoma) at the level of the cervical anastomosis following esophagectomy and gastric pull–though. Anterior FDG PET MIP image (**a**) demonstrates a large solitary focus of abnormal FDG tracer uptake in the upper mediastinum. Coronal CT (**b**) and FDG PET (**c**) images reveal a large FDG avid mass in the posterior mediastinum interposed between the trachea and left carotid artery (*arrowheads*), just caudal to the anastomotic surgical clips, corresponding to the anastomotic recurrence. There is no distant metastatic disease seen

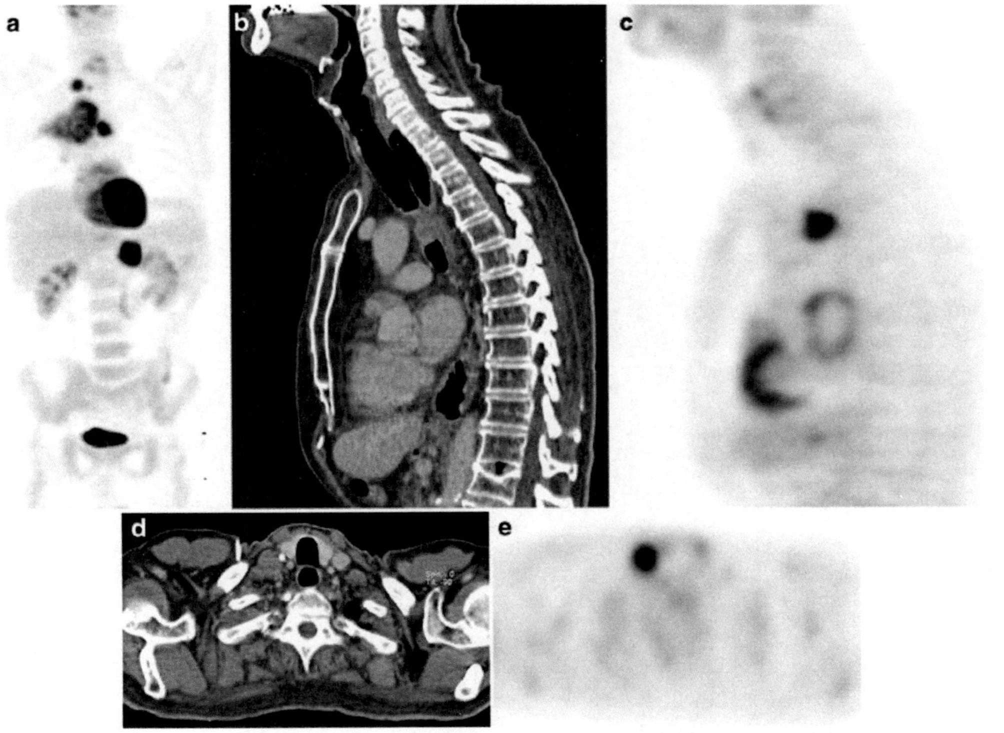

Fig. 17.10 Adenocarcinoma of the distal esophagus treated with esophagectomy and gastric pull through. Anterior FDG PET MIP image (**a**) demonstrates three discrete metastases and a large area of tracer uptake corresponding to a cavitating right upper lobe mass related to a fistula. Sagittal CT (**b**) and FDG PET (**c**) images show the focus of intense abnormal FDG tracer uptake in the left mediastinum corresponds to a 2-cm AP window lymph node metastasis. The large focus of FDG tracer uptake in the left upper abdomen seen on the whole torso MIP image corresponds to a 3-cm left adrenal metastasis (not shown). The focus of FDG tracer uptake at the right upper thorax seen on the whole torso MIP image is shown on transaxial CT (**d**) and FDG PET (**e**) to be a right 1.8-cm supraclavicular lymph node metastasis

Table 17.3 Pitfalls in the diagnosis of recurrent disease with PET-CT

Anastomotic inflammation (especially after dilatation)
Reactive hilar lymph node false-positive
Recent rib fractures (although CT findings reduce false-positives)
Focal physiologic FDG uptake at the gastroesophageal junction
Physiologic uptake in gastric pull through
Small (<1 cm) lung metastases detected by CT but not resolved with PET

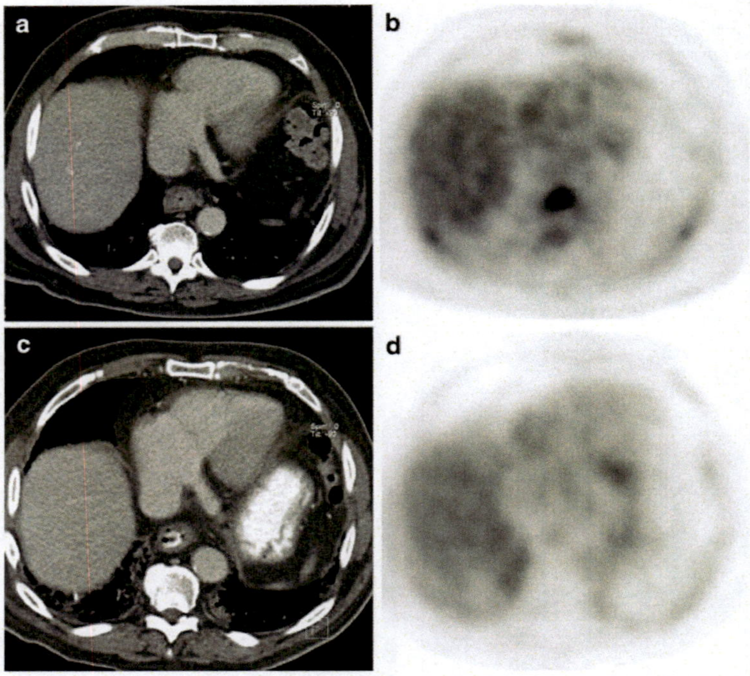

Fig. 17.11 Response of adenocarcinoma of the distal esophagus to adjuvant chemoradiation therapy. (**a**) Pretherapy transaxial CT and FDG PET, (**b**) images reveal concentric wall thickening of the distal esophagus associated with intense abnormal FDG uptake. The post therapy CT (**c**) and FDG PET (**d**) at the same transaxial level show near complete resolution of the thickened esophageal wall and complete resolution of FDG tracer uptake, consistent with responding tumor

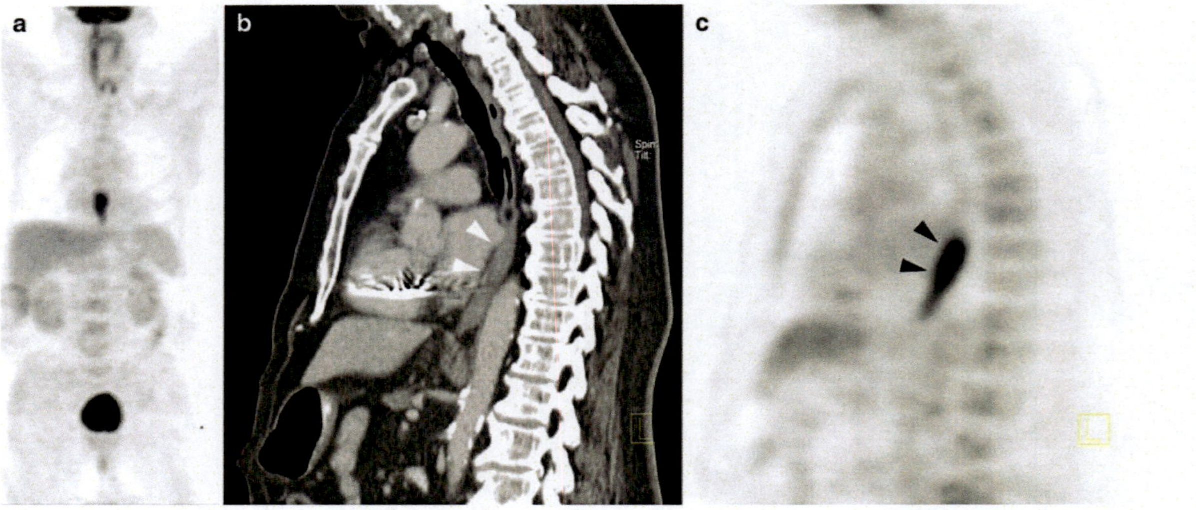

Fig. 17.12 Unfavorable response of squamous cell carcinoma of the distal esophagus to chemotherapy. Following completion of chemotherapy, the anterior FDG PET MIP image (**a**) reveals intense fusiform abnormal FDG tracer uptake in the distal esophagus. On sagittal CT (**b**) and FDG PET (**c**) images, there is a long segment of esophageal wall thickening (*arrowheads*) associated with intense abnormal FDG tracer uptake, consistent with a nonresponding tumor

functional tumor volume than morphologic methods such as CT, MRI, and EUS on their own [27, 28]. In patients who are being considered for radical radiotherapy with curative intent, a number will be found to have distant metastases or regional lymphadenopathy requiring a change to a nonradical treatment method. In patients who have local lymphadenopathy undetected by other modalities, PET may influence radiotherapy plans by increasing the field to encompass these involved nodes. It is quite likely that PET-CT will also contribute to the evaluation of the extent of primary tumor volume.

References

1. Kamel EM, Thumshirn M, Truninger K, et al. Significance of incidental 18F-FDG accumulations in the gastrointestinal tract in PET/CT: correlation with endoscopic and histopathologic results. J Nucl Med 2004;45:1804–1810.
2. Beahrs OH, Henson DE, Hutter RVP, Kennedy BJ. Manual for Staging of Cancer, 4th ed. Philadelphia: Lippincott, 1992.
3. Yeung HW, Macapinlac HA, Mazumdar M, Bains M, Finn RD, Larson SM. FDG-PET in esophageal cancer. Incremental value over computed tomography. Clin Positron Imag 1999;2: 255–260.
4. Richter E, Feyerabend T, Bondorf W (eds.). Normal Lymph Node Topography: CT Atlas. Springer: New York, 2004
5. Benhidjeb T, Hohenberger P. Oesophageal cancer. In: Souhami RL, Tannock I, Hohenberger P, Horiot J-C (eds.). Oxford Textbook of Oncology, 2nd ed. Oxford: Oxford University Press, 2002.
6. Triboulet JP. Pattern of recurrence following complete resection of esophageal carcinoma and factors predictive of recurrent disease. Cancer 2003;97:1616–1623.
7. Lerut T, Flamen P, Ectors N, et al. Histopathologic validation of lymph node staging with FDG-PET scan in cancer of the esophagus and gastroesophageal junction: a prospective study based on primary surgery with extensive lymphadenectomy. Ann Surg 2000;232:743–752.
8. Rankin SC, Taylor H, Cook GJ, Mason R. Computed tomography and positron emission tomography in the pre-operative staging of oesophageal carcinoma. Clin Radiol 1998;53:659–665.
9. Flamen P, Lerut A, Van Cutsem E, et al. Utility of positron emission tomography for the staging of patients with potentially operable esophageal carcinoma. J Clin Oncol 2000;18:3202–3210.
10. Bar-Shalom R, Guralnik L, Tsalic M, et al. The additional value of PET/CT over PET in FDG imaging of oesophageal cancer. Eur J Nucl Med Mol Imaging 2005;32:918–924.
11. Konski A, Doss M, Milestone B, et al. The integration of 18-fluoro-deoxy-glucose positron emission tomography and endoscopic ultrasound in the treatment-planning process for esophageal carcinoma. Int J Radiat Oncol Biol Phys 2005;61:1123–1128.
12. Yoon YC, Lee KS, Shim YM, et al. Metastasis to regional lymph nodes in patients with esophageal squamous cell carcinoma: CT versus FDG PET for presurgical detection prospective study. Radiology 2003;227:764–770.
13. Ott K, Weber WA, Fink U, et al. Fluorodeoxyglucose-positron emission tomography in adenocarcinomas of the distal esophagus and cardia. World J Surg 2003;27:1035–1039.
14. Choi JY, Lee KH, Shim YM, et al. Improved detection of individual nodal involvement in squamous cell carcinoma of the esophagus by FDG PET. J Nucl Med 2000;41:808–815.
15. Kole AC, Plukker JT, Nieweg OE, Vaalburg W. Positron emission tomography for staging of oesophageal and gastroesophageal malignancy. Br J Cancer 1998;78:521–527.
16. Flanagan FL, Dehdashti F, Siegel BA, et al. Staging of esophageal cancer with 18F-fluorodeoxyglucose positron emission tomography. AJR 1997;168:417–424.
17. Meyers BF, Downey RJ, Decker PA, et al. American College of Surgeons Oncology Group Z0060.The utility of positron emission tomography in staging of potentially operable carcinoma of the thoracic esophagus: results of the American College of Surgeons Oncology Group Z0060 trial. J Thorac Cardiovasc Surg 2007;133: 738–745.
18. Flamen P, Lerut A, Van Cutsem E, et al. The utility of positron emission tomography for the diagnosis and staging of recurrent esophageal cancer. J Thorac Cardiovasc Surg 2000;120: 1085–1092.
19. Weber WA, Ott K, Becker K, et al. Prediction of response to preoperative chemotherapy in adenocarcinomas of the esophagogastric junction by metabolic imaging. J Clin Oncol 2001;19: 3058–3065.
20. Wieder HA, Beer AJ, Lordick F, et al. Comparison of changes in tumor metabolic activity and tumor size during chemotherapy of adenocarcinomas of the esophagogastric junction. J Nucl Med 2005;46:2029–2034.
21. Lordick F, Ott K, Krause BJ, et al. PET to assess early metabolic response and to guide treatment of adenocarcinoma of the oesophagogastric junction: the MUNICON phase II trial. Lancet Oncol 2007;8:797–805.
22. Flamen P, Van Cutsem E, Lerut A, et al. Positron emission tomography for assessment of the response to induction radiochemotherapy in locally advanced oesophageal cancer. Ann Oncol 2002;13:361–368.
23. Brucher BL, Weber W, Bauer M, et al. Neoadjuvant therapy of esophageal squamous cell carcinoma: response evaluation by positron emission tomography. Ann Surg 2001;233:300–309.
24. Levine EA, Farmer MR, Clark P, et al. Predictive value of 18-fluoro-deoxy-glucose-positron emission tomography (18F-PET) in the identification of responders to chemoradiation therapy for the treatment of locally advanced esophageal cancer. Ann Surg 2006;243:472–478.
25. Brink I, Hentschel M, Bley TA, et al. Effects of neoadjuvant radiochemotherapy on 18F-FDG-PET in esophageal carcinoma. Eur J Surg Oncol 2004;30:544–550.
26. Nakamura R, Obara T, Katsuragawa S, et al. Failure in presumption of residual disease by quantification of FDG uptake in esophageal squamous cell carcinoma immediately after radiotherapy. Radiat Med 2002;20:181–186.
27. Vrieze O, Haustermans K, De Wever W, et al. Is there a role for FGD-PET in radiotherapy planning in esophageal carcinoma? Radiother Oncol 2004;73:269–275.
28. Leong T, Everitt C, Yuen K, et al. A prospective study to evaluate the impact of FDG-PET on CT-based radiotherapy treatment planning for oesophageal cancer. Radiother Oncol 2006;78:254–261.

Further Reading

1. Dehdashti F, Siegel BA. Neoplasms of the esophagus and stomach. Semin Nucl Med 2004;34:198–208.
2. Dobbs J. Practical Radiotherapy Planning. London: Arnold, 1999.
3. Kostakoglu L, Goldsmith SJ. PET in the assessment of therapy response in patients with carcinoma of the head and neck and of the esophagus. J Nucl Med 2004;45:56–68.
4. Rankin S. Oesophageal cancer. In: Husband JES, Reznek RH (eds.). Imaging in Oncology. Oxford: Isis Medical Media Ltd., 1998.

Chapter 18
PET-CT of Head and Neck Cancers

Barton F. Branstetter IV, Sanjay Paidisetty, Todd M. Blodgett, and Carolyn Cidis Meltzer

Cancers of the head and neck affect an estimated 48,000 Americans each year [1]. Unfortunately, these cancers are frequently fatal, even when identified early in the course of the disease. Appropriate staging is critical to proper treatment planning [2]. In fact, the need for surgery is often determined by the results of imaging. Many of the treatment regimens used for head and neck cancers have high morbidity, so it is important to assign patients to the most appropriate regimen.

Identifying tumor recurrence is similarly important for patients with cancer of the head and neck. Early recurrences can often be treated with more extensive surgery or inclusion of a new treatment modality. Recurrent tumors that are overlooked in their early stages will usually present with extensive local invasion and distant spread, and are almost uniformly fatal.

Combined PET-CT imaging has revolutionized the staging and monitoring of many cancers, but the head and neck has benefited from the new technology more than other anatomic regions [3]. The most important reason for PET-CT's critical role in the head and neck is the compact anatomy of this region. The lack of anatomic precision available with PET alone is felt most acutely in a region where many distinct anatomic structures are packed close together. Also important is the variable physiologic uptake of 18F-fluorodeoxyglucose (FDG) seen in the head and neck. Fused PET-CT images often allow the radiologist to attribute equivocal FDG uptake to normal structures such as glands or muscles.

But PET-CT imaging of the head and neck does have inherent drawbacks. As in other areas of the body, some cancers of the head and neck (particularly glandular tumors) do not uniformly accumulate FDG [4]. Thus, excluding recurrence can be difficult. In these circumstances especially, PET-CT has an advantage over PET alone – the CT will often identify lesions that would otherwise be overlooked because of poor FDG uptake [3].

Technological advances in many modalities, notably CT and MRI, have improved the ability of radiologists to identify small metastatic foci and define the extent of tumors [5, 6]. But the addition of PET-CT to the radiologist's arsenal of diagnostic examinations has had a particular impact on the imaging evaluation of head and neck cancer patients. PET-CT is poised to become the standard of care for staging and monitoring of specific cancers in the head and neck, particularly squamous cell carcinoma and lymphoma.

Imaging the Patient with Head and Neck Cancer

Staging and Restaging

Radiographic staging of head and neck tumors is designed to answer three questions: (1) What is the extent of the local tumor? (2) Are there nodal metastases? and (3) Are there distant metastases (Table 18.1)? Conventional imaging excels at answering the first question, but is notoriously poor at identifying nodal and distant metastases. PET-CT, in contrast, is most useful for assessing metastatic disease, both nodal and distant (Fig. 18.1).

Although virtually every patient with head and neck cancer will undergo radiographic imaging of some sort, not all patients would benefit from a staging PET-CT. It is important to assess the likelihood of encountering metastatic disease before performing an additional, costly, diagnostic examination.

Conventional Imaging

One of the reasons that conventional imaging suffers when assessing nodal metastases is the lack of reliable criteria for identifying metastatic cervical lymph nodes [7]. Size criteria

B.F. Branstetter (✉)
Department of Radiology, University of Pittsburgh Medical Center, Pittsburgh, PA 15213-2582, USA
e-mail: BFB1@pitt.edu

P. Shreve and D.W. Townsend (eds.), *Clinical PET-CT in Radiology: Integrated Imaging in Oncology*,
DOI 10.1007/978-0-387-48902-5_18, © Springer Science+Business Media, LLC 2011

Table 18.1 AJCC TNM staging of head and neck cancer (Used with the permission of the American Joint Committee on Cancer (AJCC), Chicago, IL. The original source for this material is the *AJCC Cancer Staging Manual*, 7th edn. New York: Springer Science and Business Media LLC, 2010. www.springer.com)

Regional Lymph Nodes (N)	
NX	Regional lymph nodes cannot be assessed
N0	No regional lymph node metastasis
N1[a]	Metastasis in a single ipsilateral lymph node, 3 cm or less in greatest dimension
N2[a]	Metastasis in a single ipsilateral lymph node, more than 3 cm but not more than 6 cm in greatest dimension; or in multiple ipsilateral lymph nodes, none more than 6 cm in greatest dimension; or in bilateral or contralateral lymph nodes, none more than 6 cm in greatest dimension
N2a[a]	Metastasis in single ipsilateral lymph node more than 3 cm but not more than 6 cm in greatest dimension
N2b[a]	Metastasis in multiple ipsilateral lymph nodes, none more than 6 cm in greatest dimension
N2c[a]	Metastasis in bilateral or contralateral lymph nodes, none more than 6 cm in greatest dimension
N3[a]	Metastasis in a lymph node more than 6 cm in greatest dimension
Distant Metastasis (M)	
M0	No distant metastasis
M1	Distant metastasis

[a]A designation of U or L may be used to indicate metastasis above the lower border of the cricoid (U) or below the lower border of the cricoid (L). Similarly, clinical/radiological extracapsular spread (ECS) should be recorded as E– or E+, and histopathologic ECS should be designated En, Em, or Eg

are most commonly reported, but experts cannot even agree on which axis (short or long) is a better determinant of malignancy [8, 9]. (At our institution, we prefer long axis because, in our experience, it correlates better with clinical assessments of the nodes.) Different thresholds for lymph node size have been studied, ranging from 5 to 15 mm. As expected, smaller thresholds result in higher sensitivities at the expense of specificity. No single size criterion is sufficient, however, because nodes less than 5 mm may still contain foci of malignancy (see Fig. 18.1).

Other criteria for malignancy have recently gained favor. The presence of central necrosis is almost always indicative of malignancy in adult patients (Fig. 18.2) [10]. Caution should be taken, however, that a central fatty hilum (indicative of benignancy) is not confused with central necrosis (indicative of malignancy).

Enhancement characteristics are also important. Lymph nodes that enhance earlier and to a greater degree than their counterparts are more likely to contain tumor [11]. The border of a suspicious node may be helpful; an ill-defined border suggests extracapsular spread [12]. Most metastatic nodes will not have progressed to extracapsular extension, however, so a well-defined border cannot be taken as a sign of benignancy. Perhaps the best characteristic for distinguishing benign from malignant nodes is the configuration of the node. Reniform nodes, especially those with an identifiable hilum, are almost always benign. Spherical nodes are worrisome.

The decision of whether to use CT or MRI for the initial evaluation of a head and neck tumor depends on the radiologist's personal preference. Some authors feel that MRI defines tumor margins better than CT, but others feel that high-resolution CT has bridged the diagnostic gap, so the added expense of MRI is not warranted [13, 14]. Clinical studies show CT to have a small but measurable advantage in the assessment of cervical lymphadenopathy [7].

In a few anatomic areas, the choice between CT and MRI is clearer. Tumors of the skull base and temporal bone are usually first imaged with CT to establish bony extent. MRI is often called upon secondarily in these cases. Tumors of the oral tongue are better evaluated with MRI. MRI is far superior for establishing the presence or absence of perineural spread. Thyroid cancer is often followed with MRI because the iodinated contrast of CT is believed to stun residual tumor and impair later attempts at radioactive iodine therapy.

Advanced Cross-sectional Techniques

In recent years, researchers in CT and MRI have tried many techniques to conclusively distinguish between benign and malignant cervical lymph nodes. These techniques represent the alternatives to PET-CT. There are no direct comparisons between advanced cross-sectional techniques and PET-CT, but PET-CT has achieved a broader acceptance than any of these alternate methods.

Dynamic contrast techniques have been studied in both CT and MRI [5]. These techniques rely on the more rapid contrast enhancement and washout of malignant nodes. Repeat images are obtained at select cross-sectional levels over the course of a contrast bolus to determine the perfusion patterns of the tissues.

Novel contrast agents, such as iron oxide particles, have been used with MRI [15]. These agents distort the magnetic field when taken up by the normal lymphatic system. Lymph nodes replaced by tumor do not take up the contrast agent, and thus have higher signal than normal nodes. Studies examining iron oxide particles for lymph node evaluation throughout the body have yielded a wide range of sensitivities and specificities dependent on contrast agent formulation [16].

MR techniques such as magnetization transfer and T1-rho imaging showed initial promise in detecting metastatic nodes, but these techniques have fallen out of favor in recent years [17, 18]. Doppler sonography has been shown to distinguish malignant nodes by their increased blood flow, but the inability to assess deep tissues and the strong operator dependence have limited the clinical utility of this technique [6].

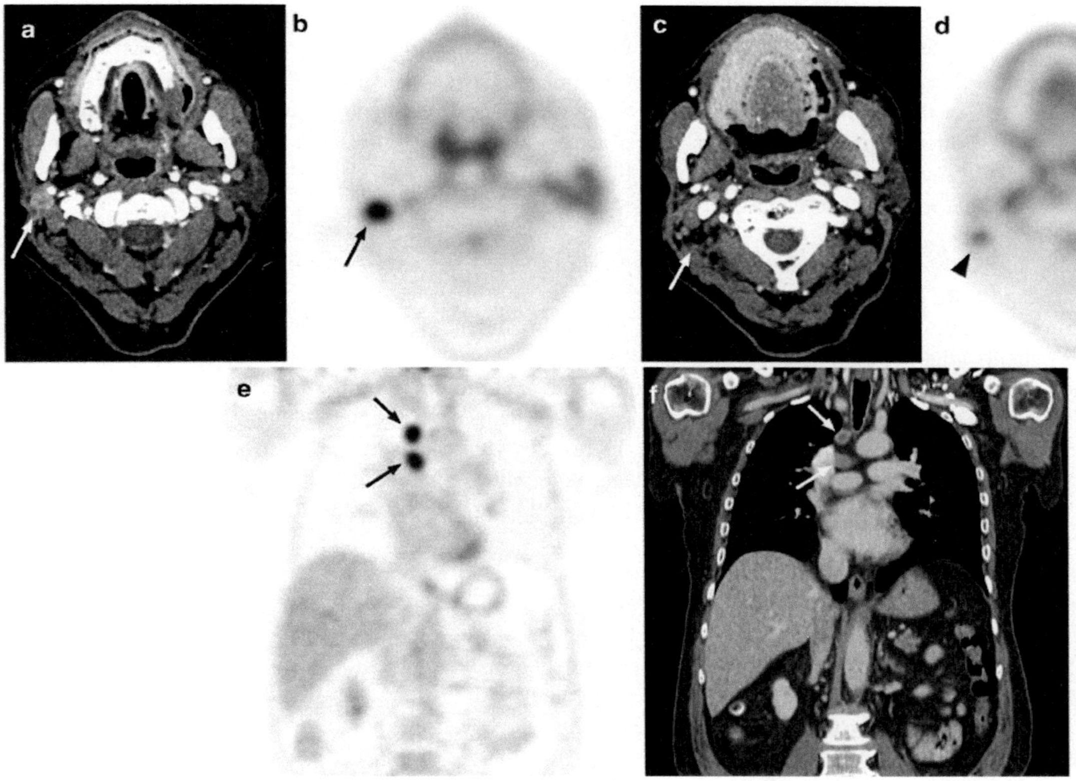

Fig. 18.1 Recurrent adenocarcinoma of the right parotid gland with local and distant lymph node metastases. Transverse contrast enhanced CT (**a**) and FDG PET (**b**) images show an area of abnormal enhancing soft tissue in the parotidectomy bed that is FDG avid (*arrow*). Just caudal to this two 4-mm right level IIb cervical lymph nodes are seen on the transaxial CT image (**c**) that are associated with abnormal FDG tracer uptake (**d**) especially given their small size (*arrowhead*). A similar size contralateral IIb node is negative of the FDG PET image. In addition to the dedicated neck PET-CT acquisition, a PET-CT acquisition of the chest and upper abdomen was performed. On the FDG PET maximum intensity projection (MIP) image (**e**), and CT (**f**) images (*arrows*)

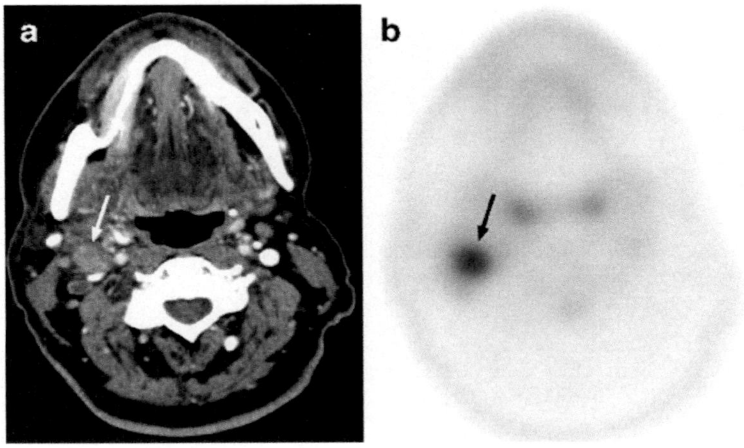

Fig. 18.2 Lymph node metastases with and without central necrosis. Cervical lymph node metastases of a primary mucosal squamous cell carcinoma.(**a**) On transaxial contrast enhanced CT image an enhancing cervical lymph node is seen that is intensely FDG avid reflecting a lymph node with metastatic neoplasm (*arrow*). Nearby there is a nonenlarged lymph node with central low attenuation and a thin enhancing rim (*arrowhead*), the characteristic appearance of a lymph node with central necrosis, indicative of metastatic involvement. Note there is no appreciable abnormal FDG tracer uptake due to the dominantly necrotic nature of the lymph node.(**b**) PET-CT involves using both CT and FDG PET findings

Role of PET-CT in Staging

Many patients who are candidates for staging PET-CT will have already undergone a CT of the neck. Patients who are seen at primary-care hospitals often begin their radiographic workup at those sites. Also, if a patient's diagnosis is in question, a CT may be performed before it is clear that a PET-CT would have been the better choice.

Not all patients who have already undergone a neck CT require an additional staging PET-CT. Because traditional cross-sectional imaging is usually sufficient to evaluate the primary lesion, only patients who are at substantial risk of nodal or hematogenous metastases should undergo PET-CT.

Patients with primary tumors that are prone to bilateral metastases are deserving of PET-CT because contralateral metastases are often less conspicuous on conventional imaging (Fig. 18.3). Primary tumors of the nasopharynx, tongue base, and supraglottis fit this category.

Patients with T3 or T4 lesions of the oral cavity, oropharynx, or larynx are at substantial risk of metastatic disease, both nodal and hematogenous. Thus, these patients merit pretreatment evaluation with PET-CT. In a study by Ha et al., 31% of patients with untreated head and neck SCC initially staged with CT or MRI had their TNM stage altered from additional information provided by PET-CT [19]. Other tumors that are prone to metastatic disease are well described in the otolaryngology literature, but a complete listing is beyond the scope of this chapter. However, it is supported, that PET-CT has greater sensitivity than conventional modalities for the detection of metastatic lesions in patients with high risk of distant metastases. While the FDG PET portion of PET-CT is most helpful in detecting unsuspected local lymph node metastases and distant metastatic involvement, the T stage of the primary neoplasm is largely determined by CT findings. Extranodal spread of local metastatic disease is also a strong negative prognostic finding, and the presence and of extranodal neoplasm spread is also primarily determined by CT findings (Fig. 18.4).

Role of PET-CT in Posttreatment Monitoring

The posttreatment evaluation of patients with head and neck cancer has changed dramatically with the introduction of PET-CT. Radiologists are no longer forced to wait for morphologic changes over time to identify recurrent or residual disease. This enables surgeons and oncologists to respond more quickly to remaining disease. No definitive protocols have been established for the use of PET-CT in this setting, but some principles can be extrapolated from the ways that cross-sectional imaging has traditionally been used for follow-up assessments.

At our institution, nonoperative patients (those treated with radiation and/or chemotherapy) undergo PET-CT every 3 months for the first year after completion of treatment. Patients with new or suspicious findings undergo a CT-guided biopsy of the area of interest. The use of combined PET-CT instead of separate PET and CT studies facilitates precise anatomic localization of the worrisome area during the biopsy. Patients with equivocal findings continue to undergo 3-month follow-up PET-CT scans until there is no longer a suspicion of tumor (Fig. 18.5). If, after 1 year, the PET-CT has normalized, routine clinical monitoring is used, and PET-CT is invoked only in patients with a concerning symptom

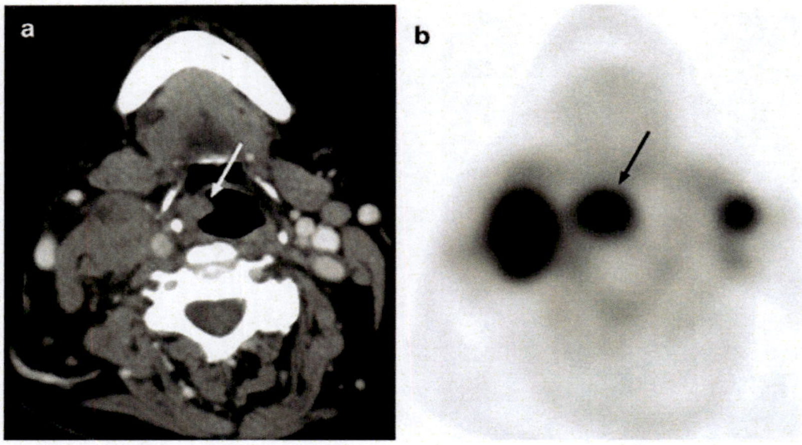

Fig. 18.3 Bilateral neck lymph metastases from squamous cell carcinoma. On the transaxial contrast enhanced CT (**a**) and FDG PET (**b**) images a primary supraglottic mucosal squamous cell carcinoma is seen as right sided mucosal thickening associated with intense abnormal FDG tracer uptake (*arrow*). Bulky ipsilateral cervical level II/III lymph node enlargement with some areas of necrosis is obvious and this is also intensely FDG avid. A 10-mm left cervical level II/III lymph node without necrosis is also seen, which by CT criteria alone would be equivocal for metastatic involvement, but this is intensely FDG avid, indicating very high likelihood of contralateral lymph node metastases

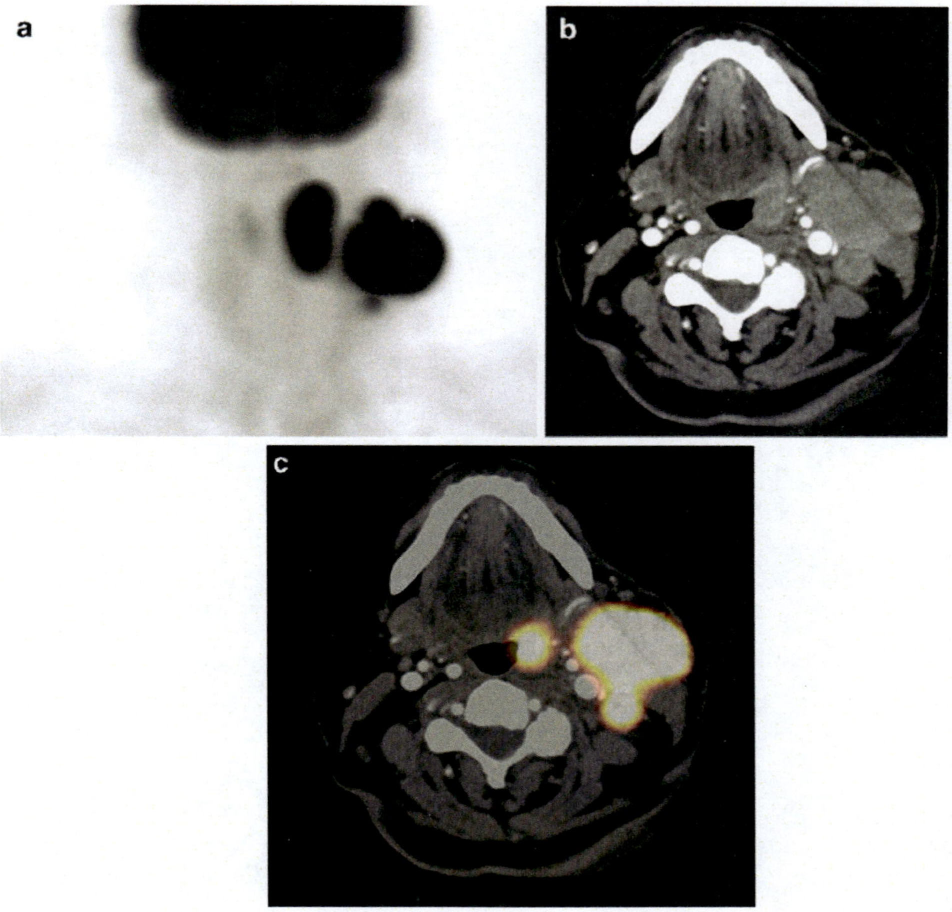

Fig. 18.4 Extranodal extension of regional metastatic disease. Left tonsillar primary squamous cell carcinoma with bulky ipsilateral nodal metastatic involvement is seen on the anterior FDG PET MIP image (**a**). The transaxial contrast enhanced CT (**b**) and FDG PET-CT fusion (**c**) images show the bulky mildly enhancing intensely FDG avid left tonsillar mass and the bulky left cervical level II nodal metastases, also mildly enhancing and intensely FDG avid. Note the extension of the large left lymph node metastasis into adjacent left submandibular gland, left sternocleidomastoid muscle

or physical exam finding. We expect that introductory protocols such as this will undergo revision as we learn more about the value of PET-CT in patients with treated head and neck cancers.

Some researchers have proposed that PET be used to assess response to therapy after the first course of radiation or chemotherapy [20]. There are currently minimal clinical data examining the use of PET for monitoring treatment response for head and neck tumors. Furthermore, the lack of anatomic localization precludes accurate detection of recu1rrent disease in the head and neck. Thus, due to its localization capabilities, this use has been extended to PET-CT. Andrade et al. examined posttreatment PET-CT scans of chemoradiotherapy treated head and neck cancer from 28 patients. The overall sensitivity and specificity of PET-CT was 77% and 93%, respectively. However, for patients with examinations greater than 8 weeks posttreatment, the sensitivity and specificity increased to 100% [21]. The results are promising, and the study brings to the forefront that optimization of the timing for posttreatment PET-CT evaluations needs to be further explored to minimize the presence of inflammation and other posttreatment physiologic effects and maximize the accuracy in identifying recurrent disease.

PET-CT in Unknown Primary Tumors

Patients with head and neck squamous cell carcinoma (SCC) will often present with an enlarging neck mass. Fine needle aspiration of the neck mass reveals metastatic SCC, but the source of the disease remains obscured (SCC does not arise de novo from lymph nodes). Usually, clinical, radiographic, and endoscopic evaluation will reveal the primary tumor that is the source of the metastatic disease. In some cases, biopsies of likely anatomic areas (tonsils, base of tongue) are used to identify the primary tumor site. Despite these efforts, unknown primary tumors account for up to 10% of head and neck SCC.

There are several possible reasons for a primary tumor to remain unknown. Tumors less than 5 mm may be difficult to

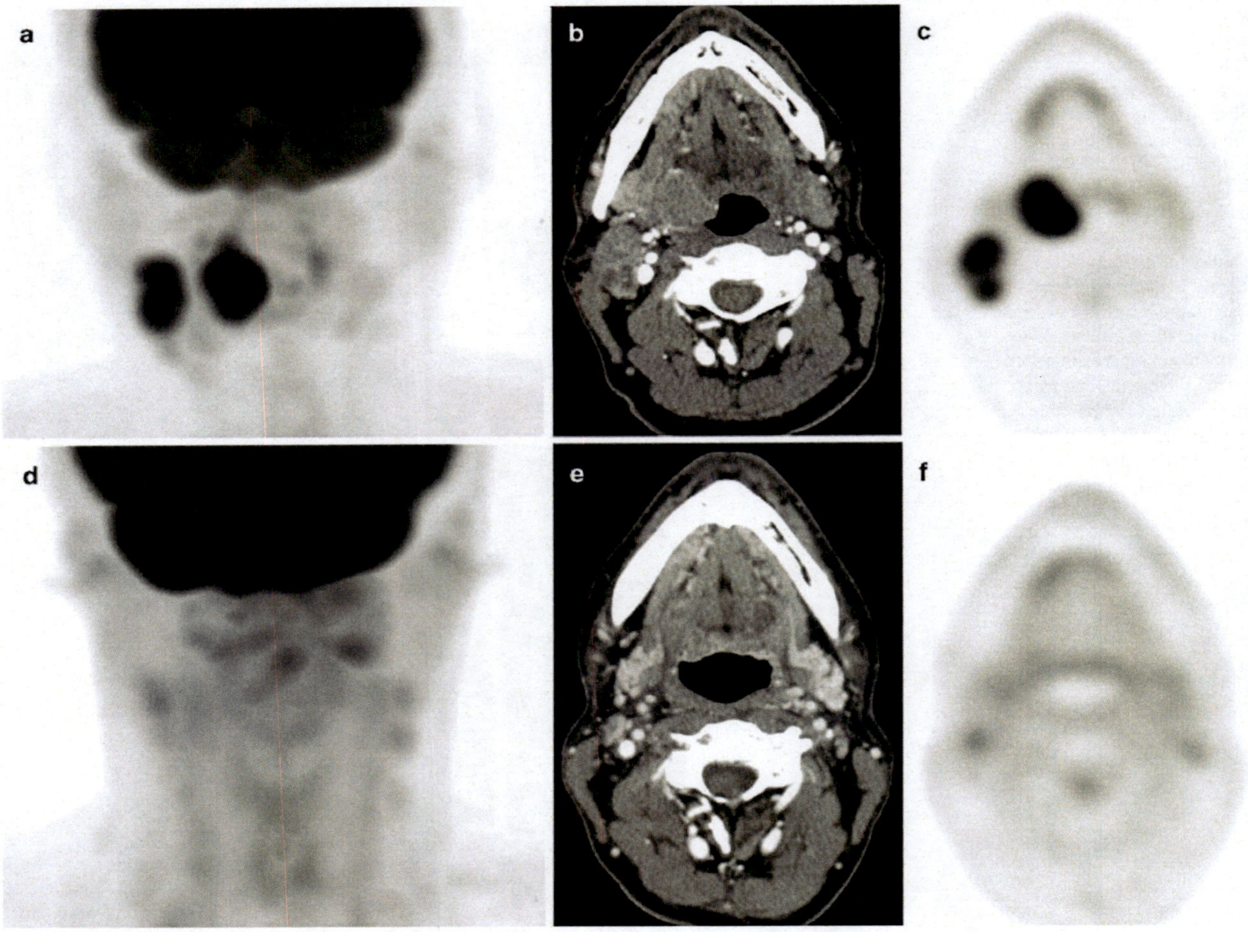

Fig. 18.5 Treatment response following completion of therapy on PET-CT. Initial staging exam FDG PET MIP image (**a**) show intense FDG tracer uptake in the primary right tongue base squamous cell carcinoma and associated right cervical lymph node metastases. On the baseline transaxial contrast enhanced CT (**b**) and FDG PET (**c**) images, the intensely FDG avid primary right tongue base mass is seen distorting the parapharyngeal space and the bulky, partially necrotic right cervical level II intensely FDG avid lymph node metastases are clearly seen. Following completion of chemoradiation therapy, the anterior FDG PET MIP image (**d**) shows resolution of the abnormal FDG tracer activity. On the corresponding transaxial contrast enhanced CT (**e**) and FDG PET (**f**) images the tongue base mass is largely resolved and there is restoration of symmetric configuration of the parapharyngeal space and no residual abnormal FDG tracer uptake at the right tongue base. The bulky right cervical lymph nodes have likewise nearly completely resolved, with only a 6 × 11 mm residual node, which is associated with only subtle FDG tracer activity

identify with endoscopy and cross-sectional imaging. Tumors embedded deep in the crypts of the palatine tonsils may escape notice (Fig. 18.6). Clinicians accustomed to evaluating the head and neck may easily overlook cutaneous primary tumors and primary tumors outside the head and neck.

It is of critical importance for a primary tumor to be identified when metastatic SCC is discovered. The treatment of head and neck SCC focuses on surgical removal of the primary tumor and/or directed radiation therapy. If a primary tumor cannot be identified, the patient must undergo radiation of the entire upper aerodigestive mucosa. This results in considerable morbidity, particularly xerostomia and stenoses of the aerodigestive tract. More advanced treatment modalities, such as intensity-modulated radiation therapy (IMRT) and cyber knife radiation, are not an option in patients with an unknown primary.

Many studies have addressed the efficacy of PET in evaluating patients with unknown primary tumors. These studies are difficult to compare because the definition of "unknown primary" varies from clinical assessment alone to a full assessment with endoscopy and cross-sectional imaging. In aggregate, the literature suggests that 24–40% of unknown primary tumors can be identified with FDG-PET [22].

The few head and neck studies focusing specifically on PET-CT in unknown primary tumors suggest that PET-CT may be of additional benefit. A meta-analysis by Dong et al.

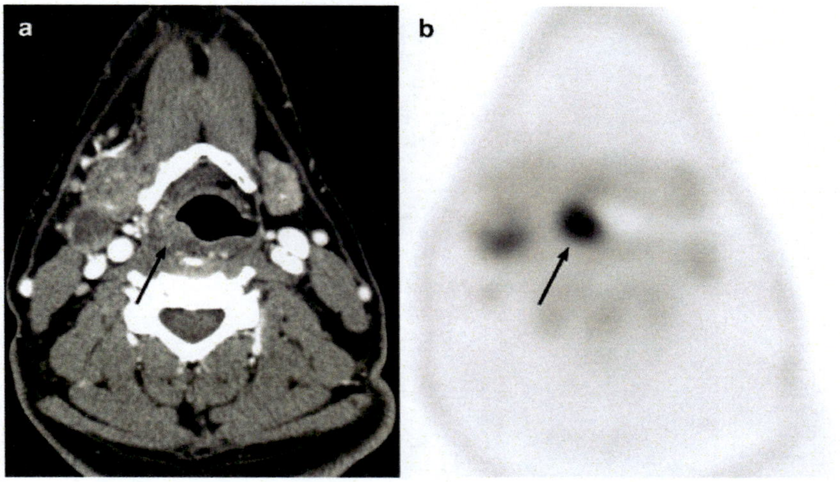

Fig. 18.6 PET-CT of neck cancer of unknown primary. PET-CT of patient presenting with needle core biopsy of a palpable right cervical lymph node positive for squamous cell carcinoma. The transaxial contrast enhanced CT (**a**) and FDG PET (**b**) images demonstrated a right cervical node with CT findings of central necrosis and with abnormal FDG tracer uptake, reflecting the known metastatic involvement. Intense focal abnormal FDG tracer uptake is also seen in the right palatine tonsil corresponding to subtle contrast enhancement and focal prominence (*arrow*) indicating the source of the cervical lymph node metastasis is a primary right tonsillar squamous cell carcinoma

evaluating studies examining the role of PET and PET-CT after physical examination and conventional workup failed to detect a primary tumor found PET-CT to have a greater pooled accuracy and specificity compared to PET evaluations [23]. A handful of small series have compared PET-CT and PET directly head to head. Gutzeit et al. demonstrated a rise in detection from 24% to 33% with PET-CT, which has been similar to our own experience [24]. However, other studies did not show a statistically significant benefit [25, 26]. Larger head to head studies are still needed to unequivocally validate the additional benefit. However, comparisons between PET and PET-CT have consistently demonstrated the superiority of PET-CT in the evaluation of head and neck lesions, so it can be expected that these advantages will also apply to the evaluation of unknown primary tumors [3, 27].

The major pitfall of identifying the primary tumor in the setting of known SCC metastases is the variable physiologic uptake of FDG in the common locations of hidden primary tumors. In particular, the palatine tonsils and the lingual tonsil at the tongue base can have variable (and asymmetric) uptake in normal individuals, and this uptake may mask an underlying lesion. In this situation, PET-CT has an advantage over PET because the presence or absence of a mass on the CT can lend credence to asymmetric FDG uptake. Alternatively, physiologic uptake may be mistaken for tumor.

The major role of PET-CT in the assessment of the unknown primary is to lead the surgeon to potential sources of tumor. These examinations should be read with high sensitivity, because the risk of a negative biopsy is worth the potential benefits of identifying the primary lesion.

Salivary Gland Malignancies

The evaluation of salivary gland malignancies is a troublesome topic in PET-CT. Unfortunately, the FDG uptake of most salivary malignancies is variable, so PET-CT is unreliable for identifying recurrence. Furthermore, many benign salivary lesions have increased FDG uptake, making the distinction between benign and malignant lesions difficult. The variable uptake of FDG within the parenchyma of the glands of the head and neck only adds to the uncertainty [3]. Yet this is an area in which PET-CT has a distinct advantage over PET alone. Even if a tumor has low FDG avidity, it may still be evident on the CT portion of the exam. Also, physiologic uptake is easier to confirm with CT correlation.

In the setting of glandular tumors, patients may benefit from pretreatment PET-CT imaging, so that the FDG-avidity of the tumor can be assessed before it is surgically removed (Fig. 18.7). This allows the radiologist to make recommendations on the utility of PET-CT for posttreatment monitoring. Patients with tumors that are not FDG-avid can be monitored with CT alone, rather than PET-CT.

PET-CT is Medicare-approved for limited use in the setting of thyroid carcinoma. Patients who have been treated with radioiodine for papillary/follicular thyroid cancer, and who have an elevated thyroglobulin level in their blood, but who have a negative radioiodine scan, are candidates for PET-CT. Tumors with low iodine avidity are more likely to be FDG avid, whereas more differentiated tumors that readily concentrate iodine are typically not well visualized with FDG-PET [28].

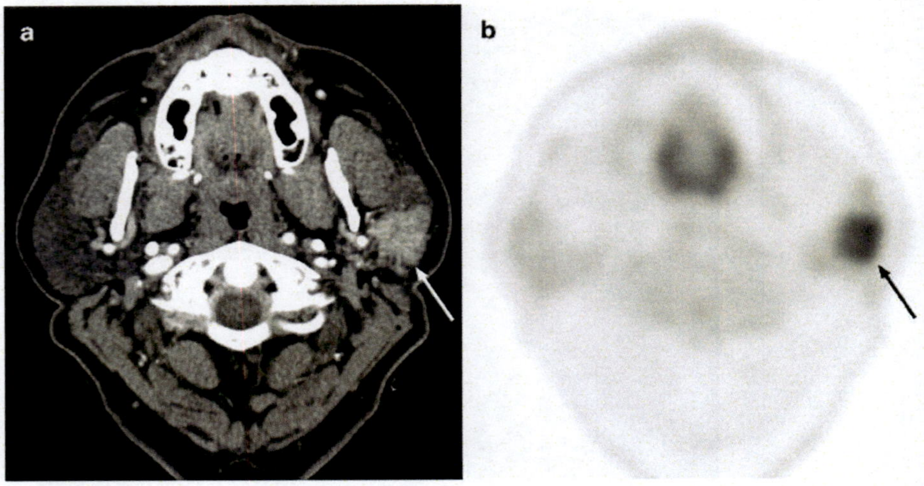

Fig. 18.7 FDG-avid salivary gland malignancy. Transaxial contrast enhanced CT (**a**) and FDG PET (**b**) images demonstrate abnormal soft tissue in the posterior aspect of the left parotid gland. The mass is well seen due to the normal low attenuation of the parotid gland and some degree of contrast enhancement of the mass. There is modest associated increased FDG tracer uptake associated with the mass, which proved to be squamous cell carcinoma on biopsy (*arrow*). Salivary gland neoplasms are variable in FDG uptake and benign salivary gland tumors such as Warthin's tumors can be FDG avid

Pretreatment PET-CT is not indicated in thyroid cancers because the physiologic uptake of the gland will prevent assessment of the primary tumor, and most of these tumors are more easily monitored with diagnostic doses of radioiodine. Only papillary/follicular cancers are included because the uptake in other forms of thyroid cancer is notoriously variable.

Treatment Planning

Coregistered contemporaneous functional and anatomic image data appear to be ideally suited to guide treatment planning. The accuracy of brain tumor biopsies has been improved by incorporating PET data into the surgical plan [29]. There is now growing evidence that radiation portals, which are typically based on anatomic image data, may be more accurately delineated with PET-CT. The addition of metabolic information with PET can alter these decisions in approximately one third of cases [30, 31].

Recently, there has been an increasing expectation that delineation of tumor targets with image-guided radiation therapy must shift toward incorporating biologic information [32, 33]. At our institution, a prospective phantom study assessed the impact of combined PET-CT relative to CT alone on radiation therapy simulation for head and neck cancer [34]. Gross tumor volumes and abnormal nodal regions were evaluated with and without the FDG PET information. This work demonstrated larger volumes for primary tumors using CT rather than PET, presumably due to the superior ability of PET to delineate normal tissue and tumor. Combined imaging with PET-CT has been demonstrated by Wang et al. to more accurately assess gross tumor volumes compared to those generated by CT scans alone [35]. However, further study is needed to assess the influence of combined imaging on long-term patient outcome.

With the advent of IMRT, precise tumor localization is vital to emphasize dose delivery to the tumor while minimizing radiation-induced damage to neighboring tissues. Schwartz and colleagues [36] showed the superiority of registered FDG PET and CT images over CT alone for geographic localization of nodal disease in 63 patients with newly diagnosed squamous cell carcinoma of the oral cavity, oropharynx, or hypopharynx. Since the magnitude of FDG uptake reflects, in part, cell proliferation rates and overall patient prognosis, preliminary work has explored the potential for tailoring IMRT dose delivery based on the FDG activity distribution [37–41]. Solberg et al. [42] reported the feasibility of using combined PET-CT to plan IMRT; selective areas with FDG-avid tumoral tissue were boosted, while dose delivery to normal structures at risk was minimized, with good results. The authors further emphasized the superiority of combined PET-CT over post hoc registration of PET and CT data sets.

Treatment Complications

PET-CT can be used to assess complications of cancer treatment, and most importantly, to distinguish complications from recurrent or residual tumor. A notable application in this category is in the assessment of the jaw. An irregular pattern of bone erosion is a nonspecific finding in the jaw of a patient who has been treated for SCC in that vicinity. The differential possibilities include tumor invasion of bone, osteoradionecrosis as a complication of treatment, and infection (osteomyelitis). Patients with radiation-treated SCC are prone to all three of these diseases. PET-CT is useful for distinguishing osteoradionecrosis, which is expected to have low FDG avidity, from infection (moderate FDG avidity) and recurrent tumor (high FDG avidity). The distinction between tumor recurrence and infection can be difficult on PET, but the diagnosis (or exclusion) of osteoradionecrosis is clinically helpful. Similar logic can be applied to chondronecrosis of the larynx after radiation therapy.

One of the most frequent complications of radiation therapy to the neck is edema of the laryngeal (and, to a lesser degree, pharyngeal) mucosa. Diffuse thickening of the mucosa is seen on both CT and MRI. Although edema should be distinguishable from tumor on the basis of inherent density and degree of enhancement, laryngeal edema is nonetheless a confusing radiographic finding that may mask a small tumor recurrence. PET also has difficulty in this setting because it may be hard to decide whether increased uptake in and around the larynx is the result of physiologic uptake in the intrinsic muscles of the larynx, or evidence of recurrent disease. The combined modality makes the identification of recurrence within an edematous postradiation larynx more reliable.

Vocal cord paralysis, another frequent complication of neck surgery, can be quite confusing on PET imaging. The contralateral vocal cord may show increased FDG avidity, presumably compensatory, while the affected side shows diminished uptake (Fig. 18.8). The resulting asymmetry can be striking, and may falsely suggest tumor recurrence. The CT portion of a combined PET-CT scan will demonstrate the paralyzed cord and prevent false-positive PET interpretation in this setting.

Pitfalls and Artifacts of PET-CT in the Head and Neck

Variable FDG uptake in normal structures such as the nasal turbinates, pterygoid muscles, extraocular muscles, parotid, and submandibular glands, and lymphoid tissue in Waldeyer's ring may confuse interpretation and result in false-positive interpretations of head and neck PET scans [43]. Although FDG uptake in primary neoplasms is usually greater than that observed in even the most metabolically active normal

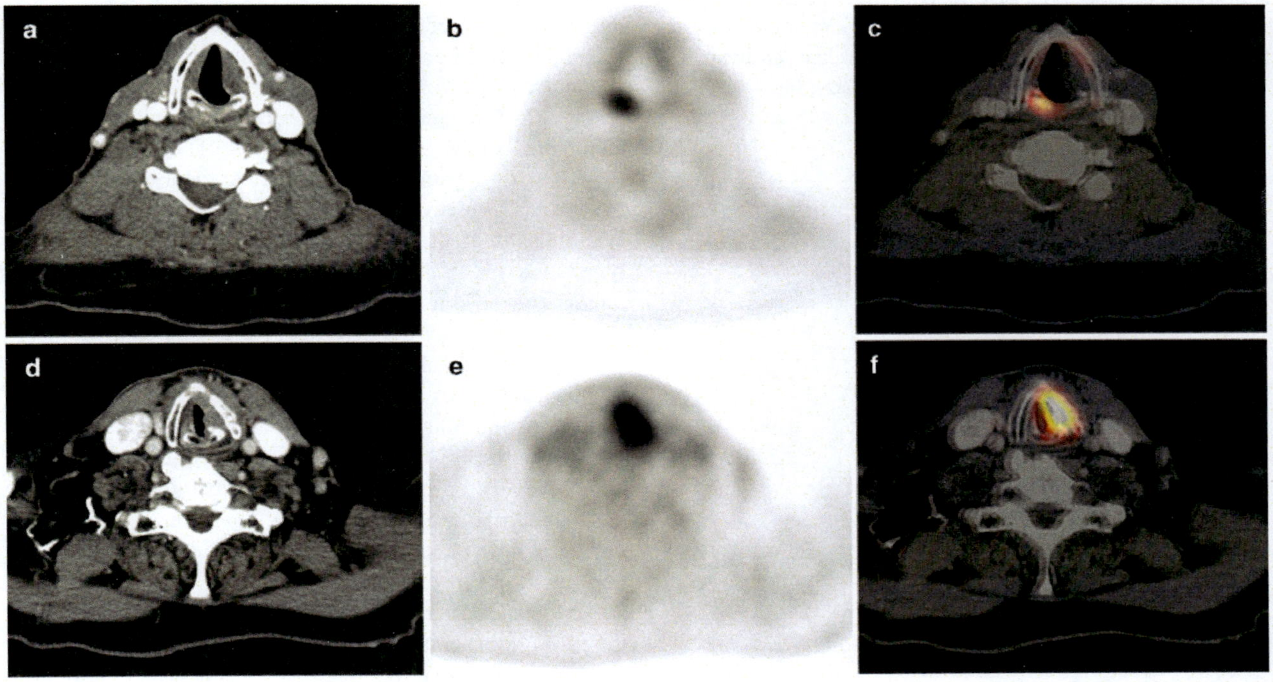

Fig. 18.8 Vocal cord asymmetry. Vocal cord paralysis can present with asymmetric vocalis or cricopharyngeal FDG tracer activity, with the normal side showing normal or increased FDG tracer uptake while the side of the palsy showing no tracer activity in the vocalis or cricopharyngeal muscles and CT signs of cord asymmetry CT (**a**), FDG PET (**b**), FDG PET-CT (**c**). Asymmetry can also be seen with vocal cord cancer, with the abnormal FDG tracer activity corresponding to vocal cord thickening or mass seen on the CT images CT (**d**), FDG PET (**e**), FDG PET-CT (**f**). With vocal cord paralysis the abnormal appearing vocal cord on CT images will not be associated with the increased FDG tracer activity while an abnormal appearing vocal cord with associated increased FDG activity is seen with primary vocal cord squamous cell carcinoma. The presence of asymmetric appearance of the muscles of vocalization on FDG PET requires careful review of the CT images

structures, overlap between tumor and physiologic uptake may confound interpretation.

Often, the interpreting physician relies on symmetry or location to differentiate between physiologic and pathologic FDG accumulations. But symmetry is not a reliable indicator of physiologic processes. Rarely, malignancies can present with symmetric FDG uptake, and conversely, physiologic uptake will often be asymmetric. Furthermore, symmetry is not reliable in postsurgical patients. For example, in patients who have undergone removal of a gland or muscle, FDG uptake in the remaining gland or muscle will typically produce an asymmetric appearance (Fig. 18.9).

Patients are generally instructed to remain quiet during the FDG uptake phase to limit physiologic vocal cord uptake. Other interventions, such as sedation or neck collars, minimize physiologic uptake in the head and neck [44, 45]. These protocols are generally inconvenient for the patient, and they do not eliminate physiologic uptake.

Several limitations of FDG PET scanning in patients with malignancies of the head and neck have been overcome with in-line sequential combined PET-CT scanners. Although this modality has undoubtedly facilitated the differentiation of physiologic and pathologic processes, there are also artifacts unique to the modality [46, 47]. Thus, in order to effectively and accurately interpret PET or combined PET-CT scans, a comprehensive knowledge of physiologic and altered physiologic FDG uptake in the head and neck, as well as an awareness of potential modality-specific artifacts, is essential.

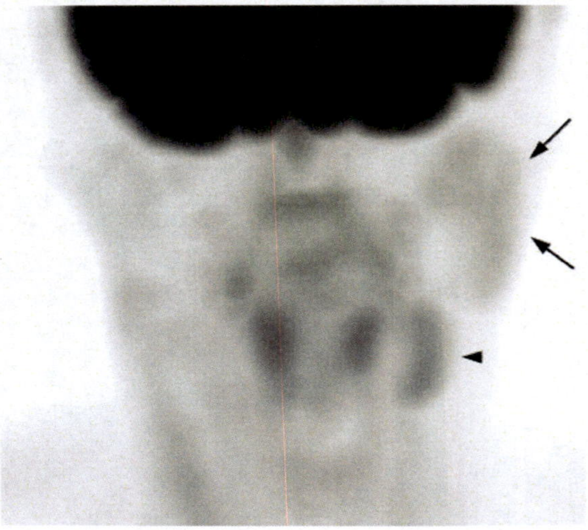

Fig. 18.9 Asymmetry of salivary gland activity due to surgery or radiation therapy. Anterior FDG PET MIP image of patient who had undergone right parotid gland resection of primary parotid gland neoplasm as well as subsequent radiation therapy to the region. Normal left parotid gland (*arrows*) and submandibular gland (*arrowhead*) FDG tracer activity is seen while the absent uptake on the right reflects the resected right parotid gland and effects on radiation therapy to the right submandibular gland which appeared normal on the CT images (not shown)

Thyroid Gland

The thyroid gland has a variable appearance on FDG PET scanning. It can demonstrate diffuse, focal, asymmetric, or virtually no FDG uptake; these uptake patterns can each be seen in physiologic, benign, and pathologic processes [44, 48–50]. Focal thyroid uptake is relatively nonspecific and has been reported in thyroid malignancies as well as in more benign entities, such as toxic thyroid adenoma (Fig. 18.10) [51]. Regardless of the primary indication for the exam, focal uptake is sufficiently concerning for primary thyroid malignancy that biopsy is often warranted [28, 52]. Biopsy is also indicated in any solitary or dominant thyroid mass greater than 1 cm. A more detailed discussion of normal thyroid uptake patterns, as well as benign and malignant thyroid pathology, is available in Chap. 19.

Salivary Glands

FDG is taken up by the salivary glands and excreted into the saliva [53]. The parotid and submandibular glands usually demonstrate symmetric mild to moderate physiologic FDG activity, but they may have little or no uptake in normal individuals. Immediately radiation therapy, the glands may become inflamed and demonstrate symmetric, increased FDG avidity (see Fig. 18.9).

Asymmetric uptake can be seen in patients who have undergone surgical removal of one of the glands (see Fig. 18.9), or in patients with primary or metastatic lesions to the glands. Relatively FDG-avid parotid tumors include Warthin's tumor, pleomorphic adenoma, and primary parotid lymphoma [54–57]. Many benign and malignant salivary tumors (oncocytoma, adenoid cystic carcinoma) have been reported to have varying degrees of FDG uptake. Nonmalignant causes of FDG uptake include infectious etiologies and granulomatous diseases such as sarcoidosis [58].

Benign and malignant parotid tumors cannot be distinguished with PET-CT alone because of high false-positive rates [56, 59]. In addition, some salivary gland malignancies have little or no FDG avidity. Therefore, lack of FDG uptake within a salivary gland mass does not exclude malignancy.

Malignancy can occasionally cause bilateral FDG uptake in the parotid or submandibular glands, or in intraparotid lymph nodes, mimicking a physiologic pattern of uptake. In summary, benign or malignant processes can cause both unilateral and bilateral FDG uptake within the salivary glands and it is necessary to consider all available clinical information, including prior oncologic and surgical history, to make an accurate diagnosis. PET-CT has a definite advantage over PET alone because of the improved surgical and anatomic information, as well as the potential to identify non-FDG-avid tumors.

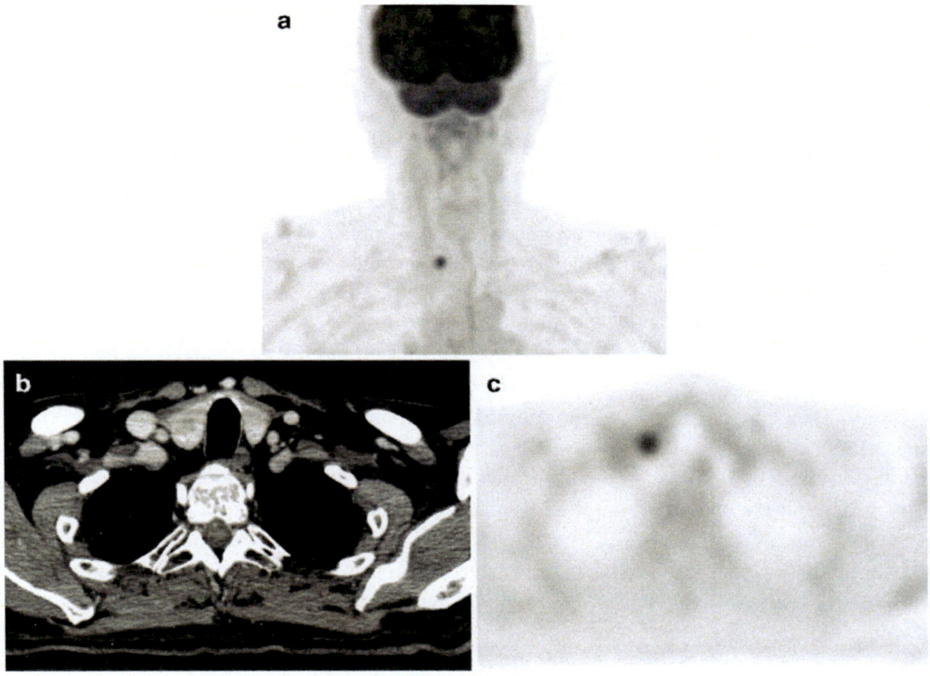

Fig. 18.10 Focal abnormality in thyroid gland on FDG PET images. (**a**) Anterior FDG PET MIP image demonstrates an intense focus of FDG tracer activity in the right lower neck. On the transaxial contrast enhanced CT (**b**) and FDG PET (**c**) images the focus of FDG tracer activity is in the right thyroid lobe and corresponds a subtle thyroid nodule. A high rate of malignancy (about 35%) is found in solitary FDG-avid thyroid masses, so biopsy is warranted

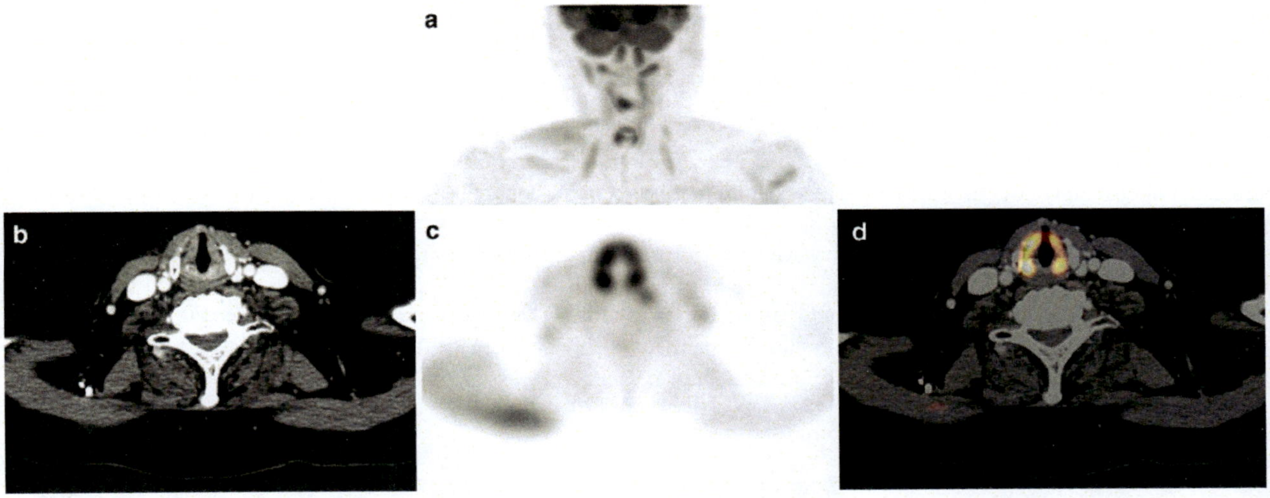

Fig. 18.11 Physiologic FDG tracer uptake in neck musculature. Anterior FDG PET MIP image (**a**) shows FDG tracer activity of vary degree and extent in neck muscles including scalene, anterior longus capitis, rectus capitis posterior, muscles of vocalization, genioglossus, and right trapezius muscles. Note that even in the neck with prior surgery, the extent of physiologic muscle uptake can be variable and asymmetric. Transaxial CT (**b**), FDG PET (**c**), and FDG PET-CT fusion (**d**) image shows intense largely symmetrical FDG tracer activity in the vocalis and cricoarytenoid muscles, a common finding unless efforts to limit talking prior to and during the FDG uptake period prior to the scan procedure

Muscles of the Neck and Face

Physiologic FDG uptake within neck muscles can be a diagnostic dilemma when interpreting PET scans [44, 60]. Frequently, muscular uptake can be distinguished from malignant nodal uptake by identifying the characteristic pattern of linear symmetric uptake. Depending on the orientation of the muscle in question, coronal or sagittal reformatted images may demonstrate this uptake pattern most convincingly. This emphasizes the importance of multiple imaging planes for assessing the configuration of a focus of increased FDG uptake.

Unfortunately, muscles often have more focal patterns of FDG uptake, which can be quite confusing on PET alone (Fig. 18.11). Fused PET-CT will confirm the source of the increased uptake in these situations. Increased uptake is most frequently associated with the myotendinous junctions. Common sites of confusing muscle uptake include the sternocleidomastoid muscle, the strap muscles in the anterior neck, and the pterygoid muscles of the jaw.

Another muscle frequently demonstrating asymmetric tracer uptake is the inferior capitis obliquus muscle. Uptake within this muscle may appear focal on coronal images, but its linear nature is evident when viewed in an axial plane. The extreme posterior position of these paraspinal muscles is also often helpful in identifying the source of the FDG uptake. Viewing the fused PET-CT image in the axial plane allows easier identification of inferior obliquus capitis muscle uptake.

The muscles of facial expression may also demonstrate linear FDG uptake. Because most muscles in the neck can display asymmetric FDG uptake, both physiologically and after strain, close inspection of all three orthogonal planes is essential to avoid misdiagnosis.

Although several methods have been used to minimize muscle uptake, including the use of soft collars and benzodiazepines during the tracer uptake period, these techniques are inconvenient to the patient and are often not completely effective [45].

Muscles of the Oropharynx and Nasopharynx

Several muscles of the oropharynx and hypopharynx demonstrate symmetric physiologic FDG uptake, including the pterygoid muscles and the muscles of the floor of mouth. These may mimic focal areas of malignancy when they are asymmetric.

Lingual FDG uptake is also common and may appear as diffuse or as bilateral symmetrical focal uptake. Lingual uptake is often inseparable from the slightly more superior palatal mucosal uptake on PET images alone, but can be differentiated on the fused PET-CT images.

Laryngeal Muscles

It is well recognized that talking during the FDG uptake period can cause tracer accumulation in the muscles of phonation and vocal cords (Fig. 18.12). Another muscle that can appear as a focal area of FDG uptake is the cricopharyngeus muscle [61]. Coughing during the uptake period produces FDG activity in the pharyngeal constrictor muscles, as well as in the vocal cords. Pronounced FDG uptake in these muscles can interfere with interpretation of PET scans in any patient, but when scans are performed in patients with head and neck malignancies, thyroid cancer, or lymphoma, it can be very difficult to distinguish physiologic muscle uptake from pathologic tracer uptake [62, 63]. PET-CT is particularly useful in these instances, because a lack of corresponding CT abnormality is reassuring.

Fat

Before the advent of PET-CT, physiologic linear and focal uptake in the neck was attributed to muscle alone. After the implementation of combined PET-CT imaging, however, it became apparent that uptake previously attributed to muscle had no definite soft tissue/muscle correlate when the fusion images were inspected. Several authors have reported intense FDG uptake within areas with fat attenuation on CT, now known to represent areas of brown fat (see Fig. 18.12) [64–66]. Although there is little clinical relevance to whether the FDG uptake is in fat or muscle, it is nonetheless an interesting pattern.

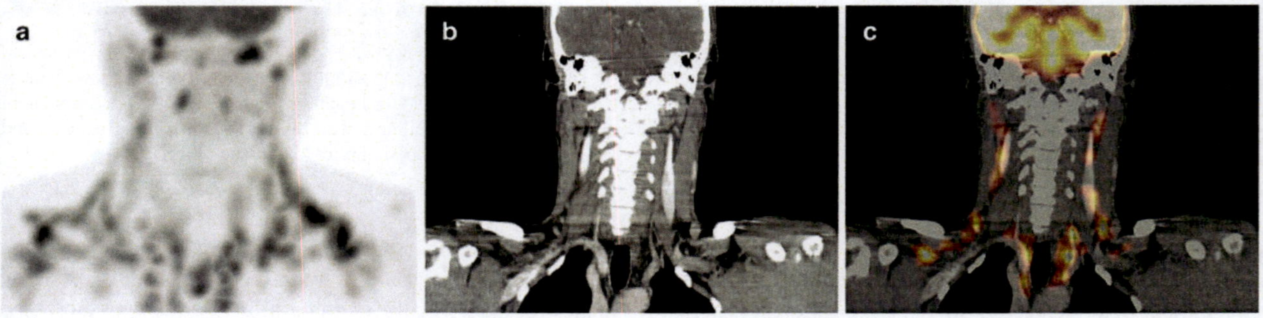

Fig. 18.12 Physiologic FDG uptake in brown fat. Anterior FDG PET MIP image (**a**) shows extensive areas of intense increased FDG uptake in the neck, shoulders, and upper mediastinum in a largely symmetric pattern. Coronal CT (**b**) and FDG PET-CT fusion (**c**) images demonstrate the FDG tracer activity is in fat rather than muscle or other soft tissue in the neck and upper shoulders and upper mediastinum

example of mislocalization of physiologic FDG accumulation solved by combined PET-CT imaging.

Lymphoid Tissue

There are many lymphatic structures in the head and neck, including Waldeyer's ring (the adenoids, palatine tonsils, and lingual tonsils), lymph nodes, and lymphatic channels. Physiologic FDG uptake can be seen in any lymphatic structure in the head and neck, due at least in part to accumulation of FDG within macrophages and lymphocytes. Several authors have described physiologic FDG uptake within these structures using dedicated PET [44, 67–69]. The interpretation is straightforward in most cases, especially when there is symmetric uptake. However, malignancy (particularly lymphoma) or hyperplasia may have a similar symmetric appearance.

It is not uncommon for the FDG uptake in Waldeyer's ring to be asymmetric, from benign pathologies such as infection or inflammation, or as a normal variant. Malignancy will usually present with asymmetric FDG uptake as well, with or without significant anatomic abnormalities. When infiltrated into the subcutaneous tissues, FDG can be transported through the lymphatic system, causing a lymphangiogram effect on the PET images. If FDG is infiltrated into the soft tissues of the upper extremity, FDG may accumulate in the lymph nodes of the axilla and supraclavicular area.

Mucosa

The mucosa of the oropharynx and nasopharynx often demonstrates physiologic FDG uptake. This uptake usually does not cause problems with interpretation because it is almost invariably superficial along the mucosal plane and linear in configuration.

PET-CT Artifacts

Several artifacts specific to PET imaging, including prominent skin activity on non-attenuation-corrected images and relative photopenic areas due to prosthetic devices, have been described [48]. These artifacts are present on combined PET-CT images as well. However, there are a number of artifacts that are unique to the combined PET-CT modality. These are not generated on PET scanners that use point-source based systems for attenuation correction because the artifacts are generated by the CT-based attenuation correction protocols.

Metallic devices, including dental implants, cause areas of photopenia on PET images. When correcting for attenuation with Germanium point sources, these areas remain photopenic on the attenuation corrected images. In contrast, when using current CT-based attenuation correction algorithms, these areas can demonstrate falsely elevated FDG uptake. This artifact is a limitation of the current CT attenuation protocols, but by using uncorrected images for comparison, misdiagnosis can be avoided.

Intravenous contrast can also cause artifacts on attenuation corrected images when using CT-based attenuation correction protocols. Dense contrast material is present in venous structures during the CT acquisition, but not during the PET portion of the exam. This mismatch causes areas of linear artifact (mimicking intense FDG accumulations) on the attenuation-corrected PET images. Occasionally, this artifact can appear focal and mimic a metastatic lymph node in the axilla or supraclavicular area [46]. Rarely a small malignant lymph node or small soft-tissue abnormality can lie within or directly beside a contrast artifact, partially or completely obscuring the abnormality. If there is any diagnostic uncertainty regarding the presence of a CT-based attenuation artifact, the emission data set (i.e., nonattenuation corrected PET image) should be examined to determine whether the apparent increase in FDG uptake is real.

Conclusion

The aggressiveness of head and neck cancer and the associated high rate of tumor recurrence and treatment-related morbidity emphasize the importance of early and accurate clinical evaluation and patient monitoring strategies. As combined PET-CT imaging has evolved to become a valuable tool in the diagnostic and prognostic assessment of cancer patients, it is clear that among its most useful roles is the role it plays in imaging head and neck tumors. Due to the complexity of anatomy in the head and neck, variability of physiologic FDG uptake in normal tissues, and the inherent difficulty in interpreting posttreatment changes with conventional anatomic imaging or FDG PET alone, PET-CT imaging has developed a useful niche for both primary assessment and therapeutic monitoring of head and neck cancer. Increasing clinical experience confirms both improved reader confidence and diagnostic accuracy with PET-CT relative to single-modality approaches, particularly in squamous cell carcinomas. However, the widespread use of PET-CT in head and neck tumor imaging necessitates an awareness of the unique artifacts that may result from CT-based attenuation correction and careful attention to details of image acquisition and processing.

References

1. Jemal A, Siegel R, Ward E, et al. Cancer statistics, 2008. CA Cancer J Clin 2008;58:71–96.
2. Pinto HA, Jacobs C. Chemotherapy for recurrent and metastatic head and neck cancer. Hematol Oncol Clin North Am 1991;5: 667–686.
3. Branstetter BF, Blodgett TM, Zimmer LA, et al. Head and neck malignancy: is PET/CT more accurate than PET or CT alone? Radiology 2005;235:580–586.
4. Keyes JW Jr, Harkness BA, Greven KM, Williams DW 3rd, Watson NE Jr, McGuirt WF. Salivary gland tumors: pretherapy evaluation with PET. Radiology 1994;192:99–102.
5. Fischbein NJ, Noworolski SM, Henry RG, Kaplan MJ, Dillon WP, Nelson SJ. Assessment of metastatic cervical adenopathy using dynamic contrast-enhanced MR imaging. AJNR Am J Neuroradiol 2003;24:301–311.
6. Eida S, Sumi M, Yonetsu K, Kimura Y, Nakamura T. Combination of helical CT and Doppler sonography in the follow-up of patients with clinical N0 stage neck disease and oral cancer. AJNR Am J Neuroradiol 2003;24:312–318.
7. Curtin HD, Ishwaran H, Mancuso AA, Dalley RW, Caudry DJ, McNeil BJ. Comparison of CT and MR imaging in staging of neck metastases. Radiology 1998;207:123–130.
8. Som PM. Lymph nodes of the neck. Radiology 1987;165: 593–600.
9. Steinkamp HJ, Cornehl M, Hosten N, Pegios W, Vogl T, Felix R. Cervical lymphadenopathy: ratio of long- to short-axis diameter as a predictor of malignancy. Br J Radiol 1995;68:266–270.
10. King AD, Tse GM, Ahuja AT, et al. Necrosis in metastatic neck nodes: diagnostic accuracy of CT, MR imaging, and US. Radiology 2004;230:720–726.
11. Ishikawa M, Anzai Y. MR imaging of lymph nodes in the head and neck. Neuroimaging Clin North Am 2004;14:679–694.
12. Yousem DM, Som PM, Hackney DB, Schwaibold F, Hendrix RA. Central nodal necrosis and extracapsular neoplastic spread in cervical lymph nodes: MR imaging versus CT. Radiology 1992;182: 753–759.
13. Yousem DM, Tufano RP. Laryngeal imaging. Neuroimaging Clin North Am 2004;14:611–624.
14. Becker M, Zbaren P, Laeng H, Stoupis C, Porcellini B, Vock P. Neoplastic invasion of the laryngeal cartilage: comparison of MR imaging and CT with histopathologic correlation. Radiology 1995;194:661–669.
15. Anzai Y, Prince MR. Iron oxide-enhanced MR lymphography: the evaluation of cervical lymph node metastases in head and neck cancer. J Magn Reson Imaging 1997;7:75–81.
16. Margolis DJ, Hoffman JM, Herfkens RJ, Jeffrey RB, Quon A, Gambhir SS. Molecular imaging techniques in body imaging. Radiology 2007;245:333–356.
17. Markkola AT, Aronen HJ, Paavonen T, et al. T1 rho dispersion imaging of head and neck tumors: a comparison to spin lock and magnetization transfer techniques. J Magn Reson Imaging 1997;7: 873–879.
18. Yousem DM, Montone KT, Sheppard LM, Rao VM, Weinstein GS, Hayden RE. Head and neck neoplasms: magnetization transfer analysis. Radiology 1994;192:703–707.
19. Ha PK, Hdeib A, Goldenberg D, et al. The role of positron emission tomography and computed tomography fusion in the management of early-stage and advanced-stage primary head and neck squamous cell carcinoma. Arch Otolaryngol Head Neck Surg 2006;132:12–16.
20. Chaiken L, Rege S, Hoh C, et al. Positron emission tomography with fluorodeoxyglucose to evaluate tumor response and control after radiation therapy. Int J Radiation Oncology Biol Phys 1993;27: 455–464.
21. Andrade RS, Heron DE, Degirmenci B, et al. Posttreatment assessment of response using FDG-PET/CT for patients treated with definitive radiation therapy for head and neck cancers. Int J Radiat Oncol Biol Phys 2006;65:1315–1322.
22. Nanni C, Rubello D, Castellucci P, et al. Role of 18F-FDG PET-CT imaging for the detection of an unknown primary tumour: preliminary results in 21 patients. Eur J Nucl Med Mol Imaging 2005;32:589–592.
23. Dong MJ, Zhao K, Lin XT, Zhao J, Ruan LX, Liu ZF. Role of fluorodeoxyglucose-PET versus fluorodeoxyglucose-PET/computed tomography in detection of unknown primary tumor: a meta-analysis of the literature. Nucl Med Commun 2008;29:791–802.
24. Gutzeit A, Antoch G, Kuhl H, et al. Unknown primary tumors: detection with dual-modality PET/CT – initial experience. Radiology 2005;234:227–234.
25. Freudenberg LS, Fischer M, Antoch G, et al. Dual modality of 18F-fluorodeoxyglucose-positron emission tomography/computed tomography in patients with cervical carcinoma of unknown primary. Med Princ Pract 2005;14:155–160.
26. Nassenstein K, Veit-Haibach P, Stergar H, et al. Cervical lymph node metastases of unknown origin: primary tumor detection with whole-body positron emission tomography/computed tomography. Acta Radiol 2007:1–8.
27. Schoder H, Yeung HW, Gonen M, Kraus D, Larson SM. Head and neck cancer: clinical usefulness and accuracy of PET/CT image fusion. Radiology 2004;231:65–72.
28. McDougall IR, Davidson J, Segall GM. Positron emission tomography of the thyroid, with an emphasis on thyroid cancer. Nucl Med Commun 2001;22:485–492.
29. Thiel A, Pietrzyk U, Sturm V, Herholz K, Hovels M, Schroder R. Enhanced accuracy in differential diagnosis of radiation necrosis by positron emission tomography-magnetic resonance imaging coregistration: technical case report. Neurosurgery 2000;46:232–234.
30. Rizzo G, Cattaneo GM, Castellone P, et al. Multi-modal medical image integration to optimize radiotherapy planning in lung cancer treatment. Ann Biomed Eng 2004;32:1399–1408.
31. Gabriele P, Malinverni G, Moroni GL, et al. The impact of 18F-deoxyglucose positron emission tomography on tumor staging, treatment strategy and treatment planning for radiotherapy in a department of radiation oncology. Tumori 2004;90:579–585.
32. Apisarnthanarax S, Chao KS. Current imaging paradigms in radiation oncology. Radiat Res 2005;163:1–25.
33. Bujenovic S. The role of positron emission tomography in radiation treatment planning. Semin Nucl Med 2004;34:293–299.
34. Heron DE, Andrade RS, Flickinger J, et al. Hybrid PET-CT simulation for radiation treatment planning in head-and-neck cancers: a brief technical report. Int J Radiat Oncol Biol Phys 2004;60:1419–1424.
35. Wang D, Schultz CJ, Jursinic PA, et al. Initial experience of FDG-PET/CT guided IMRT of head-and-neck carcinoma. Int J Radiat Oncol Biol Phys 2006;65:143–151.
36. Schwartz DL, Ford E, Rajendran J, et al. FDG-PET/CT imaging for preradiotherapy staging of head-and-neck squamous cell carcinoma. Int J Radiat Oncol Biol Phys 2005;61:129–136.
37. Haberkorn U, Strauss LG, Reisser C, et al. Glucose uptake, perfusion, and cell proliferation in head and neck tumors: relation of positron emission tomography to flow cytometry. J Nucl Med 1991;32:1548–1555.
38. Minn H, Clavo A, Grenman R, Wahl R. In vitro comparison of cell proliferation kinetics and uptake of tritiated fluorodeoxyglucose and L-methionine in squamous-cell carcinoma of the head and neck. J Nucl Med 1995;36:252–258.
39. Pugsley JM, Schmidt RA, Vesselle H. The Ki-67 index and survival in non-small cell lung cancer: a review and relevance to positron emission tomography. Cancer Journal 2002;8:222–233.
40. Schwartz DL, Rajendran J, Yueh B, et al. FDG-PET prediction of head and neck squamous cell cancer outcomes. Arch Otolaryngol Head Neck Surg 2004;130:1361–1367.

41. Das SK, Miften MM, Zhou S, et al. Feasibility of optimizing the dose distribution in lung tumors using fluorine-18-fluorodeoxyglucose positron emission tomography and single photon emission computed tomography guided dose prescriptions. Med Phys 2004;31: 1452–1461.
42. Solberg TD, Agazaryan N, Goss BW, Dahlbom M, Lee SP. A feasibility study of 18F-fluorodeoxyglucose positron emission tomography targeting and simultaneous integrated boost for intensity-modulated radiosurgery and radiotherapy. J Neurosurg 2004;101(Suppl 3):381–389.
43. Jabour BA, Choi Y, Hoh CK, et al. Extracranial head and neck: PET imaging with 2-[F-18]fluoro-2-deoxy-D-glucose and MR imaging correlation. Radiology 1993;186:27–35.
44. Shreve PD, Anzai Y, Wahl RL. Pitfalls in oncologic diagnosis with FDG PET imaging: physiologic and benign variants. Radiographics 1999;19:61–77; quiz 150–151.
45. Barrington SF, Maisey MN. Skeletal muscle uptake of fluorine-18-FDG: effect of oral diazepam. J Nucl Med 1996;37:1127–1129.
46. Antoch G, Freudenberg LS, Egelhof T, et al. Focal tracer uptake: a potential artifact in contrast-enhanced dual-modality PET/CT scans. J Nucl Med 2002;43:1339–1342.
47. Goerres GW, Hany TF, Kamel E, von Schulthess GK, Buck A. Head and neck imaging with PET and PET/CT: artefacts from dental metallic implants. Eur J Nucl Med Mol Imaging 2002;29:367–370.
48. Cook GJ, Fogelman I, Maisey MN. Normal physiological and benign pathological variants of 18-fluoro-2-deoxyglucose positron-emission tomography scanning: potential for error in interpretation. Semin Nucl Med 1996;26:308–314.
49. Gordon BA, Flanagan FL, Dehdashti F. Whole-body positron emission tomography: normal variations, pitfalls, and technical considerations. AJR Am J Roentgenol 1997;169:1675–1680.
50. Lin EC. Thyroid nodule mimicking cervical adenopathy on FDG positron emission tomographic imaging. Clin Nucl Med 2002;27:656–657.
51. Borner AR, Voth E, Wienhard K, Wagner R, Schicha H. [F-18-FDG PET in autonomous goiter]. Nuklearmedizin 1999;38:1–6.
52. Ramos CD, Chisin R, Yeung HW, Larson SM, Macapinlac HA. Incidental focal thyroid uptake on FDG positron emission tomographic scans may represent a second primary tumor. Clin Nucl Med 2001;26:193–197.
53. Stahl A, Dzewas B, Schwaiger M, Weber WA. Excretion of FDG into saliva and its significance for PET imaging. Nuklearmedizin 2002;41:214–216.
54. Horiuchi M, Yasuda S, Shohtsu A, Ide M. Four cases of Warthin's tumor of the parotid gland detected with FDG PET. Ann Nucl Med 1998;12:47–50.
55. Matsuda M, Sakamoto H, Okamura T, et al. Positron emission tomographic imaging of pleomorphic adenoma in the parotid gland. Acta Otolaryngol Suppl 1998;538:214–220.
56. Okamura T, Kawabe J, Koyama K, et al. Fluorine-18 fluorodeoxyglucose positron emission tomography imaging of parotid mass lesions. Acta Otolaryngol Suppl 1998;538:209–213.
57. Shih WJ, Ghesani N, Hongming Z, Alavi A, Schusper S, Mozley D. F-18 FDG positron emission tomography demonstrates resolution of non-Hodgkin's lymphoma of the parotid gland in a patient with Sjögren's syndrome: before and after anti-CD20 antibody rituximab therapy. Clin Nucl Med 2002;27:142–143.
58. Sagowski C, Ussmuller J. [Clinical diagnosis of salivary gland sarcoidosis (Heerfordt syndrome)]. Hno 2000;48:613–615.
59. Keyes JW, Harkness BA, Greven KM, Williams DW, Watson NE, McGuirt WF. Salivary gland tumors: pretherapy evaluation with PET. Radiology 1994;192:99–102.
60. Bar-Shalom R. Muscle uptake of 18-fluorine fluorodeoxyglucose. Semin Nucl Med 2000;30:306–309.
61. Kostakoglu L, Wong JC, Barrington SF, Cronin BF, Dynes AM, Maisey MN. Speech-related visualization of laryngeal muscles with fluorine-18-FDG. J Nucl Med 1996;37:1771–1773.
62. Igerc I, Kumnig G, Heinisch M, et al. Vocal cord muscle activity as a drawback to FDG-PET in the followup of differentiated thyroid cancer. Thyroid 2002;12:87–89.
63. Zhu Z, Chou C, Yen TC, Cui R. Elevated F-18 FDG uptake in laryngeal muscles mimicking thyroid cancer metastases. Clin Nucl Med 2001;26:689–691.
64. Virtanen KA, Peltoniemi P, Marjamaki P, et al. Human adipose tissue glucose uptake determined using [(18)F]-fluoro-deoxy-glucose ([(18)F]FDG) and PET in combination with microdialysis. Diabetologia 2001;44:2171–2179.
65. Cohade C, Osman M, Pannu HK, Wahl RL. Uptake in supraclavicular area fat ("USA-Fat"): description on 18F-FDG PET/CT. J Nucl Med 2003;44:170–176.
66. Hany TF, Gharehpapagh E, Kamel EM, Buck A, Himms-Hagen J, von Schulthess GK. Brown adipose tissue: a factor to consider in symmetrical tracer uptake in the neck and upper chest region. Eur J Nucl Med Mol Imaging 2002;29:1393–1398.
67. Stokkel MP, Bongers V, Hordijk GJ, van Rijk PP. FDG positron emission tomography in head and neck cancer: pitfall or pathology? Clin Nucl Med 1999;24:950–954.
68. Kawabe J, Okamura T, Shakudo M, et al. Physiological FDG uptake in the palatine tonsils. Ann Nucl Med 2001;15:297–300.
69. Hanasono MM, Kunda LD, Segall GM, Ku GH, Terris DJ. Uses and limitations of FDG positron emission tomography in patients with head and neck cancer. Laryngoscope 1999;109:880–885.

Chapter 19
PET-CT of Thyroid Cancer

Trond Velde Bogsrud, Val J. Lowe, and Ian D. Hay

Clinical thyroid cancer is an uncommon disease, representing only about 1% of all cancers. Microscopic papillary carcinomas, however, are very common, with an incidence reported as high as 35.6% [1]. Papillary thyroid carcinomas account for about 75%, follicular 15%, undifferentiated (anaplastic) 3%, medullary 3%, and primary thyroid lymphoma 3%. The risk of thyroid lymphoma is increased about 70-fold in Hashimoto's thyroiditis. Primary thyroid lymphoma is most frequently limited to the thyroid gland (stage IE). Papillary, follicular, and anaplastic thyroid carcinomas are thyroid follicular cell–derived cancers, while medullary thyroid carcinomas arise from the parafollicular cells or calcitonin cells (C cells), which are organized as solid nests located between the basal layer and the thyroid follicular cells. The WHO 2004 histologic classification of thyroid carcinomas is given in Table 19.1 [2].

Clinically detected metastases to the thyroid are rare. Carcinoma of the breast, cervix, colon, esophagus, kidney, lung, neuroendocrine tumors, and squamous cell carcinoma have been reported to metastasize to the thyroid gland, and involvement of non-Hodgkin's lymphoma is also seen [3, 4].

The most common clinical presentation of thyroid cancer is an asymptomatic, palpable, solitary thyroid nodule. Less commonly seen are enlarged neck lymph nodes and more rare are symptoms from bone metastases, hoarseness, dysphagia, cough, or dyspnea. For anaplastic carcinoma and thyroid lymphoma, the typical clinical manifestation is a rapidly growing thyroid tumor [5].

In the USA, a palpable thyroid nodule is found in about 5% of the general population, and the number is higher in countries with iodine deficiency. A palpable thyroid nodule is a diagnostic challenge because they are so common, but less than 5% will be malignant. Even more challenging, however, is the incidental finding of a nonpalpable thyroid nodule on ultrasound, whose prevalence is reported as high as 67%. Controversy exists about the need to evaluate these incidentally small nodules in the absence of risk factors for thyroid cancer [6, 7].

To rule out or confirm a suspicion for malignancy of a thyroid nodule, a fine needle aspiration biopsy (FNA), preferably ultrasound guided, is the diagnostic procedure of choice. An FNA can identify a papillary thyroid carcinoma with a high certainty, based on typical cytoplasmic ("ground glass" appearance) and nuclear features (clefts, grooves, and "holes"). A follicular carcinoma, however, cannot be differentiated from follicular adenoma. The diagnosis of minimally invasive follicular carcinoma is based on histopathologic demonstration of microscopic capsular invasion and/or infiltration of blood vessels immediately outside the tumor capsule. The diagnosis of minimally invasive follicular carcinoma vs. follicular adenoma is difficult with low reproducibility even in histologic samples studied by experienced pathologists. Even differentiation between minimally invasive follicular thyroid carcinoma, follicular variant of PTC, and follicular variant of medullary thyroid carcinoma may be difficult [8].

Papillary and follicular thyroid carcinomas are among the most curable of all neoplasms in humans with a 10-year survival of 98% and 92%, respectively, while anaplastic thyroid carcinoma is one of the most aggressive and lethal cancers with most patients dying within less than a year from diagnosis. Even if the prognosis is excellent for well-differentiated thyroid cancer, the disease will recur in 13–30% of the patients, and proper treatment and life-long follow up is mandatory for favorable outcome [9–11].

Ultrasound of the neck and measurement of thyroglobulin under endogenous (thyroxin withdrawal) or exogenous TSH stimulation with recombinant human TSH have been the standard in the routine followup of low-risk patients with well-differentiated thyroid cancer [12–14].

Patients at high risk for recurrent disease can be identified at the time of diagnosis through prognostic factors such as age, sex, histologic variant, tumor size, tumor extension, multicentricity/multifocally, lymph node metastases, and distant metastases. The type of primary treatment is also

T.V. Bogsrud (✉)
Department of Diagnostic Imaging, Division of Nuclear Medicine, University Clinic, The Norwegian Radium Hospital, Rikshospitalet University Hospital, Montebello, 0310 Oslo, Norway
e-mail: trondvb@klinmed.uio.no

P. Shreve and D.W. Townsend (eds.), *Clinical PET-CT in Radiology: Integrated Imaging in Oncology*,
DOI 10.1007/978-0-387-48902-5_19, © Springer Science+Business Media, LLC 2011

Table 19.1 WHO (2004) histologic classification of thyroid carcinomas (From Ref. [2]. With permission of the World Health Organization)

Papillary carcinoma
Follicular carcinomas
Poorly differentiated carcinoma
Undifferentiated (anaplastic) carcinoma
Squamous cell carcinoma
Mucoepidermoid carcinoma
Sclerosing mucoepidermoid carcinoma with eosinophilia
Mucinous carcinoma
Medullary carcinoma
Mixed medullary and follicular cell carcinoma
Spindle cell tumor with thymus-like differentiation
Carcinoma showing thymus-like differentiation

important for the outcome. For high-risk patients, there is general agreement that total thyroidectomy should be performed, followed by radioiodine ablation and thyroxine in TSH-suppressive dose.

Complications from thyroid surgery are not very common. Recurrent laryngeal nerve injury occurs in less than 1% when surgery is performed by an experienced surgeon. Unilateral nerve injury with vocal cord paralysis can result in a weak, breathy voice. Injury to the superior laryngeal nerve does not result in hoarseness, but a voice with restricted vocal range. Temporary hypoparathyroidism with moderate hypocalcemia is common after total thyroidectomy with parathyroid autotransplantation, and usually resolves within a few months. Persistent hypoparathyroidism is uncommon [15, 16].

Papillary and medullary thyroid carcinomas frequently spread early to regional lymph nodes, while follicular cancer rarely does. Without clinical evidence (including preoperative ultrasound) of lymph node metastases, lymph node dissection is normally restricted to the central compartment lymph nodes (level V), which includes the paratracheal and prelaryngeal (Delphian) lymph nodes. If lymph node metastases are demonstrated or highly suspicious, unilateral or bilateral modified lymph node dissection should be performed. A modified lymph node dissection includes Level II, III, VI, and V, with preservation of the sternocleidomastoid muscle, the internal jugular veins, and the spinal accessory nerves. In a radical neck dissection, even the sternocleidomastoid muscle, the internal jugular veins, and the spinal accessory nerves are sacrificed [15, 16]. Figures 19.1 and 19.2 and Table 19.2 show the lymphatic drainage from the thyroid gland and the standardized lymph node levels used by surgeons and oncologists.

Ultrasound-guided percutaneous ethanol injection seems to be a valuable treatment option for patients with limited cervical nodal metastases from papillary thyroid cancer who are not amendable to further surgical or radioiodine therapy [18, 19].

It is believed that most microcarcinomas do not progress into clinical cancer. A continuous debate is going on about the

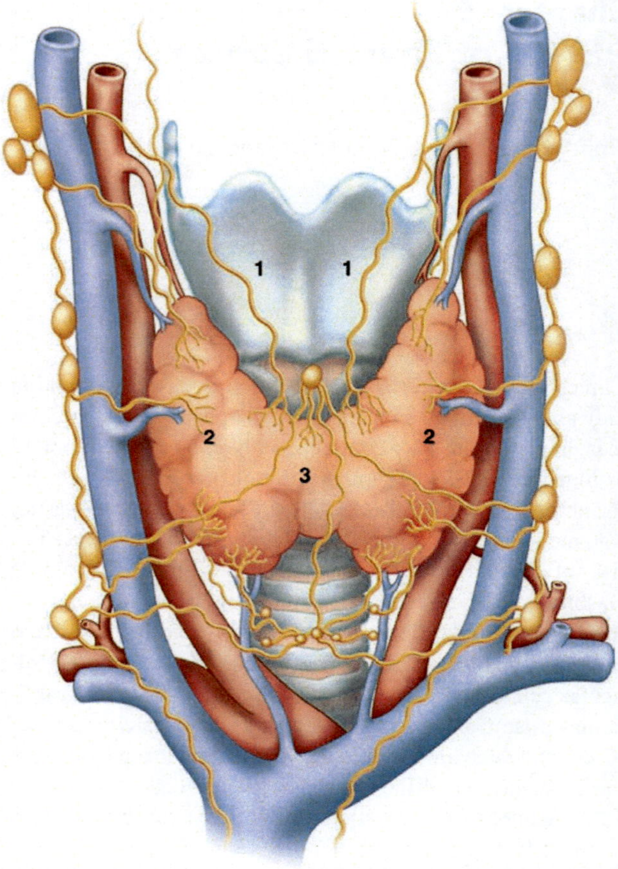

Fig. 19.1 The lymphatic drainage of the thyroid gland (From Ref. [17]. With permission)

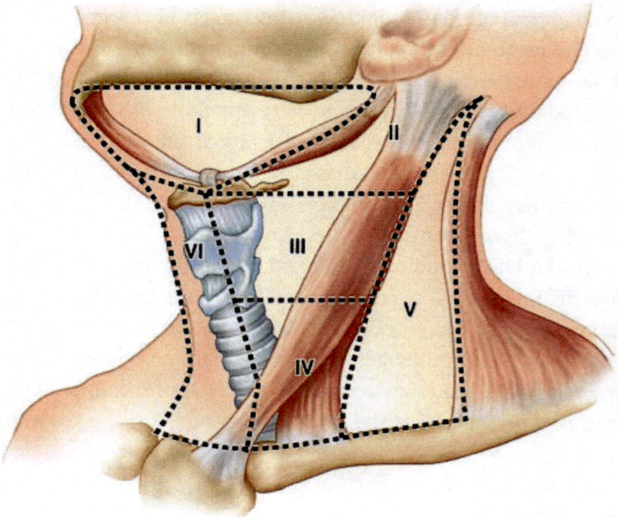

Fig. 19.2 Schematic diagram of the anatomic subsites and levels cervical lymph nodes (see also Table 19.2). (Used with permission of the American Joint Committee on Cancer [AJCC], Chicago, IL. The original source for this material is the *AJCC Cancer Staging Manual*, 6th edn. New York: Springer-Verlag, 2002. www.springer-ny.com)

Table 19.2 Classification of cervical lymph nodes into anatomical subsites and levels[a] (Used with the permission of the American Joint Committee on Cancer (AJCC), Chicago, IL. The original source for this material is the *AJCC Cancer Staging Manual*, 7th edn. New York: Springer Science and Business Media LLC, 2010. www.springer.com)

Level	Lymph nodes	Radiologic landmarks
I	Submental Submandibular	Above hyoid bone, anterior to posterior edge of submandibular gland, superficial to mylohyoid muscle, between the anterior and posterior belly of the digastric muscle.
II	Upper jugular	Extending from the base of the skull to the inferior aspect of the hyoid bone (level II as long as you can see hyoid bone), between the posterior part of the submandibular gland and the posterior border of sternocleidomastoid muscle posteriorly.
III	Mid-jugular	Extending from just below the hyoid bone (level II as long as you can see hyoid bone) to the inferior aspect of the cricoid cartilage, between the posterior border of sternocleidomastoid muscle and the sternohyoid muscle.[b]
IV	Lower jugular	Extending from below cricoid cartilage to the clavicle, between posterior border of sternocleidomastoid muscle and posterior to sternohyoid muscle.[b]
V	Posterior triangle	Extending from base of skull to clavicle, between anterior border of trapezius and posterior border of sternocleidomastoid muscle.
VI	Central compartment (prelaryngeal or Delphian, pretracheal, and paratracheal nodes)	Extending from the hyoid bone to the suprasternal notch, between the medial border of the carotid sheet/anterior border of sternocleidomastoid muscle.
Supra-clavicular	Supraclavicular	At or caudal to the clavicle, above and medial to the ribs lateral to the lower jugular chain.

[a]As recommended by American Joint Committee on Cancer (AJCC), the Union International Contre le Cancer (UICC) and the American Academy of Otolaryngology-Head and Neck Surgery (AAO-HNS)

[b]Sternohyoid muscle origin from manubrium of sternum and medial end of clavicle and inserts at the body of the hyoid bone

appropriate treatment strategies for solitary papillary microcarcinomas and smaller noninvasive follicular carcinomas.

For medullary thyroid cancer, surgery is the only curable treatment. For anaplastic thyroid carcinoma, radiation and concomitant combined chemotherapy, followed by surgery if the tumor can be completely removed, constitutes standard therapy [9–11, 16, 20].

Anatomy Relevant for PET-CT

The Thyroid Gland

The thyroid consists of two lobes joined by an isthmus. The lobes are about 4 cm in height extending from the thyroid cartilage superiorly to about the sixth tracheal ring inferiorly. The right lobe is normally somewhat larger than the left. The narrow isthmus joins the two lobes anteriorly to the second and third tracheal rings at the level of vertebra C6. A third lobe, the pyramidal lobe, is seen in about one third of people, arising from the isthmus extending upward to the thyroid cartilage. The pyramidal lobe is a remnant of the thyroglossal duct.

On cross-sectional CT at the level of C6 the main lobes appears triangular, each triangle about 3 cm in depth and 2 cm in width with a convex anterior surface. The thyroid is embedded in the visceral portion of the pretracheal layer of the deep cervical fascia. Anteriorly are the platysma, sternohyoid and sternothyroid muscles, and the anterior jugular veins. Laterally are the platysma, omohyoid (superior belly), and sternocleidomastoid muscles. Posterolaterally are the carotid sheet with the common carotid artery and internal jugular vein. Posteriorly to each lobe are the longus colli muscles. Medially is the trachea and just posterior to trachea is the esophagus. On CT the thyroid gland shows higher soft tissue attenuation than the surrounding soft tissue because of the physiologic high iodine content of the tissue. Using contrast will enhance the rich vascular thyroid tissue [21, 22]. An axial CT slice through midthyroid performed with iodinated contrast is shown in Fig. 19.3. The uptake of ^{18}F-FDG in a normal gland is the same as the surrounding soft tissue.

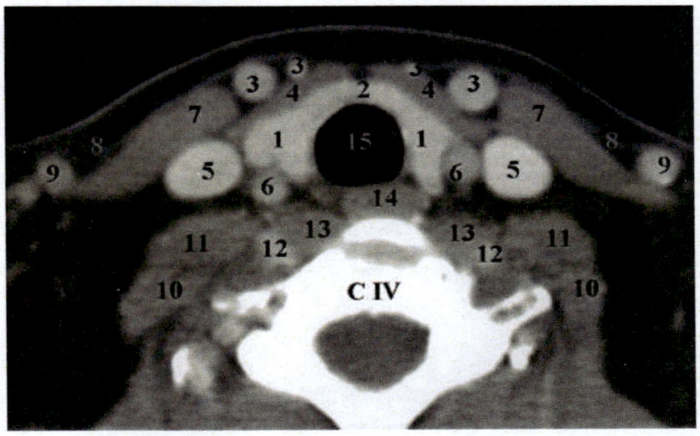

Fig. 19.3 Axial CT slice through mid-thyroid performed with iodinated contrast: (1) right and left thyroid lobe, (2) isthmus, (3) anterior jugular veins, (4) strap muscles (sternohyoid, sternothyroid, and omohyoid), (5) internal jugular veins (6) common carotid arteries, (7) sternocleidomastoid muscles, (8) platysma muscles, (9) external jugular veins, (10) middle scalenus muscles, (11) anterior scalenus muscles, (12) vertebral arteries and veins, (13) longus colli muscles, (14) esophagus, and (15) trachea

Lymphatic Drainage

The thyroid gland has a rich lymphatic drainage and lymph nodes in a number of different subsites in the neck and chest may be involved in metastatic thyroid carcinomas. It is important that the interpreting physician reporting the findings of involved lymph nodes on PET does it in a standardized way familiar to the head and neck surgeons. According to the American Joint Committee on Cancer (AJCC), the Union International Contre le Cancer (UICC), and the American Academy of Otolaryngology-Head and Neck Surgery (AAO-HNS), the lymph nodes in the neck are classified into specific groups based on anatomic and radiologic location (Figs. 19.1 and 19.2 and Table 19.2) [23–25].

The lymphatic drainage from the thyroid gland is primarily to the central compartment lymph nodes (level VI), which includes the prelaryngeal (called the Delphian nodes), pretracheal, paratracheal lymph nodes, and to lateral neck (levels III and IV), which includes the jugular lymph nodes. The lateral and superior region of each lobe drains to the internal jugular lymph nodes (levels II and III). The medial and superior regions drain to prelaryngeal nodes (level VI). The medial and inferior regions drain to the paratracheal, pretracheal, and intraglandular lymph nodes (level VI). The lateral inferior parts drain to the inferior jugular nodes (level IV). Some lymphatic vessels may drain into brachiocephalic lymph nodes and into the upper mediastinum, and these nodes are also counted as thyroid regional nodes. Involvement of upper deep jugular (level II), submandibular and submental (level I), retropharyngeal, and spinal accessory lymph nodes are less common. Bilateral lymph node involvement is common [17, 24].

Classification and Staging of Thyroid Carcinoma

The TNM system is commonly used as an expression of the anatomic extent of thyroid cancer, but other classification systems are also used. There seems, however, to be no difference in their predictability of patient outcome. Because the TNM classification of the AJCC and UICC is universally available and widely accepted for other cancers, the TNM classification is recommended for thyroid cancer as well [26]. The TNM classification and group staging for thyroid cancer are given in Tables 19.3 and 19.4.

Table 19.3 AJCC TNM classification for thyroid carcinomas (Used with the permission of the American Joint Committee on Cancer (AJCC), Chicago, IL. The original source for this material is the *AJCC Cancer Staging Manual*, 7th edn. New York: Springer Science and Business Media LLC, 2010. www.springer.com)

Primary tumor (T)*Note*: All categories may be subdivided: (s) solitary tumor and (m) multifocal tumor (the largest determines the classification)		
TX	Primary tumor cannot be assessed	
T0	No evidence of primary tumor	
T1	Tumor 2 cm or less in greatest dimension limited to the thyroid	
	T1a	Tumor 1 cm or less limited to the thyroid
	T1b	Tumor more than 1 cm but not more than 2 cm in greatest dimension, limited to the thyroid
T2	Tumor more than 2 cm but not more than 4 cm in greatest dimension limited to the thyroid	
T3	Tumor more than 4 cm in greatest dimension limited to the thyroid or any tumor with minimal extrathyroid extension (e.g., extension to sternothyroid muscle or perithyroid soft tissues)	
T4a	Moderately advanced disease.	
	Tumor of any size extending beyond the thyroid capsule to invade subcutaneous soft tissues, larynx, trachea, esophagus, or recurrent laryngeal nerve	
T4b	Very advanced disease.	
	Tumor invades prevertebral fascia or encases carotid artery or mediastinal vessels	
All anaplastic carcinomas are considered T4 tumors		
T4a	Intrathyroidal anaplastic carcinoma	
T4b	Anaplastic carcinoma with gross extrathyroid extension	
Regional lymph nodes (N)		
Regional lymph nodes are the central compartment, lateral cervical, and upper mediastinal lymph nodes.		
NX	Regional lymph nodes cannot be assessed.	
N0	No regional lymph node metastasis	
N1	Regional lymph node metastasis	
N1a	Metastasis to level VI (pretracheal, paratracheal, and prelaryngeal/Delphian lymph nodes)	
N1b	Metastasis to unilateral, bilateral, or contralateral cervical (levels I, II, III, IV, or V) or retropharyngeal or superior mediastinal lymph nodes (level VII)	
Distant metastasis (M)		
M0	No distant metastasis	
M1	Distant metastasis	

Table 19.4 Follicular or papillary carcinoma group staging (Used with the permission of the American Joint Committee on Cancer (AJCC), Chicago, IL. The original source for this material is the *AJCC Cancer Staging Manual*, 7th edn. New York: Springer Science and Business Media LLC, 2010. www.springer.com)

Papillary or follicular (differentiated)			
Under 45 years			
Stage I	Any T	Any N	M0
Stage II	Any T	Any N	M1
45 years and older			
Stage I	T1	N0	M0
Stage II	T2	N0	M0
Stage III	T3	N0	M0
	T1	N1a	M0
	T2	N1a	M0
	T3	N1a	M0
Stage IVA	T4a	N0	M0
	T4a	N1a	M0
	T1	N1b	M0
	T2	N1b	M0
	T3	N1b	M0
	T4a	N1b	M0
Stage IVB	T4b	Any N	M0
Stage IVC	Any T	Any N	M1

Table 19.5 Medullary thyroid carcinoma group staging (Used with the permission of the American Joint Committee on Cancer (AJCC), Chicago, IL. The original source for this material is the *AJCC Cancer Staging Manual*, 7th edn. New York: Springer Science and Business Media LLC, 2010. www.springer.com)

Medullary carcinoma (All age groups)			
Stage I	T1	N0	M0
Stage II	T2	N0	M0
	T3	N0	M0
Stage III	T1	N1a	M0
	T2	N1a	M0
	T3	N1a	M0
Stage IVA	T4a	N0	M0
	T4a	N1a	M0
	T1	N1b	M0
	T2	N1b	M0
	T3	N1b	M0
	T4a	N1b	M0
Stage IVB	T4b	Any N	M0
Stage IVC	Any T	Any N	M1

Because age at the time of diagnosis has such an important influence on prognosis for papillary and follicular thyroid cancer, group staging is based on both TNM classification and age at time of diagnosis. For multifocal tumor the largest tumor should determine the classification. Anaplastic and medullary carcinomas have their own group staging different from papillary and follicular carcinomas (Tables 19.5 and 19.6). Anaplastic tumors are always considered T4 [24].

Regional lymph node spread is common in papillary and medullary thyroid cancer, but the prognostic significance is

Table 19.6 Anaplastic thyroid carcinoma group staging (Used with the permission of the American Joint Committee on Cancer (AJCC), Chicago, IL. The original source for this material is the *AJCC Cancer Staging Manual*, 7th edn. New York: Springer Science and Business Media LLC, 2010. www.springer.com)

All anaplastic carcinomas are considered stage IV			
Stage IVA	T4a	Any N	M0
Stage IVB	T4b	Any N	M0
Stage IVC	Any T	Any N	M1

more important for medullary than for papillary carcinoma. The lungs are the most common site for hematogenous spread distant metastases, but bones and brain may also be involved in advanced disease.

The initial staging is based on all information available before treatment, including physical examination, diagnostic imaging (CT, MRI, US, nuclear medicine procedures including PET), FNA, biopsy, and result of surgical exploration if performed. The staging is important for selection of appropriate treatment and follow-up strategies and to facilitate the exchange of information between clinicians and scientists.

^{18}F-FDG PET in Thyroid Cancer

Normal Distribution of FDG in the Neck, Variants, and Pitfalls

A PET study of a patient with well-differentiated thyroid cancer should at least include the region from base of skull through chest. For more advanced disease and for medullary and anaplastic carcinomas, we suggest scanning from vertex through the pelvis.

The most common site for persistent disease, recurrence, and lymph node metastases is the neck. Interpretation of PET images of the neck region presents a particular challenge. The region shows substantial variations in normal uptake that can present difficulties in the identification of pathology. As already mentioned, a normal thyroid gland will not have uptake above background. Uptake in the abundant lymphoid tissue in the pharynx, forming the Waldeyer's ring (pharyngeal tonsil, palatine tonsils, lingual tonsillar tissue, and lymphoid tissue along salpingopharyngeal folds) is easily recognized. Some asymmetry of the pharyngeal and palatine tonsils is not uncommon. A V- or U-shaped high uptake in the floor of mouth along the medial borders of the mandible is the sublingual glands [27]. The sublingual gland is a predominant mucous gland, which may explain the consistently higher uptake compared to the parotid (serous gland) and submandibular glands (mixed serous and mucous).

Intense uptake of the orbital muscles is common, and with a high-resolution system, the individual eye muscles may be identified. Uptake in the intrinsic laryngeal musculature is a common finding and may be rather intense if the patient was talking during uptake of FDG. Typically finding is symmetric high uptake at the muscle origin and insertion of the arytenoid cartilage and some less intense uptake along the course of thyroarytenoid and vocalis muscle is seen. Unilateral nerve injury with vocal cord paralysis results in asymmetric vocal cord uptake. Increased uptake in skeletal muscles is rather frequent, most commonly including the sternocleidomastoid muscles, scalene muscles, longus capitis, and longus colli. Scalene muscle uptake is often particularly intense after neck dissection, where the sternocleidomastoid muscle has been removed. Especially after unilateral surgery and radiation therapy the muscle uptake may be remarkable asymmetric. The lower neck images sometimes demonstrate uptake only at the insertion sites of the neck muscles, which can be confused with bilateral supraclavicular lymph node disease. The muscle uptake is, however, usually symmetric and linear and palpation will demonstrate no nodes of sufficient size to account the amount of uptake seen on the scan. More rarely, temporalis, pterygoid, masseter, or other head and neck muscles will accumulate tracer, sometimes depending on specific use by the patient, so that obtaining a history of physical activity or chewing may be helpful. Taking steps to reduce or eliminate muscle uptake can be crucial to correct image interpretation. Ensuring that the patient is not chewing gum, chewing tobacco, reading, or talking during the uptake phase is important. Also, some have advocated the use of a benzodiazepine drug to suppress muscle uptake. Attention to the position of the head during the uptake phase is of prime importance. Experimenting with chair design and pillow placement to ensure slight head flexion and complete head relaxation is necessary to avoid unnecessary muscle uptake interference. Also, with 3D surface projections (maximum intensity projection, MIP) of PET images and careful examination of all three orthogonal views, most muscle uptake can be differentiated from disease by its anatomic pattern of distribution. PET-CT or PET fused with a diagnostic CT is of great help to differentiate between physiologic muscle uptake and pathologic uptake in tumor or metastatic lymph nodes. This should not, however, replace appropriate patient preparation. If no combined PET-CT or computer software for fusion of diagnostic CT and PET is available, CT and/or MRI images should be present for side-by-side comparison.

The cervical and upper thoracic spinal cord frequently shows mild uptake, gradually decreasing in caudal direction. Brown fat uptake is common and typically patchy, symmetric and may be very intense (Fig. 19.4). It is commonly located in neck, supraclavicular, suboccipital, and paraspinal regions in the neck and chest, and may also be located on scattered areas perivascular in the mediastinum, retrocrural, and even perirenal. Brown fat, hypermetabolic tumor, and metastatic lymph nodes may coexist, and a differentiation may be difficult without PET-CT. Increased FDG uptake in brown fat seems to be related to outdoor temperature and is thus more frequent during the colder periods of the year. Repeat imaging, making sure that the patient is warm and comfortable during injection and uptake may be needed to resolve the issue. We typically use warm blankets and keep uptake rooms warm to prevent muscle uptake as much as possible (Fig. 19.5). Benzodiazepine can be used as an extra measure to reduce fat uptake for repeated scans when necessary. Administration of low-dose propranolol may be more effective than benzodiazepine to reduce FDG uptake in brown fat [28].

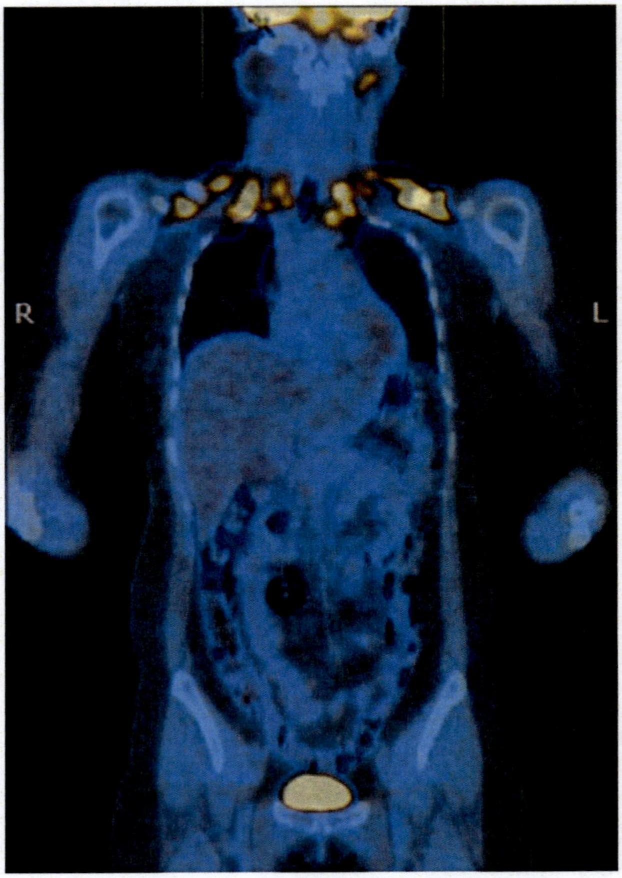

Fig. 19.4 PET-CT of young woman with no tumor, but intense uptake in brown fat in the low neck and supraclavicular regions bilaterally

Degenerative joint disease in the cervical spine is very common, and must not be mistaken for hypermetabolic lymph nodes or bone metastasis. Again, PET-CT or fusion of PET and a diagnostic CT is very useful. Degenerative joint disease uptake can be bilateral, asymmetric, and FDG uptake may be very intense.

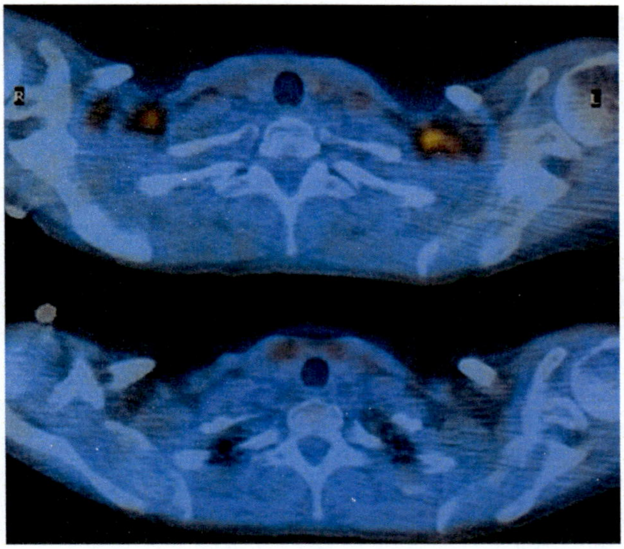

Fig. 19.5 PET-CT of young woman with intense uptake in brown fat in supraclavicular regions bilaterally (*top*). Same patients after repeated imaging (*bottom*). We made sure that patient was warm and comfortable during injection and uptake

Focal and Diffuse High Uptake in the Thyroid Gland as an Incidental Finding on FDG PET

We found focally high uptake as an incidental finding on FDG PET-CT in 79 out of 7,347 patients (1.1%) referred for oncologic whole-body PET-CT [29]. Primary and secondary thyroid malignancy was confirmed in 15/48 (35.4%) patients who had adequate follow-up (Fig. 19.6) [29]. Our results are consistent with others [30–32].

In the small series of eight patients with "hot spots" in the thyroid gland as an incidental finding on FDG PET studied by van den Bruel et al., three patients had well-differentiated thyroid cancer and two had medullary thyroid carcinomas [31]. There are some case reports of hypermetabolic nodules being autonomous thyroid nodules with subclinical hyperthyroidism [33].

There is a substantial overlap in the intensity of the FDG uptake for malignant and benign nodules, and benign nodules may be very hot. Consequently, the standardized uptake values (SUVs) in each individual are not useful to discriminate between benign and malignant nodules [29]. We usually report that the finding of a hypermetabolic focus in the thyroid gland may represent a primary or secondary thyroid cancer and we recommend follow-up with ultrasound and/or ultrasound guided FNA. Our experience is that FDG uptake in Hürthle cell (oncocytic) adenomas may be very intense.

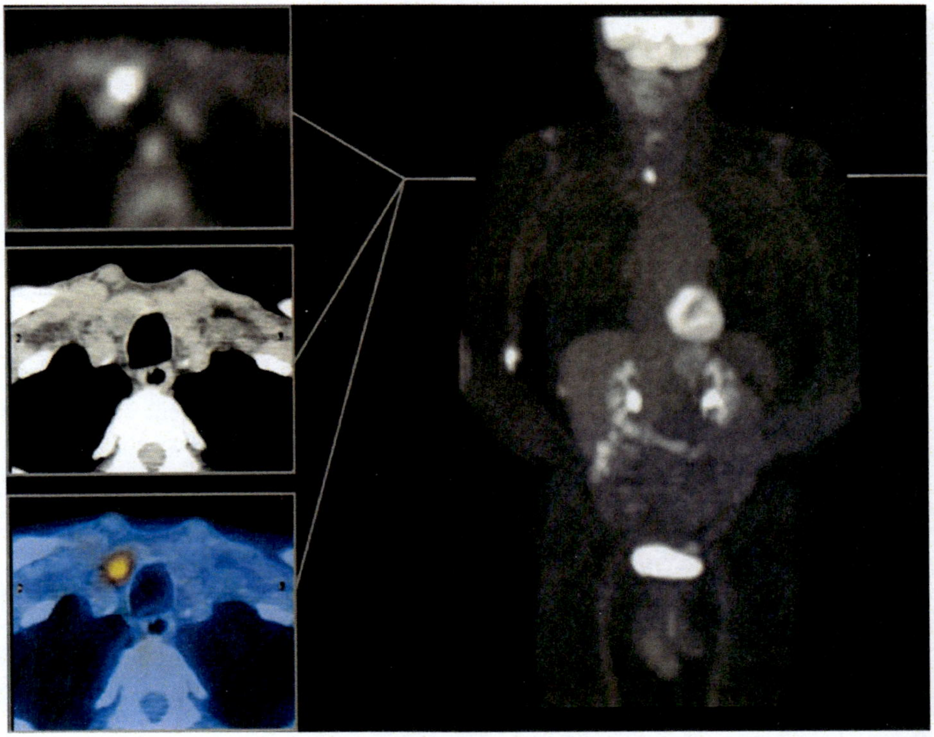

Fig. 19.6 Focally high uptake in the thyroid gland as an incidental finding on FDG PET. Ultrasound guided FNA was suspicious for Hürthle cell neoplasm. Histology after diagnostic subtotal hemithyroidectomy showed benign thyroid nodule with Hürthle cell changes and focal degeneration

Boerner et al. studied the thyroid uptake of FDG in 36 patients with Graves' disease before therapy with radioactive iodine. They found diffusely increased thyroid uptake in all the patients compared to 20 normal controls. Modeling of glucose metabolism revealed a substantial difference in thyroid FDG utilization corresponding to enhanced local metabolic rates in Graves' disease [34].

Boerner et al. also studied 30 patients with autonomous goiter with FDG PET before radioiodine therapy. The FDG uptake was increased in the areas with autonomy, determined by radionuclide scanning with ^{99m}Tc pertechnetate or ^{131}I, and the intensity correlated with the radioiodine uptake. They suggested that there is a connection between the glucose metabolism and hormone syntheses in the thyroid cells [35].

The incidental finding of diffusely increased FDG uptake in the thyroid gland is associated with chronic thyroiditis and does not seem to be affected by thyroid hormone therapy [36, 37]. The level of FDG is neither suggestive or the degree of the hypothyroidism nor correlative with the levels of TPO autoantibodies in serum [37]. In chronic thyroiditis with normal or reduced thyroid function, the increased uptake is probably caused by glucose utilization by the inflammatory cells and not by the thyroid cells. Our experience is that Hashimoto's thyroiditis may have uptake as intense as typically seen in anaplastic thyroid carcinoma and thyroid lymphoma (Fig. 19.7).

Influence of TSH Level on ^{18}F-FDG Uptake

There is evidence that TSH may stimulate FDG uptake by differentiated thyroid cancer. FDG PET under TSH stimulation may be more accurate in terms of both higher tumor to background uptake and the number of hypermetabolic foci detected. A number of authors recommend either thyroxine withdrawal or use of rhTSH routinely for FDG PET in well differentiated thyroid cancer [38–42].

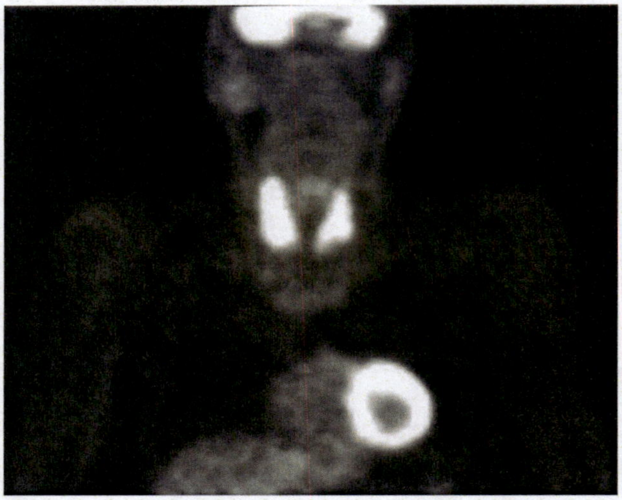

Fig. 19.7 Hypothyroid patient with Hashimoto's thyroiditis. Diffusely increased uptake in the thyroid gland is most commonly caused by chronic thyroiditis. As in this patient, the uptake may be very intense

Moog et al. compared FDG uptake on TSH suppressive therapy (TSH ≤ 0.05 mU/L) with uptake under TSH stimulation (TSH > 22 mIE/L) in ten patients with metastatic or recurrent well-differentiated thyroid cancer [38]. In 15 out of 17 lesions with increased FDG uptake, the tumor-to-background ratio was on average 63% higher TSH stimulated compared to TSH suppression. In three of the ten patients, FDG uptake consistent with malignancy was observed only on TSH stimulation. They recommend PET to be performed under TSH stimulation, and that follow-up examinations should be performed under identical TSH conditions to prevent erroneous interpretation [38].

In another intraindividual comparison, Petrich et al. compared FDG uptake on TSH suppressive therapy (TSH ≤ 0.05 mU/L) with uptake under TSH stimulation using recombinant human TSH [39]. They studied 30 patients with positive or equivocal thyroglobulin, negative or equivocal ^{131}I whole-body scan, and/or negative or equivocal conventional imaging (US, MRI, CT). The first of the two consecutive PET studies were performed on thyroxine treatment, the second after rhTSH. On thyroxine therapy, 45 foci in 9 patients were identified, compared to 82 foci in 19 patients after exogenous TSH stimulation. The tumor-to-background ratio and the SUVs were significantly higher after rhTSH than on thyroxine therapy. The authors conclude that TSH stimulates FDG uptake by differentiated thyroid carcinoma and that PET is more accurate under rhTSH than on thyroxine therapy [39].

In a small intraindividual comparison encompassing eight patients, van Tol et al. also found more lesions and that the lesion contrast was better in TSH stimulated PET compared to thyroxine therapy [40]. One patient was positive only when TSH stimulated. From another intraindividual comparison, Chin et al. concluded that rhTSH stimulation improves the detectability of occult thyroid metastases with FDG PET, compared with scans performed on TSH supression [41]. In a nicely performed in vitro study, Deiche et al., showed a strong influence of TSH on FDG uptake in differentiated thyroid cells. Their results support the clinical evidence that in well differentiated thyroid cancer, FDG PET may be more accurate at high levels of TSH [42].

No studies so far have compared the effect of thyroxin withdrawal with rhTSH on FDG uptake and no studies so far have included patients with Hürthle cell carcinomas. In dedifferentiated and anaplastic thyroid carcinoma, we would not expect high TSH to have any significant effect on FDG uptake.

^{131}I Negative/Thyroglobulin Positive Patient

Neck ultrasound is the most important and most frequently used imaging procedure in the initial diagnostic evaluation of patients with suspected or verified thyroid carcinoma and in the monitoring for residual and recurrent disease [43]. Most studies on FDG PET and thyroid cancer have been performed on patients with positive thyroglobulin but negative ^{131}I scan and this scenario is the main indication for FDG PET in differentiated thyroid cancer [43]. FDG PET-CT is an expensive procedure and is probably most useful in patients with more aggressive thyroid cancer before planned surgery or radiation therapy and to monitor such patients. Neck ultrasound, neck and chest CT, and ^{131}- or ^{123}-I scanning will normally be the first line imaging modalities [43].

Feine et al. introduced the term "flip flop" to describe the pattern of either ^{131}I or FDG uptake in metastases from thyroid cancer. When well-differentiated thyroid cancer dedifferentiate, the ability to concentrate iodine declines while the ability to concentrate FDG increases [44].

Loco-regional recurrences are common and with thyroid cancer and the patients have frequently been through multiple extensive neck surgeries with the result of modified anatomy and scarring. Conventional imaging with CT, MRI, and US is often not able to discriminate between malignant foci and changes secondary to treatment. Focal FDG uptake in the neck can help to direct ultrasound guided FNA, help the surgeon to chose the most appropriate surgery or ethanol injection, and be a guide for radiation planning (Figs. 19.8 and 19.9).

Frilling et al. prospectively analyzed 24 patients with negative ^{131}I WBS and elevated thyroglobulin [45]. They found the sensitivity for FDG PET to detect metastatic lesions to be 94.6% and an accuracy of 87.8%. The specificity was low, however, when PET without CT was used. PET resulted in changed surgical tactics in a significant number of patients [45].

In most studies evaluating PET as a diagnostic tool in thyroid cancer, the PET examinations have been performed with PET only without integrated CT. Combined PET-CT is shown to be more accurate than PET alone in the detection and anatomic localization leading to improved diagnostic accuracy in most cancers, including suspected recurrent or metastatic well-differentiated thyroid cancer [46–49]. Nahas et al. demonstrated that FDG PET-CT provided additional information that changed or supported treatment decision in 67% of 33 patients with papillary thyroid carcinoma [49].

Seiboth et al. demonstrated that neck MRI fused with FDG PET provided additional information that altered the treatment plan in 46% of 34 patients with papillary thyroid carcinoma [50]. However, FDG PET-CT and neck ultrasound will be the procedure of choice in most cases where PET is indicated. Indeed, Grant et al. in our institution demonstrated that FDG PET added valuable information to high resolution neck ultrasound in only 10% of 30 patients whom underwent surgical re-exploration after FDG PET scanning [51]. Almost all of these patients had suppressed TSH at the time of the PET scan and thyroglobulin levels were relatively low, indicating that the tumor burden was quite small. FDG PET

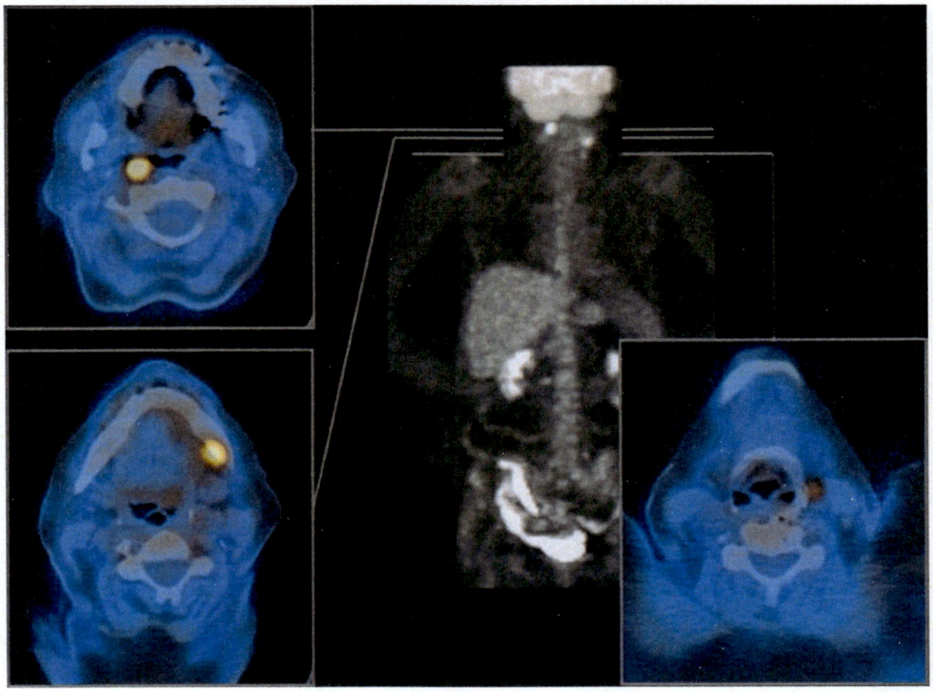

Fig. 19.8 Fifty-five year old woman with papillary thyroid cancer. ^{131}I negative. Thyroglobulin was 42 ng/mL on thyroxine. Chest CT was negative for malignancy. Ultrasound of the neck showed postoperative changes without evidence of residual disease. FDG PET-CT showed hypermetabolic lymph nodes in the right parapharyngeal, left submandibular (level I), and left high jugular (level II) regions, all confirmed to be metastasis by histology

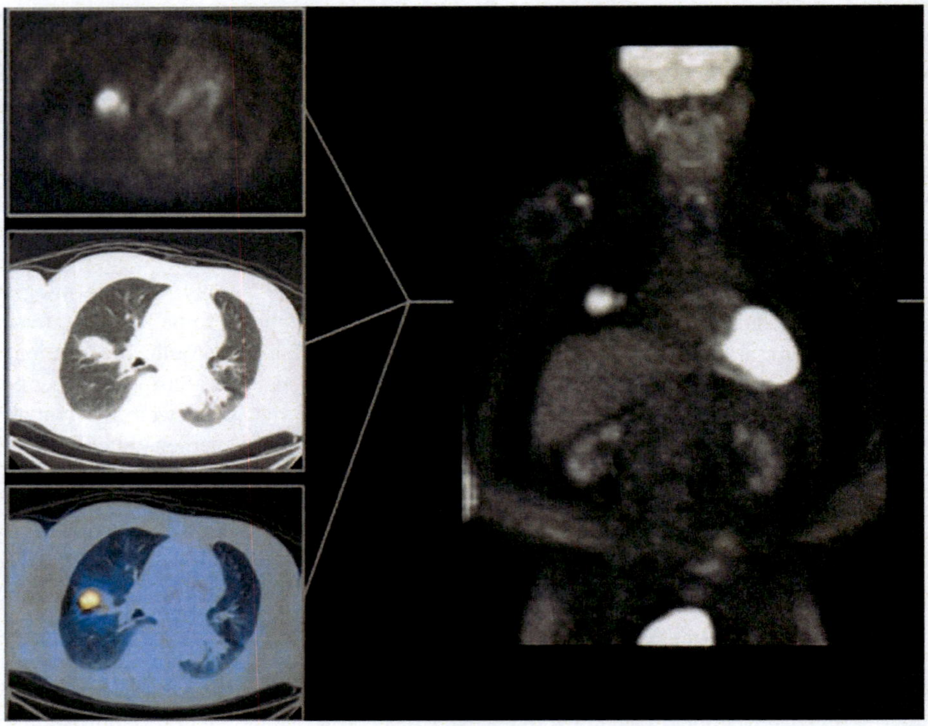

Fig. 19.9 ^{131}I negative, FDG positive metastasis from papillary thyroid carcinoma in right middle lobe of lung in a 66-year-old man. Thyroglobulin was 46 ng/mL on thyroxine

sensitivity seems to correlate with thyroglobulin blood level, and the sensitivity is low in patients with thyroglobulin level less than 10 µg/L. Not only the size of the metastases, but also the location and degree of differentiation will affect the FDG uptake. In most studies the PET examinations are performed with the patient on thyroxin. As described in a separate section, there are biological and clinical evidence that FDG PET under TSH stimulation may be more accurate in terms of both higher tumor-to-background uptake and the number of hypermetabolic foci detected [38–42]. In a small but carefully designed study Saab et al. showed that FDG PET-CT performed TSH stimulated can localize recurrent thyroid cancer in a substantial number of patients with negative neck ultrasound and chest CT, even when serum Tg is only moderately elevated [52].

Only a few studies have compared FDG PET with other non-PET nuclear medicine procedures such as ^{99m}Tc sestamibi or ^{201}Tl. In an intraindividual study encompassing 19 patients, Iwata et al. compared the ability of FDG PET, ^{131}I, and ^{99m}Tc sestamibi to detect metastatic differentiated thyroid cancer [53]. All the patients were hypothyroid when studied. There is no surprise that FDG PET detected more lesions and was found to be superior to ^{99m}Tc sestamibi. Their results on six patients with miliary lung metastases are of interest: all were negative on ^{99m}Tc sestamibi; two were positive on PET, but negative on ^{131}I; while three were positive on ^{131}I and negative on FDG PET [53]. These findings may indicate that tumor differentiation is more important for the detection of miliary lung metastases than the size of the individual lesions. FDG uptake in miliary lung metastases may indicate that ^{131}I treatment will not be useful. However, more data are needed. In another study, Hung et al., reported two patients with miliary pulmonary metastases that failed to be demonstrated on FDG PET [54]. PET scanners have limited spatial resolution and it is well known that small lung metastases less than 5 mm may be missed on PET [55, 56]. However, lesions too small to be characterized by PET, may well be detected on the low-dose CT as part of the PET-CT study.

In addition to locating recurrent or metastatic disease, there is good evidence that FDG PET is an independent prognostic indicator. Wang et al. studied 125 high-risk patients with well-differentiated thyroid cancer with known recurrent or metastatic disease [57]. During a 41-month follow-up, 14 patients died. Univariate analysis demonstrated reduced survival in those patients with FDG uptake. They found a significant correlation between survival and quantified uptake (maximum SUV), suggesting that tumors with highest metabolic activity are those with the most rapid growth potential. Survival was directly related to the total volume of FDG avid tumor mass. The larger the volume, the shorter the survival. Multivariate analysis demonstrated that the single strongest predictor of survival was the FDG avid tumor volume [57].

Robbins et al. studied 400 patients with recurrent or metastatic differentiated thyroid cancer [58]. Multivariate analysis found that only age, standard uptake value and the number of FDG avid lesions significantly correlated with survival. They found that positive PET, by itself, was associated with a 7.28-fold increased risk of death [58].

Radioactive iodine is extensively used to destroy locoregional and distant recurrent or metastatic thyroid cancer. Treatment with radioactive iodine has been shown to reduce recurrences and mortality for patients with well-differentiated thyroid cancer. Survival of patients with metastases that concentrate radioiodine is better than for patients with metastases that do not concentrate iodine. There is still a debate about how to treat thyroglobulin positive, ^{131}I negative disease. In a retrospective study of 25 patients with FDG-avid metastases, Wang et al. compared tumor volume and standard uptake values before and on average 12.9 months after treatment with ^{131}I [59]. The total volume and the standard uptake values of the FDG-avid metastases rose significantly from the PET study performed before ^{131}I treatment to the PET study performed on average 12.9 months after treatment. The thyroglobulin level increased in the same period on average to 132% of the baseline value, compared to a 32% decrease in control group with FDG negative, ^{131}I positive patients. They conclude that high-dose ^{131}I therapy has little or no effect on FDG avid thyroid metastases [59].

Serum thyroglobulin is a very sensitive and specific tumor marker used in the management of patients with well differentiated follicular and papillary thyroid carcinomas. In patients with circulating thyroglobulin autoantibodies (TgAb), however, thyroglobulin may be falsely elevated or falsely decreased dependent on the laboratory method used to quantify Tg. It is therefore important that quantification of Tg always includes measurement of TgAb as well. It is imperative that the referring physician knows how the presence of TgAb may influence the Tg measurement. Immunometric assays are the most commonly used method for measuring Tg and they always underestimate serum thyroglobulin. Paradoxically, thyroglobulin is often undetectable (false-negative Tg) in TgAb-positive patients with residual or recurrent disease. We have studied the potential value of FDG PET-CT in the management of patients with well-differentiated thyroid carcinoma and positive thyroglobulin autoantibodies (TgAb) after total thyroidectomy and radioiodine ablation [60]. Eighteen patients were included in this retrospective study. PET was true-positive in ten patients, true negative in six patients and false-negative in two patients. One of the two false-negative patients had metastatic lymph nodes in the neck, seen by US and confirmed by FNA. The other false-negative patient had known numerous tiny bilateral lung metastases too small to be characterized by PET; however, they were clearly identified on the low-dose CT. We conclude that PET may be useful in the management of patients with positive TgAb, but equivocal anatomic imaging findings.

Hürthle Cell Carcinoma

Hürthle cell carcinoma is a thyroid cancer subtype with less favorable outcome than regular follicular and papillary thyroid carcinomas [61]. The tumor is more aggressive and is more common in elderly patients, which by itself is a negative prognostic factor for well-differentiated thyroid cancer. Radioactive iodine is an important therapeutic option in a patient with metastatic differentiated thyroid carcinoma. Hürthle cell carcinomas, however, have poor iodine accumulation, and therefore iodine ablation and therapy is frequently not an option, and diagnostic scanning with ^{123}I or ^{131}I may not be useful. Hürthle cell carcinoma demonstrates intense uptake on ^{18}F FDG PET, and PET is recommended for the evaluation and clinical management of patients with this cancer (Fig. 19.10) [62–65].

Plotkin et al. studied 17 patients with Hürthle cell carcinoma [61]. They included the results from a German multicenter study encompassing 20 patients and performed a metaanalysis. They calculated an overall sensitivity of 92%, specificity of 80%, positive predictive value of 92%, negative predictive value of 80%, and accuracy of 89% [62]. It is expected that the results will be even better using PET-CT.

Lowe et al. studied retrospectively the results of 14 FDG PET studies in 12 patients with Hürthle cell carcinoma [64]. PET showed intense uptake in all known malignant lesions but one. The lesion that was false-negative by PET was a 1-cm focus in the neck. In that patient, there was a substantial nonspecific uptake in fat and muscle that obscured a moderate uptake in the region of the disease. The authors suggest that new advances with PET-CT fusion imaging may improve the accuracy of PET in such cases. Disease not identified by other imaging methods was demonstrated in 7 of the 14 PET studies, and PET provided additional information on disease extent that led to a change in patient care for 7/14 of the scans obtained [64]. Based on a retrospective study of 44 patients with Hürthle cell carcinoma, Pryma et al. found the intensity of the FDG uptake in metastatic lesions to provide important prognostic information about survival [65]. They suggest that all patients with Hürthle cell thyroid cancer should undergo FDG PET as part of their initial postoperative staging and periodically to screen for occult recurrence, particularly in patients with elevated thyroglobulin.

Medullary Thyroid Cancer

The role of FDG PET in the diagnosis and follow-up medullary thyroid cancer is not well defined. Based on the results from a recently published prospective study in 55 patients with MTC and elevated calcitonin after primary treatment, Giraudet et al. concluded that FDG PET has no

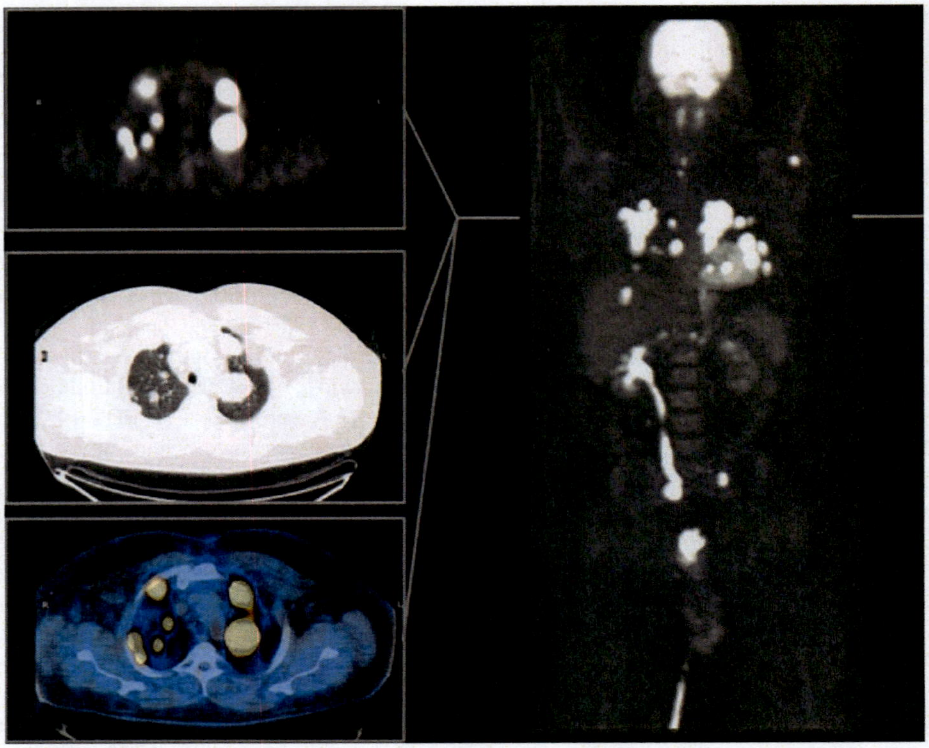

Fig. 19.10 Extensive metastases from Hürthle cell carcinoma

place in routine imaging of MTC [66]. However, a number of other studies indicate that FDG PET may be useful complementary to ultrasound of the neck, CT of the chest and abdomen, and MRI of liver and bone in a patient with elevated basal or stimulated calcitonin levels after surgery when residual or recurrence disease is suspected (Fig. 19.11) [67–71]. The higher the calcitonin, the higher the probability of having a positive PET. Ong et al. concluded that a meaningful sensitivity for FDG PET seems to achieved only for calcitonin levels greater than about 1,000 pg/mL [71]. However, PET may detect disease even with very low calcitonin levels [66]. The level of calcitonin is important, however, the blood calcitonin doubling time is important as well. CEA blood levels do not correlate very well with findings on FDG PET.

^{68}Ga-D-Phe(1)-Tyr(3)-octreotide (DOTATOC) is a PET radiopharmaceutical highly specific for somatostatin receptors and seems to be promising for MTC [72, 73]. Öksüz et al. have reported that high differentiated neuroendocrine tumors showed high uptake of 68Ga-DOTATOC and low ^{18}F-FDG uptake, while in low differentiated tumors the ^{18}F-FDG uptake was the highest [72]. They suggest that 68Ga-DOTATOC and ^{18}F-FDG may be used to characterize the grade of differentiation of neuroendocrinetumorsincludingMTC. ^{18}F-Dihydroxyphenylalanine (FDOPA) is another PET radiopharmaceutical reported potential useful in MTC as well [74–76].

Our own experience (unpublished data) is that ^{18}F FDG PET seems to be a strong prognostic indicator in patients with suspected residual or recurrent MTC. Patients with elevated calcitonin but negative PET seems to have an indolent disease, while positive PET seems to indicate less favorable prognosis.

Anaplastic Thyroid Carcinoma

Anaplastic thyroid carcinoma (ATC) is one of the most aggressive solid tumors in humans with a very poor prognosis [77, 78]. We have studied the potential contribution of FDG PET to the clinical management of patients with ATC in a retrospective study of 16 patients [79]. We found that ATC demonstrates intense uptake on ^{18}F-FDG PET images (Fig. 19.12). It should be noted that primary thyroid lymphoma, sometimes Hashimoto thyroiditis, and metastatic high-grade malignancy to the thyroid may also show very intense uptake (Fig. 19.13). We found that PET-CT localized more metastatic or residual foci than ultrasound and CT combined. In 8 of the 16 patients (50%) the medical records reported an impact of the PET findings on the clinical management of the patients. A negative PET-scan after completed therapy may be indicative of extended survival. ATC does

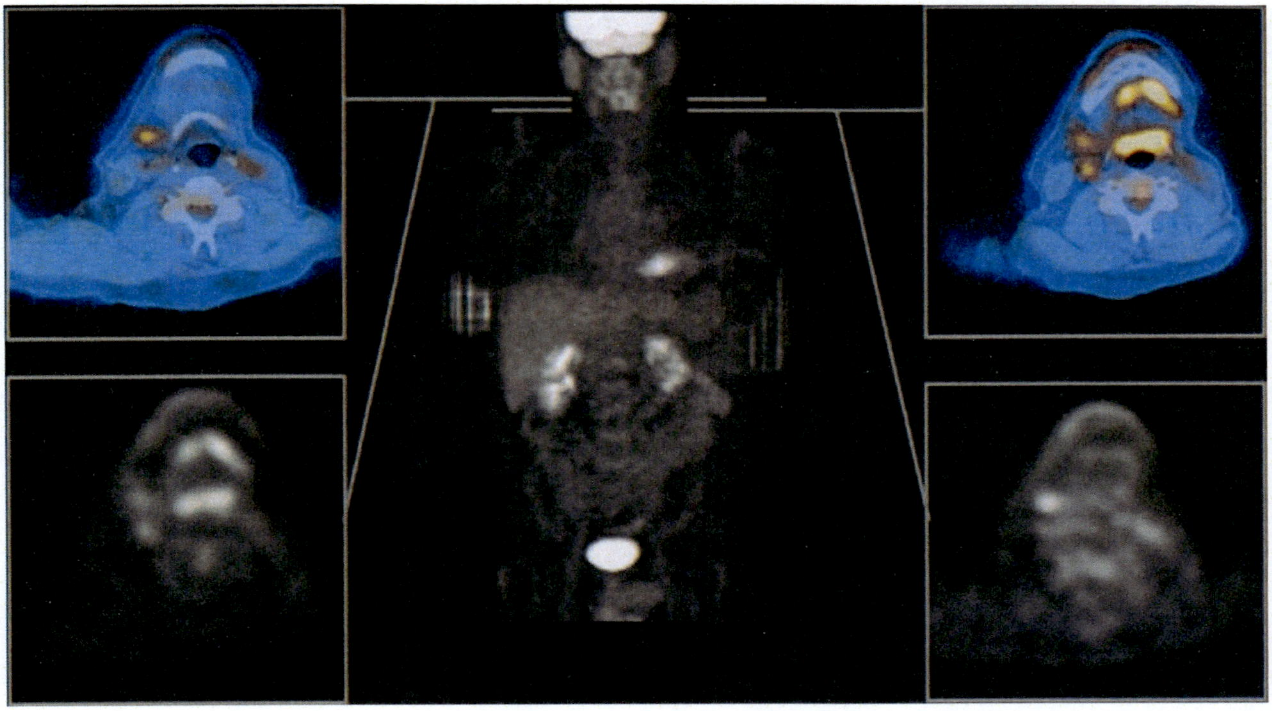

Fig. 19.11 Patient with medullary thyroid carcinoma and increased basal calcitonin. Chest CT was negative for metastasis. Ultrasound of the neck showed postoperative changes without evidence of residual disease. PET-CT shows hypermetabolic lymph nodes in the tight upper jugular chain (level II)

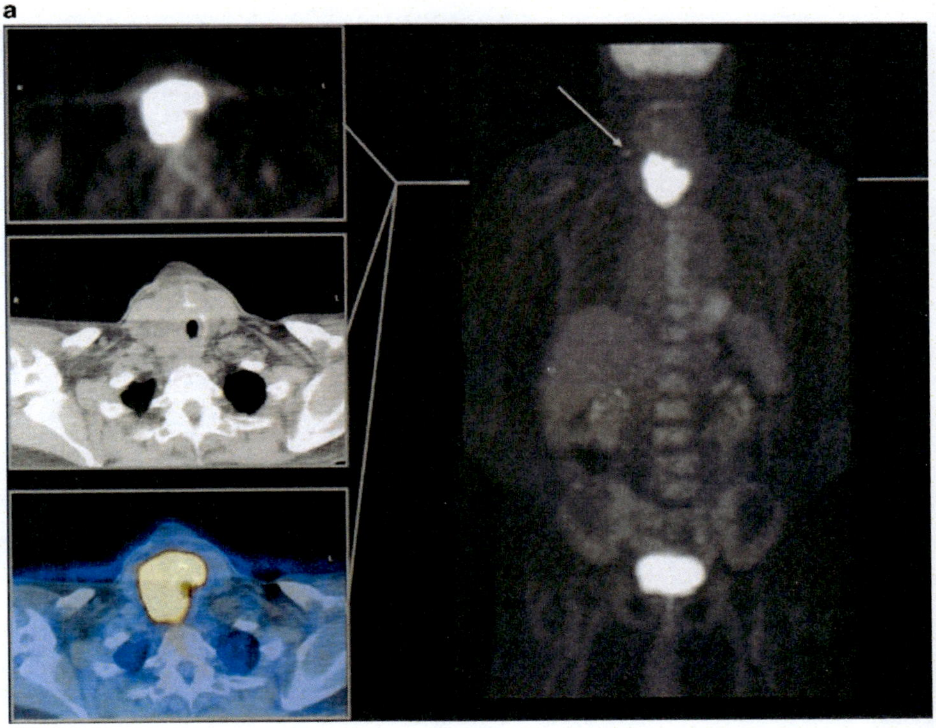

Fig. 19.12 (**a**) Anaplastic thyroid carcinoma with a hypermetabolic, metastatic right upper jugular (level II) lymph node (*arrow*)

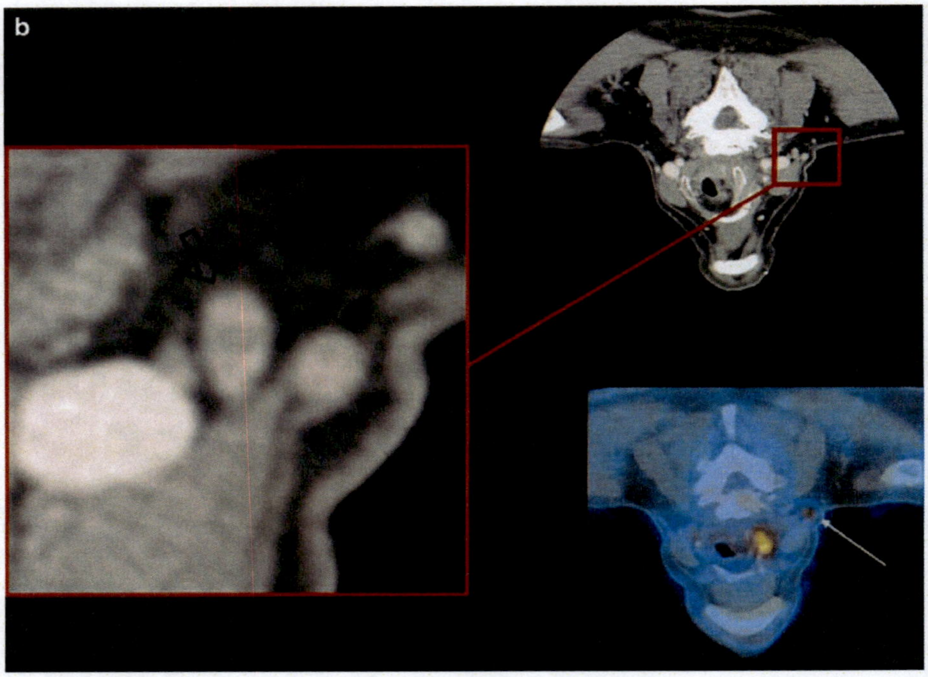

Fig. 19.12 (continued)
(**b**) Hypermetabolic lymph nodes of normal size can easily be missed on CT. However, the CT magnification shows inhomogeneous structure, consistent with metastases (*bold arrow*)

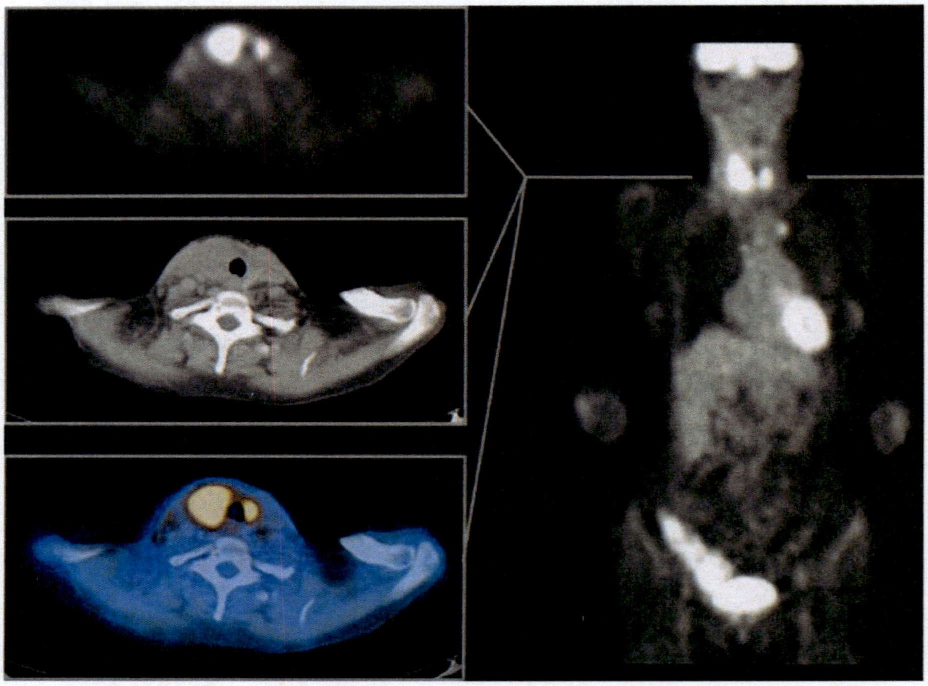

Fig. 19.13 Metastasis from poorly differentiated adenocarcinoma to the thyroid gland, most likely lung primary. The patient died shortly after diagnosis

not produce thyroglobulin; therefore, PET may also be useful for early detection of recurrent disease. It is concluded that PET may improve disease detection and have an impact on patient management in patients with ATC relative to other imaging modalities.

References

1. Harach HR, Franssila KO, Wasenius VM. Occult papillary carcinoma of the thyroid. A "normal" finding in Finland. A systematic autopsy study. Cancer 1985;56:531–538.

2. DeLellis RA, Lloyd RV, Heitz PU, Eng C, eds. Tumours of the thyroid and the thyroid gland. In: World Health Organization Classification of Tumours: Pathology and genetics of tumors of endocrine organs. Lyon: IARC Press, 2004, pp. 49–133.
3. Carlson EH. Endocrine neoplasms. In: Casciato DA, ed. Manual of clinical oncology, 5th edn. Philadelphia: Lippincott Williams & Wilkins, 2004, pp. 333–354.
4. Leboulleux S, Baudin E, Young J, Caillou B, Lazar V, Pellegriti G, Ducreux M, Schaison G, Schlumberger M. Gastroenteropancreatic neuroendocrine tumor metastases to the thyroid gland: differential diagnosis with medullary thyroid carcinoma. Eur J Endocrinol 1999;140:187–191.
5. Schlumberger M, Tubiana M, Chanson P, Schaison G. Cancer of the endocrine glands. In: Rubin P, ed. Clinical oncology, 8th edn. Philadelphia: Saunders, 2001, pp. 648–684.
6. Silver RJ, Parangi S. Management of thyroid incidentalomas. Surg Clin North Am 2004;84:907–919.
7. Hegedus L. Clinical practice. The thyroid nodule. NEJM 2004;351: 1764–1771.
8. Franc B, Salmonière PDL, Lange F, Hoang C, Louvel A, Roquanucourt, Vildè F, Hejblum G, Chevret S, Chastang C. Interobserver and intraobserver reproducibility in the histopathology of follicular thyroid carcinoma. Hum Pathol 1993;34:1092–1100.
9. Samaan NA, Schultz PN, Hickey RC, Goepfert H, Haynie TP, Johnston DA, Ordonez NG. The results of various modalities of treatment of well differentiated thyroid carcinomas: a retrospective review of 1599 patients. J Clin Endocrinol Metab 1992;75:714–720.
10. Mazzaferri EL, Jhiang SM. Long-term impact of initial surgical and medical therapy on papillary and follicular thyroid cancer. Am J Med 1994;97:418–428.
11. Hay ID, Thompson GB, Grant CS, Bergstralh EJ, Dvorak CE, Gorman CA, Maurer MS, McIver B, Mullan BP, Oberg AL, Powell CC, van Heerden JA, Goellner JR. Papillary thyroid carcinoma managed at the Mayo Clinic during six decades (1940–1999): temporal trends in initial therapy and long-term outcome in 2444 consecutively treated patients. World J Surg 2002;26:879–885.
12. Mazzaferri EL, Robbins RJ, Spencer CA, Braverman LE, Pacini F, Wartofsky L, Haugen BR, Sherman SI, Cooper DS, Braunstein GD, Lee S, Davies TF, Arafah BM, Ladenson PW, Pinchera A. A consensus report of the role of serum thyroglobulin as a monitoring method for low-risk patients with papillary thyroid carcinoma. J Clin Endocrinol Metab 2003;88:1433–1441.
13. Schlumberger M, Berg G, Cohen O, Duntas L, Jamar F, Jarzab B, Limbert E, Lind P, Pacini F, Reiners C, Sanchez Franco F, Toft A, Wiersinga WM. Follow-up of low-risk patients with differentiated thyroid carcinoma: a European perspective. Eur J Endocrinol 2004;150:105–112.
14. Torlontano M, Attard M, Crocetti U, Tumino S, Bruno R, Costante G, D'Azzo G, Meringolo D, Ferretti E, Sacco R, Arturi F, Filetti S. Follow-up of low risk patients with papillary thyroid cancer: role of neck ultrasonography in detecting lymph node metastases. J Clin Endocrinol Metab 2004;89:3402–3407.
15. Brenner DL, Breau RL, Suen JY. Cancer of the thyroid. In: Myers EN, Suen JY, Myers JN, Hanna EYN, eds. Cancer of the head and neck, 4th edn. Philadelphia: Saunders, 2003, pp. 431–464.
16. Clark OH, Noguchi S, eds. Thyroid cancer. St. Louis: Quality Medical Publishing, 2000.
17. Richter E, Feyerabend T. Normal lymph node topography CT atlas. Berlin: Springer Verlag, 2004, pp. 7–39.
18. Lewis BD, Hay ID, Charboneau JW, McIver B, Reading CC, Goellner JR. Percutaneous ethanol injection for treatment of cervical lymph node metastases in patients with papillary thyroid carcinoma. Am J Roentgenol 2002;178:699–704.
19. Lim CY, Yun JS, Lee J, Nam KH, Chung WY, Park CS. Percutaneous ethanol injection therapy for locally recurrent papillary thyroid carcinoma. Thyroid 2007;17:347–350.
20. Mazzaferri EL, Kloos RT. Current approaches to primary therapy for papillary and follicular thyroid cancer. J Clin Endocrinol Metab 2001;86:1447–1463.
21. Ryan S, McNicholas M, Eustace S. Head and neck. In: Ryan S, McNicholas M, Eustace S, eds. Anatomy for diagnostic imaging, 2nd edn. Philadelphia: Saunders, 2004, pp. 1–47.
22. Phelps PD. The pharynx and the larynx: The neck. In: Sutton D, ed. Textbook of radiology and imaging, 7th edn. London: Churchill Livingstone, 2003, pp. 1489–1517.
23. Myers EN, Suen JY, Myers JN, Hanna EYN, eds. Cancer of the head and neck, 4th edn. Philadelphia: Saunders, 2003.
24. Greene, FL, Page DL, Fleming ID, Fritz AG, Balch CM, Haller DG, Morrow M, eds. AJCC cancer staging handbook, 6th edn. New York: Springer-Verlag, 2002, pp. 27–87.
25. Harnsberger HR. Handbook of head and neck imaging, 2nd edn. St. Louis: Mosby, 1995.
26. Brierley JD, PanzarellaT, Tsang RW, Gospodarowitz MK, ÓSullivan B. A comparison of different staging systems predictability of patient outcome, Thyroid carcinoma as an example. Cancer 1997; 79:2414–2423.
27. Bogsrud TV, Karantanis D, Lowe VJ. Normal uptake of F-18 FDG in the sublingual gland. Clin Nucl Med 2006;31:50.
28. Parysow O, Mollerach AM, Jager V, Racioppi S, San Roman J, Gerbaudo VH. Low-dose oral propranolol could reduce brown fat adipose tissue F-18 uptake in patients undergoing PET scans. J Nucl Med 2007;32:351–357.
29. Bogsrud TV, Karantanis D, Nathan MA, Mullan BP, Wiseman GA, Collins DA, Kasperbauer J, Scott E, Strome S, Reading C, Hay ID, Lowe VJ. The value of quantifying ^{18}F-FDG uptake in thyroid nodules found incidentally on whole-body PET-CT. Nucl Med Commun 2007;28:373–381.
30. Cohen MS, Arslan N, Dehdashti F, Doherty GM, Lairmore TC, Brunt LM, Moley JF. Risk of malignancy in thyroid incidentalomas identified by fluorodeoxyglucose-positron emission tomography. Surgery 2001;130:941–946.
31. Van den Bruel A, Maes A, De Potter T, Mortelmans L, Drijkoningen M, Van Damme B, Delaere P, Bouillon R. Clinical relevance of thyroid fluorodeoxyglucose-whole body positron emission tomography incidentaloma. J Clin Endocrinol Metab 2002;87:1517–1520.
32. Kang KW, Kim SK, Kang HS, Lee ES, Sim JS, Lee IG, Jeong SY, Kim SW. Prevalence and risk of cancer of focal thyroid incidentaloma identified by 18F-fluorodeoxyglucose positron emission tomography for metastasis evaluation and cancer screening in healthy subjects. J Clin Endocrinol Metab 2003;88:4100–4104.
33. Gianoukakis AG, Karam M, Cheema A, Cooper JA. Autonomous thyroid nodules visualized by positron emission tomography with 18F-fluorodeoxyglucose: a case report and review of the literature. Thyroid 2003;13:395–399.
34. Boerner AR, Voth E, Theissen P, Wienhard K, Wagner R, Schicha H. Glucose metabolism of the thyroid in Graves' disease measured by F-18-fluoro-deoxyglucose positron emission tomography. Thyroid 1998;8:765–772.
35. Boerner AR, Voth E, Theissen P, Wienhard K, Wagner R, Schicha H.Glucose metabolism of the thyroid in autonomous goiter measured by F-18-FDG-PET. Exp Clin Endocrinol Diab 2000;108:191–196.
36. Yasuda S, Shohtsu A, Ide M, Takagi S, Takahashi W, Suzuki Y, Horiuchi M. Chronic thyroiditis: diffuse uptake of FDG at PET. Radiology 1998;207:775–778.
37. Karantanis D, Bogsrud TV, Wiseman GA, Mullan BP, Subramaniam RM, Nathan MA, Peller PJ, Bahn RS, Lowe VJ. Clinical significance of diffusely increased ^{18}F-FDG uptake in the thyroid gland. J Nucl Med 2007;48:896–901.
38. Moog F, Linke R, Manthey N, Tiling R, Knesewitsch P, Tatsch K, Hahn K. Influence of thyroid-stimulating hormone levels on uptake of FDG in recurrent and metastatic differentiated thyroid carcinoma. J Nucl Med 2000;41:1989–1995.

39. Petrich T, Börner AR, Otto D, Hofmann M, Knapp WH. Influence of rhTSH of [^{18}F]fluorodeoxyglucose uptake by differentiated thyroid carcinoma. Eur J Nucl Med 2002;29:641–647.
40. van Tol KM, Jager PL, Piers DA, Pruim J, de Vries EG, Dullaart RP, Links TP. Better yield of (18)fluorodeoxyglucose-positron emission tomography in patients with metastatic differentiated thyroid carcinoma during thyrotropin stimulation. Thyroid 2002;12:381–387.
41. Chin BB, Patel P, Cohade C, Ewertz M, Wahl R, Ladenson P. Recombinant human thyrotropin stimulation of fluoro-D-glucose positron emission tomography uptake in well-differentiated thyroid carcinoma. J Clin Endocrinol Metab 2004;89:91–95.
42. Deichen JT, Schmidt C, Prante O, Maschauer S, Papadopoulos T, Kuwert T. Influence of TSH on uptake of [18F]fluorodeoxyglucose in human thyroid cells in vitro. Eur J Nucl Med Mol Imaging 2004;31:507–512.
43. Leboulleux S, Schroeder PR, Schlumberger M, Ladenson PW. The role of PET in follow-up of patients treated for differentiated epithelial thyroid cancers. Nature Clin Pract Endocrinol Metab 2006;3:112–121.
44. Feine U, Lietzenmayer R, Hanke JP, Wohrle H, Muller-Schauenburg W. [18FDG whole-body PET in differentiated thyroid carcinoma. Flipflop in uptake patterns of 18FDG and 131I] Nuklearmedizin 1995;34:127–134.
45. Frilling A, Tecklenborg K, Gorges R, Weber F, Clausen M, Broelsch EC. Preoperative diagnostic value of [(18)F] fluorodeoxyglucose positron emission tomography in patients with radioiodine-negative recurrent well-differentiated thyroid carcinoma. Ann Surg 2001;234:804–811.
46. Schoder H, Yeung HW, Gonen M, Kraus D, Larson SM. Head and neck cancer: clinical usefulness and accuracy of PET/CT image fusion. Radiology 2004;231:65–72.
47. Zoller M, Kohlfuerst S, Igere I, Kresnik E, Gallowitsch H-J, Gomez I, Lind P. Combined PET/CT in the follow-up of differentiated thyroid carcinoma: what is the impact of each modality? Eur J Nucl Med Mol Imaging 2006;34:487–495.
48. Shammas A, Degirmenci B, Mountz JM, McCook BM, Branstetter B, Bencherif BB, Joyce JM, Carty SE, Kuffner HA, Avril N. 18F-FDG PET/CT in patients with suspected recurrent or metastatic well-differentiated thyroid cancer. J Nucl Med 2007;48:221–226.
49. Nahas Z, Goldenberg D, Fakhry C, Ewertz M, Zeiger M, Ladenson PW, Wahl R, Tufano RP. The role of positron emission tomography/computed tomography in the management of recurrent papillary thyroid carcinoma. Laryngoscope 2006;115:237–243.
50. Seiboth L, Van Nostrand D, Wartofsky L, Ousman Y, Jonklaas J, Butler C, Atkins F, Burman K. Utility of PET/neck MRI digital fusion images in the management of recurrent or persistent thyroid cancer. Thyroid 2008;18:103–111.
51. Grant CS, Thompson GB, Farley DR, Richards ML, Mullan BP, Hay ID. The value of positron emission tomography in the surgical management of recurrent papillary thyroid carcinoma. World J Surg 2008;32:708–715.
52. Saab G, Driedger AA, Pavlosky W, McDonald T, Wong CY, Urbain JL. Thyroid-stimulating hormone-stimulated fused positron emission tomography/computed tomography in the evaluation of recurrence in 131I-negative papillary thyroid carcinoma. Thyroid 2006;16:267–272.
53. Iwata M, Kasagi K, Misaki T, Matsumoto K, Iida Y, Ishimori T, Nakamoto Y, Higashi T, Saga T, Konishi J. Comparison of whole-body 18F-FDG PET, 99mTc-MIBI SPET, and post-therapeutic 131I-Na scintigraphy in the detection of metastatic thyroid cancer. Eur J Nucl Med Mol Imag 2004;31:491–498.
54. Hung MC, Wu HS, Kao CH, Chen WK, Changlai SP. F18-fluorodeoxyglucose positron emission tomography in detecting metastatic papillary thyroid carcinoma with elevated human serum thyroglobulin levels but negative I-131 whole body scan. Endocr Res 2003;29:169–175.
55. Dietlein M, Scheidhauer K, Voth E, Theissen P, Schicha H. Fluorine-18 fluorodeoxyglucose positron emission tomography and iodine-131 whole-body scintigraphy in the follow-up of differentiated thyroid cancer. Eur J Nucl Med 1997;24:1342–1348.
56. Palmedo H, Bucerius J, Joe A, Strunk H, Hortling N, Meyka S, Roedel R, Wolff M, Wardelmann E, Biersack HJ, Jaeger U. Integrated PET/CT in differentiated thyroid cancer: diagnostic accuracy and impact on patient management. J Nucl Med 2006;47:616–624.
57. Wang W, Larson SM, Fazzari M, Tickoo SK, Kolbert K, Sgouros G, Yeung H, Macapinlac H, Rosai J, Robbins RJ. Prognostic value of [18F]fluorodeoxyglucose positron emission tomographic scanning in patients with thyroid cancer. J Clin Endocrinol Metab 2000;85: 1107–1113.
58. Robbins RJ, Wan Q, Grewal RK, Reibke R, Gonen M, Strauss W, Tuttle RM, Drucker W, Larson SM. Real-time prognosis for metastatic thyroid carcinoma based on 2-[18F]Fluoro-2-deoxy-D-glucose-positron emission tomography scanning. J Clin Endocrinol Metab 2006;91:498–505.
59. Wang W, Larson SM, Tuttle RM, Kalaigian H, Kolbert K, Sonenberg M, Robbins RJ. Resistance of [18f]-fluorodeoxyglucose-avid metastatic thyroid cancer lesions to treatment with high-dose radioactive iodine. Thyroid 2001;11:1169–1175.
60. Bogsrud TV Karantanis D, Nathan MA, Mullan BP, Wiseman GA, Hay ID, Kasperbauer JL, Reading CC, Lowe VJ. FDG PET in the management of patients with well differentiated thyroid carcinoma and positive thyroglobulin autoantibodies [abstract 14]. Eur J Nucl Med Mol Imag 2007;34(Suppl 2):S122.
61. Stojadinovic A, Hoos A, Ghossein RA, Hürthle cell carcinoma: a 60 year experience. Ann Surg Oncol 2002;9:197–203.
62. Plotkin M, Hautzel H, Krause BJ, Schmidt D, Larisch R, Mottaghy FM, Boemer AR, Herzog H, Vosberg H, Muller-Gartner HW. Implication of 2-18fluor-2-deoxyglucose ,positron emission tomography in the follow-up of Hürthle cell thyroid cancer. Thyroid 2002;12:155–1561.
63. Grünwald F, Kälicke Th, Feine U, Lietzenmayer R, Scheidhauer K, Dietlein M, Schober O, Lerch H, Brandt-Mainz K, Burchert W, Hiltermann G, Cremerius U, Biersack HJ. Fluorine-18 fluorodeoxyglucose positron emission tomography in thyroid cancer: results of a multicenter study. Eur J Nucl Med 1999;26:1547–1552.
64. Lowe VJ, Mullan BP, Hay ID, McIver B, Kasperbauer JL. 18F-FDG PET of patients with Hürthle cell carcinoma. J Nucl Med 2003;44:1402–1406.
65. Pryma DA, Schröder H, Gönen M, Robbins RJ, Larson SM, Yeung HWD. Diagnostic accuracy and prognostic value of ^{18}F-FDG PET in Hürthle cell thyroid cancer patients. J Nucl Med 2006;47:1260–1266.
66. Giraudet, AL, Vanel D, Leboulleux S, Aupérin A, Dromain C, Chami L, Tovo NN, Lumbroso J, Lassau N, Bonniaud G, Hartl D, Travagli J-P, Baudin E, Schlumberger M. Imaging medullary thyroid carcinoma with persistent elevated calcitonin levels. J Endocrinol Metabol 2007;92:4185–4190.
67. Diehl M, Risse JH, Brandt-Mainz K, Dietlein M, Bohuslavizki KH, Matheja P, Lange H, Bredow J, Korber C, Grunwald F. Fluorine-18 fluorodeoxyglucose positron emission tomography in medullary thyroid cancer: results of a multicentre study. Eur J Nucl Med 2001;28:1671–1676.
68. de Groot JW, Links TP, Jager PL, Kahraman T, Plukker JT. Impact of 18F-fluoro-2-deoxy-D-glucose positron emission tomography (FDG-PET) in patients with biochemical evidence of recurrent or residual medullary thyroid cancer. Ann Surg Oncol 2004;11:786–794.
69. Brandt-Mainz K, Muller SP, Gorges R, Saller B, Bockisch A. The value of fluorine-18 fluorodeoxyglucose PET in patients with medullary thyroid cancer. Eur J Nucl Med 2000;27:490–496.
70. Szakall S Jr, Esik O, Bajzik G, Repa I, Dabasi G, Sinkovics I, Agoston P, Tron L. 18F-FDG PET detection of lymph node metastases in medullary thyroid carcinoma. J Nucl Med 2002;43:66–71.

71. Ong SC, Schröder H, Patel SG, Tabangay-Lim IM, Doddamane I, et al. Diagnostic accuracy of ^{18}F-FDG PET in restaging patients with medullary thyroid carcinoma and elevated calcitonin levels. J Nucl Med 2007;48:501–507.
72. Öksüz MÖ, Aschoff P, Kemke B, Rauch D, Zhernosekov K, et al. 68Ga-DOTATOC-PET/CT versus 18F-FDG-PET/CT: the flip-flop-phenomenon in the imaging of somatostatin-receptor expressing neuroendocrine tumors [abstract]. Eur J Nucl Med Mol Image 2005;32:S54.
73. Koukouraki S, Strauss LG, Georgoulias V, Eisenhut M, Haberkorn U, Dimitrakopoulou-Strauss A. Comparison of the pharmacokinetics of 68Ga-DOTATOC and [18F]FDG in patients with metastatic neuroendocrine tumours scheduled for 90Y-DOTATOC therapy. Eur J Nucl Med Mol Imaging 2006;33: 1115–22.
74. Hoegerle S, Altehoefer C, Ghanem N, Brink I, Moser E, Nitzsche E. 18F-DOPA positron emission tomography for tumour detection in patients with medullary thyroid carcinoma and elevated calcitonin levels. Eur J Nucl Med 2001;28:64–71.
75. Gourgiotis L, Sarlis N, Reynolds J, VanWaes C, Merino M, Pacak K. Localization of medullary thyroid carcinoma metastasis in multiple endocrine neoplasia type 2A patient by 6-[18F]-fluorodopamine positron emission tomography. J Clin Endocrinol Metab 2003;88: 637–641.
76. Beuthien-Baumann B, Strumpf A, Zessin J, Bredow J, Kotzerke J. Diagnostic impact of PET with (18)F-FDG , (18)F-DOPA and 3-O-methyl-6-[(18)F]-fluoro-DOPA in recurrent or metastatic medullary thyroid carcinoma. Eur J Nucl Med Mol Imaging 2007;34: 1604–1609.
77. Ara C, Shaha AR. Anaplastic thyroid carcinoma: biology, pathogenesis, prognostic factors, and treatment. Ann Surg Oncol 2006;13:453–464.
78. Comett WR, Shama AK, Day TA, Richardson MS, Hoda RS, van Heerden JA, Femandes JK. Anaplastic thyroid carcinoma: an overview. Curr Oncol Rep 2007;9:152–158.
79. Bogsrud TV, Karantanis D, Nathan MA, Mullan BP, Wiseman GA, Kasperbauer JL , Reading CC, Hay ID, Lowe VJ. ^{18}F-FDG PET in the management of patients with anaplastic thyroid carcinoma. Thyroid 2008;18(7):713–719.

Chapter 20
PET-CT in Breast Cancer

Mehmet S. Erturk, Rick Tetrault, and Annick D. Van den Abbeele

Breast carcinomas are classified generally into noninvasive (in situ) and invasive carcinomas, and further subdivided into ductal and lobular types [1, 2]. Invasive carcinomas also include relatively infrequent histologic subtypes such as medullary carcinoma, mucinous carcinoma, and tubular carcinoma. The growth pattern of noninvasive breast tumors is characterized by intraductal the tumor extension without invasion of the basement membrane. If the malignant cells break through the basement membrane, the tumor becomes invasive. Noninvasive ductal carcinoma or ductal carcinoma in situ (DCIS) was previously considered a rare lesion. However, with the extended use of mammography, it constitutes approximately 20–30% of carcinomas today. In 50% of cases, DCIS produces microcalcifications, which can be recognized on mammograms. Lobular carcinoma in situ (LCIS) typically does not present as a palpable mass and is often diagnosed incidentally in breast biopsies. DCIS is traditionally considered as a precancerous stage that can convert into invasive cancer. Initially, LCIS was also thought to be a premalignant condition that behaves in a similar fashion to DCIS. Today, LCIS is considered a benign lesion that does confer an increased risk for future development of breast cancer [3].

Invasive ductal carcinoma is the most frequently encountered tumor entity among breast cancers, accounting for nearly 65–80% of all breast malignancies. Invasive lobular carcinoma is diagnosed less frequently (10–20%). Approximately 50% of breast carcinomas arise in the upper outer quadrant, 10% in each of the other three quadrants, and 20% in the central or subareolar region. Breast cancers can also be present as more than one solid tumor. In cases with multiple cancers, multifocal tumor growth is defined as the presence of two different tumor sites in one quadrant of the breast, whereas multicentric tumor growth is defined as tumor involving two different quadrants of the breast.

A.D. Van den Abbeele (✉)
Department of Imaging and Center for Biomedical Imaging in Oncology, Dana-Farber Cancer Institute, 44 Binney Street, Boston, MA, 02115, USA
e-mail: abbeele@dfci.harvard.edu

Breast cancer is often curable at early stages. For localized cancer, survival is high, with an estimated 96% 5-year survival rate [4]. Unfortunately, survival decreases dramatically with the presence of regional or distant metastatic disease. While surgery provides the best chance at a cure, the importance of the roles of chemotherapy and radiotherapy is increasing as adjuvant therapies, both before and after surgery [5]. Considering the side effects and cost of chemoradiotherapy, it is also clear that imaging methods are required to monitor the response of the tumor to the therapy as well.

Role of PET-CT in Initial Diagnosis of Breast Cancer

There is no clearly defined role for PET-CT in the initial diagnosis of breast cancer. Mammography is currently the most widely accepted and established modality for the detection of occult breast carcinoma. Mammography, however, has a limited accuracy in distinguishing benign from malignant lesions and a low sensitivity for detecting cancer in women with dense breast tissue. In fact, using mammography, diagnosis of a malignant tumor will be confirmed by histopathology in only about 30% of patients with suspected breast cancer. In about 10% of cases, mammography is negative, even if the carcinoma is palpable [6]. Ultrasound has a better detection rate for palpable breast masses, but its sensitivity is not optimal for excluding breast cancer. MRI with dynamic intravenous contrast enhancement is highly sensitive but lacks specificity and is employed most often as a problem-solving technique in dense breasts or the postoperative with suspicious clinical, sonographic or mammographic findings. As a result of the above-mentioned limitations of conventional imaging methods, aspiration, core needle, or open biopsies of the tumor are still necessary in most patients for the ultimate diagnosis of a primary breast cancer.

FDG-PET has reported sensitivity and specificity for the presence of disease ranging from 66% to 100% and 83% to 100%, respectively [1, 4]. There are studies in the current literature reporting that PET was twofold more sensitive (63%)

P. Shreve and D.W. Townsend (eds.), *Clinical PET-CT in Radiology: Integrated Imaging in Oncology*,
DOI 10.1007/978-0-387-48902-5_20, © Springer Science+Business Media, LLC 2011

than combined mammography and US (32%) for detecting multifocal or multicentric disease without a significant difference in specificity [7]. FDG uptake can be affected by many factors such as tumor size and histopathologic type, resulting in limitations for PET imaging of primary breast cancer. In particular, lesion detection is clearly related to lesion size. For lesions smaller than 1 cm, FDG-PET has a relatively low sensitivity for detection of a primary breast cancer. Lobular carcinomas have been reported to be metabolically less active than invasive ductal carcinomas and therefore may not be visualized with standard FDG-PET techniques. Similarly, well-differentiated and slow-growing tumors such as tubular carcinomas may not accumulate FDG above the background level of normal breast tissue and may therefore cause false-negative results. Although FDG tracer uptake is higher in dense breast tissue than in non-dense breast tissue, the difference in uptake does not seem to affect the detection of primary breast cancer with the exception of focal asymmetric uptake mimicking focal malignant processes [8]. Inflammatory and infectious lesions of breast, however, may show an increased accumulation of FDG, resulting in false-positive findings [1, 5].

Considering the previously mentioned limitations and the cost of a PET-CT study, there is a general agreement that PET-CT should not be considered as a primary screening tool or first choice in the diagnostic workup of palpable breast masses. PET-CT has diagnostic value in determining multicentricity and multifocality, although breast MRI with dynamic contrast technique has clearly established value in this setting as well. The high positive predictive value of the FDG-PET images are however helpful in a select group of patients in which biopsy is not a desirable option, and PET-CT is useful in localizing the primary tumor in those patients with metastases of breast origin when the conventional imaging methods are indeterminate. Finally, any focal FDG uptake seen in the breast of a patient undergoing a PET-CT for other reasons, should be further investigated by mammography and/or ultrasound or biopsy, since it may represent an unsuspected primary breast cancer (Fig. 20.1).

Staging

Breast cancer metastasizes through the lymphatic and hematogenous routes. The primary lymphatic routes are to axillary lymph nodes, supraclavicular lymph nodes and the internal mammary chain lymph nodes in the mediastinum (Fig. 20.2). The majority of breast carcinomas first metastasize in the axillary lymph nodes. Axillary lymph nodes are divided into three regions regarding their anatomical location: level 1 is the lymphatic region located laterally to the pectoralis minor muscle; level 2 includes all the nodes located between the pectoralis major and minor muscles;

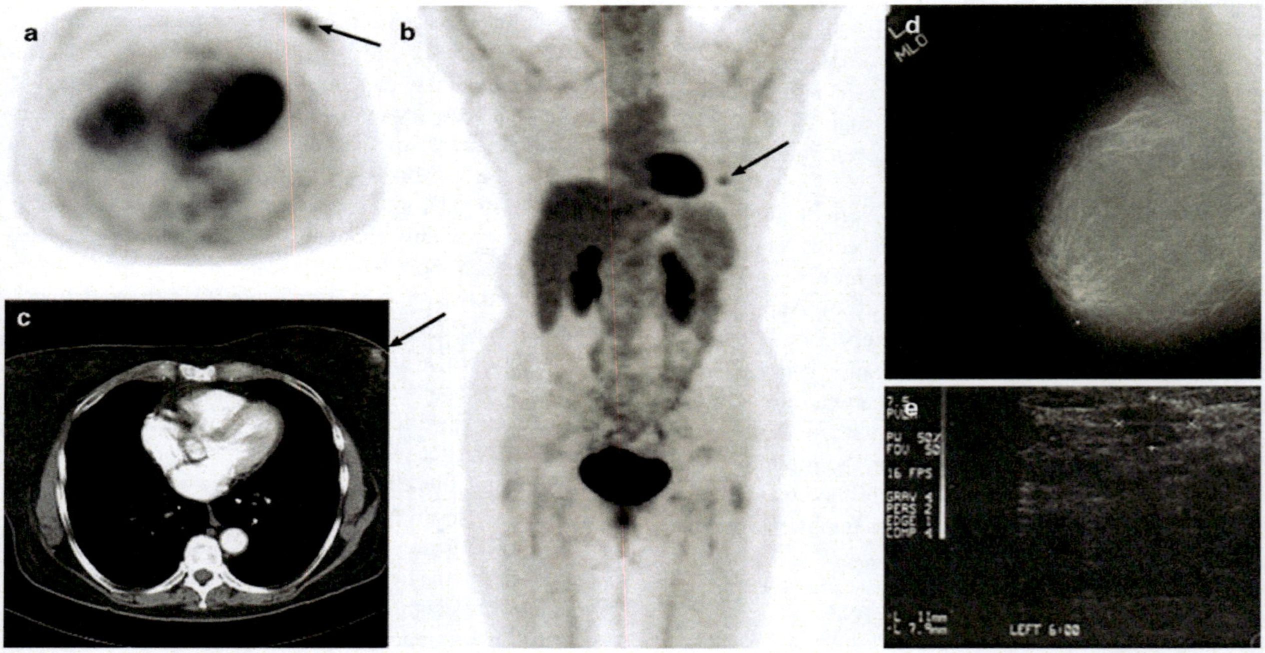

Fig. 20.1 On PET-CT scan performed for evaluation of a left upper lobe pulmonary nodule, focal increased FDG tracer uptake was observed in the left breast (**a**, **b**) corresponding to a small nodule in the breast on the CT image (**c**, *arrow*). Correlative mammography (**d**) and breast ultrasound (**e**) demonstrate an 8 × 11 mm poorly marginated soft tissue mass, which was confirmed on biopsy to be invasive ductal carcinoma

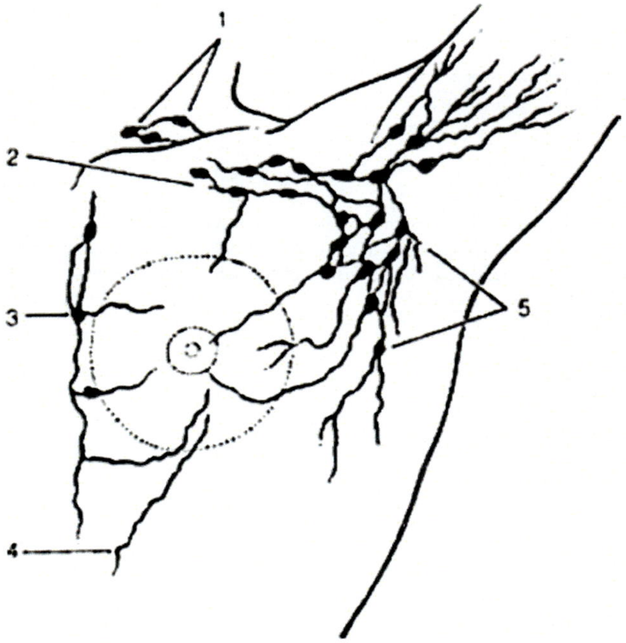

Fig. 20.2 Primary lymphatic drainage routes of the breast. The principal nodal basins for lymphatic route metastases of breast cancer are the axillary, supraclavicular, and internal mammary chains. Classification of axillary lymph nodes: superficial (Level 1) axillary lymph nodes are low and lateral to the pectoralis muscle; central (Level 2) lymph axillary lymph nodes are at the level of the axillary vasculature between the pectoralis major and minor muscles; and, deep axillary lymph nodes (Level III) are high in the axilla medial to the pectoralis muscle (From Ref. [9]. With permission)

level 3 is the lymphatic region located medially to the pectoralis minor muscle. Tumor cells typically start to metastasize to level 1 and spread to the next level. The internal mammary and infraclavicular and supraclavicular nodes are the second and the third most favored sites of the nodal involvement, respectively. Metastases to these lymph nodes are stage II and III disease (Table 20.1). Hematogenous sites of breast cancer metastases include lung, bone, liver, adrenal glands, brain and meninges most commonly, and is stage IV disease.

The presence of ipsilateral axillary lymph node metastases is the most important prognostic factor in early stage breast cancer patients [5]. Regarding the involvement of the axillary lymph nodes, patients are classified based on clinical findings which is defined as findings on physical examination and imaging studies and additionally, as a further refinement, known as pathologic classification which includes lymph node histopathologic findings. The clinical classification distinguishes between the presence (N1) or absence (N0) of abnormal axillary lymph nodes (on palpation or imaging studies) and further between abnormal axillary lymph nodes that are abnormally enlarged only (N1), and axillary lymph nodes which are fixed or matted together (N2). The pathologic classification further bases N staging of axillary lymph nodes on the presence of microscopic disease and the extent of confluent neoplasm in the lymph nodes. In the pathologic classification pN1 is 1–3 non-enlarged axillary lymph nodes with microscopic metastases, pN2 is 4–9 positive nodes with at least one confluent tumor deposit >2 mm, and pN3 is 10 or more positive nodes with at least one confluent tumor deposit >2 mm. Prognosis typically becomes worse following the order of increasing axillary lymph metastases; patients with four or more axillary lymph node metastases have a significantly increased risk for both distant metastasis and recurrence [10].

In order to accurately stage the patient, axillary lymph node dissection used to be routinely performed in all breast cancer patients who undergo breast surgery for a primary invasive breast cancer. In this procedure at least ten lymph nodes were sampled and histopathologically evaluated to definitively stage the axilla for lymph node metastases. Such axillary lymph node dissection is associated with considerable morbidity, including upper extremity lymphedema. Axillary lymph node dissection has been replaced by sentinel lymph node dissection in early stage breast cancer. In this technique, the node is marked using radioactively labeled colloid filtered sulfur and/or blue dye to localize it for resection [11]. Using the radioactive labeling method, the sentinel node may be identified preoperatively by scintigraphy and a hand-held gamma probe that also helps the surgeon to localize the node intraoperatively. The sentinel lymph node is the first lymph node in the nodal basin receiving lymphatic drainage from the portion of the breast with the cancer. The status of the sentinel node reflects the status of the remaining nodes obviating the need to dissect other lymph nodes and thus operation-related morbidity is significantly reduced. This approach also allows use of more thorough sectioning of the lymph node, immunohistochemical staining, and molecular biological detection by means of reverse transcriptase chain reaction to examine the dissected nodes in more detail since only one or two nodes are removed in each case.

Although distant metastases of breast cancer may affect virtually any organ of the body via the bloodstream, as mentioned earlier, the favored sites for dissemination for breast cancer on initial staging are the lungs, bones, liver, adrenals, brain, and meninges. Breast cancer can also spread to the brachial plexus. Conventional preoperative evaluation of symptomatic patients has typically included bone scintigraphy, contrast MRI of the brain or brachial plexus, and CT of the chest and abdomen. However, PET-CT can provide whole body evaluation of metastatic involvement of the bone marrow, skeleton, and all soft tissues in one setting and is the preferred method for evaluation of extracranial metastatic disease.

Table 20.1 American Joint Committee on Cancer Stage Grouping and TNM classification for breast carcinoma (Used with permission from the *AJCC Cancer Staging Manual*, 7th edn, 2010, published by Springer Science+Business Media, New York. www.springer.com. Used with permission)

TX	Primary tumor cannot be assessed		
T0	No evidence of primary tumor		
Tis	Carcinoma in situ		
Tis (DCIS)	Ductal carcinoma in situ		
Tis (LCIS)	Lobular carcinoma in situ		
Tis (Paget's)	Paget's disease of the nipple NOT associated with invasive carcinoma and/or carcinoma in situ (DCIS and/or LCIS) in the underlying breast parenchyma. Carcinomas in the breast parenchyma associated with Paget's disease are categorized based on the size and characteristics of the parenchymal disease, although the presence of Paget's disease should still be noted		
T1	Tumor ≤20 mm in greatest dimension		
T1mi	Tumor ≤1 mm in greatest dimension		
T1a	Tumor >1 mm but ≤5 mm in greatest dimension		
T1b	Tumor >5 mm but ≤10 mm in greatest dimension		
T1c	Tumor >10 mm but ≤20 mm in greatest dimension		
T2	Tumor >20 mm but ≤50 mm in greatest dimension		
T3	Tumor >50 mm in greatest dimension		
T4	Tumor of any size with direct extension to the chest wall and/or to the skin (ulceration or skin nodules). *Note*: Invasion of the dermis alone does not qualify as T4		
T4a	Extension to the chest wall, not including only pectoralis muscle adherence/invasion		
T4b	Ulceration and/or ipsilateral satellite nodules and/or edema (including peau d'orange) of the skin which do not meet the criteria for inflammatory carcinoma		
T4c	Both T4a and T4b		
T4d	Inflammatory carcinoma (see Rules for Classification)		
Regional lymph nodes (N)			
Clinical			
NX	Regional lymph nodes cannot be assessed (e.g., previously removed)		
N0	No regional lymph node metastases		
N1	Metastases to movable ipsilateral level I, II axillary lymph node(s)		
N2	Metastases in ipsilateral level I, II axillary lymph nodes that are clinically fixed or matted; or in clinically detected[a] ipsilateral internal mammary nodes in the *absence* of clinically evident axillary lymph node metastases		
N2a	Metastases in ipsilateral axillary lymph nodes fixed to one another (matted) or to other structures		
N2b	Metastases only in clinically detected[a] ipsilateral internal mammary nodes and in the *absence* of clinically evident axillary lymph node metastases		
N3	Metastases in ipsilateral infraclavicular (level III axillary) lymph node(s) with or without level I, II axillary lymph node involvement; or in clinically detected[a] ipsilateral internal mammary lymph node(s) with clinically evident level I, II axillary lymph node metastases; or metastases in ipsilateral supraclavicular lymph node(s) with or without axillary or internal mammary lymph node involvement		
N3a	Metastases in ipsilateral infraclavicular lymph node(s)		
N3b	Metastases in ipsilateral internal mammary lymph node(s) and axillary lymph node(s)		
N3c	Metastases in ipsilateral supraclavicular lymph node(s)		
Distant metastases (M)			
M0	No clinical or radiographic evidence of distant metastases		
cM0(i+)	No clinical or radiographic evidence of distant metastases, but deposits of molecularly or microscopically detected tumor cells in circulating blood, bone marrow or other nonregional nodal tissue that are no larger than 0.2 mm in a patient without symptoms or signs of metastases		
M1	Distant detectable metastases as determined by classic clinical and radiographic means and/or histologically proven larger than 0.2 mm		
Anatomic stage • Prognostic groups			
Stage IA	T1[b]	N0	M0
Stage IB	T0	N1mi	M0
	T1[b]	N1mi	M0
Stage IIA	T0	N1[c]	M0
	T1[b]	N1[c]	M0
	T2	N0	M0
Stage IIB	T2	N1	M0
	T3	N0	M0

(continued)

Table 20.1 (continued)

Stage IIIA	T0	N2	M0
	T1[b]	N2	M0
	T2	N2	M0
	T3	N1	M0
	T3	N2	M0
Stage IIIB	T4	N0	M0
	T4	N1	M0
	T4	N2	M0
Stage IIIC	Any T	N3	M0
Stage IV	Any T	Any N	M1

[a]Clinically detected is defined as detected by imaging studies (excluding lymphoscintigraphy) or by clinical examination and having characteristics highly suspicious for malignancy or a presumed pathologic macrometastasis based on fine needle aspiration biopsy with cytologic examination. Confirmation of clinically detected metastatic disease by fine needle aspiration without excision biopsy is designated with an (f) suffix, e.g., cN3a(f). Excisional biopsy of a lymph node or biopsy of a sentinel node, in the absence of assignment of a pT, is classified as a clinical N, e.g., cN1. Information regarding the confirmation of the nodal status will be designated in site-specific factors as clinical, fine needle aspiration, core biopsy, or sentinel lymph node biopsy. Pathologic classification (pN) is used for excision or sentinel lymph node biopsy only in conjunction with a pathologic T assignment

[b]T1 includes T1mi

[c]T0 and T1 tumors with nodal micrometastases only are excluded from stage IIA and are classified stage IB

- M0 includes M0(i+)
- The designation pM0 is not valid; any M0 should be clinical
- If a patient presents with M1 prior to neoadjuvant systemic therapy, the stage is considered stage IV, and remains stage IV regardless of response to neoadjuvant therapy
- Stage designation may be changed if postsurgical imaging studies reveal the presence of distant metastases, provided that the studies are carried out within 4 months of diagnosis in the absence of disease progression and provided that the patient has not received neoadjuvant therapy

Postneoadjuvant therapy is designated with "yc" or "yp" prefix. Of note, no stage group is assigned if there is a complete pathologic response (CR) to neoadjuvant therapy, for example, ypT0ypN0cM0.

Malignant breast tumors are classified according to the tumor-node-metastasis (TNM) classification of the American Joint Committee on Cancer (see Table 20.1). Stage 0 includes in situ carcinomas without nodal or distant metastasis. Stage I involves tumors less than 2 cm in diameter without nodal or distant metastases. Tumors less than 5 cm in diameter with involved but movable axillary nodes and without distant metastases and tumors greater than 5 cm in diameter without nodal involvement and distant metastases are included in stage II. Stage IIIA includes tumors either smaller than 5 cm in diameter but with fixed ipsilateral axillary lymph node metastases or greater than 5 cm in diameter with movable or fixed ipsilateral axillary lymph node metastases. In stage IIIB disease, direct extension of the tumor to chest wall or skin is present. Stage IIIC describes tumors metastasized to ipsilateral infraclavicular or supraclavicular lymph nodes. Finally, any form of breast cancer with or without nodal involvement, and direct extension to chest wall and/or skin, but having disseminated metastases, is included in stage 4 [12].

Historically, the treatment of noninvasive ductal carcinoma, or ductal carcinoma in situ (DCIS) was mastectomy. The rational for this approach was based on the 30% incidence of multicentric disease, the 40% prevalence of residual tumor at mastectomy following wide excision alone, and a 25–50% incidence of recurrence following limited surgery for palpable tumor [13]. However, breast-conserving surgery and radiation therapy, with or without tamoxifen are considered as a relatively conservative alternative to mastectomy today. A large clinical trial indicated that local excision and breast irradiation is an acceptable therapy approach for localized DCIS [14]. The treatment options for patients with lobular carcinoma in situ (LCIS) include observation after diagnostic biopsy and tamoxifen to decrease the incidence of subsequent breast cancers [15]. The other option is bilateral prophylactic total mastectomy, although this is considered to be an overly aggressive approach by many breast surgeons.

Stage I, II, IIIA, and operable IIIC breast tumors require a multimodality treatment strategy. Options for surgical management of the primary tumor include breast-conserving surgery with radiotherapy, mastectomy and reconstruction, and mastectomy alone [10]. Adjuvant radiotherapy including postoperative chest wall and regional lymph node irradiation is given to patients considered at high risk for locoregional recurrence [16], such as patients with four or more positive axillary nodes, grossly evident extracapsular nodal extension, large primary tumors, and very close or positive deep margins of resection of primary tumor. In general, following the resection of the primary tumor and sentinel node evaluation, the oncologist decides whether or not an adjuvant systemic therapy such as chemotherapy or hormonal therapy must be performed. For this decision, prognostic factors such as tumor size and differentiation, axillary lymph node status, expression of estrogen and progesterone receptors, and the menopausal status of the patient are evaluated.

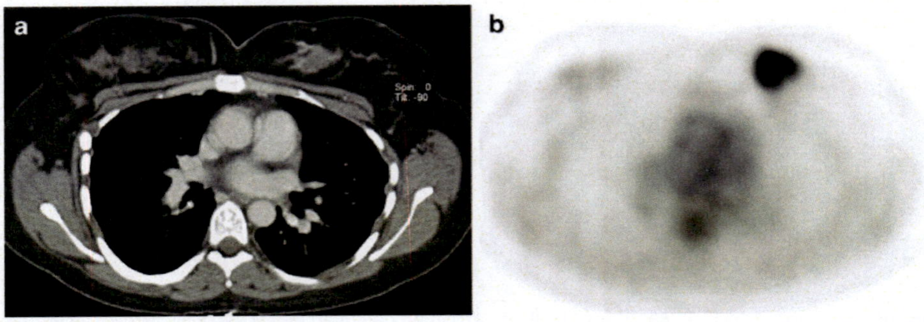

Fig. 20.3 Invasive ductal carcinoma of the left breast is not easily defined within normal glandular tissue on CT (a), although asymmetry of the glandular tissue in the upper inner quadrants of the breasts is evident. FDG-PET images (b) demonstrate intense focal abnormal tracer uptake within the glandular tissue of the left breast corresponding to the neoplasm, which was up to 2.5 cm in diameter on resection

Today, delivery of multimodality therapy with curative intent is the standard of care for patients with up to stage IIIB disease [17]. If the patient responds, adjuvant chemotherapy is followed by mastectomy and axillary lymph node dissection with postoperative radiotherapy to the chest wall and regional lymph nodes. In patients with a good partial or complete response to neoadjuvant chemotherapy, breast-conserving therapy is also an alternative. Subsequent systemic therapy with or without hormonal therapy is usually included in the regimen. Patients with locoregional recurrence may become long-term survivors when treated properly. For the patients with only local chest wall recurrence following mastectomy, surgery and/or radiotherapy may be curative. Systemic therapy should be considered in all patients with recurrence because of the high risk of distant metastases. Regarding stage IV disease, treatment is palliative and aims to prolong life and improve the quality of life, although durable complete responses of advanced metastatic disease in response to Herceptin are now being seen and encouraging results are emerging regarding novel targeted therapies in combination with other therapeutic agents.

T Staging

Most patients will have the primary breast tumor T stage and axillary lymph node status determined at the time of the initial breast surgery and sentinel lymph node biopsy. T staging is also estimated on clinical exam based on the palpable size and mobility of the primary tumor and evidence of skin involvement. Patients considered at high risk of metastatic disease based on initial clinical evaluation and core needle biopsy results often will, however, have a complete imaging and laboratory evaluation for staging prior to breast surgery. In such cases the T staging will be based on the CT portion of the PET-CT imaging study. In postmenopausal women the size of the primary mass, especially when large, is a relatively straightforward CT based measurement due to the paucity of glandular tissue, and the relevant distinction will be whether the primary tumor is greater than 2 cm but less than 5 cm greatest dimension (T2) or greater than 5 cm (T3). In younger women with dense breasts, however, it may not be possible to directly measure the diameter of the primary breast mass based on CT findings to directly determine whether the tumor is greater than or less than 2 cm in its greatest dimension (Fig. 20.3). In any case, contiguous involvement of the skin or chest wall musculature is an important finding as this elevates T stage to T4 (Fig. 20.4). As noted above, FDG-PET has been reported as twice as sensitive as combined mammography and ultrasound for detecting multifocal or multicentric tumor growth in the breast [7], and thus the PET images can be particularly useful in locating separate macroscopic foci of breast cancer, particularly in dense breasts (Fig. 20.5).

N Staging

As discussed, axillary lymph node stage is the most important prognostic factor for most patients with a new diagnosis of breast cancer. Sentinel node biopsy is the standard diagnostic procedure for staging axillary lymph nodes for metastases, and the AJCC TNM classification contains specific criteria for N staging based on lymph node biopsy results. Micrometastases in lymph nodes cannot be detected on FDG-PET, and hence PET-CT is not a substitute for sentinel node biopsy for determination of metastatic disease to ipsilateral axillary lymph nodes [31]. Macroscopic deposits of metastatic breast cancer 7–8 mm or larger can however be detected on the FDG-PET images and the specificity of FDG-PET for axillary lymph node metastases of breast cancer has been reported to be on the order of 90% [5]. In a recent series about 236 patients, 103 had axillary nodes (44%), 93 (39%) being staged pT1c, 86 (37%) pT2 and 14 (6%) of pT3. Sensitivity in this series for detection of axillary lymph nodes was low (37%) but specificity and positive predictive value were quite high, 96% and 88%. PET is unable to detect micrometastasis and sensitivity is very low for small

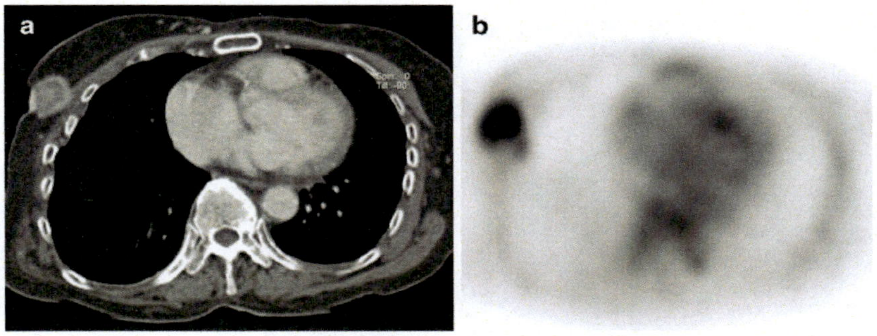

Fig. 20.4 Infiltrating ductal adenocarcinoma of the right breast is clearly delineated on CT images (**a**) by surrounding fat. The 2.5-cm mass has spiculated margins, and is extending to the overlying skin laterally where there is contiguous skin thickening. Medially the mass extends into the pectoralis muscle. The mass and its extension into the muscle is associated with intense abnormal FDG tracer uptake on FDG-PET images (**b**)

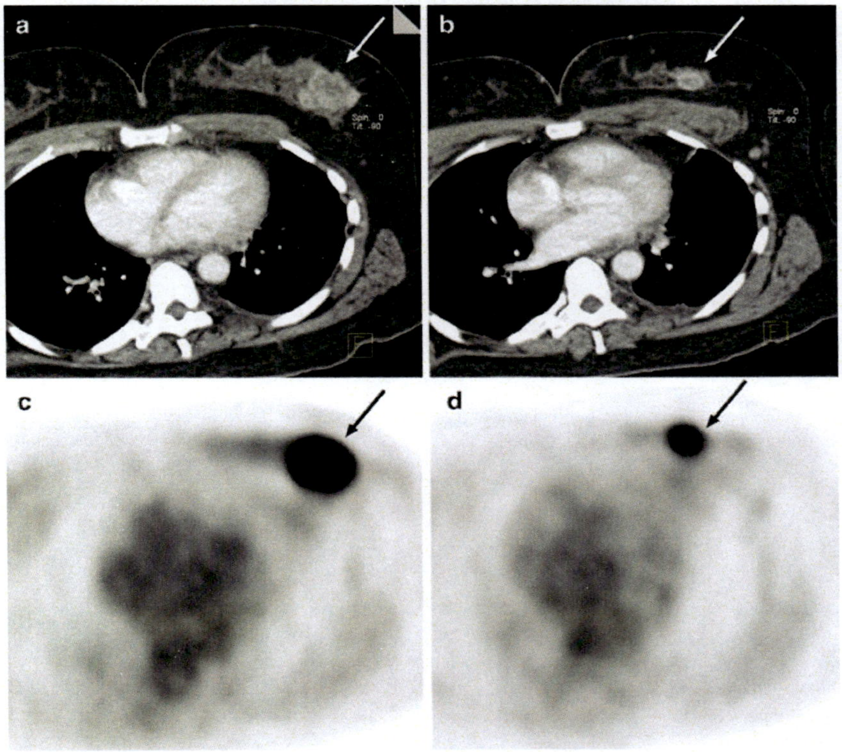

Fig. 20.5 Multifocal breast cancer. Left breast mass positive for invasive ductal carcinoma on needle biopsy. PET-CT reveals two discrete masses within the glandular tissue of the upper outer left breast defined by abnormal contrast enhancement on CT images (**a**, **b**) and intense abnormal FDG tracer uptake on corresponding FDG-PET images (**c**, **d**), including a large mass approximately 3.5-cm maximum diameter (*arrow*), and nearby, medial and superior, a smaller separate mass (*arrowhead*) approximately 1.5 cm maximum diameter

lesion (<5 mm) [20]. Hence, despite its limitations in detecting lymph node metastases compared with sentinel lymph node dissection, this high specificity warrants use of whole body PET-CT during the preoperative staging of patients with breast cancer, especially in those with large tumors [5], and aggressive cancers such as inflammatory breast cancers (Fig. 20.6). Of note, FDG-PET has the ability to detect disease in normal size lymph nodes. In addition to the detection of lymph node metastases based on the FDG-PET image findings, CT and FDG-PET findings of extracapsular spread are an important prognostic finding included in the N staging (Fig. 20.7).

N staging with PET-CT is particularly advantageous for the evaluation of lymph nodes outside of the axilla, which are not routinely sampled for histological evaluation, such as the

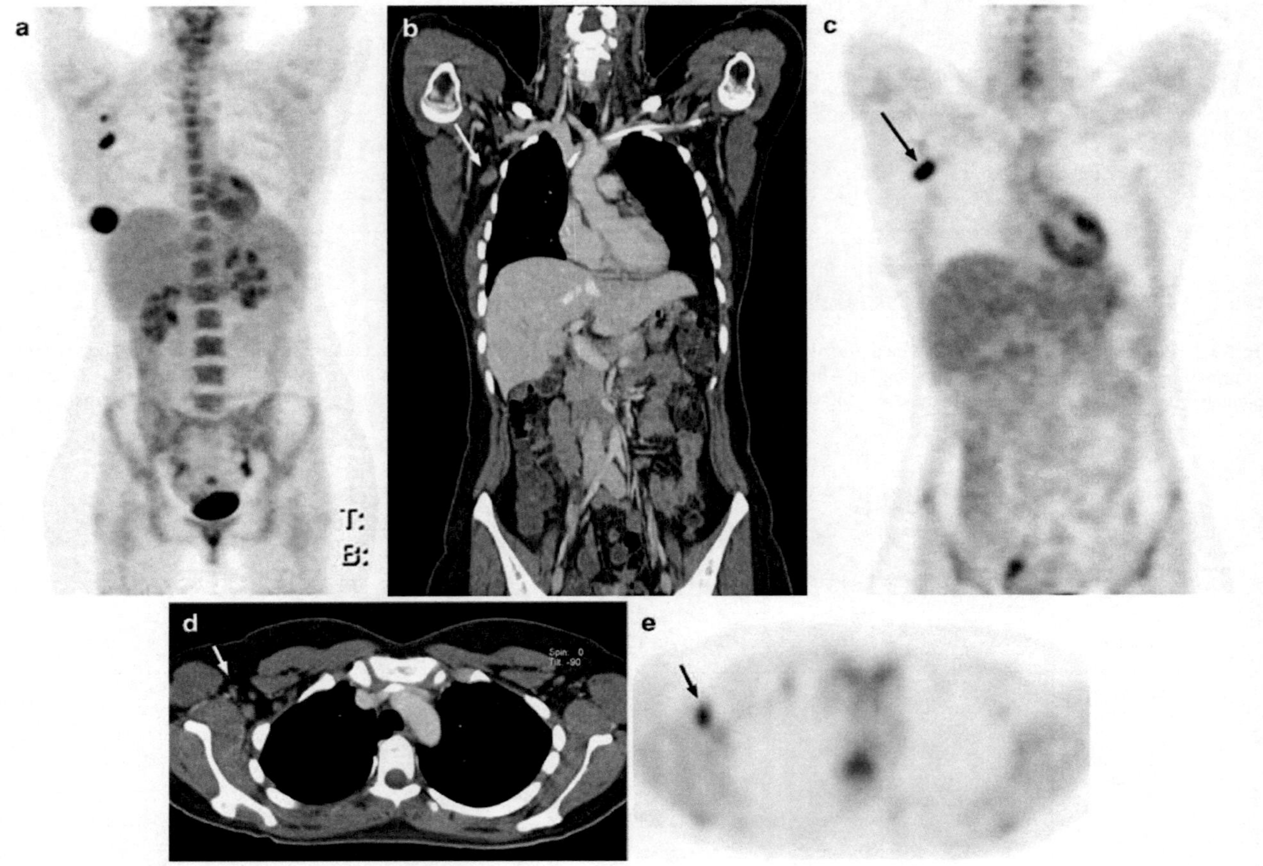

Fig. 20.6 Axillary lymph node metastases in a patient with a new diagnosis of high-grade infiltrating ductal carcinoma of the right breast. The FDG-PET anterior MIP image (**a**) shows intense focal abnormal tracer uptake in the lower outer quadrant of the right breast corresponding to a 3-cm primary breast cancer, and two additional foci of abnormal tracer uptake in the right axilla. Coronal CT (**b**) and FDG-PET images (**c**) show a 10 × 14 mm axillary node associated with intense abnormal tracer uptake (*arrow*). Transaxial CT (**d**) and FDG-PET images (**e**) show the nonenlarged (7-mm) additional lymph node with associated abnormal FDG uptake (*arrow*)

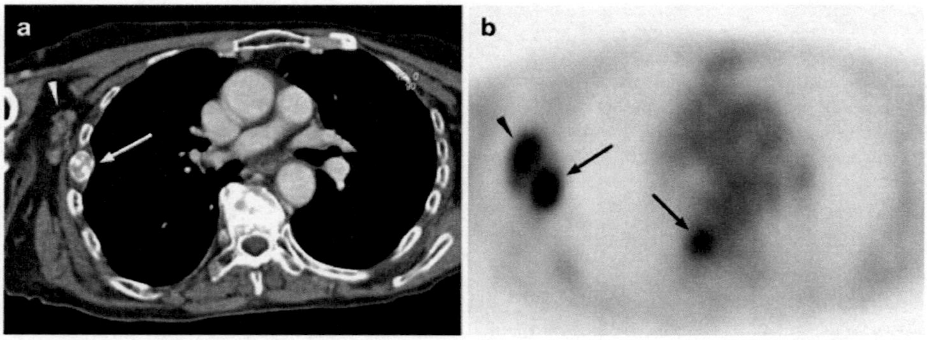

Fig. 20.7 Axillary lymph node metastases. Transaxial CT (**a**) and FDG-PET (**b**) images show right axillary lymph nodes that are associated with abnormal FDG tracer uptake consistent with metastatic lymphadenopathy (*small arrow*). While the nodes are not individually enlarged, they are FDG-avid and seen on CT to be matted together rendering N stage N2. Rib and vertebral body osseous metastases are also present (*large arrows*)

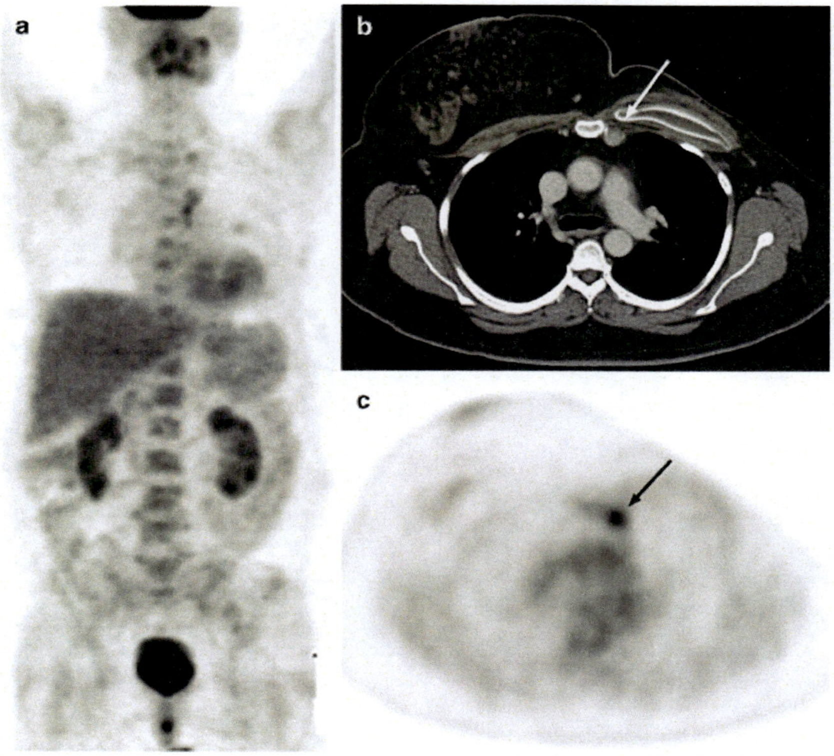

Fig. 20.8 Internal mammary chain lymph node metastases. On anterior FDG-PET MIP image (**a**) left parasternal increased FDG tracer uptake is present. On transaxial CT (**b**) and FDG-PET (**c**) images a 1-cm anterior mediastinal lymph node, just below the chest wall, is present (*arrow*) and is associated with abnormal FDG tracer uptake

internal mammary node chain (Fig. 20.8) and supraclavicular and infraclavicular nodes (Fig. 20.9). PET-CT may be particularly appropriate when the sentinel node biopsy is positive indicating higher risk of other regional lymph node involvement or in patients at high risk of locoregional and distant metastatic disease based on size and histologic grade of the primary tumor. Lymphatic spread of tumor to the internal mammary nodes occurs in up to 25% of patients at the time of initial diagnosis. FDG-PET has significantly higher sensitivity, specificity and accuracy than CT size-based criteria alone (85%, 90%, and 88% vs 54%, 85%, and 73%, respectively) [18]. Metastases to internal mammary and axillary nodes are usually synchronous and prognosis becomes significantly worse in case of involvement of internal mammary lymph nodes or supraclavicular lymph nodes [19].

Detection of unsuspected internal mammary nodal involvement also can change patient management such as modification of the radiation therapy field. Neoplastic spread to mediastinal nodes is also common in patients with advanced disease. As with internal mammary nodes, mediastinal nodes are rarely sampled in breast cancer patients, but mediastinal lymph node involvement is detectable by the combined PET-CT modality due to the higher sensitivity of PET in detecting mediastinal nodal metastasis compared with CT.

M Staging

PET-CT is especially useful in detection of distant metastatic disease. FDG-PET has been shown to be superior to conventional CT alone for detecting distant metastases in breast cancer. In a recent study of FDG-PET for the detection of distant metastases or recurrence in patients with breast cancer, the authors reported sensitivity, specificity, positive predictive value, negative predictive value, and accuracy of 97%, 82%, 87%, 96%, and 90%, respectively, for FDG-PET, compared with 84%, 60%, 73%, 75%, and 74%, respectively, for conventional CT alone [20]. By combining FDG-PET and CT the accuracy for the detection of visceral metastases is significantly improved, particularly for bone marrow, skeletal, hepatic and other visceral metastases and distant lymph node metastases (Figs. 20.7–20.10). Hepatic metastases, even when large, can be difficult to detect on even contrast-enhanced CT, and the addition of FDG-PET improves sensitivity for hepatic metastases. Contrast-enhanced MRI, however, remains more sensitive for very small hepatic metastases.

In patients with breast cancer, particular attention should be paid to skeletal involvement since approximately 10% of breast cancer patients develop skeletal metastases in the course of their disease (Fig. 20.10), and the frequency of bone

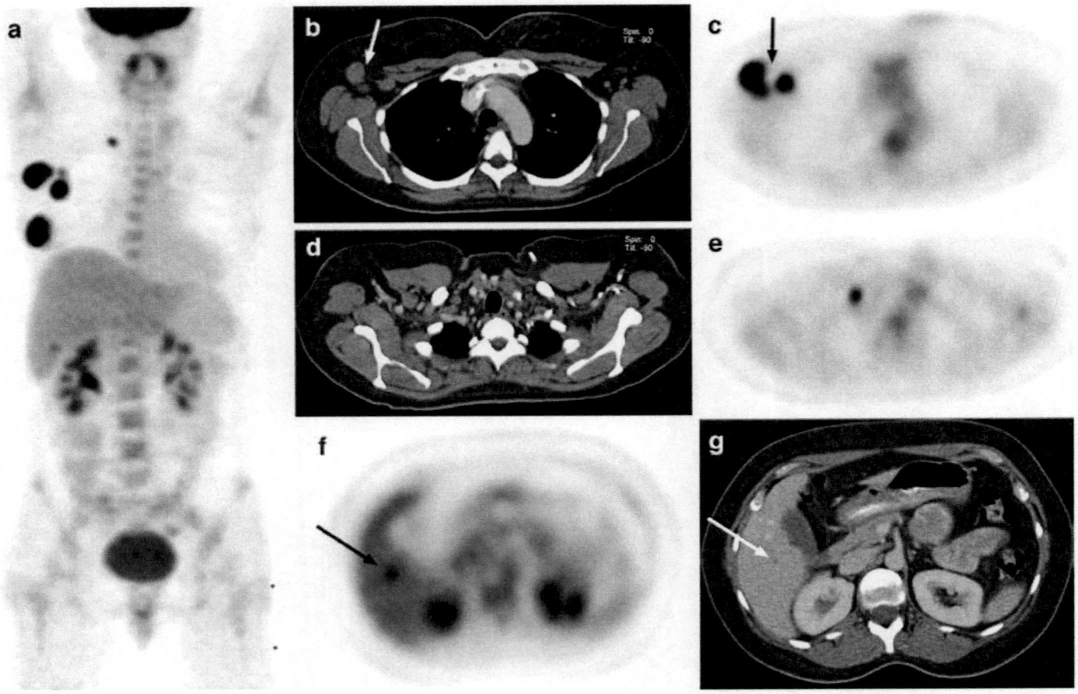

Fig. 20.9 Initial staging of right breast poorly differentiated ductal carcinoma on PET-CT. Anterior FDG-PET MIP image (**a**) demonstrates the primary breast cancer, right axillary lymph node metastases, an isolated right supraclavicular nodal metastasis and an isolated liver metastasis. On transaxial CT (**b**) and FDG-PET (**c**) images axillary level I and II enlarged and highly FDG-avid nodes (*arrows*) are identified and are without extracapsular extension. A nonenlarged right supraclavicular node (**d**, **e**) is associated with clearly abnormal FDG tracer uptake. The solitary focus of abnormal FDG tracer activity in the right hepatic lobe is clearly present on FDG-PET images (**f**), corresponding to a subtle 4 mm low attenuation lesion (*arrow*) seen on the portal venous phase contrast enhanced CT images (**g**)

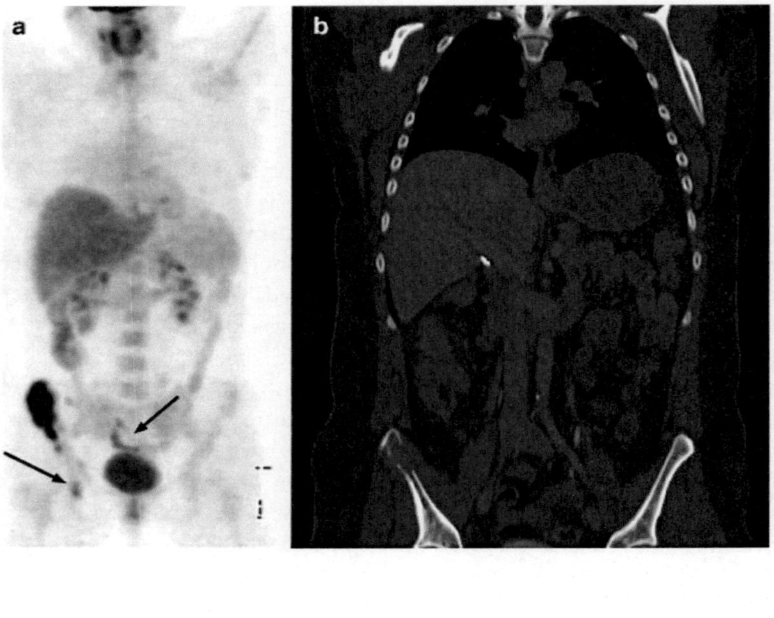

Fig. 20.10 Osseous metastatic disease following lumpectomy for ductal adenocarcinoma. The anterior FDG-PET MIP image (**a**) shows intense tracer uptake in the right iliac wing corresponding to destructive changes seen on the coronal CT image (**b**) as well as extension of metastatic involvement into the inferior right acetabulum and in a focal lesion in the right parasacral region (*arrows*). Aside from the right pelvis osseous metastases, no other metastatic disease is present

metastases is nearly 70% in patients with advanced disease. Skeletal involvement portends poor prognosis, as the median survival of patient with skeletal metastases is 2 years and the 5-year survival rate does not exceed 20% [11]. FDG-PET alone has revealed variable results compared with the conventional bone scintigraphy, mainly depending on the stage and state of the disease activity. In general, bone scintigraphy visualizes the osteoblastic response to bone destruction by the cancer cells, while PET visualizes largely the metabolic activity of the cancer cells themselves. Sensitivity of bone scintigraphy is limited in the detection of purely lytic lesions or metastases confined to the marrow cavity due to a lack of sufficient osteoblastic activity while FDG-PET readily identifies these lesions. On the other hand, FDG-PET is reported to have a higher false-negative rate than bone scanning for sclerotic lesions seen on CT. Although there is evidence in the current literature that PET is able to detect more lesions than a conventional bone scan, this is especially true for osteolytic metastases and bone marrow metastases. It remains to be determined, in further controlled prospective trials, whether in treated patients, the low level or absence of FDG uptake seen in lesions that appear sclerotic on CT is actually a true reflection of healing and response to therapy rather than a false negative finding. Considering this, at least currently it can be assumed that PET-CT and conventional bone scan should not be considered as substitutes, but rather complementary methods for assessing skeletal involvement.

Pitfalls in imaging breast cancer with PET-CT include the specificity limitations of FDG-PET and CT in the detection of lymph node metastases. Inflammatory response of lymph nodes can cause increased FDG tracer uptake indistinguishable from lymph node metastases. Morphologic characterization of lymph nodes, including loss of fatty hilus and increased contrast enhancement are nonspecific findings regarding tumor infiltration vs. inflammation, and CT-based size criteria for lymph node metastases is nonspecific and inferior to FDG-PET criteria both in terms of specificity and sensitivity. Both axillary and mediastinal lymph nodal basins are important sites for local and distant metastatic breast cancer, respectively, but these are also regions prone to inflammatory response due to their respective origins of lymphatic drainage. Hence, FDG-avid lymph nodes should be interpreted with caution and with careful consideration of possible inflammatory etiologies. For example, PET-CT scans performed shortly after lumpectomy can result in false-positive ipsilateral axillary lymph nodes on the FDG-PET images (Fig. 20.11). Similarly, positive mediastinal lymph nodes, especially as an isolated finding in the initial staging of breast cancer, should be interpreted with caution; convincingly abnormal nodes on the FDG-PET images, even when enlarged, may require histologic proof of metastases due to the false-positive rate of 15% or higher in these lymph nodes.

Histologies such as lobular carcinoma may not be as FDG-avid as other breast cancer histologies such as ductal breast carcinoma hence, the sensitivity of the FDG-PET images will be somewhat less for the detection of small metastatic deposits from these tumors as well. Mucinous breast cancer in particular can be associated with low levels of FDG uptake, and hence in patients with such histology careful attention to the CT images for hepatic metastases and lymph node enlargement must be maintained. As noted, FDG-PET may have limitations relative to conventional bone scintigraphy for osseous metastases that are primarily sclerotic and, at the very least, careful review of the CT images in bone window image settings should be routine.

The CT imaging component of a PET-CT study improves diagnostic accuracy both by providing precise anatomic localization of PET abnormalities and further CT morphologic characterization of the localized PET findings. In addition, some lesions not detected or equivocally delineated on FDG-PET such as a mucin-producing breast cancer or sclerotic bone metastasis may be depicted chiefly on the CT images. Although few PET-CT studies have been performed in breast cancer, studies in other malignancies showed that PET-CT provided additional information in nearly half of the patients who are previously examined with FDG-PET or CT

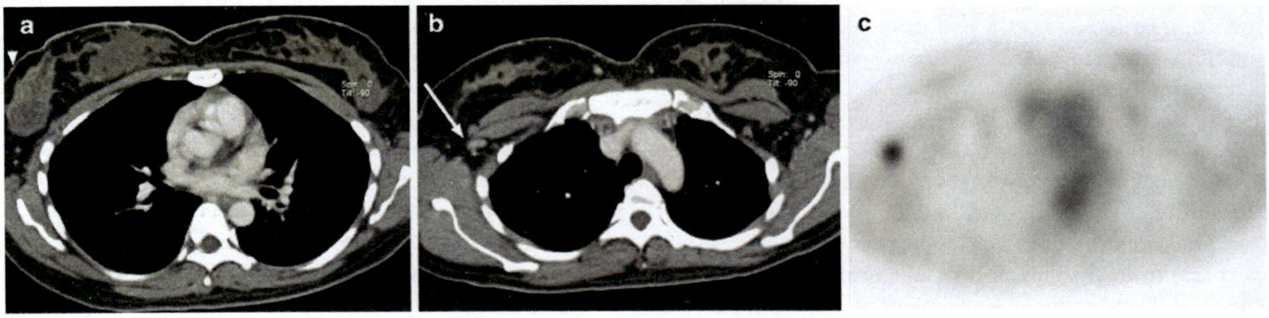

Fig. 20.11 False-positive axillary lymph node due to inflammation in a patient 10 days following lumpectomy. Resolving hematoma is seen in the medial right breast on CT (**a**, *arrow*). In the ipsilateral axilla there is a 7 × 12 mm lymph node seen (*arrow*) on CT (**b**), which is associated with abnormal FDG tracer uptake on the corresponding FDG-PET image (**c**)

alone [21, 22]. It has been reported that PET-CT had better diagnostic accuracy in cancer in comparison with FDG-PET alone, CT alone, and even side-by-side visual correlation of PET and CT [22].

In conclusion, in the primary diagnosis and preoperative staging of breast cancer, PET-CT has a very important complementary role, but is not the primarily diagnostic technique or tool of choice. PET-CT is not of sufficiently high sensitivity to take the place of histologic lymph node or sentinel node evaluation. But in suspected high-risk disease or when the sentinel node biopsy is positive for metastases, it can provide critical information by detecting additional locoregional lymph node metastases and distant metastases.

Restaging

Following primary treatment of breast cancer, locoregional and distant recurrence occurs in approximately 35% of patients within 10 years after initial surgery. Early detection of recurrence or metastasis is essential for instituting a proper treatment plan to prevent further progression and tumor-related symptoms. While local recurrences and lymph node metastases may be treated surgically or with radiation therapy, the presence of distant metastases make the disease incurable, and aggressive therapeutic approaches are no longer indicated. The breast, the skin of the breast, axillary nodes, the chest wall, and supraclavicular lymph nodes are the most common sites of first locoregional recurrence after primary surgical resection. Mediastinal lymph node metastases are more commonly encountered in breast cancer patients on restaging and are considered distant metastases. Common distant metastatic sites on recurrence of breast cancer include the skeleton, liver, and brain primarily, and less commonly lung, pleura, adrenal glands. Overall reported sensitivity, specificity, and accuracy of FDG-PET for detecting relapse in cancer patients in one study was 89%, 84%, and 87%, respectively [23]. Interestingly, the authors also concluded that FDG-PET is more sensitive than the serum tumor marker CA15-3 level in detecting breast cancer relapse.

The more common use of breast-conserving surgery and local radiation therapy for early breast cancer in recent years has heightened concern over locoregional recurrence. The ability of mammography to diagnose local recurrences following breast-conserving surgery can be limited by surgical scar formation and fibrosis as a result of radiotherapy. The overall sensitivity and specificity of mammography for the detection of local recurrence was found to be 52% and 84%, respectively [24]. Similarly, ultrasound is also inadequate for the detection of recurrent disease. Chest wall invasion occurs by direct local extension of tumor through the pectoral fascia or extranodal extension from interpectoral nodes into the pectoral muscles. The other important site of locoregional recurrence is supraclavicular lymph nodes. Although involvement of this group of lymph nodes is technically considered stage IV disease, patients with only supraclavicular lymph node involvement as disseminated disease, may still benefit from aggressive local radiation therapy. Lymphatic drainage to the internal mammary nodal chain is also an important pathway of spread of disease after primary treatment of breast cancer. The prognosis of patients with internal mammary and axillary nodal metastases is significantly worse than that of patients with only axillary nodal disease, indicating that the internal mammary nodal chain is a "gateway" for more widespread dissemination of the disease [19]. Recent studies have suggested benefit from aggressive regional nodal irradiation following lumpectomy or mastectomy even in patients with limited spread to axilla, and have raised more interest in developing methods to identify patients who are at risk for internal mammary involvement. FDG-PET has been shown to be superior in detecting mediastinal or internal mammary lymph node involvement in recurrent disease in comparison with conventional CT alone (88% accuracy for PET, vs 73% for CT) [18].

Another important site of locoregional recurrence of breast cancer is the brachial plexus region. (Fig. 20.12). Recurrence involving the brachial plexus is treated with local radiation therapy; however, brachial plexopathy may be due to posttreatment fibrosis or to new or recurrent malignant disease. FDG-PET has also been found superior in detecting brachial plexus involvement when compared to conventional CT alone [5]. Moreover, in a study comparing MR imaging with FDG-PET in breast cancer patients with a clinical suspicion of local involvement of the axilla or brachial plexus, FDG-PET was found more accurate and detected additional metastases [25]. Hence PET-CT is the preferred method for evaluation of breast cancer patients with clinical suspicion of recurrence involving the brachial plexus.

The skeleton is the most common site of distant metastases in patients treated with mastectomy and adjuvant chemotherapy (Fig. 20.13). As mentioned before, PET-CT and conventional bone scintigraphy are presently considered as complementary methods in the detection of skeletal metastases. Also as mentioned before, because osseous metastases of breast, and especially recurrent osseous metastases, can have a dominant sclerotic component, careful review of the CT images of the skeleton is particularly important in the setting of recurrence. An important pitfall on restaging breast cancer patients with osseous metastases after chemotherapy

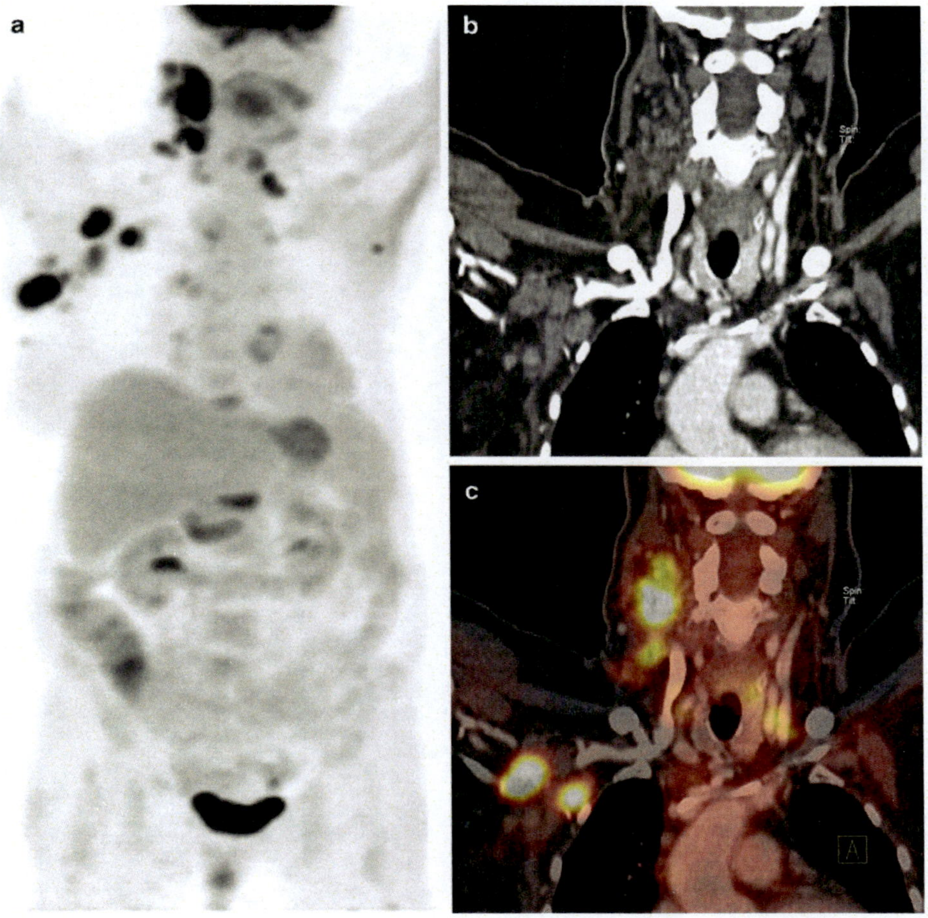

Fig. 20.12 Recurrent breast cancer involving the brachioplexus. Anterior FDG-PET MIP image (**a**) demonstrates right axillary and supraclavicular lymph node metastases, left supraclavicular, axillary and mediastinal metastases, and a cluster of intense large FDG-avid foci of abnormal in the right neck. Coronal CT (**b**) and FDG-PET-CT fusion images (**c**) demonstrate discrete and conglomerate FDG-avid lymphadenopathy in the brachioplexus region

is the effect of hemapoietic stimulates such as colony stimulating factor on bone marrow FDG tracer uptake. The elevated bone marrow tracer activity obscures the tracer activity of the metastatic deposits in the marrow space, and consequently it is frequently not possible to directly determine on the FDG-PET images whether the osseous metastases have responded to treatment. Changes in the CT appearance can be helpful, however, replacement of dominantly lytic lesions by sclerotic changes can also reflect bone growth in response to tumor regression, the underlying process of the "flare phenomenon" seen on conventional bone scintigraphy.

Liver metastases usually occur later than locoregional recurrences and typically are associated with a much worse prognosis. It is not uncommon for liver metastases of breast cancer to be clearly depicted on the FDG-PET images while remaining quite subtle or entirely occult on the contrast-enhanced CT images of the liver (see Fig. 20.11). Pleural and lung parenchymal metastases are seen with more widely disseminated disease. Finally, metastasis to the brain occurs near the end of the course of the disease, and as with other cancers, cerebral metastases are most accurately diagnosed on contrast-enhanced MRI or CT. Inclusion of the brain on PET-CT restaging of breast cancer patients suspected of having cerebral metastases may thus be worthwhile especially when Contrast-enhanced CT technique is used.

The follow-up of patients with breast cancer is still a subject of discussion. The current tendency is to reduce the number of instrumental examinations during follow-up in asymptomatic patients. Due to its whole-body imaging capability and combined metabolic and anatomic imaging potential, PET-CT may become an essential tool in the follow-up of breast cancer patients, particularly when recurrence is suspected because of an increase in biochemical

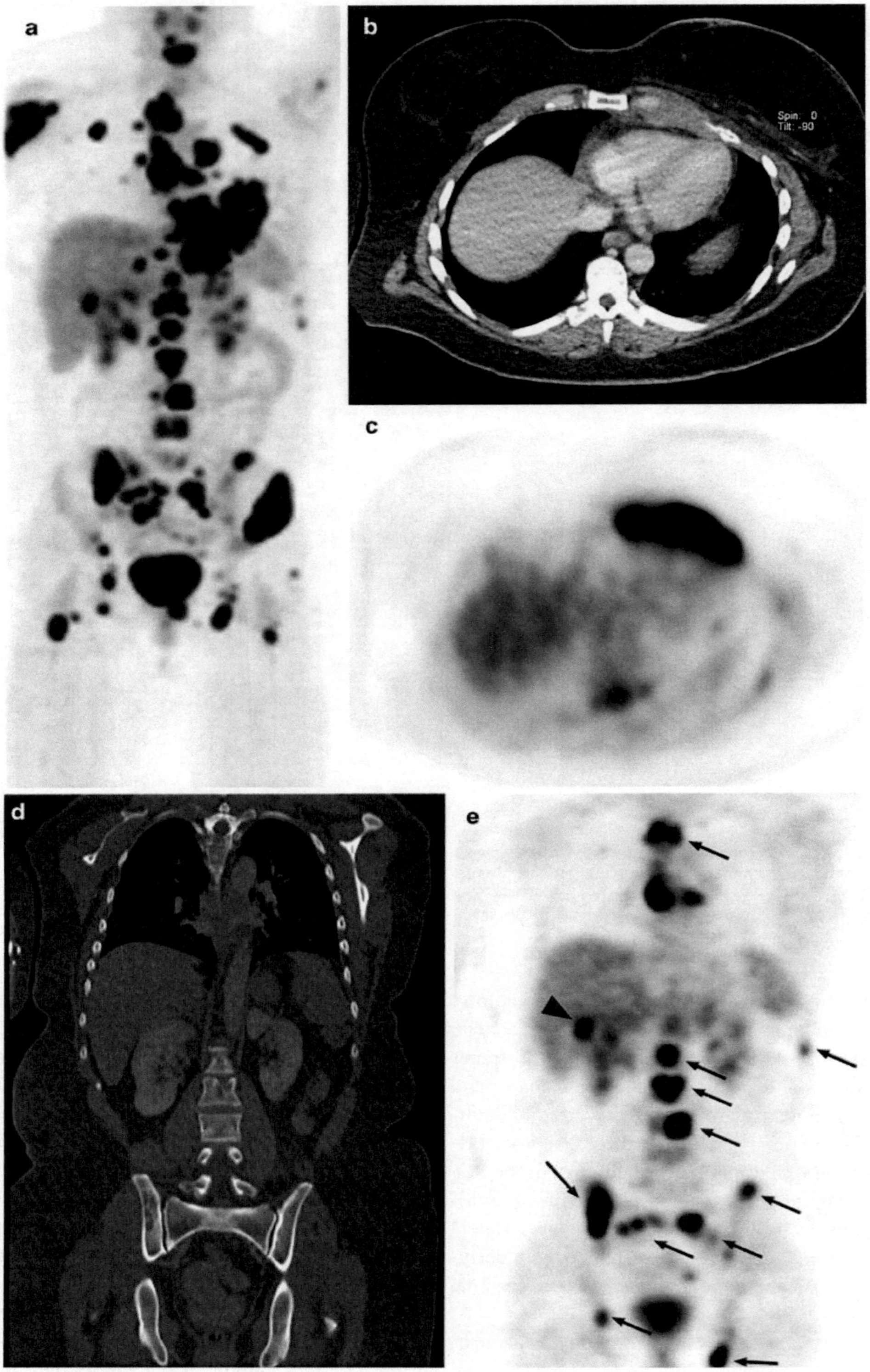

Fig. 20.13 Recurrent breast cancer 4 years following left mastectomy and chemotherapy. Anterior FDG-PET MIP image (**a**) shows extensive intense abnormal FDG tracer uptake at multiple sites throughout the skeleton as well as the left chest, mediastinum, axilla and liver. Transaxial CT (**b**) and FDG-PET (**c**) images reveal local recurrence in the left chest wall with full thickness involvement and associated rib destruction. Coronal CT (**d**) and FDG-PET images (**e**) demonstrate multiple lytic and mixed osseous and marrow metastases (*arrowhead*), mediastinal lymph node metastases and a liver metastasis (*arrowhead*)

tumor markers (CA15-3, CEA) or because of clinical symptoms. In these cases, PET-CT may be considered a very efficient diagnostic tool and has been reported to be 90% sensitive in diagnosing recurrent disease in patients with elevated tumor marker levels, and to affect clinical management in 51% of patients [32]. In conclusion, PET-CT has shown great accuracy in the evaluation of patients both during restaging after primary treatment and during follow-up, clearly surpassing the use of other conventional imaging modalities for whole-body detection.

Therapy Monitoring

For patients with locally advanced breast cancer, neoadjuvant chemotherapy is the standard of care. It is associated with a good response rate in more than 70% of patients. Following successful neoadjuvant chemotherapy, surgery and/or radiotherapy are available as therapeutic options. Therefore, it is essential to assess the actual state of the tumor after therapy. In contrast to morphologic imaging modalities, FDG-PET has been shown to detect metabolic changes in breast cancer as early as 8 days after initiation of chemotherapy. Moreover, the effectiveness of PET in evaluating response to treatment has also been demonstrated in breast cancer. The uptake of FDG by the tumor after one or two cycles of chemotherapy has been shown to be predictive of therapeutic response, as evaluated by CT at the end of therapy [26]. In reported studies, the reduction in tumor metabolic activity correlated with the degree of clinical response. Early assessment of response is critical for planning of management of patients receiving neoadjuvant chemotherapy by assuring continuance of the regimen in those who respond and allowing an early evaluation of alternative therapeutic approaches in those who do not (Fig. 20.14). Rousseau et al reported on the efficacy of FDG- PET for evaluating early response to neoadjuvant chemotherapy in 64 patients with stages II and III breast cancer who underwent FDG-PET after the first, second, third, and sixth courses of chemotherapy. Using a 60% decrease in baseline standardized uptake value (SUV) as their threshold for response, they found that FDG-PET was 61% sensitive and 96% specific after a single cycle. This increased to a 89% sensitivity and a 95% specificity after two cycles of therapy. The negative predictive value of FDG-PET rose from 68% after a single cycle to 85% after the second cycle[33]

FDG-PET has been shown to be useful in predicting response to chemotherapy after its completion. FDG-PET is more accurate than combined conventional imaging techniques for predicting the outcome of patients who had previously undergone primary therapy, with positive and negative predictive values of 93% and 84%, respectively for FDG-PET, and 85% and 59%, respectively for combined conventional imaging [27]. Disease-free survival showed statistically significant differences between FDG-PET-positive and FDG-PET-negative patients in this study.

There is also evidence that using FDG-PET to monitor response to treatment in sites other than the primary tumor may be useful. For example, using quantification, Smith et al. showed that a significant reduction in axillary nodal uptake of FDG after neoadjuvant chemotherapy can predict complete histopathologic response in a small group of patients [28]. Furthermore, in a study of nine patients with breast cancer metastatic to the liver, lung, and soft tissues, an average decrease in lesion SUV of 72% was reported after chemotherapy among patients who showed clinical response to treatment compared with no change in nonresponders [29]. Moreover, the drop in lesion SUV was detectable even after the first cycle of chemotherapy. Finally, considering the usefulness of FDG-PET in monitoring breast cancer response to chemotherapy and the already mentioned additional advantages of combined modality PET-CT, it can be clearly assumed, that PET-CT will improve the accuracy in the evaluation of treatment response, because of its ability to define metabolic and morphologic changes within the tumor following the chemotherapy.

Radiation Therapy Planning

Early studies of FDG-PET and coregistered CT imaging demonstrated that the addition of FDG-PET data to the standard CT protocol significantly changed radiation treatment planning. In 22–100% of patients, changes of 22–64% in the target volume have been already reported for patients with locally advanced lung cancer [30]. Studies of FDG-PET-CT for radiation treatment planning for breast cancer are not yet available; however, as noted above, the importance of locoregional lymph node involvement in determining the extent of radiation treatment field and precise location of the involved lymph nodes requiring inclusion in the treatment field suggests that FDG-PET-CT will have an important role in radiation therapy planning in the treatment of regionally advanced breast cancer.

Acknowledgments The authors gratefully acknowledge the help of Yulia Melenevsky, MD, and Agnieszka Szot Barnes, MD, in the preparation of the figures.

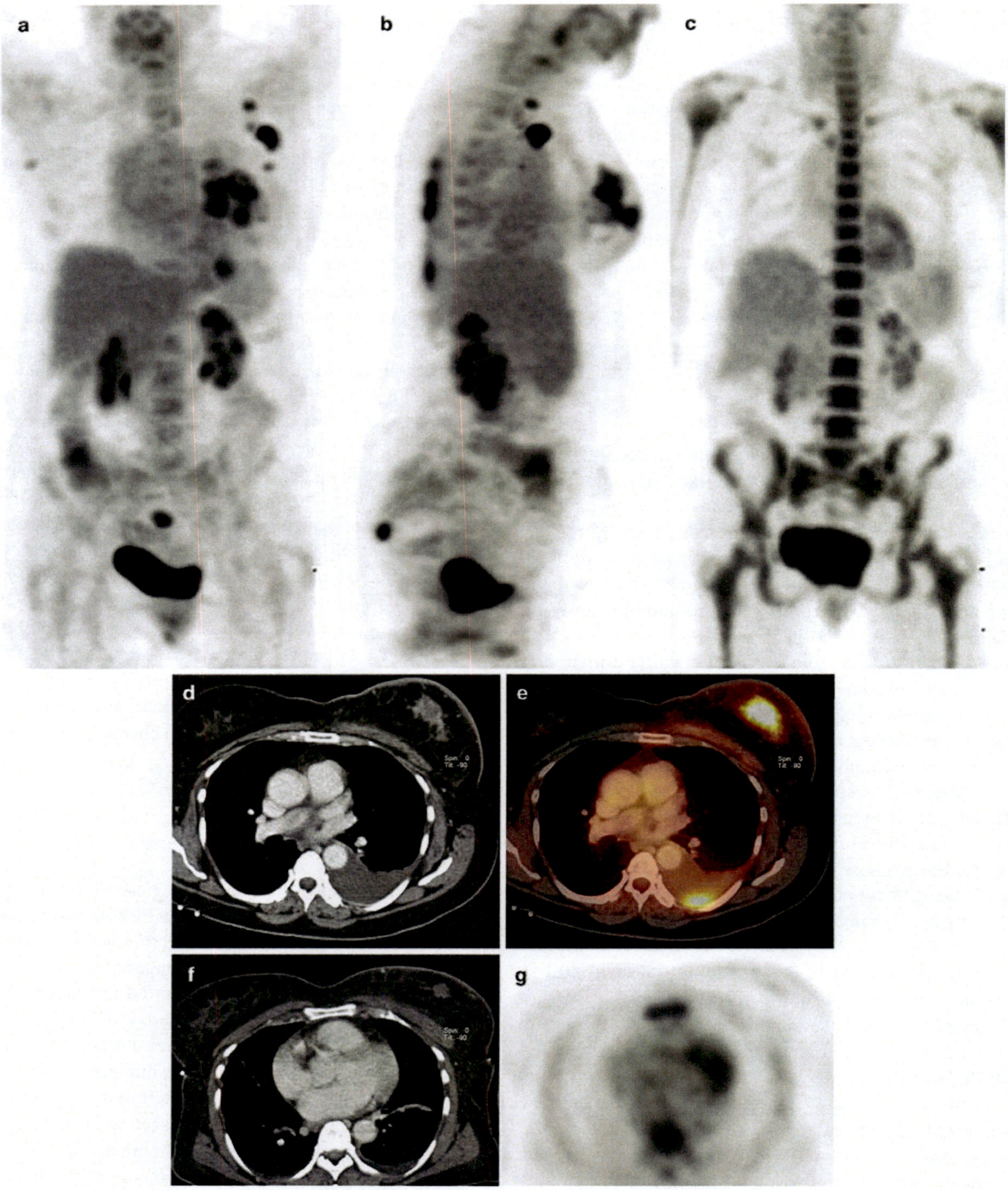

Fig. 20.14 Response of primary left breast cancer and metastases to neoadjuvant chemotherapy. Pretreatment anterior and lateral FDG-PET MIP images (**a**, **b**) show abnormal FDG tracer activity in the primary tumor in the left breast, in posterior metastatic left axillary lymphadenopathy, in left posterior pleural metastases, as well as in a small focus in the sacrum reflecting an isolated osseous metastasis. The posttherapy anterior FDG-PET MIP image (**c**) demonstrates resolution of the pretreatment abnormal areas of tracer uptake and diffused bone marrow FDG uptake related to treatment-related hemopoietic stimulation. Transaxial CT (**d**) and FDG-PET-CT fusion image pretreatment (**e**) demonstrates the 3-cm primary left breast mass and associated abnormal FDG tracer uptake and a left pleural effusion with abnormal pleural contrast enhancement. The abnormal FDG tracer uptake seen on the fusion image demonstrates that the focal abnormal area is within the pleura and not within the rib and is smaller than the associated pleural effusion seen on CT. The posttherapy transaxial CT (**f**) and FDG-PET images (**g**) demonstrate resolution of the FDG uptake in the primary breast mass and reduction in the size of the breast mass on CT, resolution of the abnormal FDG tracer uptake previously seen at the pleural surface and reduction in the size of the pleural effusion

References

1. Eubank WB, Mankoff DA. Evolving role of positron emission tomography in breast cancer imaging. Semin Nucl Med 2005;35(2):84–99.
2. Jemal A, Murray T, Ward E, Samuels A, Tiwari RC, Ghafoor A, Feuer EJ, Thun MJ. Cancer statistics, 2005. CA Cancer J Clin 2005;55(1):10–30.
3. Garreau JR, Nelson J, Look R, Walts D, Mahin D, Homer L, Johnson N. Risk counseling and management in patients with lobular carcinoma in situ. Am J Surg 2005;189(5):610–614.
4. Rohren EM, Turkington TG, Coleman RE. Clinical applications of PET in oncology. Radiology 2004;231(2):305–332.
5. Kumar R, Alavi A. Fluorodeoxyglucose-PET in the management of breast cancer. Radiol Clin North Am 2004;42(6):1113–1122.
6. Kopans DB. The positive predictive value of mammography. AJR Am J Roentgenol 1992;158(3):521–526.
7. Schirrmeister H, Kuhn T, Guhlmann A, Santjohanser C, Horster T, Nussle K, Koretz K, Glatting G, Rieber A, Kreienberg R, Buck AC, Reske SN. Fluorine-18 2-deoxy-2-fluoro-D-glucose PET in the preoperative staging of breast cancer: comparison with the standard staging procedures. Eur J Nucl Med 2001;28(3):351–358.
8. Kumar R, Mitchell S, Alavi A. 18F-FDG uptake and breast density in women with normal breast tissue. J Nucl Med 2004;45(8):14–23.
9. Richter E, Feyerabend T, Bondorf W (eds.). Normal Lymph Node Topography: CT Atlas. New York: Springer, 2004.
10. Fisher B, Anderson S, Bryant J, Margolese RG, Deutsch M, Fisher ER, Jeong JH, Wolmark N. Twenty-year follow-up of a randomized trial comparing total mastectomy, lumpectomy, and lumpectomy plus irradiation for the treatment of invasive breast cancer. NEJM 2002;347(16):1233–1241.
11. Buscombe JR, Holloway B, Roche N, Bombardieri E. Position of nuclear medicine modalities in the diagnostic work-up of breast cancer. Q J Nucl Med Mol Imag 2004;48(2):109–118.
12. Singletary SE, Allred C, Ashley P, Bassett LW, Berry D, Bland KI, Borgen PI, Clark GM, Edge SB, Hayes DF, Hughes LL, Hutter RV, Morrow M, Page DL, Recht A, Theriault RL, Thor A, Weaver DL, Wieand HS, Greene FL. Staging system for breast cancer: revisions for the 6th edition of the AJCC Cancer Staging Manual. Surg Clin North Am 2003;83(4):803–819.
13. Fonseca R, Hartmann LC, Petersen IA, Donohue JH, Crotty TB, Gisvold JJ. Ductal carcinoma in situ of the breast. Ann Intern Med 1997;127(11):1013–1022.
14. Julien JP, Bijker N, Fentiman IS, Peterse JL, Delledonne V, Rouanet P, Avril A, Sylvester R, Mignolet F, Bartelink H, Van Dongen JA. Radiotherapy in breast-conserving treatment for ductal carcinoma in situ: first results of the EORTC randomised phase III trial 10853. EORTC Breast Cancer Cooperative Group and EORTC Radiotherapy Group. Lancet 2000;355(9203):528–533.
15. Fisher B, Costantino JP, Wickerham DL, Redmond CK, Kavanah M, Cronin WM, Vogel V, Robidoux A, Dimitrov N, Atkins J, Daly M, Wieand S, Tan-Chiu E, Ford L, Wolmark N. Tamoxifen for prevention of breast cancer: report of the National Surgical Adjuvant Breast and Bowel Project P-1 Study. J Natl Cancer Inst 1998;90(18):1371–1388.
16. Favourable and unfavourable effects on long-term survival of radiotherapy for early breast cancer: an overview of the randomised trials. Early Breast Cancer Trialists' Collaborative Group. Lancet 2000;355(9217):1757–1770.
17. Brito RA, Valero V, Buzdar AU, Booser DJ, Ames F, Strom E, Ross M, Theriault RL, Frye D, Kau SW, Asmar L, McNeese M, Singletary SE, Hortobagyi GN. Long-term results of combined-modality therapy for locally advanced breast cancer with ipsilateral supraclavicular metastases: The University of Texas M.D. Anderson Cancer Center experience. J Clin Oncol 2001;19(3):628–633.
18. Eubank WB, Mankoff DA, Takasugi J, Vesselle H, Eary JF, Shanley TJ, Gralow JR, Charlop A, Ellis GK, Lindsley KL, Austin-Seymour MM, Funkhouser CP, Livingston RB. 18fluorodeoxyglucose positron emission tomography to detect mediastinal or internal mammary metastases in breast cancer. J Clin Oncol 2001;19(15):3516–3523.
19. Eubank WB, Mankoff DA, Vesselle HJ, Eary JF, Schubert EK, Dunnwald LK, Lindsley SK, Gralow JR, Austin-Seymour MM, Ellis GK, Livingston RB. Detection of locoregional and distant recurrences in breast cancer patients by using FDG-PET. Radiographics 2002;22(1):5–17.
20. Gallowitsch HJ, Kresnik E, Gasser J, Kumnig G, Igerc I, Mikosch P, Lind P. F-18 fluorodeoxyglucose positron-emission tomography in the diagnosis of tumor recurrence and metastases in the follow-up of patients with breast carcinoma: a comparison to conventional imaging. Invest Radiol 2003;38(5):250–256.
21. Lardinois D, Weder W, Hany TF, Kamel EM, Korom S, Seifert B, von Schulthess GK, Steinert HC. Staging of non-small-cell lung cancer with integrated positron-emission tomography and computed tomography. NEJM 2003;348(25):2500–2507.
22. Bar-Shalom R, Yefremov N, Guralnik L, Gaitini D, Frenkel A, Kuten A, Altman H, Keidar Z, Israel O. Clinical performance of PET/CT in evaluation of cancer: additional value for diagnostic imaging and patient management. J Nucl Med 2003;44(8):1200–1209.
23. Kamel EM, Wyss MT, Fehr MK, von Schulthess GK, Goerres GW. [18F]-Fluorodeoxyglucose positron emission tomography in patients with suspected recurrence of breast cancer. J Cancer Res Clin Oncol 2003;129(3):147–153.
24. Kolasinska AD, Buscombe JR, Cwikla JB, Holloway B, Parbhoo SP, Davidson T, Hilson AJ. The role of scintimammography and mammography in recurrent breast cancer. Evaluation of their accuracy using ROC curves. Nucl Med Rev Cent East Eur 2001;4(2):77–82.
25. Goerres GW, Michel SC, Fehr MK, Kaim AH, Steinert HC, Seifert B, von Schulthess GK, Kubik-Huch RA. Follow-up of women with breast cancer: comparison between MRI and FDG-PET. Eur Radiol 2003;13(7):1635–1644.
26. Wahl RL, Zasadny K, Helvie M, Hutchins GD, Weber B, Cody R. Metabolic monitoring of breast cancer chemohormonotherapy using positron emission tomography: initial evaluation. J Clin Oncol 1993;11(11):2101–2111.
27. Vranjesevic D, Filmont JE, Meta J, Silverman DH, Phelps ME, Rao J, Valk PE, Czernin J. Whole-body (18)F-FDG-PET and conventional imaging for predicting outcome in previously treated breast cancer patients. J Nucl Med. 2002;43(3):325–329.
28. Smith IC, Welch AE, Hutcheon AW, Miller ID, Payne S, Chilcott F, Waikar S, Whitaker T, Ah-See AK, Eremin O, Heys SD, Gilbert FJ, Sharp PF. Positron emission tomography using [(18)F]-fluorodeoxy-D-glucose to predict the pathologic response of breast cancer to primary chemotherapy. J Clin Oncol 2000;18(8):1676–1688.
29. Gennari A, Donati S, Salvadori B, Giorgetti A, Salvadori PA, Sorace O, Puccini G, Pisani P, Poli M, Dani D, Landucci E, Mariani G, Conte PF. Role of 2-[18F]-fluorodeoxyglucose (FDG) positron emission tomography (PET) in the early assessment of response to chemotherapy in metastatic breast cancer patients. Clin Breast Cancer 2000;1(2):156–161.
30. Zangheri B, Messa C, Picchio M, Gianolli L, Landoni C, Fazio F. PET/CT and breast cancer. Eur J Nucl Med Mol Imaging. 2004;31(Suppl 1):S135–142.
31. Avril N, Dose J, Janicke F, Ziegler S, Romer W, Weber W, Herz M, Nathrath W, Graeff H, Schwaiger M. Assessment of axillary lymph node involvement in breast cancer patients with positron emission tomography using radiolabeled 2-(fluorine-18)-fluoro-2-deoxy-D-glucose. J Natl Cancer Inst 1996;88(17):1204–1209.
32 Radan L, Ben-Haim S, Bar-Shalom R, Guralnik L, Israel O. The role of FDG-PET/CT in suspected recurrence of breast cancer. Cancer. Dec 1 2006;107(11):2545-2551.
33 Rousseau C, Devillers A, Sagan C, et al. Monitoring of early response to neoadjuvant chemotherapy in stage II and III breast cancer by [18F]fluorodeoxyglucose positron emission tomography. J Clin Oncol. Dec 1 2006;24(34):5366-5372.

Chapter 21
PET-CT in Colorectal Carcinoma

Michael Blake, James Slattery, Owen O'Connor, Dushyant Sahani, and Mannudeep Kalra

Colorectal cancer is a common cancer and a major cause of mortality particularly in Western countries. It is the third most commonly diagnosed cancer, with an estimated 146, 970 new cases diagnosed in the USA during 2009 and accounted for 53, 219 deaths in 2007 [1]. In 2007, the annual mortality rate from colorectal cancer was 20.0 and 14.1 per 100,000 in men and women, respectively accounting for 53,219 deaths [2]. Approximately 80% of patients present with locoregional disease and 20% with metastatic disease [1]. Therapy is chosen that will optimize the chance for cure, minimize the possibility of local recurrence, and provide the best possible functional result.

Current Management of Colorectal Cancer

Surgery remains the mainstay of treatment. The aim of surgery should be to achieve cure and avoid locoregional recurrence. Chemotherapy and radiation therapy, both adjunctive and palliative, also play important roles in the current management of patients with colorectal cancer. Adjuvant chemotherapy can prolong survival in patients with disease that has reached the lymph nodes. Both systemic and locoregional chemotherapy (e.g., intrahepatic intraarterial chemotherapy for liver metastases) are used in patients with metastatic colon cancer. Radiotherapy is used in patients with rectal cancer to reduce the risk of local recurrence.

Surgical Treatment of Rectal Cancer

Surgical therapeutic options include local therapy for early stage tumors, total mesorectal excision for tumors with early local spread, and pelvic exenteration or radical en bloc pelvic resection for locally advanced tumors. Surgery also plays a role in advanced disease because of the risks of obstruction, perforation, and hemorrhage that can occur with invasive tumors.

M. Blake (✉)
Department of Abdominal Imaging and Intervention, Massachusetts General Hospital, 55 Fruit Street, Boston, MA, USA
e-mail: Mblake2@partners.org

Local therapy, such as transanal endoscopic microsurgery, is generally reserved for patients with early stage tumors with favorable prognostic factors. Advantages of local therapy include avoidance of a colostomy, improved quality of life, and avoidance of urinary and sexual dysfunction that can complicate pelvic surgery. Total mesorectal excision (TME), as described by Heald [2, 3] is now the standard of operative management for surgical resection of rectal carcinoma. The sharp dissection technique along the plane of the visceral fascia surrounding the mesorectum used in TME ensures a specimen with intact mesorectum and negative tumor margins in the majority of resectable rectal cancers. As most rectal cancers are confined to the mesorectum at the time of presentation, TME has resulted in a dramatic drop in local recurrence rates. TME also allows for better preservation of autonomic function compared to traditional surgical techniques. In patients with high rectal cancer (located in the upper one third of the rectum) or rectosigmoid tumors, TME is considered not necessary, as metastatic involvement of the mesorectum will rarely be found more than 3 cm distal to the macroscopic primary tumor. Partial mesorectal excision may suffice in this situation.

Abdominoperineal resection (APR) is performed for patients who have cancers that overlap or abut the sphincter or who are incontinent of feces. Recurrent disease is managed on an individual patient basis. Patients with resectable local recurrence can benefit from surgery, and for patients with advanced disease, surgical intervention may be helpful in palliative care of bleeding or obstruction. Partial hepatectomy for colorectal cancer metastases limited to the liver is a therapeutic option for a subset of patients with recurrent colorectal cancer confined to the liver. Some studies have reported increased median survival duration in highly selected patients.

Surgical Treatment of Colon Cancer

The classic surgical operation for patients with colon cancer is an anterior resection that involves a so called "no touch"

P. Shreve and D.W. Townsend (eds.), *Clinical PET-CT in Radiology: Integrated Imaging in Oncology*,
DOI 10.1007/978-0-387-48902-5_21,

isolation technique. The abdomen is first explored to determine whether the tumor is indeed resectable, and resection if indicated is then performed in a segmental fashion (e.g., right or left hemicolectomy) with an end-to-end anastomosis. Total colonic resection is performed when patients have a familial polyposis syndrome with multiple colonic polyps. Laparoscopic techniques can now be employed to achieve colon resection. Recent studies have reported favorable results with over 5 years of follow-up. Surgery plays a similar role in patients with recurrent and metastatic colon cancer as for rectal cancer as outlined in the preceding paragraph.

Because of the role of surgery in both limited and advanced disease, colorectal cancer staging classifications have been developed on the basis of surgical and pathologic criteria. Currently the American Joint Committee on Cancer recommends the standard TNM classification (Tables 21.1 and 21.2). The depth of tumor invasion through the bowel wall (T staging) and the presence of lymph nodes (N staging) and distant metastases (M staging) are the major factors that influence prognosis. Pericolic, perirectal, and adjacent mesenteric nodes are considered regional, whereas metastases in the common iliac or external iliac nodes are considered distant

Table 21.1 AJCC *definitions of TNM* for colorectal cancer (Used with the permission of the American Joint Committee on Cancer (AJCC), Chicago, IL. The original source for this material is the *AJCC Cancer Staging Manual*, 7th edn (2010) published by Springer Science + Business Media LLC. www.springer.com)

The same classification is used for both clinical and pathologic staging		
Primary tumor (T)		
TX	Primary tumor cannot be assessed	
T0	——No evidence of primary tumor	
Tis	Carcinoma in situ: intraepithelial or invasion of lamina propria[a]	
T1	——Tumor invades submucosa	
T2	——Tumor invades muscularis propria	
T3	Tumor invades pericolorectal tissues	
T4a	Tumor penetrates the visceral peritoneum[b]	
T4b	Tumor directly invades or is adherent to other organs or structures[b,c]	
Regional lymph nodes (N)		
NX	Regional lymph nodes cannot be assessed	
N0	——No regional lymph node metastasis	
N1	——Metastasis in 1–3 regional lymph nodes	
	N1a	Metastasis in 1 regional lymph node
	N1b	Metastasis in 2–3 regional lymph nodes
	N1c	Tumor deposit(s) in the subserosa, or non-peritonealized pericolic or perirectal tissues without regional nodal metastasis
N2	——Metastasis in 4 or more regional lymph nodes	
	N2a	Metastasis in 4–6 regional lymph nodes
	N2b	Metastasis in 7 or more regional lymph nodes

Note: A satellite peritumoral nodule in the pericolorectal adipose tissue of a primary carcinoma without histologic evidence of residual lymph node in the nodule may represent discontinuous spread, venous invasion with extravascular spread (V1/2) or a totally replaced lymph node (N1/2). Replaced nodes should be counted separately as positive nodes in the N category, whereas discontinuous spread or venous invasion should be classified and counted in the Site-Specific Factor category Tumor Deposits (TD).

Distant metastasis (M)		
M0	No distant metastasis	
M1	Distant metastasis	
	M1a	Metastasis confined to one organ or site (e.g., liver, lung, ovary, nonregional node)
	M1b	Metastases in more than one organ/site or the peritoneum

[a]Tis includes cancer cells confined within the glandular basement membrane (intraepithelial) or mucosal lamina propria (intramucosal) with no extension through the muscularis mucosae into the submucosa

[b]Direct invasion in T4 includes invasion of other organs or other segments of the colorectum as a result of direct extension through the serosa, as confirmed on microscopic examination (for example, invasion of the sigmoid colon by a carcinoma of the cecum) or, for cancers in a retroperitoneal or subperitoneal location, direct invasion of other organs or structures by virtue of extension beyond the muscularis propria (i.e., respectively, a tumor on the posterior wall of the descending colon invading the left kidney or lateral abdominal wall; or a mid or distal rectal cancer with invasion of prostate, seminal vesicles, cervix, or vagina)

[c]Tumor that is adherent to other organs or structures, grossly, is classified cT4b. However, if no tumor is present in the adhesion, microscopically, the classification should be pT1–3 depending on the anatomical depth of wall invasion. The V and L classifications should be used to identify the presence or absence of vascular or lymphatic invasion whereas the PN 320-detector row site-specific factor should be used for perineural invasion

Table 21.2 Comparison of AJCC and Dukes staging systems The *AJCC Cancer Staging Manual*, 7th edn (2010) published by Springer Science+Business Media LLC.

Staging	TNM	Dukes	Treatment principles
Stage 0	TisN0M0	–	–
Stage I	T1N0M0	A	Surgery
	T2N0M0	A	Surgery
Stage IIa	T3N0M0	B	Surgery + ?chemotherapy
Stage IIb	T4N0M0	B	Surgery + ?chemotherapy
Stage IIIa	T1–2N1M0	C	Surgery + chemotherapy
Stage IIIb	T3–4N1M0	C	Surgery + chemotherapy
Stage IIIc	AnyTN2M0	C	Surgery + chemotherapy
Stage IV	AnyTAnyNM1	–	Chemotherapy + ?surgery

metastases (M1). Common metastatic sites thus include distant nodal disease in the retroperitoneum and liver metastases with lung, bony, brain, and adrenal metastases generally occurring later. Lung and bony metastases are seen more commonly and earlier in patients with rectal cancers compared to colonic cancers due to the unique dual venous drainage of the rectum, which allows blood to reach the systemic circulation without entering the portal circulation. An alternative drainage route for rectosigmoid cancer is via the vertebral venous system of Batson to the lumbar and pelvic bones and up to the thoracic and cervical vertebrae. This system carries blood from rectosigmoid tumors to the paravertebral venous plexus and then to the vertebral venous system, including the internal vertebral veins, intraosseous vertebral veins, and paravertebral veins. Survival after onset of bone metastases is very poor, with a reported median survival of approximately 5 months and a 20% survival rate at 1 year.

Adjuvant therapy plays an important role in the treatment of colorectal cancer (Tables 21.3 and 21.4). Several trials of both postoperative and Preoperative radiotherapy for rectal cancer have indicated a significant reduction in local recurrence with the use of either modality [5, 6]. Postoperative adjuvant chemotherapy with 5-fluorouracil/leucovorin reduces local recurrence and improves survival [7]. Preoperative chemoradiotherapy combined with total mesorectal excision has helped reduce local recurrence rates to less than 10% at 5 years and has also increased disease free survival and overall survival rates[1, 2, 3].

Distant metastases, and particularly liver metastases, represent the major cause of death in patients with colorectal carcinoma. Depending on tumor stage, liver metastases occur in 20–70% of patients and lung metastases in 10–20%. Surgical resection offers the only hope for cure for patients with liver or lung metastases.

Treatment outcomes in colorectal carcinoma are generally related to stage at presentation. Detection of colorectal carcinoma before breach of the muscularis propria (stage T1 and T2) and before lymph node metastases have occurred offers the best prognosis for the patient (Table 21.5).

Table 21.3 Current recommendation for adjuvant therapy for colon cancer (From Ref. [4]. With permission)

Stage	Recommendation
I	No adjuvant therapy
IIA	Observation or clinical trial
IIA[a]	Consider 5-FU/leucovorin or clinical trial or observation
IIB	Consider 5-FU/leucovorin (radiation or clinical trial or observation)
III	5-FU/leucovorin or clinical trial incorporating 5-FU/leucovorin
IV[b]	Colectomy and mastectomy followed by adjuvant 5-FU/leucovorin, irinotecan or oxaliplatin; or colectomy, neoadjuvant chemotherapy, staged resection, and adjuvant chemotherapy
IV[c]	Palliative combination chemotherapy or clinical trial

[a]Patients with poor prognostic factors such as poorly or undifferentiated tumors, perforated or obstructing tumors, or tumors with lymphatic, vascular, or perineural invasion

[b]Patients with respectable liver or lung metastases

[c]Patients with unresectable metastatic disease

Table 21.4 Current recommendations for adjuvant therapy for rectal cancer (From Ref. [4]. With permission)

Stage	Recommendation
I	No adjuvant therapy
II/III	Neoadjuvant 5-FU and radiation therapy, then surgery, then adjuvant 5-FU/leucovorin or adjuvant combination of 5-FU/leucovorin and radiation therapy
IV[a]	Resection of primary tumor and mastectomy followed by adjuvant 5-FU/leucovorin, irinotecan or oxaliplatin; or resection neoadjuvant chemotherapy, staged resection, concurrent 5-FU and radiation therapy and adjuvant chemotherapy
IV[b]	Palliative combination chemotherapy or concurrent 5-FU and radiation therapy then palliative combination chemotherapy

[a]Patients with resectable liver or lung metastases

[b]Patients with unresectable metastatic disease. Consider palliative resection or bypass surgery

Table 21.5 Risk of positive lymph nodes by T stage (Modified from Ref. [8]. With permission of Elsevier)

T stage	Positive lymph nodes risk (%)
T1	6–12%
T2	17–22%
T3	Up to 66%

Accurate preoperative staging is essential to determine prognosis and correctly assign patients to an appropriate treatment strategy. Imaging-based methods for locoregional staging of colorectal cancer include transrectal ultrasound, magnetic resonance imaging (MRI), and computed tomography (CT) while metastatic disease is best assessed with CT, MRI, FDG PET, and more recently PET-CT. Successful locally targeted therapy can increase life expectancy and current data indicate that liver resection can regularly produce long-term survival with the chance of cure in patients with hepatic metastatic colorectal carcinoma. A five year disease-free survival of 28% has been reported among patients with colorectal liver metastases treated with surgical resection [6]. An overall five year survival rate of 32% has been reported in this group [6]. In addition, it appears that resection of recurrent disease may also increase survival [6]. Although a number of clinical or pathologic factors are associated with a poor outcome, the only absolute contraindications to this surgery are general health incompatible with recovery from major hepatic resection or evidence of widespread dissemination of disease. The resection of synchronous liver metastases in patients with six or more regional lymph node metastases is relatively contraindicated. Important areas for future study include the potential role of adjuvant regional chemotherapy after resection and cryoablation of "close" margins. Less invasive alternatives to surgical resection include percutaneous tumor ablation by using methods such as radiofrequency (RF) ablation, cryosurgery, or interstitial laser thermotherapy. The efficacy of radiofrequency ablation has been compared with that of hepatic resection for the treatment of patients with single liver metastases from colorectal cancer [7]. It has been shown that rates of local recurrence-free survival and tumor free survival were comparable following treatment of lesions measuring less than 3cm in size. The rates of overall survival were 56.1% vs 55.4% ($P = 0.451$) and local recurrence-free survival were 95.7% vs 85.6% ($P = 0.304$) among patients with lesions of less than 3cm treated with either hepatic resection or ablation, respectively [7]. For lesions of all sizes, however, surgical resection offered better local recurrence-free survival and five year survival rates compared with radiofrequency ablation. Local recurrence-free survival and five year survival rates after hepatic resection were 89.7% and 50.1%, respectively, and 69.7% and 25.5%, respectively after radiofrequency ablation [7]. For patients with unresectable disease, operative therapy also plays an important role. Multiple operative and interventional modalities hold promise in palliative treatment in the setting of clinically incurable disease. Pulmonary resection for metastases from colorectal cancer may help survival in selected patients. Single metastasis, DFI greater than 36 months, normal preoperative CEA levels are important prognostic factors. When feasible, reoperation is a safe procedure with satisfactory long-term results.

Role of PET/CT in the Initial Diagnosis of Colorectal Carcinoma

In clinical practice, FDG PET is rarely specifically used for the diagnosis of colorectal cancer. There are, however, circumstances where PET-CT may make the initial diagnosis, particularly with increased incidental detections with its more widespread use (Fig. 21.1). In addition, precancerous adenomatous polyps can be detected incidentally on whole body images performed for other indications, sensitivity increasing with polyp size [9, 10]. CT can help distinguish the causes of abnormal FDG uptake and PET-CT clearly performs better than either modality in isolation. Conventional CT is limited in the detection of subtle colonic polyps and tumors, although contrast-enhanced CT with oral contrast can be helpful in detecting gross masses and assessing their complications. In addition CT colonography with a distended, clean colon is now accepted as a screening test for colorectal cancer with a high accuracy for detecting both adenomatous polyps and malignant tumors [11]. The sensitivity of CT colonography is approximately 95%. This compares very favorably with the sensitivities of barium enema (94%) and optical colonoscopy (92%) [11]. PET-CT colonography, while an intriguing prospect, may have too great a radiation load for a screening study. This combination may yet prove to be appropriate for other selected indications. CT colonography and indeed all CT applications have benefited from the recent dramatic advances in CT technology with multidetector scanners now up to 320-detector row allowing increased speed, resolution, and impressive 3D reconstructions. CT radiation dose optimization is also now a more realizable goal with the development of various dose reduction strategies such as beam current modulation.

Staging of Colorectal Carcinoma with PET/CT

Patterns of Regional Colorectal Cancer Spread and Metastases

The lymphatic and venous drainage pathways determine the pattern of metastatic spread of colorectal cancer. The lymphatic drainage of the colon starts as a network of vessels within the muscularis mucosa, which drain into pericolic and mesenteric nodes of the extramural system. Thus, the ability of a tumor to metastasize begins once the tumor has invaded through the muscularis mucosa. The extramural lymphatic vessels and nodes of the colon along with the upper two thirds of the rectum follow the arteries to their origins at the superior and inferior mesenteric vessels (Fig. 21.2). Similarly, the venous drainage of the colon and the upper two thirds of the rectum is via the inferior mesenteric vein to the portal vein, and thus the liver is a common site of metastases (Fig. 21.3). Although lymph from the lower rectum may also drain into the inferior mesenteric system, it may drain to the systems along the middle and inferior rectal arteries, posteriorly along the middle sacral artery, and anteriorly through channels in the retrovesical or rectovaginal septum. These drain to the internal iliac nodes and ultimately to the paraaortic nodes. Venous drainage of the lower rectum is via the

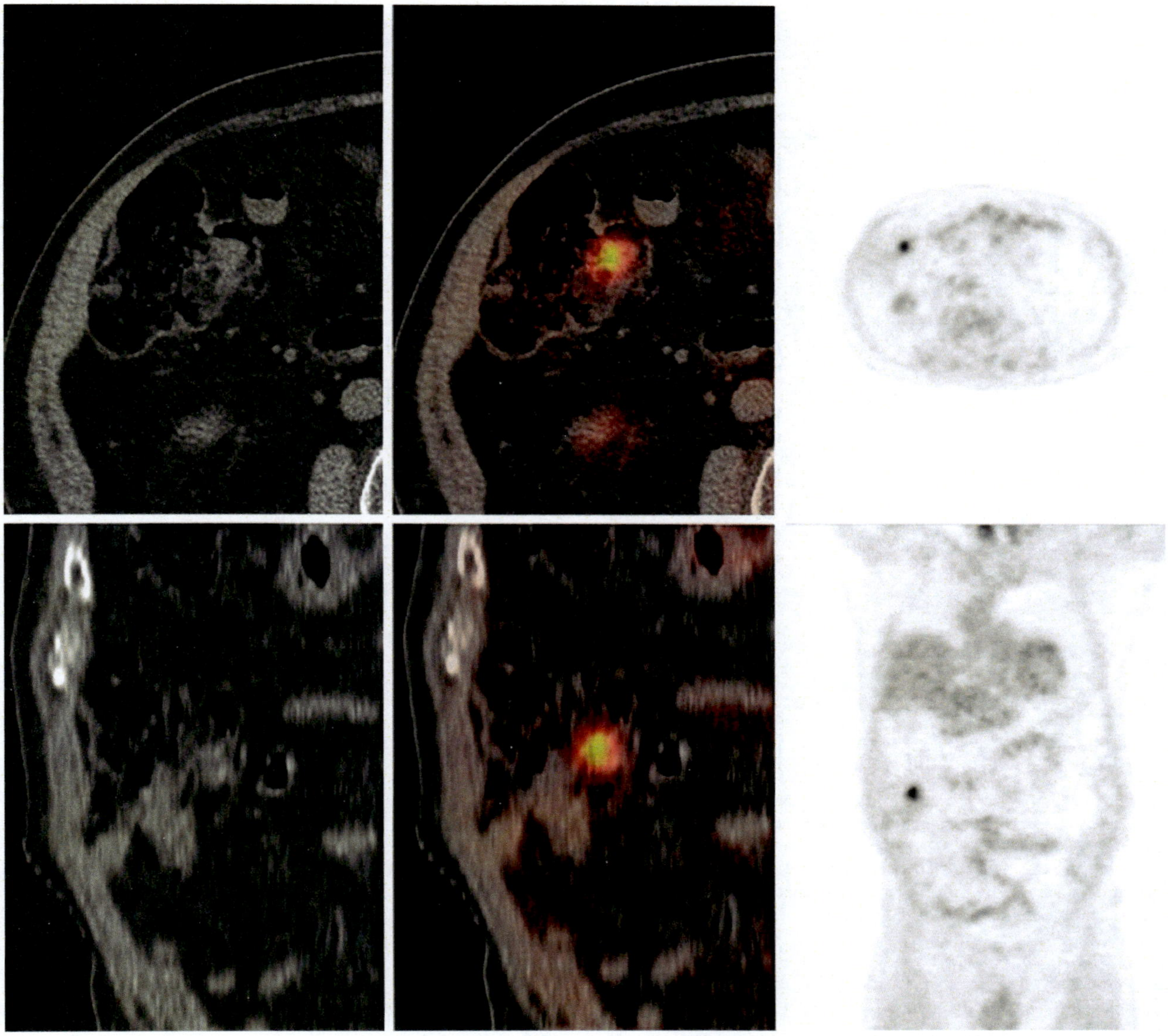

Fig. 21.1 Incidental abnormal finding in colon. Composite axial (*upper row of images*) and coronal (*lower row of images*) CT (*left*), PET-CT fusion images (*center*), and FDG PET images (*right*). Incidental colon polyp on PET-CT performed for evaluation of solitary pulmonary nodule in a 91-year-old man. Focal FDG activity was also noted in the region of the cecum, which coregistered to a soft tissue mass. Colonoscopy revealed a 1.7 × 1.5 × 1.4 cm polyp that was resected. Pathology revealed a tubulovillous adenoma

middle and inferior rectal veins, into the pelvic veins, and then directly into the inferior vena cava. This drainage pattern explains why distal rectal cancer can produce isolated pulmonary metastases without hepatic metastases. Lymphatics from the anal canal above the dentate line drain via the superior rectal lymphatics to the inferior mesenteric lymph nodes and laterally to the internal iliac nodes. Below the dentate line drainage occurs primarily to the inguinal nodes, but can also occur to the inferior rectal lymph nodes. Other common sites of metastases from colon cancer include the lungs, adrenal glands, and bones. Mucinous adenocarcinoma of the colon are also particularly prone to cause widespread intraperitoneal metastases.

Greater than 75% of patients with colorectal cancer have disease limited to the bowel or regional pericolic or mesenteric lymph nodes at the time of diagnosis [13] and most surgeries for colon cancer are, therefore, performed with intent to cure. The dependence of staging schemes on surgical and pathologic information limits the ability of imaging to provide the complete staging information before surgery. Because of its limited spatial resolution, FDG PET is unsuited to providing the precise information needed for

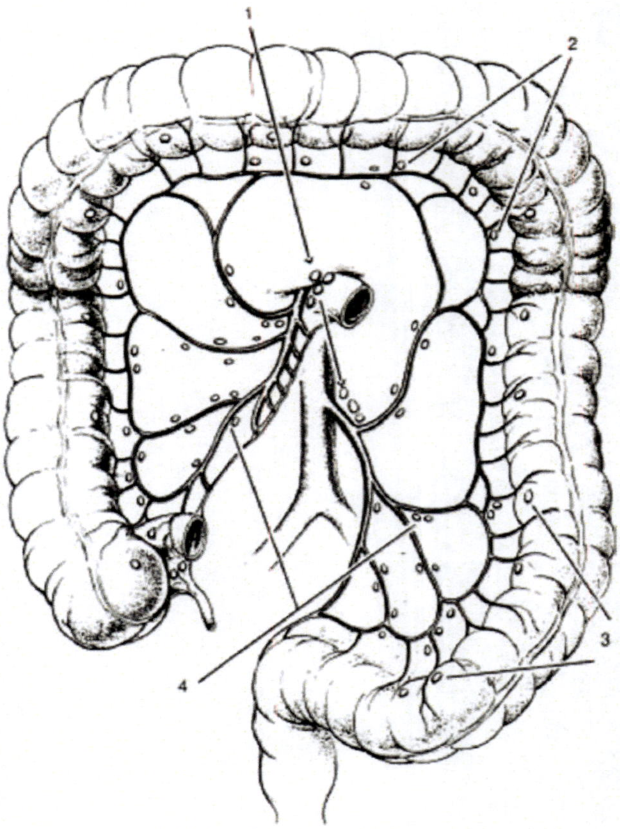

Fig. 21.2 Regional lymph nodes of the colon. N staging in colon cancer is determined by involvement of these regional lymph nodes and is primarily a surgical-pathologic rather than imaging based diagnosis. Lymph node metastases beyond mesenteric nodes such as retroperitoneal lymph nodes are considered distant metastatic disease (From Ref. [12]. With permission)

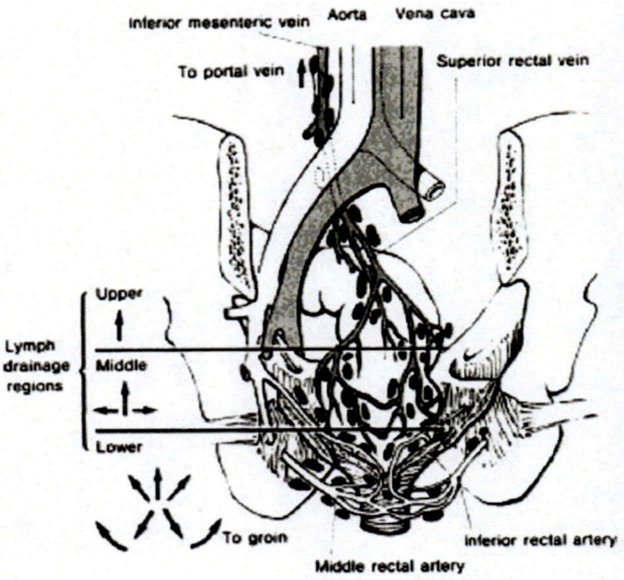

Fig. 21.3 Lymphatic drainage of the rectum. High rectal cancers have lymphatic drainage to the inferior mesenteric vein resulting in paraaortic lymph node and hepatic metastatic routes. Middle and low rectal cancer have lymphatic drainage to the inferior mesenteric chain as well as drainage to middle and inferior rectal and pelvic veins, resulting in perirectal and iliac lymph node metastases. Since the pelvic veins drain directly into the inferior vena cava, low rectal cancers can produce isolated pulmonary metastases without hepatic metastases (From Ref. [12]. With permission)

local and regional staging. In the TNM nomenclature, PET is of little use for the determination of T stage, where precise depth of invasion is the primary determinant. Only in cases of gross serosal penetration and invasion of adjacent structures might PET be accurate. CT gives more precise structural information but usually cannot discriminate the bowel wall layers.

Assignment of N stage requires numeric assessment of pericolic and mesenteric nodes. Regional lymph nodes in colorectal carcinoma are frequently small and lie in proximity to the primary tumor mass. In addition, pericolic nodes often contain small quantities of tumor cells, which are apparent only at the time of histopathologic evaluation. In a recent study, the sensitivity of both PET and CT in detecting involved regional lymph nodes was low at 29%, whereas the specificity of FDG PET was higher (96% vs 85%) [14, 15]. False-negative PET findings in regional metastatic lymph nodes are in part due to the intense FDG uptake by the primary site, which obscures the immediately adjacent structures. For these reasons, FDG PET has a sensitivity of approximately 29-30% for regional lymph node metastases from colorectal cancer [14].

Distinction of small malignant nodes from reactive nodes is problematic with CT also. FDG uptake in pericolic nodes is a good predictor of disease, however, and FDG PET is highly specific for regional lymph node metastases with a reported specificity of 96-100%. The depth of bowel wall infiltration and spread to regional lymph nodes is thus frequently obtained only intraoperatively or histopathologically. The local regional nodes are taken regardless in a mesorectal excision but nevertheless, an attempt to detect nodal or organ metastases is important in planning the general therapeutic approach (i.e., palliation vs. curative tumor resection).

T Staging

A meta-analysis from 2004 comparing CT, MRI, and US for perirectal tissue invasion of colorectal carcinoma reported sensitivity estimates for US, CT, and MR imaging were 90%, 79%, and 82%, respectively, with a significantly higher sensitivity estimate for US than for CT ($p < 0.001$) and MR imaging ($p = 0.003$), indicating understaging of T3 (or higher) tumors with CT and MR imaging. The specificity estimates for US, CT, and MR imaging were comparable: 75%, 78%, and 76%, respectively. For adjacent organ invasion sensitivity estimates of all imaging modalities were comparable: 70% for US, 72% for CT, and 74% for MR imaging. Specificity estimates were also comparable: 97% for US, 96% for CT, and 96% for MR imaging [16].

Because of its limited spatial resolution, FDG PET alone is unsuited to providing the precise information needed for local and regional staging. T staging of colorectal cancer by PET-CT is almost exclusively CT dependent. Only in cases of gross serosal penetration and invasion of adjacent structures (T4 stage) might PET be accurate. T staging of rectal malignancy has seen many advances in recent years. In the setting of rectal cancer endorectal ultrasound is very accurate for staging superficial T1 and T2 tumors but less so for T3 and T4 tumors [13]. The imaging of T3 and T4 tumors is better performed with either MRI or CT. Recent studies have shown MRI using a phased array coil to be highly accurate and the imaging method of choice for staging primary rectal tumors and assessing for involvement of the mesorectal fascia [14]. Preoperative MRI is not feasible in all patients and multislice CT offers the potential to examine the mesorectum and identify distant metastases during a single examination. The accuracy of multislice CT for the evaluation of mesorectal extension by rectal carcinoma is dependent on the site of the primary tumor. Overall sensitivity and specificity for predicting mesorectal fascial involvement is 74% and 94%, respectively. For tumors in the lower third of the rectum the sensitivity and specificity are 66% and 82%, respectively. Sensitivity and specificity of CT for assessing mesorectal extension are much better for tumors of the upper two-thirds of the rectum (76% and 96%, respectively) [15]. The role of combined PET-CT scanning has not yet been adequately assessed for this indication and has been limited by the poor spatial resolution of PET. Both modalities may benefit from being combined in PET-CT, as soft tissue attenuation on CT alone may represent scar or tumor but if it is positive on the FDG PET images, then there is increased confidence that there is a tumor mass.

Regional Lymph Node Staging (N Staging)

Determination of regional lymph node involvement is primarily surgical-pathologic for colorectal cancer. Assignment of N stage requires numeric assessment of pericolic and mesenteric nodes with evidence of metastatic disease. Regional lymph nodes in colorectal carcinoma are frequently small and lie in proximity to the primary lesion and thus can be obscured by increased FDG activity. In addition, pericolic nodes often contain small quantities of tumor cells, which are apparent only at the time of histopathologic evaluation. Enlarged and nonenlarged FDG avid lymph nodes can be identified in the mesentery on PET-CT, indicating the presence of regional lymph node metastases, but this is more commonly encountered on restaging patients with colorectal cancer rather than on initial staging. The presence of only regional lymph nodes metastases on PET-CT evaluation for initial staging would not in any case preclude resection of the primary lesion and surgical staging of regional lymph node metastases. Nevertheless, it has been demonstrated that PET-CT has been shown in one study to alter the staging of colorectal carcinoma compared with conventional imaging in 31% of cases[1]. Altered staging as a result of PET-CT changed treatment intent in 8% of cases. This was mainly due to the redesignation of nodal staging.

Metastatic Disease

Disease spread beyond the regional pericolic or mesenteric lymph nodes is considered to be metastatic disease. These include liver, lymph nodes such as retroperitoneal and iliac nodes, bone, adrenal glands, and soft tissue. FDG-PET images or PET-CT can clarify abnormal CT findings and may depict unsuspected metastases such as nonenlarged lymph nodes (Fig. 21.4). PET-CT can find unidentified sites of disease in patients with abnormal carcinoembryonic antigen levels and a negative workup with conventional diagnostic modalities. A recent study of the role of PET-CT for the detection of recurrent or metastatic disease in patients with a history of colorectal and raised carcinoembryonic antigen found PET-CT to be considerably better than multislice CT alone [1]. The sensitivities and specificities of PET-CT and multislice CT for tumor detection were 98.1% and 66.7% ($p < 0.0001$), and 75% and 62.5% ($p = 0.056$), respectively. The use of combined PET-CT for preoperative staging has been shown to improve survival in patients with hepatic metastases deemed suitable for hepatic resection by primarily demonstrating the presence extrahepatic metastases, thus appropriately eliminating ineffective surgery in patients with inoperable disease [17]. Indeed, imaging with FDG in patients with colorectal cancer has also been proven to be a cost-effective technique that often leads to a change in patient management [18].

Hepatic Metastases

Early identification of liver metastases provides the opportunity for neoadjuvant chemotherapy and resection, which may prolong survival for patients with colorectal carcinoma [19, 20]. In many institutions, contrast-enhanced multidetector-row CT is the primary imaging modality for the detection, localization, and characterization of focal liver lesions [21]. In a PET-CT

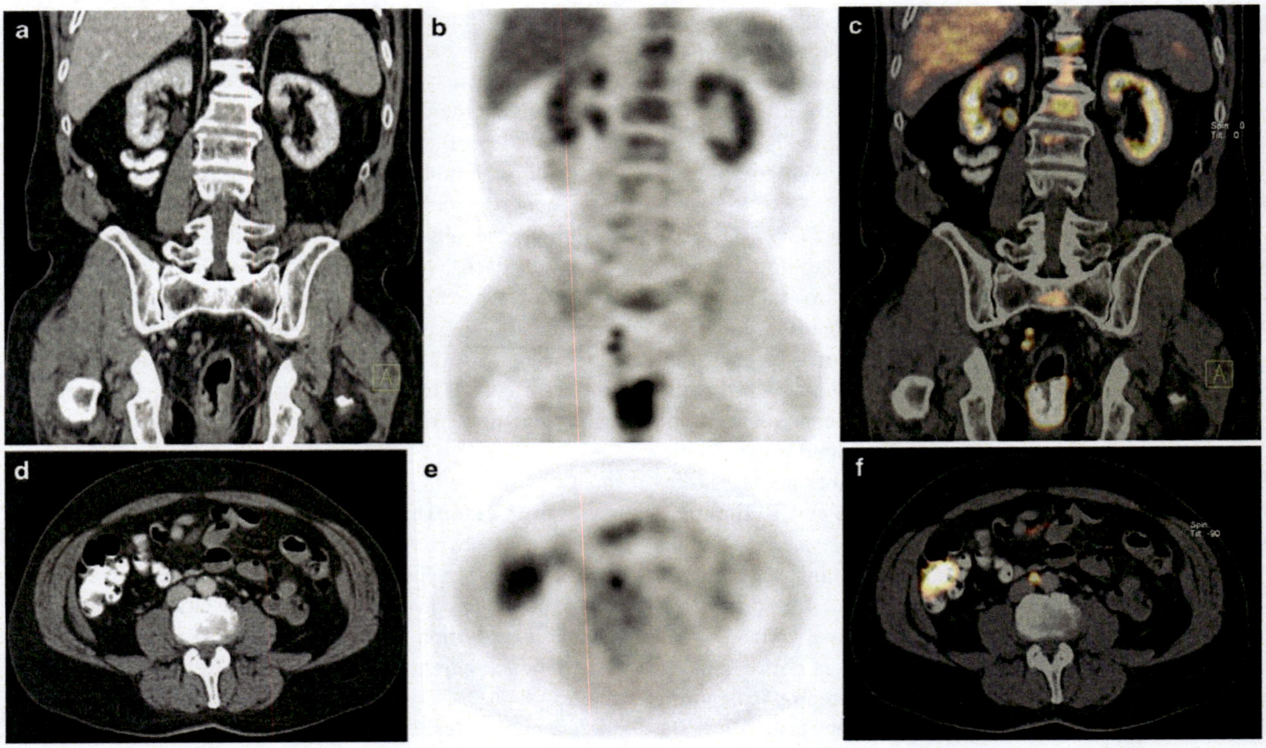

Fig. 21.4 Nonenlarged lymph node metastases. Adenocarcinoma of the rectum for initial staging. Coronal CT (**a**), FDG PET (**b**), and FDG PET-CT fusion (**c**) images demonstrate right perirectal FDG avid lymph nodes slightly larger than 5 mm. On transaxial CT (**d**), FDG PET (**e**), and FDG PET-CT fusion (**f**) images an 8-mm aortocaval retroperitoneal FDG avid lymph node is identified

protocol, the authors advocate a contrast-enhanced portal-venous phase CT scanning be included in the PET-CT acquisition. This provides maximal contrast for detection of relatively low attenuation hepatic metastases, which is lacking in the low-dose noncontrast CT. This is of particular importance in mucinous metastases which can be poorly FDG avid. Moreover portal venous phase contrast-enhanced CT provides better delineation of the vessels and hepatic segments should the patient be a candidate for liver resection surgery.

Several studies have demonstrated that FDG PET is highly sensitive for the detection of liver metastases [22–24]. A recent meta-analysis demonstrated the sensitivities of CT, MR and FDG PET for the detection of hepatic metastases from colorectal carcinoma to be 83.6%, 88.2%, and 94.1%, respectively. The sensitivity of MR has improved over the past 5 years with the development of newer MR technologies, and MR is superior to CT for the detection of lesions measuring less than 1cm in size. These finding are supported by other studies that have demonstrated that PET is accurate for identification of hepatic metastases greater than 1 cm in diameter but is limited in its ability to demonstrate lesions smaller than 1 cm [25–27]. PET-CT imaging may be particularly useful in patients with several hypodense or hypoenhancing liver lesions that are not clearly characterized by CT alone and in patients in whom standard CT fails to detect metastases in the setting of a rising serum CEA. In these cases, PET-CT has the ability to directly affect patient management by guiding biopsies or directing surgical resections of liver metastases.

The greatest influence of PET-CT imaging in patients with hepatic metastases is in detection of extrahepatic sites of disease that would preclude a curative procedure (Fig. 21.5). Several investigators have examined the incremental value of FDG PET as a supplement to CT and found that FDG PET offers information beyond that from CT alone, and that this information often affects patient care. Investigators have found that when FDG PET is added to CT alone in preoperative planning for patients with hepatic metastases, additional sites of extrahepatic disease are identified in 11–32% of patients [17, 28, 29]. This frequently leads to a change in therapeutic management from localized therapy to a more systemic approach with chemotherapy.

Lymph Node Metastases

Spread of colorectal cancer to lymph nodes beyond regional pericolic or mesenteric lymph nodes is considered metastatic

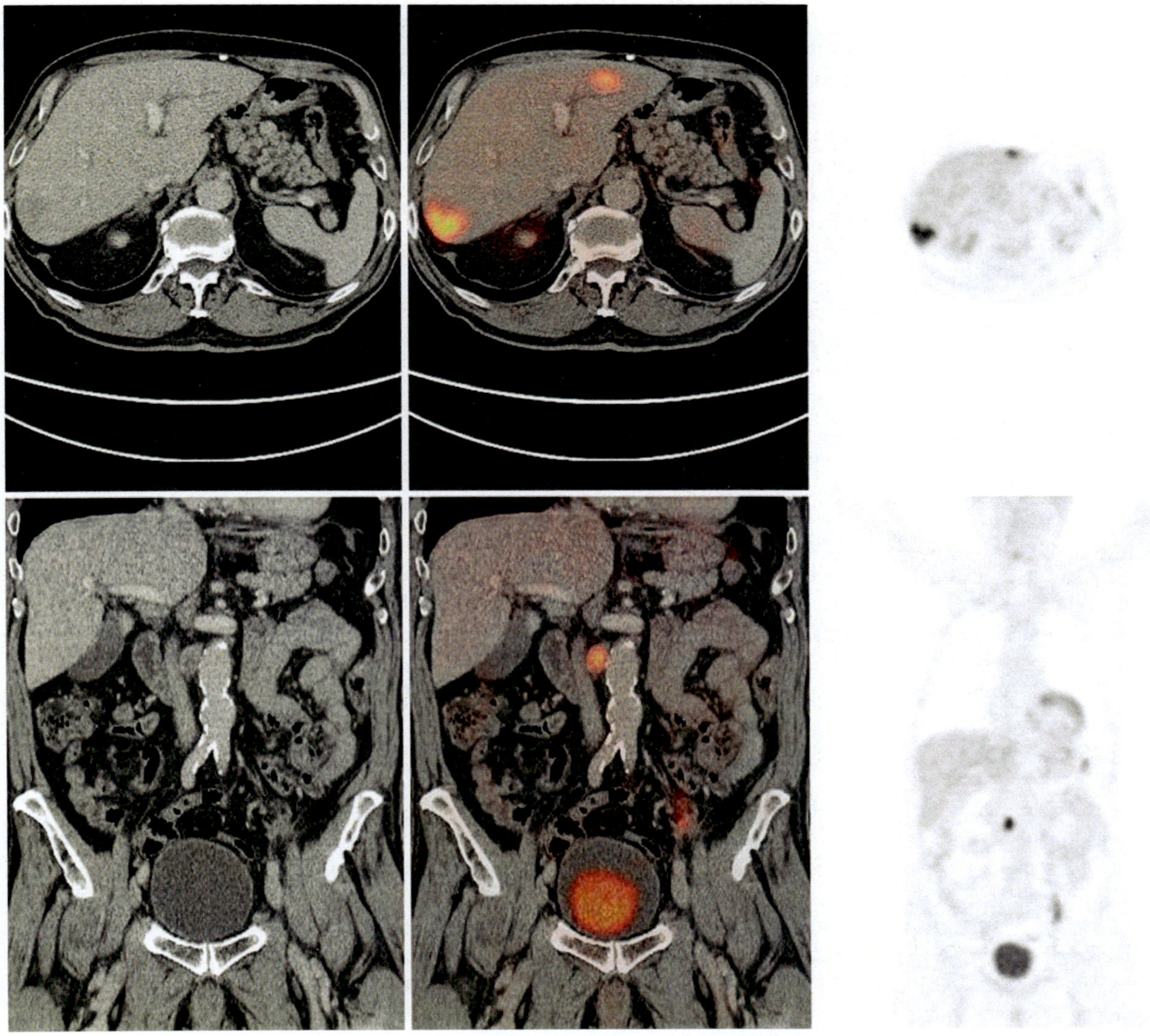

Fig. 21.5 Extrahepatic metastases in recurrent colorectal cancer. Composite axial (*upper row of images*) and coronal (*lower row of images*) CT (*left*), PET-CT fusion images (*center*), and PET images (*right*). Rising CEA 1 year after resection of an adenocarcinoma of the transverse colon. Two hepatic lesions are demonstrated, one each in the right and left hepatic lobes. The metastasis in the right hepatic lobe is depicted on the portal venous contrast enhanced CT images while the metastasis in the left hepatic lobe is only clearly seen on the FDG PET images. In addition, moderately increased FDG activity in seen in an enlarged aortocaval node in the region of the origin of the mesenteric vessels (*coronal images*) indicative of extrahepatic metastases. Such a finding would preclude hepatic metastases resection

spread (M1 disease). The lymphatic vessels of the ascending and transverse parts of the colon terminate, after traversing the right colic and mesocolic nodes, in the superior mesenteric nodes. Those of the descending and sigmoid colon are interrupted by the small nodes on the branches of the left colic and sigmoid arteries, and terminate in the preaortic nodes around the origin of the inferior mesenteric artery. The lymphatics from the anus pass forward and end with those of the perineum and scrotum in the superficial inguinal lymph nodes; those from the anal canal accompany the middle and inferior rectal arteries, and end in the hypogastric lymph nodes; while the vessels from the rectum traverse the pararectal nodes and pass to the sigmoid mesocolon which in turn terminate in the preaortic lymph nodes around the origin of the inferior mesenteric artery.

The strengths of CT are its accuracy for the detection of anatomic abnormalities and its ability to define structures that are below the resolution of nuclear medicine imaging. However, the limitation of CT is its reliance on anatomic criteria in order to identify pathologic conditions, such as a

1-cm short-axis dimension threshold for pathologic lymphadenopathy. Although this criterion results in an acceptable balance between sensitivity and specificity for disease, nodes smaller than 1 cm can contain malignant cells and, in addition, reactive or inflammatory processes can result in nodes larger than 1 cm. Other overlapping CT nodal features that can be seen with lymph node metastases and inflammatory conditions include low density (as in mucinous metastases) and calcifications.

By assessing metabolic activity within a node, FDG PET is not directly reliant on nodal size to determine the presence or absence of malignancy (Figs. 21.4 and 21.5). Nodes that are not enlarged can be shown to contain tumor on FDG PET images, and nodes that are enlarged can be shown to be reactive in nature. For this reason, PET has been shown to be more sensitive and specific than CT alone for identification of sites of lymph node metastatic disease [30]. However, PET also has limitations regarding size and false-positives may occur due to inflammation. In addition some cystic or mucinous nodal metastases may not show significant FDG uptake, and hence the FDG PET images cannot be entirely relied upon to exclude lymph node metastases in the setting of colorectal cancer.

Pulmonary Metastases

Apart from the liver, the lung is among the most prominent target organs for metastatic disease of colorectal tumors. Possible manifestations of pulmonary metastatic disease include pulmonary nodules, lymphangitic carcinomatosis, and pleural involvement. Ten percent of patients with colorectal cancer will develop lung metastases, usually in association with other extrathoracic systemic disease. But 2–4% will have isolated lung metastases and 50% of these will be amenable to resection [31, 32]. The sensitivity and specificity of PET-CT for the detection of malignant solitary pulmonary nodules are 96% and 83%, respectively [1]. Perioperative morbidity is low and 5-year survival ranges from 28% to 40% after successful resection [31–34].

The CT component of PET-CT provides the most sensitive detection of pulmonary metastases, although the FDG PET images can provide additional specificity for nodules generally greater than 8 mm. Routine chest CT is now able to delineate pulmonary nodules as small as 2–3 mm. This facilitates the diagnosis of even the smallest pulmonary nodules, leading to a therapeutic dilemma [35] because the low specificity of findings (most pulmonary nodules will be benign) remains a problem.

Typical findings of pulmonary metastases in CT include multiple, round, variably sized nodules and diffuse thickening of the pulmonary interstitium. In daily practice, however, atypical imaging features of metastases are often encountered making a distinction of metastases from other benign pulmonary diseases based on CT findings alone difficult. Due to limited spatial resolution, a negative PET scan cannot exclude pulmonary metastases with certainty, while a positive FDG-PET will confirm suspicious abnormalities detected on the CT images [36]. A standardized uptake value (SUV) of greater than 2.5 defines a solitary pulmonary nodule as malignant with a relatively high degree of sensitivity and specificity [1]. One method that shows potential for better spatial resolution on FDG-PET and therefore the potential for better correlation between nodule SUV values and nodule size is the use of respiratory gating during the acquisition of PET-CT [2].

Osseous Metastases

Osseous metastases from colorectal carcinoma are a relatively rare event. One retrospective review of over 5,000 cases reported an incidence of 6.6% for osseous metastases in combination with visceral metastases, while the incidence of skeletal metastases only was 1.1% [37]. Osseous metastases may be overlooked on CT particularly if early metastatic disease is confined to the skeleton. Typical appearances of visible bone metastases on CT include lytic or mixed lytic/sclerotic lesions. Metastatic osseous lesions may become sclerotic with treatment.

FDG uptake in bone marrow is usually relatively, roughly equivalent to, or slightly greater than that of liver background tracer activity. FDG uptake in marrow of the vertebral bodies can appear focal on axial imaging and could be misinterpreted as metastatic disease. However, a repeating pattern, which is most evident on sagittal or coronal images, is characteristic of physiologic FDG uptake in vertebral marrow. Metastases can be distinguished by the greater intensity of FDG uptake and nonuniform distribution. Patients undergoing treatment with hematopoietic stimulates as part of their chemotherapy regimen will have demonstrate uniformly high levels of accumulation of FDG tracer in bone marrow [38].

Studies suggest that PET-CT is both sensitive and specific for diagnosing malignant bone lesions [39]. For example, one study of 712 patients, 59 of whom had bone metastases demonstrated PET/CT to have a positive predictive value of 98% when findings on PET and CT were concordant [1a]. The PET focal finding often draws the reviewer's attention to the site of disease on the CT images and facilitates detection of subtle bony changes resulting from early metastasis. Indeed, occasionally no corresponding CT abnormality is detected and if necessary for confirmation an MRI of the suspicious area can clarify the discordant PET and CT findings.

Other Soft Tissue Metastases

Peritoneal implants can occur with colon cancer, and are difficult to detect on CT alone without careful attention to CT technique and interpretation. The FDG PET images can be very useful in locating peritoneal implants 7–8 mm or greater in size, and the CT images essential in confirming the presence of a nodular implant (Fig. 21.6). Other favored sites for colorectal metastases include the adrenal glands. PET imaging of the adrenals is very sensitive for the detection of malignant adrenal lesions. Adrenal adenomas can uncommonly exhibit increased FDG activity and all of the reported cases of PET positive adenomas have been indeterminate by CT criteria (>10 HU). However, analysis using CT contrast washout analysis may be useful for further lesion characterization. Ultimately adrenal biopsy may be the final arbiter if histologic confirmation is critical.

Restaging of Colorectal Cancer

Locoregional pelvic recurrence and liver metastases are the major sites of relapse after resection of colorectal cancer. Recurrence occurs in one third of patients in the first 2 years after resection. Patterns of recurrence are different in colon cancer than in rectal cancer. Local recurrence is more common with rectal cancers than colon cancer ranging from 7% to 33%, and 1–19%, respectively [40]. Only 20% of local recurrences can be completely resected, and the majority of patients who develop local recurrence will die from their disease [40]. Sites of distant metastasis are influenced by the venous drainage of the primary site. As mentioned, the venous drainage of the colon and upper rectum is via the portal vein, and thus the liver is a common site of metastases. However, the lower rectum, again as noted before, has a dual drainage pattern which explains why distal rectal cancer can produce isolated pulmonary metastases without hepatic metastases.

Several studies have reported on the patterns and survival statistics with respect to local, locoregional and metastatic recurrence. In a review by Willett et al. [41] of local recurrence in colon carcinoma, 20% of the recurrences were local only and 43% were concurrent local and distant failures. Pilipshen et al. [42] reviewed patterns of recurrent rectal cancer in which 30% of the recurrences were pelvic recurrences alone and 58% of the recurrences were pelvic with concomitant distant disease. Obrand and Gordon [43] reported patterns

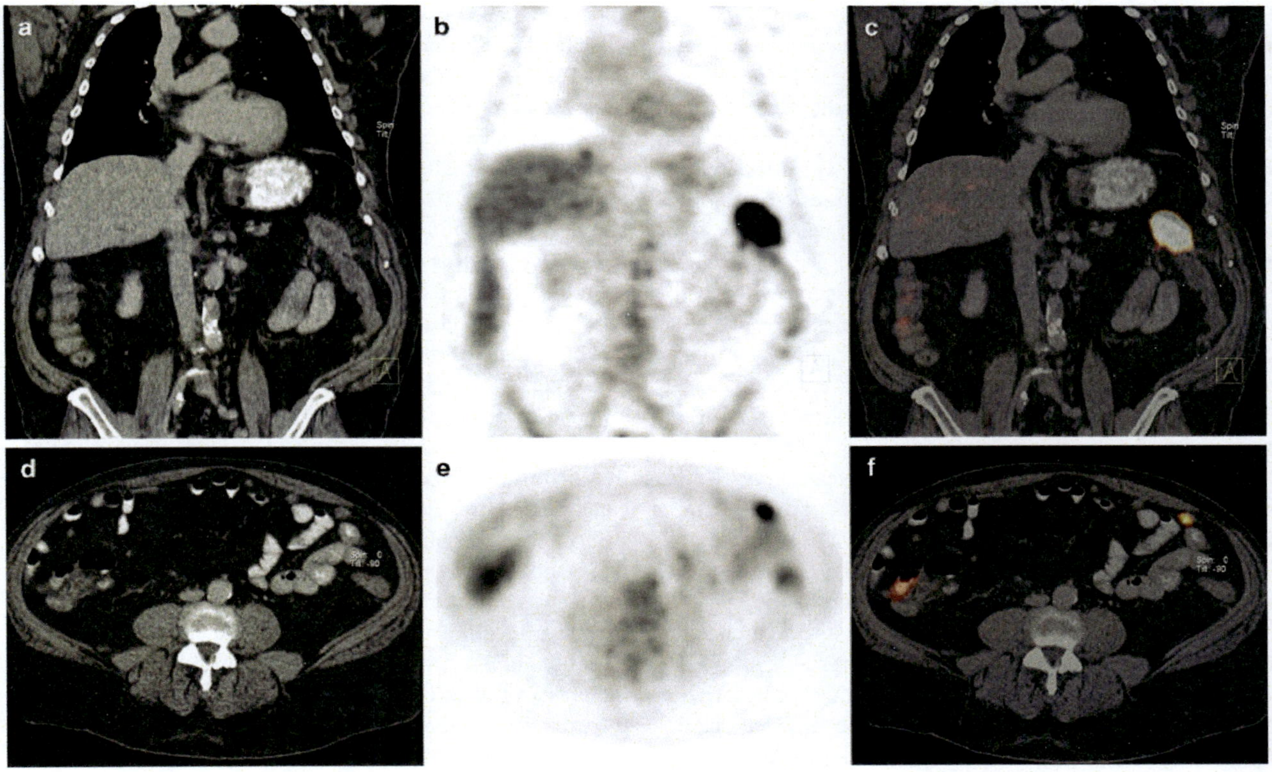

Fig. 21.6 Peritoneal implant metastases of colon caner. The primary colon cancer is seen at the splenic flexure region as thickening of the colon wall on coronal CT (**a**) image which is associated with intense focal abnormal FDG tracer uptake on the coronal FDG PET (**b**) and FDG PET-CT fusion (**c**) images. Transaxial CT (**d**), FDG PET (**e**), and FDG PET-CT fusion images (**f**) depict small peritoneal nodules, the larger of which is clearly FDG avid while smaller peritoneal metastatic deposits are seen only on the CT images. While the PET images are very helpful in identifying the location of peritoneal implants, very small implants may only be seen on the CT images

of recurrence for 146 patients with colorectal primaries in which 46% of the recurrences were locoregional alone, 52% had locoregional as a component, and 52% had a distant component at the time of recurrence. Obrand also found that stage, perforation, local invasion, and rectal carcinoma were positive predictors of recurrence.

Brethauer et al. reported 54% of recurrences [44] had distant metastases alone at the time of recurrence and 67% had distant metastases as a component of failure. The most common site of distant metastases (isolated and as a component of all distant metastases) was the liver. Similar findings were reported by other investigators [45–48].

As demonstrated by Brethauer et al. and others [42, 47, 49] approximately one fifth of patients with recurrence will have isolated liver metastases. Untreated, patients with limited metastases to the liver have a 5-year survival rate of 28% [50, 51] and long-term survival with chemotherapy alone is equally dismal. Surgical treatment is the only hope for cure in these patients and can offer 5-year survival rates from 25% to 37% [52–54] and 10-year survival rates of 20% [54].

Resection of isolated or limited pulmonary metastases of colorectal cancer is frequently considered for patients with resectable lesions. Approximately 20% of patients with colorectal cancer will eventually develop pulmonary metastases but a much smaller percentage will be candidates for resection. Twelve patients (25%) with recurrence in Brethauer's study [44] developed pulmonary metastases. Seven patients (15%) had pulmonary metastases only at the time of recurrence and three patients (6%) underwent reoperation with curative intent. These three recurrences were detected by standard chest x-ray. Five-year disease-free survival rates after resection of pulmonary metastasis for colorectal cancer range from 16% to 40% [40, 45, 55].

Resection of locally recurrent rectal cancer, with preoperative or postoperative radiation therapy, can provide palliation and may be curative. Suzuki et al. [56] reported a 34% 5-year survival rate after resection of locally recurrent rectal cancer. The cumulative probability of local re-recurrence and distant metastases at 5 years, however, were 47% and 62%, respectively. Wiggers et al. [57] reported a 5-year survival after reoperation for locally recurrent rectal cancer of 20% and a high success rate for curative operations (77% of curative intent operations successfully completed). Local re-recurrence occurred in 59% of patients after reoperation.

When there is a rising CEA, we thus focus or search to the common sites of local and distant recurrence. Focal FDG uptake can guide us to look for corresponding CT abnormalities such as a soft tissue mass or bone erosion on CT. Correlation with the patient's clinical status is always important in PET-CT interpretation particularly as there is some imaging features overlap between abscess and cystic metastatic disease. Mucinous adenocarcinoma of the colon can also cause widespread intraperitoneal metastases, which can be detected with CT only if they produce thickening of the peritoneal surfaces or peritoneal nodules. Microscopic seeding of the peritoneal surfaces will not be detected by either CT or PET. However the combination of CT and PET together helps to identify macroscopic peritoneal implants more accurately (Fig. 21.6).

A particular challenge in patients with prior colorectal carcinoma is differentiation of the sequelae of prior therapy, including surgical scarring and radiation fibrosis, from disease recurrence. This is most problematic with distal colon and rectal tumors, where presacral scarring and pelvic changes are common. With conventional imaging, serial examinations are frequently required, before slowly developing changes can be appreciated. With FDG PET performed 6 months postsurgery, the presence of metabolic activity in the presacral space is indicative of tumor recurrence, while post-surgical change is not hypermetabolic. FDG PET has been shown to be accurate for differentiation of benign from malignant presacral changes and to be superior to CT and MR imaging in this regard [58]. Metabolic imaging has a further advantage in that only a single study is necessary to make this determination, rather than the serial morphologic studies often required with conventional imaging. However, PET alone has limitations given the anatomical changes in appearance and position seen resulting from surgery. Even-Sapir et al. [58] have documented the additional value of PET-CT in the detection of pelvic recurrence after surgical removal of rectal cancer. Sensitivity, specificity, positive-predictive value, negative predictive value, and accuracy for differentiating malignant from benign 18F FDG uptake in the pelvis were 98%, 96%, 90%, 97%, and 93% for PET/CT and 82%, 65%, 73%, 75%, and 74% for PET alone, respectively. Overall, it is currently believed that PET-CT imaging should be the preferred imaging modality in these patients, because it identifies and localizes the disease in one setting and can guide diagnostic or therapeutic interventions.

Surgical management of local recurrence depends on the site and extent of the disease. Wound recurrences are rare and, although resectable when isolated, are usually indicative of diffuse intraabdominal disease. Isolated recurrence can occur at the site of prior resection of metastases and PET-CT can be helpful in precisely locating and characterizing such recurrences (Fig. 21.7). Similarly, anastomotic recurrences may be resected but can be associated with more extensive local or metastatic disease which would preclude resection. PET-CT can be particularly useful in determining the present and extent of local recurrence of rectal cancer in the presacral region (Figs. 21.8 and 21.9). Recurrent rectal cancer can involve the adjacent pelvic organs, pelvic sidewalls, or sacrum, and may require pelvic exenteration, en bloc resection, or a palliative diversion procedure.

Liver metastases from colorectal carcinoma represent 50% of all recurrences. The size and number of hepatic

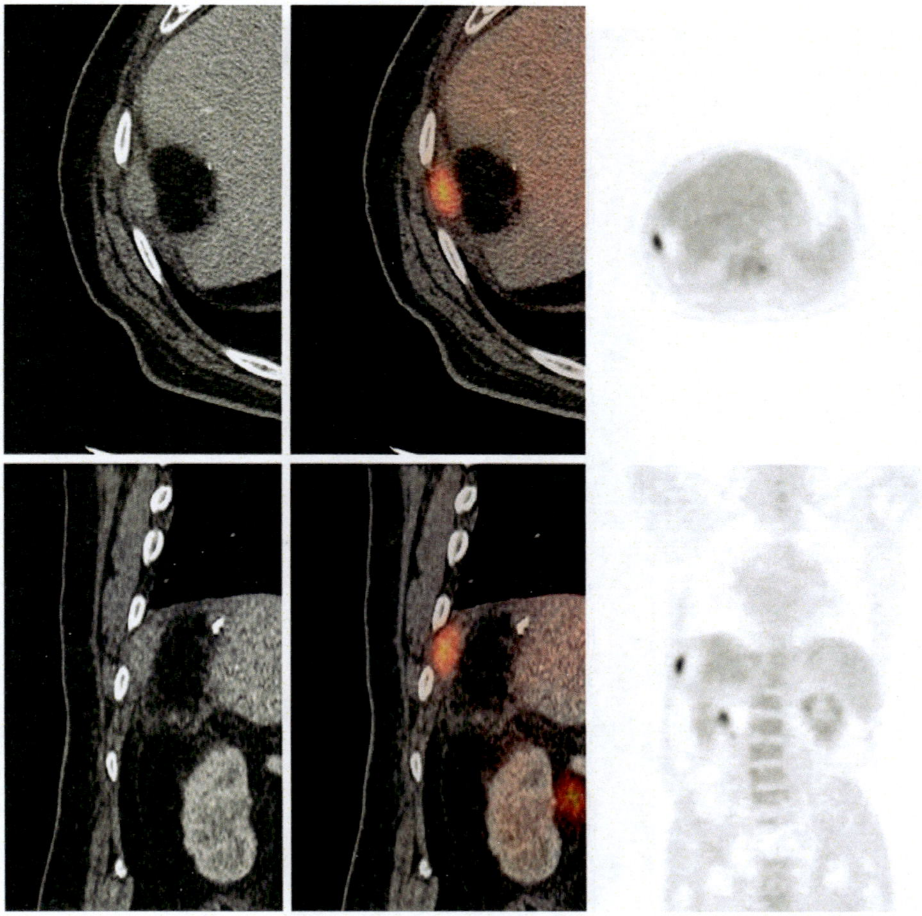

Fig. 21.7 Localized soft tissue recurrence following wedge resection of hepatic metastasis. Composite axial (*upper row of images*) and coronal (*lower row of images*) CT (*left*), PET-CT fusion (*center*), and PET images (*right*). Patient is 4 years postsigmoid colectomy for adenocarcinoma and 3 years post-wedge excision of an isolated hepatic metastasis. Surveillance PET-CT demonstrates increased FDG uptake in a subtle soft tissue mass (*arrow*) abutting the lateral abdominal wall. Biopsy of this region confirmed recurrent isolated disease

metastases and the presence of extrahepatic disease affect the prognosis. Surgical resection is the only curative therapy in these patients. Patients most suited to undergo liver resection are those with fewer than four lesions; smaller than 5 cm; and without extrahepatic disease [59]. Recurrence rates after resection of liver metastases are high and there is significant associated morbidity and mortality.

Pitfalls and Issues in Reporting PET-CT of Colorectal Cancer

Fashioning a concise and pertinent PET-CT report with regard to colorectal cancer patients firstly requires that a detailed and accurate clinical history be available. Relevant issues include the patient's preoperative or postoperative status, prior imaging and colonoscopic findings if any. The oncologist will want to know any finding that is pertinent to the patient's staging or restaging and any complication that might have resulted from the tumor or need intervention for such as abscess, venous thrombosis, bowel obstruction, or perforation or urinary tract obstruction. In addition to these general findings, the surgeon will also want to know of any specific factors that will influence any future operation including vascular relationships or specific complications of surgery. Relevant nonneoplastic findings should also be recorded. Pertinent negatives and positives should be detailed in the body of the report, and specific issues, conclusions, and recommendations stated in the impression.

In patients without a known history of colorectal carcinoma, it is important to be aware that the large bowel FDG uptake may be quite avid in the absence of pathology particu-

a

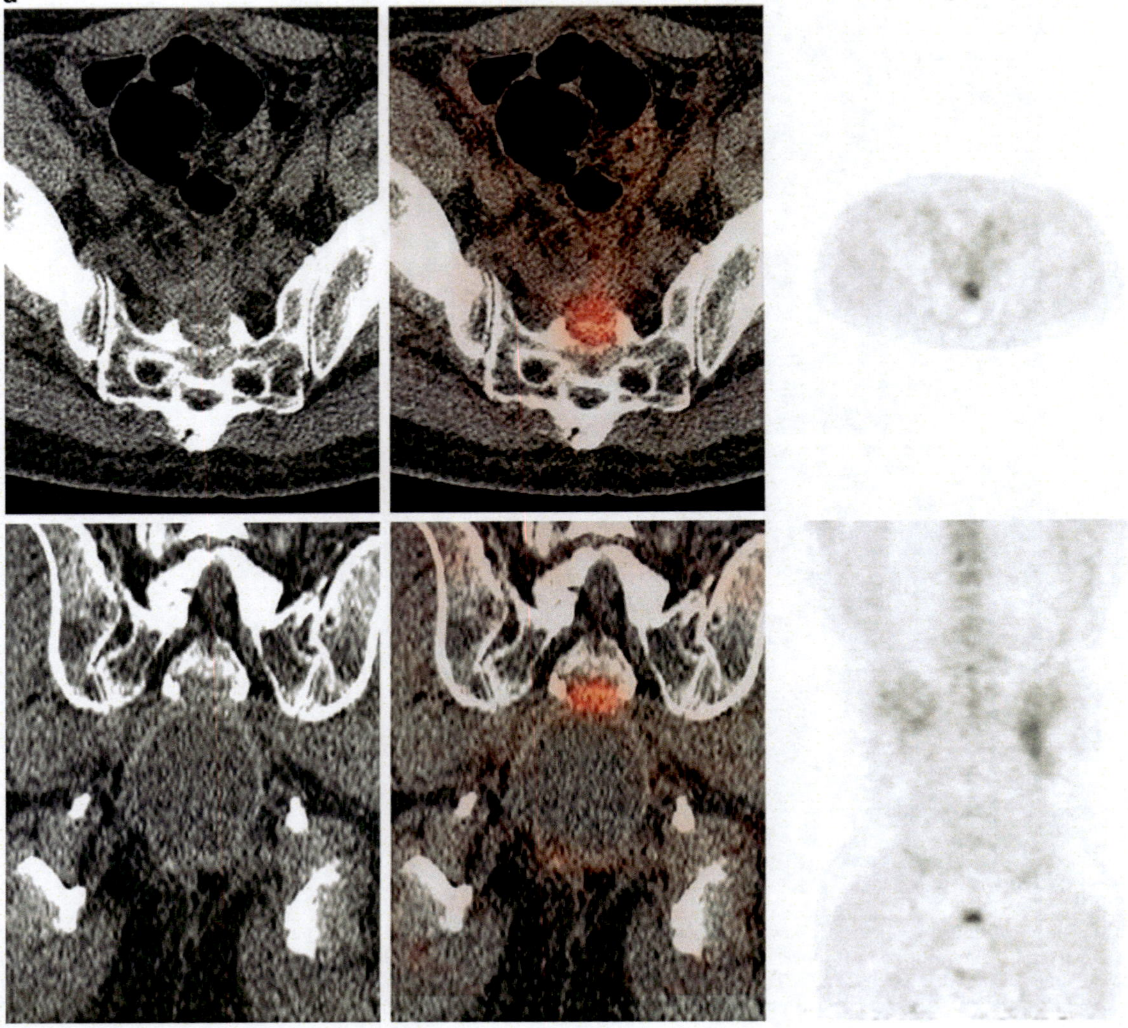

Fig. 21.8 Localized recurrence of rectal cancer. Composite axial (*upper row of images*) and coronal (*lower row of images*) CT (*left*), PET-CT fusion images (*center*), and PET images (*right*). Patient is 5 years post-abdominoperineal resection for recurrent adenocarcinoma of the rectum and despite persistently elevated CEA all previous CT examinations were reported as normal save for a presacral fluid collection. However, the PET-CT examination reveals increased FDG activity corresponding to a subtle enhancing soft tissue mass (*arrow*) in the presacral space (**a**), associated with erosion of the sacrum (**b**). Biopsy of the small soft tissue mass revealed adenocarcinoma

larly in the cecum/ascending colon and within the rectoanal region. Moreover, inflammatory conditions such as Crohn's disease, ulcerative colitis, typhlitis, and diverticulitis can all lead to increased colonic FDG activity (Fig. 21.10). However, regardless of etiology, focal large bowel activity greater than hepatic activity is unusual and should always alert the interpreting physician to the possible presence of pathology. A thorough regional review of the coregistered CT images is warranted to look for focal masses or neighboring signs of inflammation bearing in mind that peristalsis, patient motion, and breathing may lead to misregistration of the PET and CT images. A long segment of colon of diffusely increased FDG uptake should not be interpreted as inflammatory bowel disease unless there are CT findings of such as this finding is not uncommonly seen in normal colon on FDG PET. In the absence of specific corresponding CT findings, focal intense colonic activity on PET however certainly warrants further investigation such as colonoscopy.

False-Negative FDG-PET Findings

False-negative FDG PET findings have been reported with mucinous adenocarcinoma and for this and other diagnostic reasons standard evaluation of the entire colon on the CT interpretation is still required. Whiteford and coworkers [60] reported that the sensitivity of FDG-PET

b

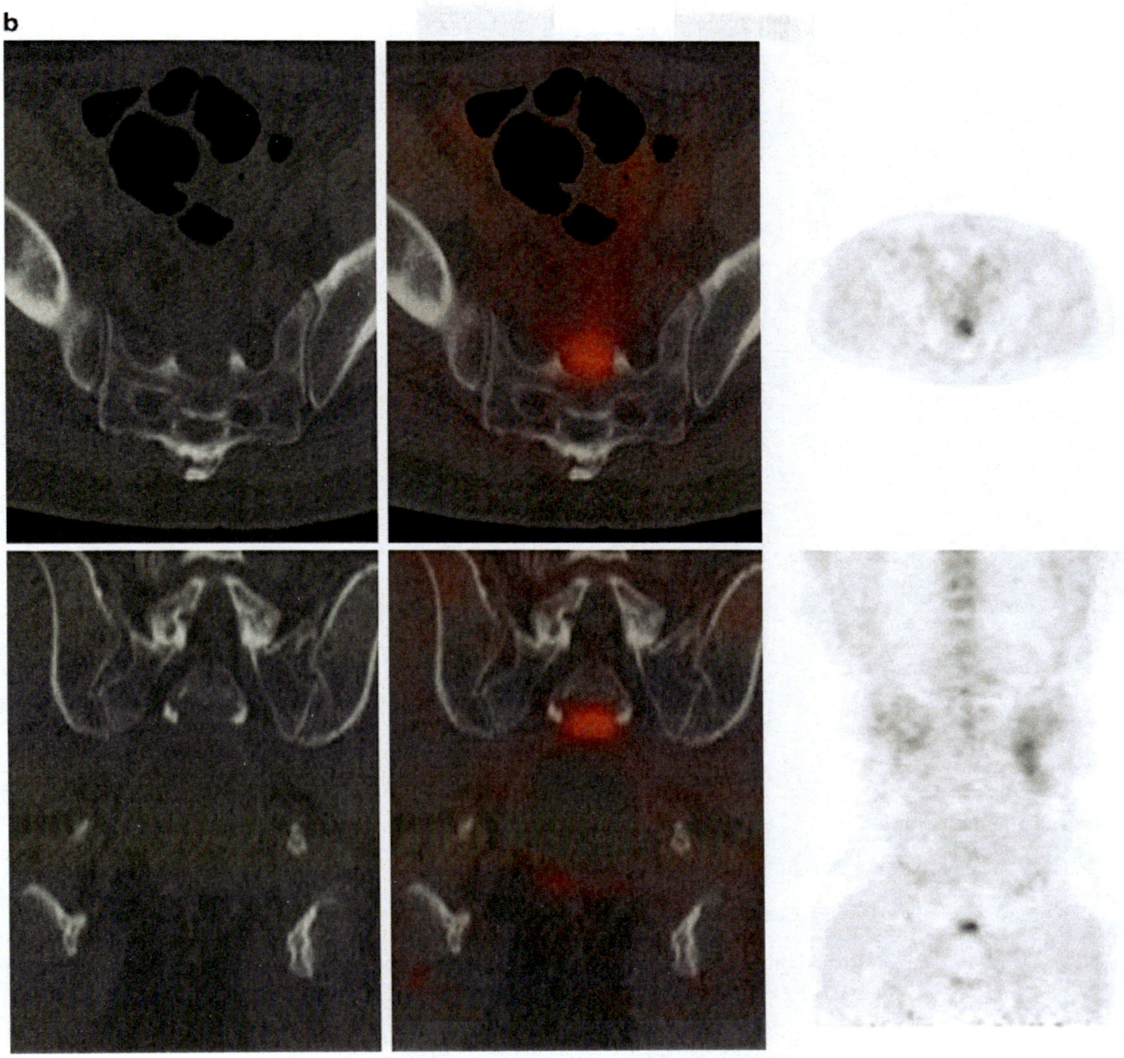

Fig. 21.8 (continued)

imaging for detection of mucinous adenocarcinoma is significantly lower than the nonmucinous adenocarcinoma (Fig. 21.11).

PET-CT readers should also be cognizant of the impact different degrees of rectal distention can have particularly on pelvic disease coregistration. Similarly caution must be exercised when interpreting liver metastases, as dome lesions can be erroneously projected in the lung base due to respiratory artifact.

False negative results on FDG PET are particularly common within 4 months of chemotherapy. This is thought to be due to chemotherapy induced cessation of metabolic activity resulting in apoptosis and cell death. A recent study of 224 patients with colorectal hepatic metastases demonstrated that FDG PET within 4 weeks of chemotherapy had a negative predictive value of 13% and a positive predictive value of 94% [1].

Fistulous tracts, sinus tracts, and abscess will typically be associated with intense abnormal FDG tracer uptake, and careful review of the CT images in important in the setting of abnormalities in the region of anastomoses of colon or rectum, and in general in the presacral region in the setting of treated rectal cancer. When a fistula is suspected or questioned, oral contrast becomes particularly important to differentiate neoplasm from physiologic inflammatory tracer uptake.

Therapy Monitoring with PET-CT

For colorectal cancers, PET-CT is now considered the standard of care both to detect recurrence, and monitor treatment response. FDG PET imaging has been used to monitor tumor

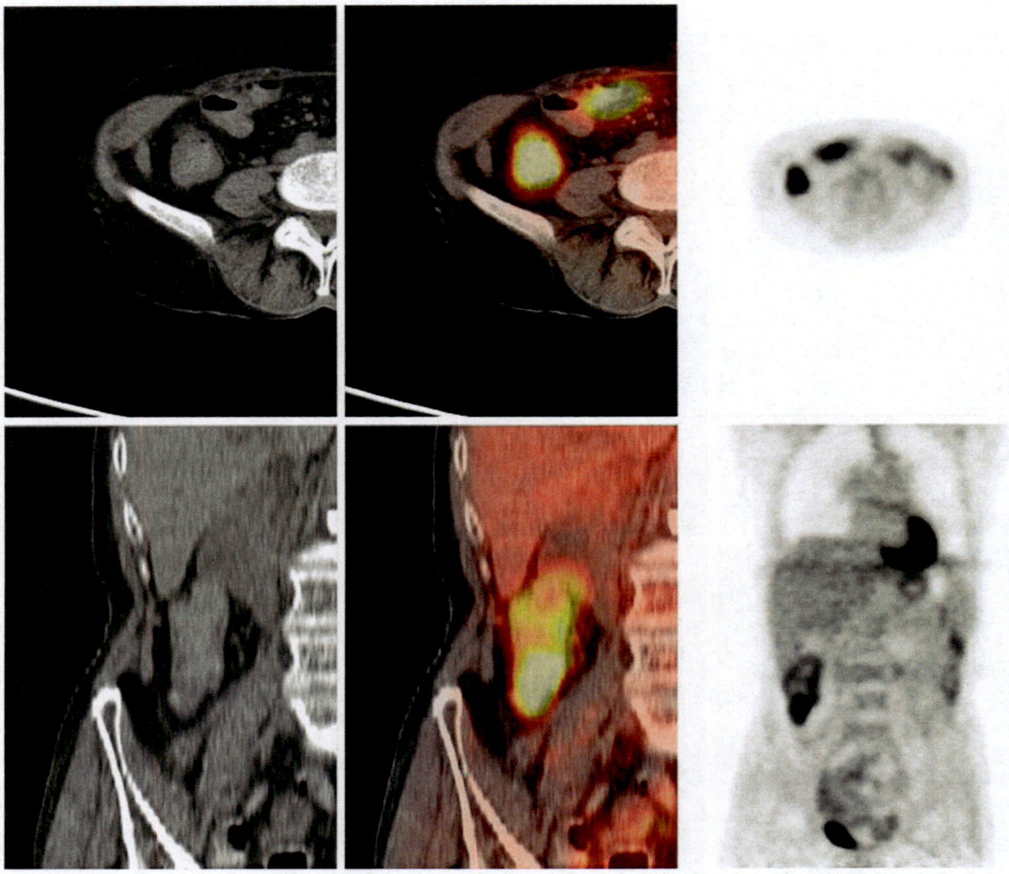

Fig. 21.10 False-positive FDG uptake in colon. Composite axial (*upper row of images*) and coronal (*lower row of images*) CT (*left*), PET-CT fusion images (*center*), and PET images (*right*). This PET-CT scan was performed in a 72-year-old woman for surveillance postresection of lung cancer. Intense FDG activity is noted in the cecum and ascending colon. However, the patient had a history of Crohn's disease. The clinical history and diffuse nature of the FDG uptake should suggest normal physiologic FDG uptake or inflammatory bowel disease in this instance

Fig. 21.11 False-negative FDG PET due to mucinous adenocarcinoma of the colon. Transaxial CT (**a**) and FDG PET (**b**) images show low attenuation lesions in the liver (arrows) on portal venous contrast enhanced CT images which are without clearly abnormal FDG tracer uptake

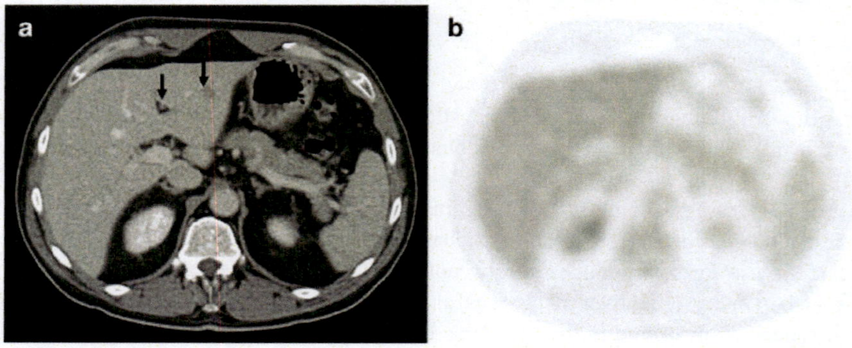

response following chemotherapy as well as radiation therapy [61, 62]. Complete resolution of abnormal glucose metabolism in primary and metastatic lesions of colon cancer can be observed following chemotherapy (Fig. 21.12). Studies have shown that FDG-PET can be used to predict response to chemotherapy and radiofrequency ablation in patients with hepatic metastases from colorectal cancer [63, 64]. However, many issues, including optimal time for imaging, criteria for response, and the decision-making and cost-effective benefits of PET-CT imaging for monitoring therapy response in patients with colorectal cancer have not yet been fully established.

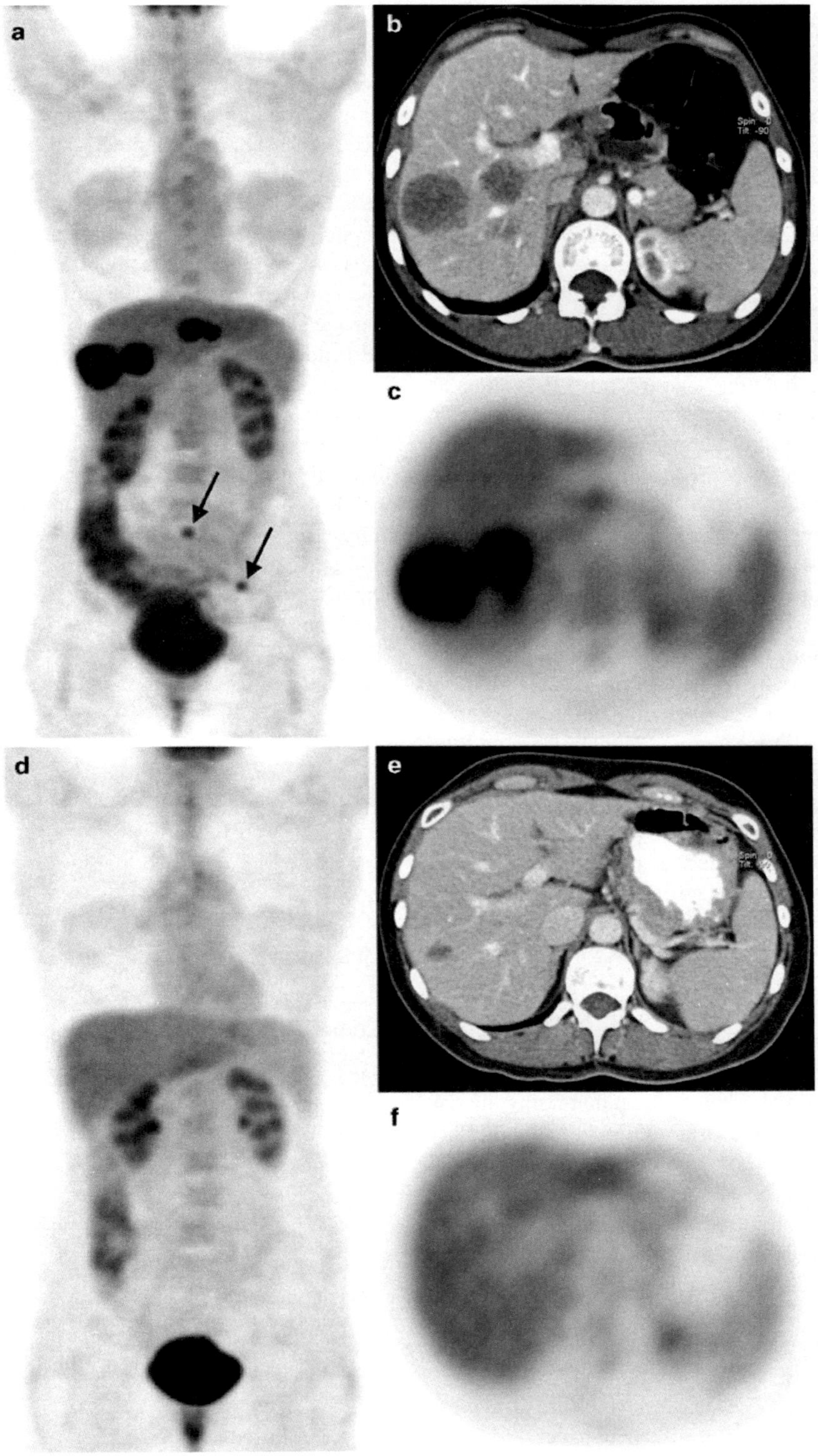

Fig. 21.12 Response of metastatic colorectal cancer to chemotherapy. Postsigmoid colon resection for moderately differentiated adenocarcinoma, but with hepatic and osseous metastases. (**a**) Pretherapy anterior FDG PET MIP demonstrate four hepatic metastases and a small isolated osseous metastasis at the left supraacetabular pelvis and the sacrum (arrows). Transaxial (**b**) and FDG PET (**c**) show two of the hepatic metastases are intensely FDG avid. Two months following eight cycles of chemotherapy, the anterior FDG PET MIP image (**d**) reveals complete resolution of the abnormal glucose metabolism in the liver and in the osseous pelvis. Transaxial CT (**e**) and FDG PET (**f**) images reveal only minimal residual low attenuation in the liver with no corresponding abnormal FDG tracer activity

Radiation Therapy Planning for Colorectal Cancer with PET-CT

Radiation along with surgery and chemotherapy is employed for patients with stage II and III rectal cancer. Radiation is associated with a reduced rate of local recurrence but also increases the risks of sexual dysfunction, postoperative mortality in older patients and perineal dehiscence [65]. Cross-sectional structural imaging techniques such as CT and MR imaging are the most common methods for planning of radiation therapy in patients with colorectal cancer. The structural imaging techniques provide anatomic delineation of tumor mass and adjacent structures as well as an estimation of tumor volume in three-dimensions. However, these techniques can be limited by several inabilities: First to differentiate a primary or recurrent malignant lesion from surrounding inflammatory changes or fibrosis; secondly to correctly represent time-averaged position and shape of the tumor for patient motion and finally to accurately take into account the metabolic and biologic features of cancer.

PET-CT imaging for radiation therapy planning has been found to be useful in patients with brain, lung, head, and neck, as well as pelvic cancers (including colorectal cancer) [66]. In this study, the influence of PET data from an integrated PET-CT system, in addition to the CT images for defining the gross tumor volume (GTV) and as a consequence the clinical tumor volume (CTV) and planning target volume (PTV), were investigated. Six patients with rectal cancer treated in a preoperative setting were included in the patient population. GTV increases were observed in three of six patients. The mean changes of the GTV were 50% (±22%), translating into a changes of the PTV of 20% (±8%). The impact of PET in volume definition for RT before surgery is on GTV, thereby improving on the rate of negative margins after surgery. PET-CT–based RT planning may allow minimized portal field sizes without increasing the risk of missing macroscopic tumor tissue adjacent to the primary tumor. The CT for RT planning is obtained in RT treatment position before surgery. The authors also conclude that PET-defined GTV is potentially useful for planning of the boost volume for adjuvant radiation therapy after tumor resection of rectal cancer, if PET-CT is obtained in RT position before surgery.

PET-CT imaging is useful to plan laser-induced thermotherapy for liver metastases from colorectal cancer [67]. Metastases with increased FDG uptake, which are difficult to localize on PET images alone, can be better identified with fused PET-CT image data. Detection of lesions not seen on CT images can facilitate in planning of laser-induced thermotherapy for liver metastases as well as in the identification of patients with extra-hepatic metastases, who may not profit from the procedure.

18F-FDG PET and PET-CT can provide added diagnostic information compared with conventional imaging in patients after radiofrequency ablation of liver metastases and can be useful in guiding repeat ablation procedures [68]. Areas of focal FDG accumulation greater than background activity in the region of the treated lesion are interpreted as being pathologic. On CT an irregular, hypoattenuated area around the margins of the ablated tumor that increases in size on follow-up scans is interpreted as residual tumor Donckier et al. [69] have reported that in 4 of 17 patients whose unresectable liver metastases were treated by RFA, FDG-PET at 1 week and 1 month showed peripheral hypermetabolic residue after RFA, whereas CT did not reveal the residual tumor. FDG-PET appears to accurately monitor the local efficacy of RFA for treatment of liver metastases, as it recognizes incomplete tumor ablation, earlier than detectable on CT. Langenhoff et al. [70] has reported a similar experience but we consider comparison of the PET findings with CT essential and preferably as part of a PET-CT examination. These studies and others support the use of FDG PET in combination with CT scan in the followup of RF ablated colorectal metastases and PET-CT may lead to earlier detection of tumor recurrence than conventional imaging modalities.

References

1. Jemal A, Siegel R, Ward E, et al. Cancer statistics, 2009. CA Cancer J Clin 2009;59:225–249.
2. Heald RJ. A new approach to rectal cancer. Br J Hosp Med 1979; 22:277–281.
3. Heald RJ. Total mesorectal excision is optimal surgery for rectal cancer: a Scandinavian consensus. Br J Surg 1995;82: 1297–1299.
4. Cameron JL. Current Surgical Therapy, 8th ed. Philadelphia: Elsevier Mosby, 2004.
5. Kapiteijn E, Marijnen CA, Nagtegaal ID, et al. Preoperative radiotherapy combined with total mesorectal excision for resectable rectal cancer. NEJM 2001;345:638–646.
6. Camma C, Giunta M, Fiorica F, Pagliaro L, Craxi A, Cottone M. Preoperative radiotherapy for resectable rectal cancer: a meta-analysis. JAMA 2000;284:1008–1015.
7. Anonymous Levamisole and fluorouracil for adjuvant therapy of resected colon carcinoma. NEJM 1990;323:197–198.
8. Moore HG, Guillem JG. Local therapy for rectal cancer. Surg Clin North Am 2002;82:967.
9. Agress H Jr, Cooper BZ. Detection of clinically unexpected malignant and premalignant tumors with whole-body FDG PET: histopathologic comparison. Radiology 2004;230:417–422.
10. Yasuda S, Fujii H, Nakahara T, et al. 18F-FDG PET detection of colonic adenomas. J Nucl Med 2001;42:989–992.
11. Pickhardt PJ, Choi JR, Hwang I, et al. Computed tomographic virtual colonoscopy to screen for colorectal neoplasia in asymptomatic adults. NEJM 2003;349:2191–2200.
12. Richter E, Feyerabend T, Bondorf W (eds.). Normal Lymph Node Topography: CT Atlas. New York: Springer, 2004.
13. Skibber JM, Minsky BD, Hoff PM. Spread of colorectal cancer. In: DeVita VT, Hellman S, Rosenberg SA (eds.). Cancer: principles

and practice of oncology. 6th ed. Philadelphia: Lippincott Williams & Wilkins, 2001:1229–1230.
14. Abdel-Nabi H, Doerr RJ, Lamonica DM, et al. Staging of primary colorectal carcinomas with fluorine-18 fluorodeoxyglucose whole-body PET: correlation with histopathologic and CT findings. Radiology 1998;206:755–760.
15. Mukai M, Sadahiro S, Yasuda S, et al. Preoperative evaluation by whole-body 18F-fluorodeoxyglucose positron emission tomography in patients with primary colorectal cancer. Oncol Rep 2000;7:85–87.
16. Bipat S, Glas AS, Slors FJ, Zwinderman AH, Bossuyt PM, Stoker J. Rectal cancer: local staging and assessment of lymph node involvement with endoluminal US, CT, and MR imaging – a meta-analysis. Radiology 2004;232:773–783.
17. Strasberg SM, Dehdashti F, Siegel BA, Drebin JA, Linehan D. Survival of patients evaluated by FDG-PET before hepatic resection for metastatic colorectal carcinoma: a prospective database study. Ann Surg 2001;233:293–299.
18. Valk PE, Abella-Columna E, Haseman MK, et al. Whole-body PET imaging with [18F]fluorodeoxyglucose in management of recurrent colorectal cancer. Arch Surg 1999;134:503–511; discussion 511–513.
19. Adam R. Chemotherapy and surgery: new perspectives on the treatment of unresectable liver metastases. Ann Oncol 2003;14(Suppl 2):ii13–6.
20. Tanaka K, Adam R, Shimada H, Azoulay D, Levi F, Bismuth H. Role of neoadjuvant chemotherapy in the treatment of multiple colorectal metastases to the liver. Br J Surg 2003;90:963–969.
21. Valls C, Andia E, Sanchez A, et al. Hepatic metastases from colorectal cancer: preoperative detection and assessment of resectability with helical CT. Radiology 2001;218:55–60.
22. Vitola JV, Delbeke D, Sandler MP, et al. Positron emission tomography to stage suspected metastatic colorectal carcinoma to the liver. Am J Surg 1996;171:21–26.
23. Imdahl A, Reinhardt MJ, Nitzsche EU, et al. Impact of 18F-FDG-positron emission tomography for decision making in colorectal cancer recurrences. Langenbecks Arch Surg 2000;385:129–134.
24. Boykin KN, Zibari GB, Lilien DL, McMillan RW, Aultman DF, McDonald JC. The use of FDG-positron emission tomography for the evaluation of colorectal metastases of the liver. Am Surg 1999;65:1183–1185.
25. Fong Y, Saldinger PF, Akhurst T, et al. Utility of 18F-FDG positron emission tomography scanning on selection of patients for resection of hepatic colorectal metastases. Am J Surg 1999;178:282–287.
26. Rohren EM, Paulson EK, Hagge R, et al. The role of F-18 FDG positron emission tomography in preoperative assessment of the liver in patients being considered for curative resection of hepatic metastases from colorectal cancer. Clin Nucl Med 2002;27:550–555.
27. Sahani DV, Kalva SP, Fischman AJ, et al. Detection of liver metastases from adenocarcinoma of the colon and pancreas: comparison of mangafodipir trisodium-enhanced liver MRI and whole-body FDG PET. AJR Am J Roentgenol 2005;185:239–246.
28. Huebner RH, Park KC, Shepherd JE, et al. A meta-analysis of the literature for whole-body FDG PET detection of recurrent colorectal cancer. J Nucl Med 2000;41:1177–1189.
29. Lai DT, Fulham M, Stephen MS, et al. The role of whole-body positron emission tomography with [18F]fluorodeoxyglucose in identifying operable colorectal cancer metastases to the liver. Arch Surg 1996;131:703–707.
30. Stumpe KD, Urbinelli M, Steinert HC, Glanzmann C, Buck A, von Schulthess GK. Whole-body positron emission tomography using fluorodeoxyglucose for staging of lymphoma: effectiveness and comparison with computed tomography. Eur J Nucl Med 1998;25:721–728.
31. McCormack PM, Attiyeh FF. Resected pulmonary metastases from colorectal cancer. Dis Colon Rectum 1979;22:553–556.
32. Goya T, Miyazawa N, Kondo H, Tsuchiya R, Naruke T, Suemasu K. Surgical resection of pulmonary metastases from colorectal cancer. 10-year follow-up. Cancer 1989;64:1418–1421.
33. Mori M, Tomoda H, Ishida T, et al. Surgical resection of pulmonary metastases from colorectal adenocarcinoma. Special reference to repeated pulmonary resections. Arch Surg 1991;126:1297–1301; discussion 1302.
34. Cahan WG, Castro EB, Hajdu SI. Therapeutic pulmonary resection of colonic carcinoma metastatic to lung. Dis Colon Rectum 1974;17:302–309.
35. Shaffer K. Role of radiology for imaging and biopsy of solitary pulmonary nodules. Chest 1999;116:519S–522S.
36. Franzius C, Daldrup-Link HE, Sciuk J, et al. FDG-PET for detection of pulmonary metastases from malignant primary bone tumors: comparison with spiral CT. Ann Oncol 2001;12:479–486.
37. Kanthan R, Loewy J, Kanthan SC. Skeletal metastases in colorectal carcinomas: a Saskatchewan profile. Dis Colon Rectum 1999; 42:1592–1597.
38. Sugawara Y, Fisher SJ, Zasadny KR, Kison PV, Baker LH, Wahl RL. Preclinical and clinical studies of bone marrow uptake of fluorine-1-fluorodeoxyglucose with or without granulocyte colony-stimulating factor during chemotherapy. J Clin Oncol 1998;16:173–180.
39. Even-Sapir E, Metser U, Flusser G, et al. Assessment of malignant skeletal disease: initial experience with 18F-fluoride PET/CT and comparison between 18F-fluoride PET and 18F-fluoride PET/CT. J Nucl Med 2004;45:272–278.
40. Turk PS, Wanebo HJ. Results of surgical treatment of nonhepatic recurrence of colorectal carcinoma. Cancer 1993;71:4267–4277.
41. Willett C, Tepper JE, Cohen A, Orlow E, Welch C, Donaldson G. Local failure following curative resection of colonic adenocarcinoma. Int J Radiat Oncol Biol Phys 1984;10:645–651.
42. Pilipshen SJ, Heilweil M, Quan SH, Sternberg SS, Enker WE. Patterns of pelvic recurrence following definitive resections of rectal cancer. Cancer 1984;53:1354–1362.
43. Obrand DI, Gordon PH. Incidence and patterns of recurrence following curative resection for colorectal carcinoma. Dis Colon Rectum 1997;40:15–24.
44. Brethauer SA, Magrino TJ, Riffenburgh RH, Johnstone PA. Management of recurrent colorectal carcinoma. Colorectal Dis 2002;4:246–253.
45. Goldberg RM, Fleming TR, Tangen CM, et al. Surgery for recurrent colon cancer: strategies for identifying resectable recurrence and success rates after resection. Eastern Cooperative Oncology Group, the North Central Cancer Treatment Group, and the Southwest Oncology Group. Ann Intern Med 1998;129:27–35.
46. Welch JP, Donaldson GA. Detection and treatment of recurrent cancer of the colon and rectum. Am J Surg 1978;135:505–511.
47. Dawson LE, Russell AH, Tong D, Wisbeck WM. Adenocarcinoma of the sigmoid colon: sites of initial dissemination and clinical patterns of recurrence following surgery alone. J Surg Oncol 1983; 22:95–99.
48. Minsky BD, Mies C, Rich TA, Recht A, Chaffey JT. Potentially curative surgery of colon cancer: the influence of blood vessel invasion. J Clin Oncol 1988;6:119–127.
49. Russell AH, Tong D, Dawson LE, Wisbeck W. Adenocarcinoma of the proximal colon. Sites of initial dissemination and patterns of recurrence following surgery alone. Cancer 1984;53:360–367.
50. Wood CB, Gillis CR, Blumgart LH. A retrospective study of the natural history of patients with liver metastases from colorectal cancer. Clin Oncol 1976;2:285–288.
51. Wagner JS, Adson MA, Van Heerden JA, Adson MH, Ilstrup DM. The natural history of hepatic metastases from colorectal cancer. A comparison with resective treatment. Ann Surg 1984;199:502–508.
52. Adson MA, van Heerden JA, Adson MH, Wagner JS, Ilstrup DM. Resection of hepatic metastases from colorectal cancer. Arch Surg 1984;119:647–651.
53. Fong Y, Cohen AM, Fortner JG, et al. Liver resection for colorectal metastases. J Clin Oncol 1997;15:938–946.

54. Scheele J, Stang R, Altendorf-Hofmann A, Paul M. Resection of colorectal liver metastases. World J Surg 1995;19:59–71.
55. Brister SJ, de Varennes B, Gordon PH, Sheiner NM, Pym J. Contemporary operative management of pulmonary metastases of colorectal origin. Dis Colon Rectum 1988;31:786–792.
56. Suzuki K, Dozois RR, Devine RM, et al. Curative reoperations for locally recurrent rectal cancer. Dis Colon Rectum 1996;39:730–736.
57. Wiggers T, de Vries MR, Veeze-Kuypers B. Surgery for local recurrence of rectal carcinoma. Dis Colon Rectum 1996;39:323–328.
58. Even-Sapir E, Parag Y, Lerman H, et al. Detection of recurrence in patients with rectal cancer: PET/CT after abdominoperineal or anterior resection. Radiology 2004;232:815–822.
59. Penna C, Nordlinger B. Colorectal metastasis (liver and lung). Surg Clin North Am 2002;82:1075–1090, x-xi.
60. Whiteford MH, Whiteford HM, Yee LF, et al. Usefulness of FDG-PET scan in the assessment of suspected metastatic or recurrent adenocarcinoma of the colon and rectum. Dis Colon Rectum 2000;43:759–767; discussion 767–70.
61. Haberkorn U, Strauss LG, Dimitrakopoulou A, et al. PET studies of fluorodeoxyglucose metabolism in patients with recurrent colorectal tumors receiving radiotherapy. J Nucl Med 1991;32:1485–1490.
62. Guillem JG, Puig-La Calle J, Jr, Akhurst T, et al. Prospective assessment of primary rectal cancer response to preoperative radiation and chemotherapy using 18-fluorodeoxyglucose positron emission tomography. Dis Colon Rectum 2000;43:18–24.
63. Findlay M, Young H, Cunningham D, et al. Noninvasive monitoring of tumor metabolism using fluorodeoxyglucose and positron emission tomography in colorectal cancer liver metastases: correlation with tumor response to fluorouracil. J Clin Oncol 1996;14:700–708.
64. Anderson GS, Brinkmann F, Soulen MC, Alavi A, Zhuang H. FDG positron emission tomography in the surveillance of hepatic tumors treated with radiofrequency ablation. Clin Nucl Med 2003;28: 192–197.
65. Janjan NA, Crane C, Feig BW, et al. Improved overall survival among responders to preoperative chemoradiation for locally advanced rectal cancer. Am J Clin Oncol 2001;24:107–112.
66. Ciernik IF, Dizendorf E, Baumert BG, et al. Radiation treatment planning with an integrated positron emission and computer tomography (PET/CT): a feasibility study. Int J Radiat Oncol Biol Phys 2003;57:853–863.
67. Hosten N, Kreissig R, Puls R, et al. Fusion of CT and PET data: methods and clinical relevance for planning laser-induced thermotherapy of liver metastases. Rofo 2000;172:630–635.
68. Barker DW, Zagoria RJ, Morton KA, Kavanagh PV, Shen P. Evaluation of liver metastases after radiofrequency ablation: utility of 18F-FDG PET and PET/CT. AJR Am J Roentgenol 2005;184:1096–1102.
69. Donckier V, Van Laethem JL, Goldman S, et al. F-18] fluorodeoxyglucose positron emission tomography as a tool for early recognition of incomplete tumor destruction after radiofrequency ablation for liver metastases. J Surg Oncol 2003;84:215–223.
70. Langenhoff BS, Oyen WJ, Jager GJ, et al. Efficacy of fluorine-18-deoxyglucose positron emission tomography in detecting tumor recurrence after local ablative therapy for liver metastases: a prospective study. J Clin Oncol 2002;20:4453–4458.

Suggested Reading

1. Jemal A, Siegel R, Ward E et al (2009) Cancer statistics, 2009. CA Cancer J Clin 59:225–249
2. . State Cancer Profiles (2007) Death rate report by state, death years through 2003. Available at: http://statecancerprofiles.cancer.gov. Accessed 5 October 2010
3. Gerard JP, Conroy T, Bonnetain F et al (2006) Preoperative radiotherapy with or without concurrent fluorouracil and leucovorin in T3-4 rectal cancers: results of FFCD 9203. J Clin Oncol 24:4620–4625
4. Bosset JF, Collette L, Calais G et al (2006) Chemotherapy with preoperative radiotherapy in rectal cancer. N Engl J Med 355: 1114–1123
5. Krook JE, Moertel CG, Gunderson LL et al (1991) Effective surgical adjuvant therapy for high-risk rectal carcinoma. N Engl J Med 324:709–715
6. Gomez D, Sangha VK, Morris-Stiff G, Malik HZ, Guthrie AJ, Toogood GJ, Lodge JP, Prasad KR (2010) Outcomes of intensive surveillance after resection of hepatic colorectal metastases. Br J Surg 97(10):1552–1560
7. Hur H, Ko YT, Min BS, Kim KS, Choi JS, Sohn SK, Cho CH, Ko HK, Lee JT, Kim NK (2009) Comparative study of resection and radiofrequency ablation in the treatment of solitary colorectal liver metastases. Am J Surg 197(6):728–736
8. Sabanli M, Balasingam A, Bailey W, Eglinton T, Hider P, Frizelle FA (2010) Computed tomographic colonography in the diagnosis of colorectal cancer. Br J Surg 97(8):1291–1294
9. Veit P, Kühle C, Beyer T, Kuehl H, Herborn CU, Börsch G, Stergar H, Barkhausen J, Bockisch A, Antoch G (2006) Whole body positron emission tomography/computed tomography (PET/CT) tumour staging with integrated PET/CT colonography: technical feasibility and first experiences in patients with colorectal cancer. Gut 55(1):68–73
10. Kalra MK, Maher MM, Toth TL, Schmidt B, Westerman BL, Morgan HT, Saini S (2004) Techniques and applications of automatic tube current modulation for CT. Radiology 233(3): 649–657
11. American Joint Committee on Cancer (2010) *The AJCC Cancer Staging Manual*, 7th edn. Springer Science+Business Media LLC, New York
12. Ono K, Ochiai R, Yoshida T, Kitagawa M, Omagari J, Kobayashi H, Yamashita Y (2009) Comparison of diffusion-weighted MRI and 2-[fluorine-18]-fluoro-2-deoxy-D-glucose positron emission tomography (FDG-PET) for detecting primary colorectal cancer and regional lymph node metastases. J Magn Reson Imaging 29(2):336–340
13. Garcia-Aguilar J, Pollack J, Lee SH et al (2002) Accuracy of endorectal ultrasonography in preoperative staging of rectal tumors. Dis Colon Rectum 45:10–15
14. MERCURY Study Group (2007) Extramural depth of tumor invasion at thin-section MR in patients with rectal cancer: results of the MERCURY study. Radiology 243:132Y9
15. Wolberink SV, Beets-Tan RG, de Haas-Kock DF, van de Jagt EJ, Span MM, Wiggers T (2009) Multislice CT as a primary screening tool for the prediction of an involved mesorectal fascia and distant metastases in primary rectal cancer: a multicenter study. Dis Colon Rectum 52(5):928–934
16. Davey K, Heriot AG, Mackay J, Drummond E, Hogg A, Ngan S, Milner AD, Hicks RJ (2008) The impact of 18-fluorodeoxyglucose positron emission tomography-computed tomography on the staging and management of primary rectal cancer. Dis Colon Rectum (7):997–1003
17. Metser U, You J, McSweeney S, Freeman M, Hendler A (2010) Assessment of tumor recurrence in patients with colorectal cancer and elevated carcinoembryonic antigen level: FDG PET/CT versus contrast-enhanced 64-MDCT of the chest and abdomen. Am J Roentgenol 194(3):766–771
18. Niekel MC, Bipat S, Stoker J (2010) Diagnostic imaging of colorectal liver metastases with CT, MR imaging, FDG PET, and/or FDG PET/CT: a meta-analysis of prospective studies including patients who have not previously undergone treatment. Radiology 9 Sep 2010 [Epub ahead of print]

19. Bar-Shalom R, Kagna O, Israel O, Guralnik L (2008) Noninvasive diagnosis of solitary pulmonary lesions in cancer patients based on 2-fluoro-2-deoxy-D-glucose avidity on positron emission tomography/computed tomography. Cancer 113(11):3213–3221
20. Lowe VJ, Fletcher JW, Gobar L et al (1998) Prospective investigation of positron emission tomography in lung nodules. J Clin Oncol 16:1075–1084
21. Werner MK, Parker JA, Kolodny GM, English JR, Palmer MR (2009) Respiratory gating enhances imaging of pulmonary nodules and measurement of tracer uptake in FDG PET/CT. Am J Roentgenol 193(6):1640–1645
22. Taira AV, Herfkens RJ, Gambhir SS, Quon A (2007) Detection of bone metastases: assessment of integrated FDG PET/CT imaging. Radiology 243(1):204–211
23. Glazer ES, Beaty K, Abdalla EK, Vauthey JN, Curley SA (2010) Effectiveness of positron emission tomography for predicting chemotherapy response in colorectal cancer liver metastases. Arch Surg 145(4):340–345
24. Kuehl H, Antoch G, Stergar H, Veit-Haibach P, Rosenbaum-Krumme S, Vogt F, Frilling A, Barkhausen J, Bockisch A (2008) Comparison of FDG-PET, PET/CT and MRI for follow-up of colorectal liver metastases treated with radiofrequency ablation: initial results. Eur J Radiol 67(2):362–371
25. Coenegrachts K, De Geeter F, ter Beek L, Walgraeve N, Bipat S, Stoker J, Rigauts H (2009) Comparison of MRI (including SS SE-EPI and SPIO-enhanced MRI) and FDG-PET/CT for the detection of colorectal liver metastases. Eur Radiol 19(2): 370–379

Chapter 22
PET-CT Imaging of Lymphoma

Lale Kostakoglu

Effective combination therapy protocols can produce prolonged disease-free and overall survival in the majority of patients with Hodgkin's disease (HD) and certain subtypes of non-Hodgkin's lymphoma (NHL). Even in patients with advanced-stage HD and aggressive NHL, complete remission can be achieved in up to 75% of patients at first presentation with proper management [1, 2]. Accurate risk factor profiling using staging and established predictors of outcome, including gene profiting as well as effective restaging and response evaluation during or following therapy are prerequisites in the determination of optimal treatment. This may also lead to selection of a proper subset of patients in whom radiation therapy (RT) could be avoided. Anatomic imaging modalities such as computed tomography (CT) lack the ability to identify lymphoma in normal size lymph nodes and are unable to differentiate nodes which are enlarged due to other therapy-related benign causes [3]. Similar to CT, magnetic resonance imaging (MRI) findings are not specific for viable tumor and cannot differentiate active lymphoma from infectious or inflammatory processes including radiation fibrosis [4, 5]. Ga-67 scintigraphy, despite its proven prognostic value as a predictor of therapy response during or after therapy, suffers from low spatial resolution, lack of specificity, low sensitivity in infradiaphragmatic lesions, and low-grade lymphoma [6, 7]. Ga-67 scintigraphy has now largely been superseded by positron emission tomography imaging using [F-18]fluorodeoxyglucose (FDG PET).

FDG PET has become an integral part of the initial staging and response evaluation algorithm for lymphoma, providing vital information regarding tumor biology and metabolism. There is now convincing evidence that FDG PET is a more accurate imaging modality in the staging and evaluation of treatment response in lymphomas compared to conventional imaging techniques [8–20], including both CT and Ga-67 scintigraphy. Furthermore, persistent FDG uptake during and after chemotherapy has proven highly sensitive and specific in the differentiation of residual viable disease from benign posttherapy changes. This superior feature can potentially alter patient management and outcome by identifying the subset of patients requiring additional therapy or a change in treatment regimen. The accuracy of FDG PET imaging has significantly improved with the recent introduction of combined modality PET-CT [19]. PET-CT provides a comprehensive examination that combines morphologic diagnosis and functional/metabolic information in the same imaging session [21].

This chapter summarizes the data on the proven and potential utility of FDG PET imaging in combination with CT at staging, restaging, and predicting response to therapy as well as the current limitations of this combined imaging modality in patients with lymphoma.

Pathologic and Clinical Classification of Lymphomas

The current lymphoma classification system is based on both morphologic and biologic characteristics of lymphomas. The Revised European-American Classification of Lymphoid Neoplasms (REAL) system was developed in 1994 to incorporate morphology, clinical features, immunophenotype and cytogenetics [22]. The World Health Organization (WHO) classification subsequently updated the REAL system with minor modifications [23]. This integrated system – WHO/REAL classification – is currently in clinical use for both HD and NHL [24]. Despite the complexity and diversity of this integrated system, lymphomas are traditionally subdivided into two broad categories: Hodgkin's disease (HD) and non-Hodgkin's lymphomas (NHL). Also for practical purposes NHL can be classified into indolent (low-grade) and aggressive lymphomas. NHL accounts for more than 85% of the lymphomas. Aggressive lymphomas constitute approximately 60% of NHL series, while indolent lymphomas account for approximately 40% of new diagnoses. The vast majority of NHL (~90%) are of B-cell origin. Early stage lymphoma is

L. Kostakoglu (✉)
Section of Nuclear Medicine, Department of Radiology, Mt. Sinai Medical Center, New York, NY 10029, USA
e-mail: lale.kostakoglu@mountsinai.org

P. Shreve and D.W. Townsend (eds.), *Clinical PET-CT in Radiology: Integrated Imaging in Oncology*,
DOI 10.1007/978-0-387-48902-5_22, © Springer Science+Business Media, LLC 2011

curable in greater than 75% of patients; however, advanced stage disease is curable in only 50% of patients [25].

HD accounts for 10–15% of lymphomas and composed of two different entities, classical HD representing 95% of cases, and nodular lymphocyte-predominant HD that makes up 5% of cases. Classical HD is further subdivided into nodular sclerosis (accounts for 65–80% of all cases), mixed cellularity, lymphocyte rich, and lymphocyte depletion types. With polychemotherapy the cure rate for HD is greater than 80% of patients with first-line therapy. Patients with nodular lymphocyte-predominant HD, usually present with isolated peripheral lymph node involvement. These patients have a clinical course resembling NHL with an indolent growth pattern with single and multiple relapses as well as late relapses. Diffuse large cell lymphoma, most common type of aggressive NHL, sometimes occurs concurrently or subsequently in patients with nodular lymphocyte-predominant HD with a cumulative risk of 9% at 10 years [26].

Staging of Lymphomas

The TNM (tumor, node, metastasis) system is not applicable in lymphomas because usually the specific origin of tumor is not clearly identified. The Ann Arbor staging system remains the most widely used staging system which was introduced for HD and a modified version of this system is adopted for the use in NHL (Table 22.1) [27, 28]. There are basically four stages of lymphomas as demonstrated in Table 22.1. Subscript suffixes are affixed to any stage for more detailed staging. The constitutional symptoms (B) (Fever higher than 100.5°F, night sweats, and weight loss) and bulky disease (X) (tumor >10 cm) portend worse prognosis for each stage of HD. The subscript is "E" denotes extranodal disease contiguous or proximal to the known nodal site: Stages I and IIA are considered early-stage disease although up to 35% of patients with early-stage HD have occult abdominal nodal or splenic involvement [29]. Stages IIB (particularly bulky), III, and IV are considered advanced-stage disease.

Table 22.1 Ann Arbor staging system of lymphomas

Stage I
Involvement of a single lymph node region or involvement of a single extralymphatic organ
Stage II
Involvement of two or more lymph node regions on the same side of the diaphragm or localized involvement of an extralymphatic organ or site plus an involved lymph node region on the same side of the diaphragm
Stage III
Involvement of lymph nodes involved on both sides of the diaphragm can be accompanied by extralymphatic organ involvement including the spleen
Stage IV
Diffuse or disseminated involvement of one or more extralymphatic organs with or without associated lymph node involvement
The presence or absence of the following symptoms should be noted with each stage designation
A = asymptomatic
B = fever, sweats, or weight loss greater than 10% of body weight

Staging Workup of Lymphomas

Recommended procedures for a thorough staging workup include medical history and physical examination, laboratory procedures (complete blood cell count with differential, peripheral blood smear, lactate dehydrogenase, β_2 microglobulin, serum protein electrophoresis, sedimentation rate, and blood chemistries), bone marrow biopsy in patients with B symptoms and advanced stage disease. The imaging studies typically include chest radiograph, chest, abdomen, and pelvis CT, and may also involve ultrasonography, endoscopy, and MRI, and lately whole-body FDG PET. Ga-67 SPECT imaging can still be used, although it has been replaced by FDG PET imaging in most centers. Other studies, including organ biopsy and CSF sampling, are considered in certain clinical situations.

Role of Imaging in Management of Lymphoma

Aggressive NHL and HD

At initial staging, an accurate and objective imaging modality is of particular importance in guiding therapeutic approach, especially the use of radiation therapy (RT). Although staging is clinically important, studies of immunophenotype and molecular genetics are essential to refine diagnosis and management, particularly in NHL. Until recently, extended field RT has been considered the standard treatment for early stage HD. There is, however, an increasing trend to employ chemotherapy and most groups adopted a strategy using short duration chemotherapy combined with involved field RT (restricted to involved lymph nodes) in this group of patients [30]. Advanced stage (stages III–IV) disease is invariably treated with multiple chemotherapy protocols. Thus, staging still holds its critical position in the management of lymphoma even with the latest changes in therapeutic approach. In patients with HD or aggressive NHL (mostly DLCL), the therapy objective is the complete eradication of disease while minimizing adverse short- or long-term complications of therapy, particularly related to the RT. Unnecessary use of RT could result in excess toxicity such as secondary malignancies and cardiac disease, while appropriate use can potentially decrease risk of disease recurrence and allow for shorter courses of chemotherapy cycles attendant reduction of chemotherapy toxicity [31]. Hence, segregating patients who could achieve cure without the need of RT is an important management strategy involving imaging.

Perhaps the most clinically relevant issue surrounding aggressive NHL and HD is the ability to perform prognostic determination. FDG PET findings can be an independent predictor of tumor response or complementary to the established prognostic factors; international prognostic index in NHL and international prognostic score in HD, and potentially contribute to, or single-handedly, direct a change in management. For this concept to be of practical value, however, alternative treatment options should be available and also establishment of prognosis as favorable or poor must be followed up with a treatment change that is necessary and sufficiently effective to improve outcomes.

Mantle Cell Lymphoma

Mantle cell lymphoma is a rare and distinct entity of lymphomas which accounts for 5–10% of all lymphoma cases. Patients usually present with advanced stage disease (Ann Arbor stages II and IV) with generalized lymphadenopathy and extranodal involvement (90%) (BM, liver spleen GIT) similar to other indolent lymphomas. The prognosis is invariably poor, however, due to aggressive and progressive clinical course with no curative conventional therapy generally available. Imaging for staging purposes does not have major influence on management due to disseminated nature of disease; however, evaluation of therapy response is important for potential therapeutic alterations. PET-CT may have a niche in the posttherapy period for evaluating residual masses and therapy response. Nonetheless, in the absence of effective alternative therapy options, the role for imaging in the management of mantle cell lymphoma is relatively limited.

Indolent (Low-Grade) NHL

Low-grade lymphomas are incurable with current treatment modalities. The treatment in indolent lymphomas is defined by clinical symptoms rather than disease extent; therefore, determination of extent of disease or therapy response may not lead to improved outcomes. With current therapeutic strategies, identification of additional disease sites using PET-CT in the staging of indolent NHL is not an important determinant of management, as 80–90% of patients initially present with advanced-stage disease with generalized nodal and extranodal disease (mainly BM) involvement. New approaches combining classical dose-intense chemotherapy with "tumor-specific" antibody targeting may lead to a survival benefit [32], potentially increasing the role of imaging in the management of low-grade NHL. Nonetheless, imaging currently has a limited role in the management of indolent lymphoma owing to specific features of the disease. A characteristic of indolent lymphomas is the phenomenon of spontaneous regression. Such spontaneous regression is usually partial and short-lived, and imaging findings can help determine the disease status which may prompt therapy during the active course of disease. Other characteristics of indolent lymphomas include synchronous discordant lymphomas (20–30% of newly diagnosed patients) and transformation to an aggressive subtype (30–50%) during the first 10 years following diagnosis [33]. In these situations, PET-CT has a definite role to determine the sites of discordant lymphomas as well as transformation for biopsy guidance and subsequent effective management.

PET-CT for Diagnosis and Staging of Lymphoma

The diagnosis of lymphoma requires adequate tissue for histopathologic diagnosis, and imaging can direct the site of biopsy when such is not clinically obvious. Accurate initial staging of patients with lymphoma can be crucial for determining treatment strategy, including the use of RT. Advanced-stage HD or NHL is treated with combination chemotherapy. Early-stage HD patients (stage I and II) are generally divided into favorable or unfavorable groups based on prognostic factors. The patients in the favorable group are managed with treatment reduction strategies; the patients in the unfavorable group are managed with combined modality therapy.

Traditionally the imaging modality of choice for the diagnosis and staging of lymphoma has been CT, in some instances accompanied by sonography or endoscopy. MRI is a competitive anatomic imaging technique which can provide images of the abdomen of somewhat comparable diagnostic quality with the advent of faster acquisition sequences, particularly the turbo spin-echo (TSA) or fast spin-echo sequences. Additionally, MRI offers advantages including better tissue discrimination, lack of ionizing radiation and use of contrast agents with less risk of systemic effects [34–36]. Nevertheless, the diagnostic accuracy of both CT and MRI depends largely on lymph node enlargement and multiplicity. Thus, false-negative results occur in normal size lymph nodes that harbor lymphoma and lymph nodes that are enlarged due to reactive changes can give rise to false-positive findings.

FDG PET as a metabolic imaging modality and more recently PET-CT as a combined morphologic and metabolic

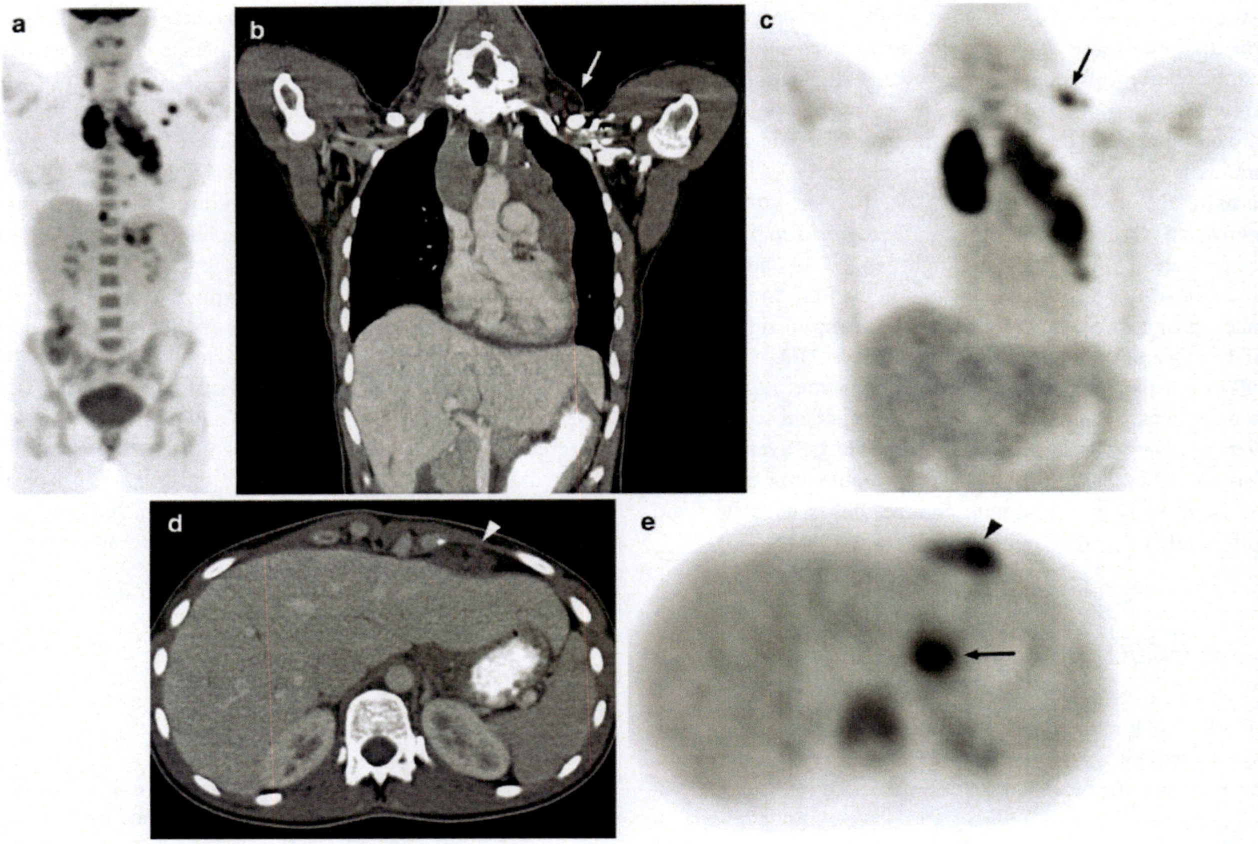

Fig. 22.1 Hodgkin's lymphoma on left supraclavicular lymph node biopsy. Anterior FDG PET (**a**) maximum intensity projection image (MIP) shows mediastinal FDG uptake as well as small foci in the left axilla, left supraclavicular fossa, and in the upper abdomen. Coronal contrast enhanced CT (**b**) and FDG PET (**c**) images demonstrate the confluent bulky intensely FDG avid mediastinal soft tissue and a 1.2-cm FDG avid left supraclavicular lymph node (*arrow*). Transaxial contrast-enhanced CT (**d**) and FDG PET (**e**) images demonstrate an FDG avid 1.3-cm lymph node just below the gastroesophageal junction (*arrow*) and FDG avid nodal mass at the anterior cardiophrenic sulcus (*arrowhead*). The cardiophrenic nodal involvement is still considered above the diaphragm disease; however the gastrohepatic ligament node involvement, not readily apparent on CT images alone, is below the diaphragm and renders the patient stage III

modality has been integrated into the diagnostic algorithm of staging for both HD and NHL. The findings of FDG PET are usually concordant with those of CT at initial staging, even though, PET detects additional tumor sites and also can upstage or downstage disease in some patients (Fig. 22.1) [10–12]. One should also realize, however, that although the additional information derived from an imaging modality can upstage or downstage disease, the findings may not lead to management changes unless early stage disease is upstaged to advanced stage disease or vice versa.

Nodal Lymphoma

HD and NHL have different presentations both in the chest and abdomen, including different morphologic and metabolic features (Tables 22.2 and 22.3). Lymph node involvement is a central feature of diseases.

CT in Nodal Lymphoma

At initial staging, CT is usually performed with oral and intravenous contrast and in the follow-up evaluation is performed without the use of intravenous contrast at some centers. Most mediastinal lymph nodes can be detected without intravenous contrast, but are more reliably measured on contrast enhanced scans. Inclusion of the neck in the CT or MRI evaluation yields a more accurate staging as lymphoma, particularly with HD, which accounts for 10% of the head and neck tumors. When lymphoma involves cervical lymph nodes they can be either enlarged or numerous. In general cervical, axillary, and mediastinal lymph nodes are considered abnormal when their

Table 22.2 PET-CT imaging features of Hodgkin's disease

Lymphoma type	General characteristics and PET-CT findings
Classical HD	• Contiguous involvement along lymph node regions • Initial disease located in the chest in ≥70% • Superior mediastinal LN's involved in the most of patients (>90%) • Coronal scans are useful in defining mediastinal disease • Bulky mediastinal HD defined as tumor mass greater than one third of intrathoracic diameter at T5–T6 • Bulky mediastinal HD is denoted as "X" in staging, associated with worse prognosis • Bulky mediastinal disease has to be specifically reported for a proper management • Isolated lung involvement does not occur in the absence of mediastinal disease • Pulmonary and chest wall involvement is often the result of direct extension • Posterior mediastinal involvement is usually associated with infradiaphragmatic disease • Pleural effusions usually occur with bulky disease • In the abdomen, HD is mostly located in upper abdomen and retroperitoneal LNs • PET is particularly important in evaluating the abdomen as LN enlargement may not occur in retroperitoneal nodal compartment • Majority of recurrences occur within 2 years of completion of therapy • Patients treated with combination of chemo and RT are at a higher risk of developing secondary tumors including leukemia, NHL, solid tumors
Lymphocyte-predominant Hodgkin's disease	• Involvement of mediastinum and hilar regions is not as common as in classical HD • Skip areas are more common compared to contiguous pattern seen with classical HD • Recurrences are usually late, development of NHL is more common than classical HD

LN lymph node, *RT* radiation therapy

Table 22.3 PET-CT imaging features of non-Hodgkin's lymphoma

Lymphoma type	General characteristics and PET-CT findings
Aggressive	• PET-CT defines the lung parenchyma for excluding involvement in patients with lower mediastinal and hilar lymphoma • Disease distribution is more even in the involved parts of the body compared to HD • Pulmonary lymphoma is a part of advanced stage disease • In the abdomen, disease can be at any LN station including mesenteric LNs • Mesenteric LN involvement is usually associated with encasement of the vessels • In abdominal disease, LNs are almost always enlarged unlike HD • Majority of recurrences occur within 2 years of completion of therapy • In evaluating Waldeyer's ring PET should be accompanied with contrast CT or MRI, as physiologic uptake in lymphatic tissues especially in tonsils may be prominent • Lymphoma in Waldeyer's ring is with cervical LN involvement in 50% of patients • Salivary gland involvement is invariably the result of systemic disease • Lymphoma of the thyroid gland presents as a thyroid nodule and usually affects women with Hashimoto's thyroiditis
Indolent Follicular	• Low-grade FDG uptake in multiple LN stations, both in supradiaphragmatic and infradiaphragmatic sites • Hilar and mediastinal LNs are often involved but large mediastinal masses are rare • Heterogenous uptake with at times focal lesions in the BM suggests BM involvement • Lesions with FDG uptake in the liver, spleen indicate lymphoma involvement • Hepatosplenomegaly is diffuse rather than with discrete lesions • During waxing and waning periods FDG uptake may disappear and reappear in various sites
CLL/SLL	• Low-grade to undetectable FDG uptake in massively enlarged LNs in a widespread fashion • Hepatosplenomegaly is diffuse rather than with discrete lesions
Marginal zone/MALT	• Primary pulmonary lymphoma is often of MALT type NHL • MALT lesions if positive on initial staging should be followed by PET-CT after treatment of H. pylori with antibiotics if applicable
Mantle cell	• Heterogenous uptake with at times focal lesions in the BM suggests BM involvement • Extranodal involvement of the liver and GIT is not rare

BM bone marrow, *CLL/SLL* chronic lymphocytic leukemia/small lymphocytic lymphoma, *GIT* gastrointestinal tract, *LN* lymph nodes

short axis diameter exceeds 10 mm. This size criterion of 6 mm has been advocated for prevascular, internal mammary, posterior mediastinal, and anterior diaphragmatic lymph nodes [37].

In patients with HD, thoracic disease, mediastinal nodes, particularly those in the superior mediastinal location, is more frequently involved (≥85%), while intrathoracic lymphoma in NHL is an extension of widespread disease process (Tables 22.2 and 22.3). Mediastinal HD is characterized by the presence of a discrete anterior superior mediastinal mass with surface lobulation due to involvement and coalescence of multiple lymph nodes (Fig. 22.2), while characteristic features of mediastinal aggressive NHL, mainly diffuse large cell type, included regular contour and absence of associated cervical and abdominal lymphadenopathy [38]. In general, extranodal involvement of the lung parenchyma, pleura, and pericardium is more common with NHL than with HD because of the frequent vascular invasion and hematogenous spread associated with the former [39]. Although CT and MRI are equally sensitive in the evaluation of mediastinal involvement, CT is usually preferred for its availability and relatively lower cost. MRI is spared for patients with iodine allergies and poor renal function. CT plays a significant role for recognizing bulky mediastinal HD as these patients have worse prognosis due to higher risk of disease recurrence compared to those with nonbulky disease. Bulky disease is defined as a mediastinal mass exceeding one third of the chest diameter or greater than 10 cm in diameter.

In the abdomen, lymph node enlargement of greater than 10 mm, most often retroperitoneal, are generally considered pathologic. It should be noted that with HD, retroperitoneal lymph nodes may be involved without enlargement compromising the sensitivity of CT scans with a reported false-negative rate of 20–80% [40]. With NHL, bulky and usually confluent retroperitoneal lymph node involvement is more common (Fig. 22.3) and mesenteric disease is seen in approximately 50% of the patients, unlike in HD (~15%) [36]. Lymph node calcification at initial presentation is very rare. MRI with a T2-weighted TSE sequence is considered equivalent to multidetector helical CT and represents an alternative morphologic method of examination in abdominal lymphoma [35].

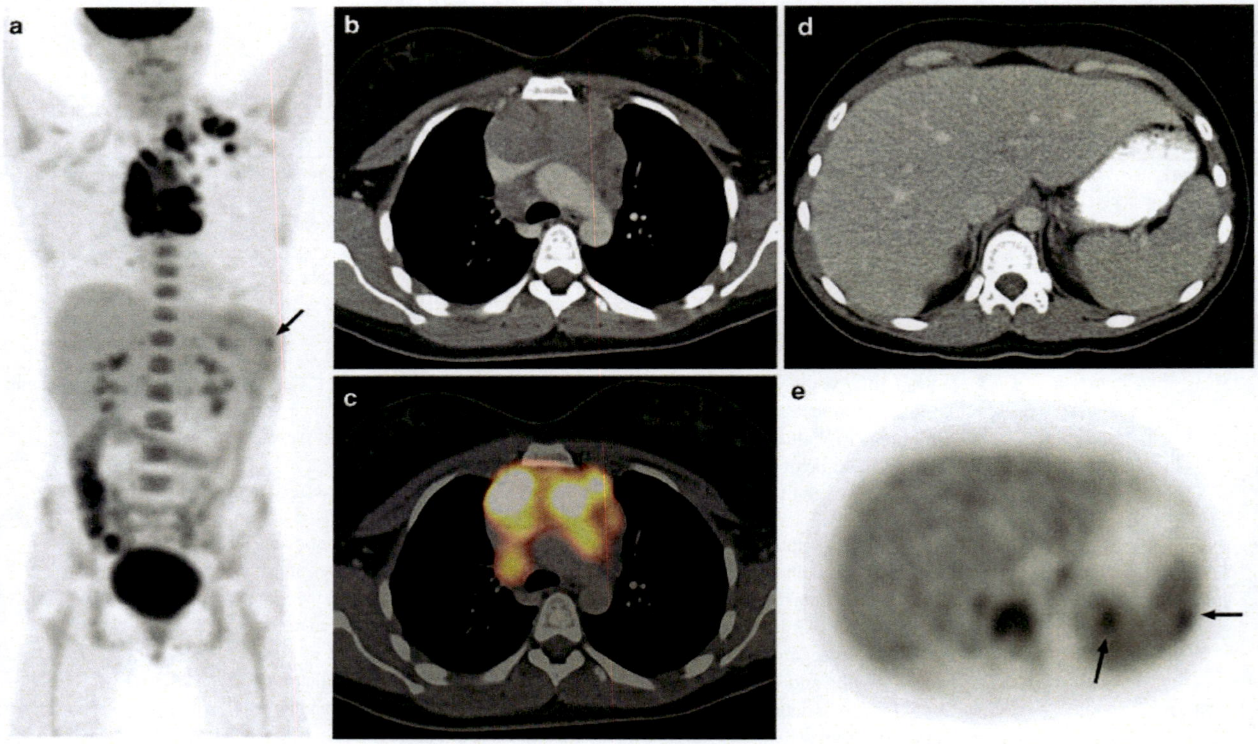

Fig. 22.2 Nodular sclerosing Hodgkin's lymphoma. Anterior FDG PET MIP image (**a**) shows bulky mediastinal disease and left supraclavicular lymph node involvement. Transaxial contrast-enhanced CT (**b**) and FDG PET-CT fusion (**c**) images of the chest reveal surface lobulation of the mediastinal mass due to coalescence of enlarging lymph nodes as typically seen with Hodgkin's lymphoma. Transaxial contrast enhanced CT (**d**) and FDG PET (**e**) images of the abdomen demonstrate two small foci of FDG tracer uptake in the spleen (*arrows*), only seen as subtle findings on the FDG PET MIP image, and without corresponding abnormality on the portal venous phase contrast enhanced CT images, corresponding to splenic involvement, rendering the patient stage III

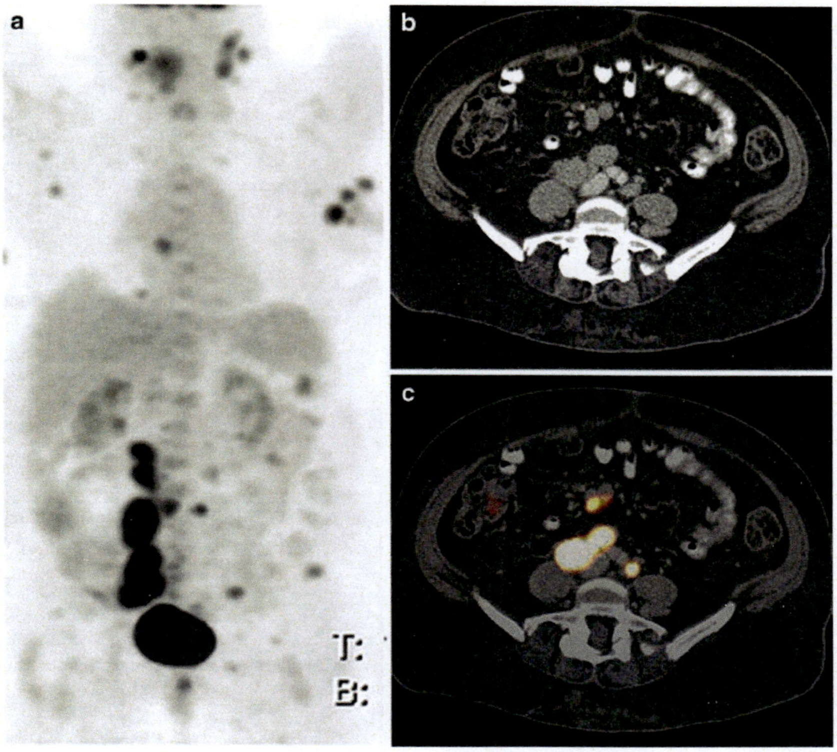

Fig. 22.3 Non-Hodgkin's lymphoma. Anterior FDG PET MIP image (**a**) shows multiple foci of widely distributed nodal disease including lymph node involvement in cervical, axillary, mediastinal, mesenteric, and retroperitoneal nodal basins. Unlike classic Hodgkin's lymphoma, disease is not centripetally extending from a dominant focus. Transaxial contrast enhanced CT (**b**) and FDG PET-CT fusion (**c**) images reveal enlarged FDG avid right common iliac lymph nodes and nonenlarged FDG avid left common iliac and mesenteric lymph nodes. Aside from the right iliac lymphadenopathy, the involved lymph nodes elsewhere are, at most, borderline enlarged, and thus largely diagnosed as disease involvement based on the abnormal FDG tracer uptake depicted on the FDG PET images

FDG PET in Nodal Lymphoma

Although FDG accumulates in the majority of lymphomas, because of the differences in immunophenotype and cytogenetics, glucose utilization may vary as evidenced by FDG uptake characteristics among various subtypes (Table 22.4). In a review of 172 patients, FDG PET detected disease in at least one site in 94% of patients, including 100% of patients with aggressive NHL (diffuse large cell lymphoma) and 98% of patients with HD. In contrast, FDG PET detected disease in only 67% of marginal zone and 40% of peripheral T-cell lymphoma [41]. Our experience has been in line with these findings with regard to sensitivity of FDG PET in different subtypes of lymphoma.

The lower typical FDG tracer uptake in certain indolent lymphomas diminishes the sensitivity advantage of FDG PET images relative to conventional morphologic criteria such as used by CT. Nonetheless, several studies have reported a potential role for FDG PET in staging low-grade NHL, particularly follicular cell and nodal marginal zone lymphoma [8, 11, 14, 20, 42, 43]. In contrast to marginal zone lymphoma, however, FDG PET is considerably less reliable in the detection of extranodal marginal zone lymphoma of mucosa-associated lymphoid tissue (MALT) where FDG tracer uptake in involved lymph nodes is usually very low to undetectable (Fig. 22.4) [43, 44]. These differences support other recent data suggesting that nodal and extranodal marginal zone lymphomas may be distinctive entities rather than nodal lymphoma being a more advanced stage of MALT [45].

Small lymphocytic subtype (SLL) is also typically associated with low to undetectable FDG tracer uptake in involved lymph nodes resulting in diminished sensitivity relative to CT [42]. SLL and chronic lymphocytic leukemia (CLL) are closely related and in WHO classification wherein SLL is considered as the tissue infiltrate of CLL; this disease is referred to as CLL/SLL. In this entity, the most consistent clinical finding is diffuse lymphadenopathy and the corresponding FDG PET finding is varying degrees (usually low to undetectable) of FDG uptake (Fig. 22.5). A diminished sensitivity for small lymphocytic lymphomas is interestingly seen with Ga-67 imaging as well [46].

Mantle cell lymphoma is a rare type subentity of lymphoma associated with aggressive clinical behavior, but with

Table 22.4 FDG PET imaging in subtypes (REAL/WHO classification) of lymphomas

Subtype	Clinical course	FDG uptake patterns
HD		
Classical HD (most common)	Aggressive	High FDG uptake ≥95% positive
Lymphocyte-predominance HD	Aggressive	FDG uptake may be < classical HD
NHL		
DLCL (most common)	Aggressive	High FDG uptake ≥95% positive
Follicular (second most common)	Low-grade	Moderate to low FDG uptake ≤90% positive
Transformed follicular	Aggressive	High FDG uptake ≥95% positive
Small lymphocytic lymphoma/chronic *Lymphocytic leukemia (CLL/SLL)*	Low-grade	Low to undetectable FDG uptake 60–70% positive
Extranodal Marginal zone/MALT	Low-grade	Varies from low-to-undetectable to high ≤70% positive
Nodal Marginal Zone	Low-grade	High FDG uptake ≥95%
Burkitt's	Aggressive	High FDG uptake ≥95% positive
T/natural killer cell	Aggressive	High FDG uptake ≥95% positive
Peripheral T-cell	Aggressive	Low-to-undetectable FDG uptake ≤50%
Mantle cell	Aggressive	High-to-moderate FDG uptake ≥90% positive
CNS lymphoma	Aggressive	High FDG uptake (> adjacent gray matter) ≥95% positive

Bone marrow involvement may not be reliably assessed by PET imaging; however, FDG PET is highly reliable in primary or bone involvement of advanced stage disease.

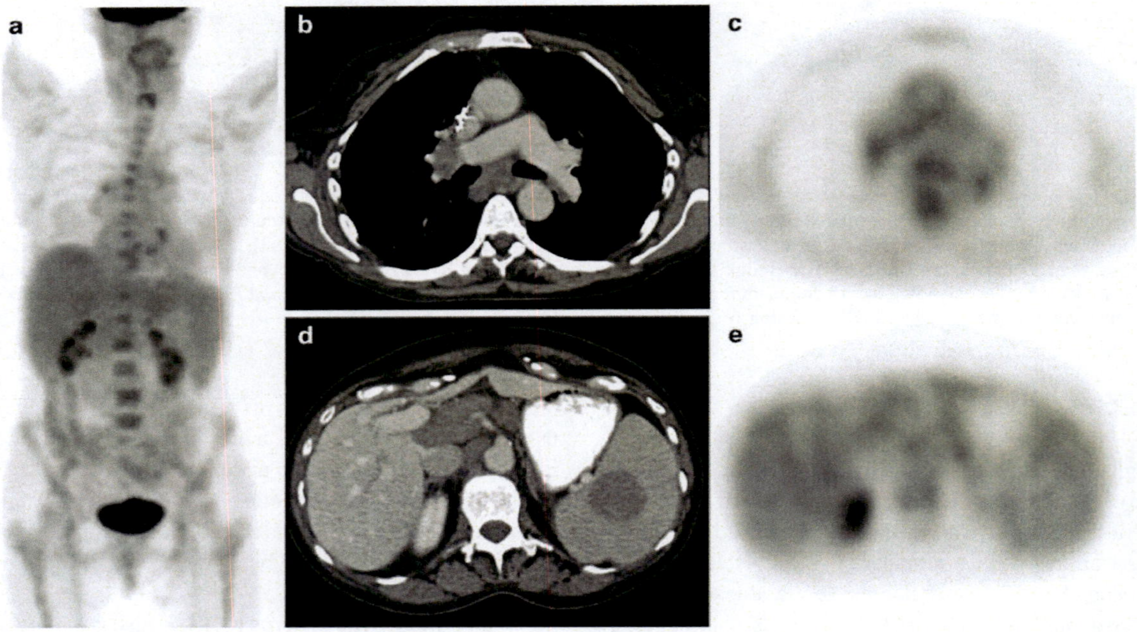

Fig. 22.4 Non-Hodgkin's lymphoma on left axillary lymph node biopsy, found consistent with marginal zone of mucosa associated lymphoid tissue (MALT). Anterior FDG PET MIP image (**a**) shows no appreciable abnormal FDG tracer uptake on the whole torso image. Transaxial contrast enhanced CT; (**b**) and FDG PET (**c**) images reveal subcarinal and right hilar lymphadenopathy which is associated with no abnormal FDG tracer uptake. Transaxial contrast-enhanced CT (**d**) and FDG PET (**e**) images of the upper abdomen reveal bulky para celiac and porta hepatic lymphadenopathy as well as a large mass in the spleen, none of which is associated with appreciable abnormal FDG tracer uptake

molecular features of low-grade lymphomas. The diagnostic sensitivity of FDG PET for mantle cell lymphoma is high, reported to be 90–100% [43, 47]. In this subtype FDG uptake characteristics are more or less similar to that seen in follicular low-grade lymphoma. Also in this patient population, one should be mindful of extranodal involvement, which is found in approximately 90% of patients and may involve unusual areas such as skin, GIT, breast, and lung (Fig. 22.6).

On initial staging the CT and FDG PET findings will be in agreement for the majority of cases, although the FDG PET images have been reported to manifest additional disease sites in about 10–28% of patients with aggressive NHL or HD (10–17). Overall, FDG PET is more sensitive and specific than CT in identifying lymphoma involved lymph nodes, except in the case of indolent lymphomas, which demonstrate low level or absent FDG tracer uptake [9, 48–52]. In general, FDG

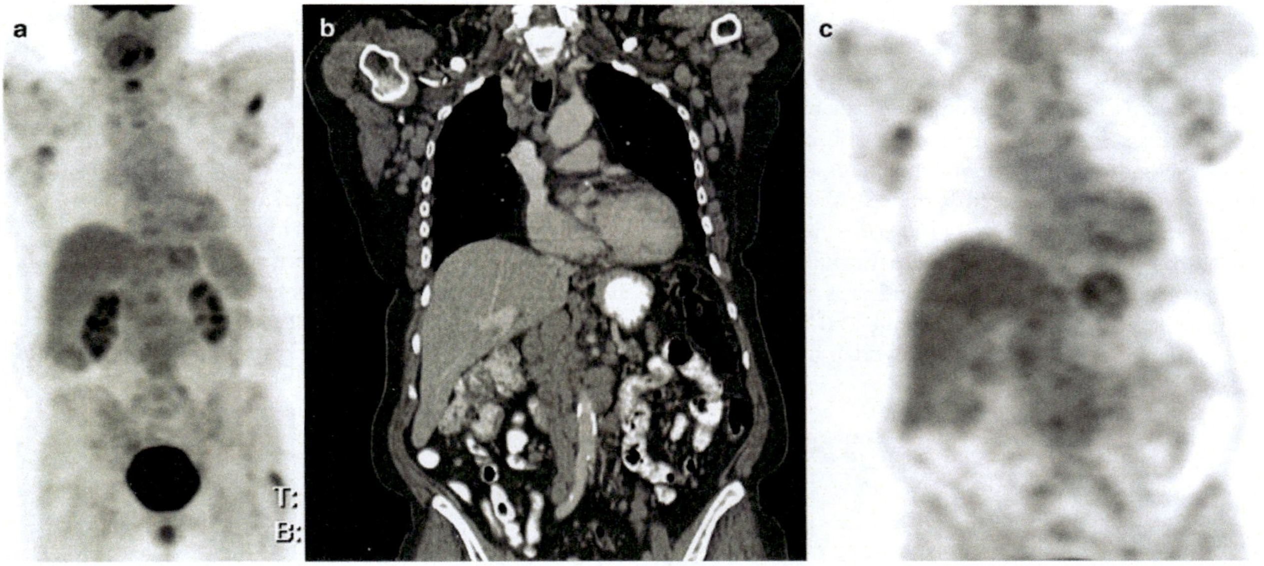

Fig. 22.5 Non-Hodgkin's lymphoma, small lymphocyte subtype. Patient with history of chronic lymphocytic leukemia presenting with axillary lymphadenopathy. Anterior FDG PET MIP image (**a**) shows only faint FDG tracer uptake in the bulky axillary lymphadenopathy and subtle increased FDG tracer activity in the bulky retroperitoneal lymphadenopathy. Coronal contrast-enhanced CT (**b**) and FDG PET (**c**) images demonstrate the extensive discrete enlarged retroperitoneal and axially lymph nodes with very little associated FDG tracer uptake

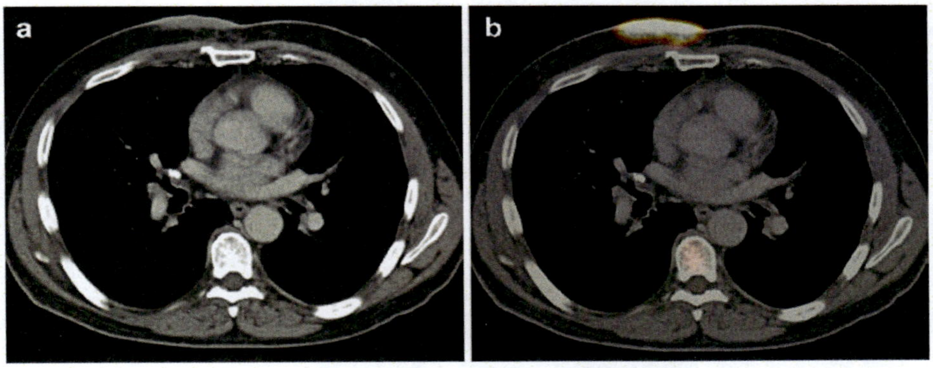

Fig. 22.6 Cutaneous involvement of non-Hodgkin's lymphoma (mantle cell lymphoma). Transaxial contrast-enhanced CT (**a**) and FDG PET-CT fusion image (**b**) demonstrates intense FDG tracer uptake by the soft tissue centered in the skin over the right anterior chest. Such extranodal involvement is commonly seen with mantle cell lymphoma and can also include gastrointestinal tract, breast, and lung

PET has been superior to CT alone in the detection of nodal disease except in the abdomen and pelvis, in which the two methods have produced equivalent results. However, combined PET-CT systems can improve the sensitivity and specificity of the FDG PET image further, particularly in the neck, abdomen and pelvis. In a small study of 19 patients with nodal disease (either HD or aggressive NHL) evaluated by both PET-CT and separately acquired contrast enhanced CT studies [53], PET-CT demonstrated additional lesions in four patients which were not detected on contrast-enhanced CT, while contrast-enhanced CT did not depict any nodal involvement that was undetectable on PET-CT [53]. As noted, however, when the lymphoma subtype is one with characteristically low or absent FDG tracer uptake, such as MALT, CLL/SLL, peripheral T cell, and low-grade follicular lymphoma, the CT findings based on lymph node size will be the chief criterion for nodal involvement.

Regarding size criteria for abnormal lymph nodes, in a study comparing one-, two-, and three-dimensional measurements of nodal involvement in lymphoma, there were no significant differences in staging between the three groups, although three-dimensional methods were most accurate and reproducible [54]. Regarding FDG PET criteria for abnormal lymph nodes, tracer uptake greater than mediastinal background activity is considered abnormal, with tracer uptake greater than liver tracer activity definitely abnormal. By semiquantitative measurement of standardized uptake value (SUV), this has generally corresponded to SUV measured values greater than 2–2.5 in the earlier literature. It should be noted that due to rapid changes in scanner design, image acquisition protocols, and image reconstruction methods, measured uptake values referred to as SUVs are no longer reliably comparable.

Differences in FDG tracer uptake observed between aggressive and indolent lymphoma expressed semiquantitatively by SUVs have been reported; SUV = 11.8 ± 4.7 for aggressive lymphomas and SUV = 6.4 ± 5.3 for indolent lymphomas [8, 11, 14, 20]. Our experience has been such that the mean SUVs are 4.5 ± 2.0 (range, 1.5–9.5) in indolent lymphomas and 12.5 ± 5.5 (range, 3.0–36) in aggressive lymphomas with a significant overlap in small lesions (unpublished data). Segregating SUVs into two distinct categories for the differentiation of aggressive and indolent lymphomas may be accurate for majority of cases, but not for all due to the high and low outliers for both groups. Also one of the inherent problems is the inaccurate SUV measurements in small tumors and the need for specification of standardization parameters.

In cases of transformation to a more aggressive subtype of lymphoma FDG uptake characteristics may help identify an area of high-grade transformation in indolent disease and thereby influence management (Fig. 22.7). While the capability of FDG PET has not been prospectively assessed for

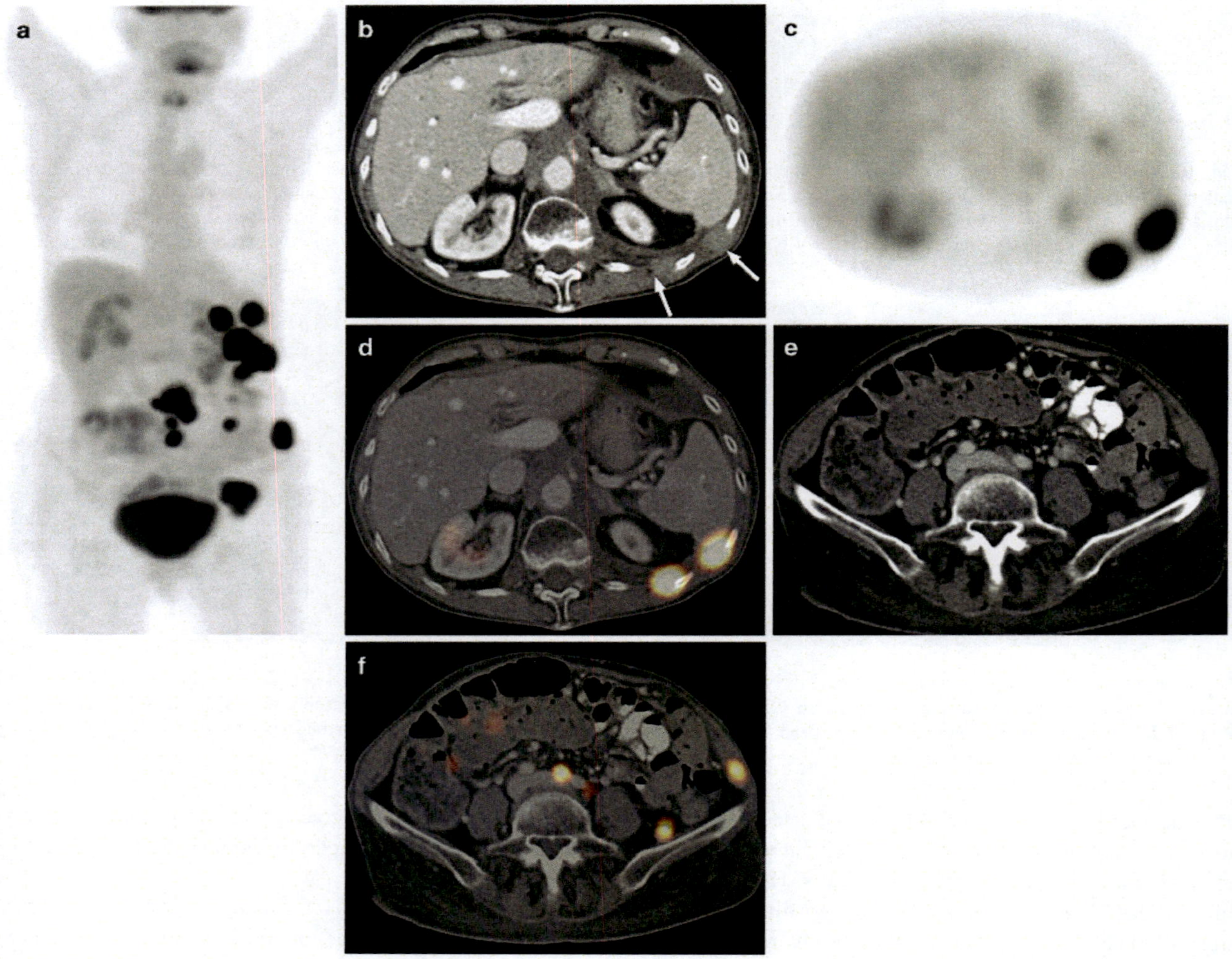

Fig. 22.7 Transformation to high grade lymphoma. Patient with original diagnosis of low grade follicular lymphoma treated 15 years prior, now presents with left sided abdominal pain. Anterior FDG PET MIP image (**a**) reveals intense foci of FDG tracer uptake in the abdomen and pelvis, not in an entirely nodal distribution. Transaxial contrast-enhanced CT (**b**), FDG PET (**c**), and FDG PET-CT fusion (**d**) images reveal the residual retroperitoneal soft tissue from the original lymphoma encasing the aorta is without any FDG tracer uptake, but enhancing soft tissue nodules (*arrows*) are seen in the lower posterior chest wall musculature that are intensely FDG avid. Transaxial contrast enhanced CT (**e**) and FDG PET-CT (**f**) fusion images at the level of the pelvis reveal both lymph node involvement and extranodal involvement in the abdominal wall musculature. Such recurrent disease presenting with extranodal involvement will typically be of higher grade than the original disease and requires biopsy for histopathological classification of the new disease. PET-CT findings identify sites of high-grade transformation most suitable for biopsy

this purpose, based on the disparate SUVs between high- and low-grade lymphomas, FDG PET may offer clinically valuable information by directing biopsy to the sites with highest FDG tracer uptake relative to other sites of disease involvement.

Extranodal Lymphoma

The exact definition of extranodal lymphoma remains controversial, but generally extranodal definition indicates presentation outside lymph node areas (i.e., extranodal lesion is the presenting site and constitutes the predominant disease bulk). Extranodal NHL can arise in any organ and encompasses a heterogeneous group of disease presentations. The most common extranodal sites include: central nervous system (CNS), gastrointestinal tract (GIT), especially stomach, Waldeyer's ring (palatine and lingual tonsils/tongue base, nasopharyngeal lymphoid tissue), liver, spleen, bone, and bone marrow (BM). HD usually involves extranodal sites by direct invasion from nodal sites. The therapeutic strategy in patients with primary extranodal lymphomas is in general analogous to that of nodal lymphomas. In stage I and II disease local therapy is administered, however, detection of occult distant disease necessitates the use of chemotherapy. In state III or IV disease the mainstay of treatment is chemotherapy.

CT and MRI in Extranodal Lymphoma

In the head and neck, the most common site for extranodal lymphoma involvement is the Waldeyer's ring (Fig. 22.8). Lymphoma of the head and neck cannot be distinguished from squamous cell cancer although necrosis is more common in the latter and calcification is rare with lymphoma. This is followed by sinus, nasal cavity, nodal sites, salivary glands (mostly parotid), and orbit. Almost 50% of extranodal head and neck lymphoma is associated with nodal disease. Patients with Waldeyer's ring involvement have a slightly worse prognosis [55].

The gastrointestinal tract can be involved by primary NHL or by extension of nodal or adjacent organ involvement of NHL or HD (Fig. 22.9). The most common site is the

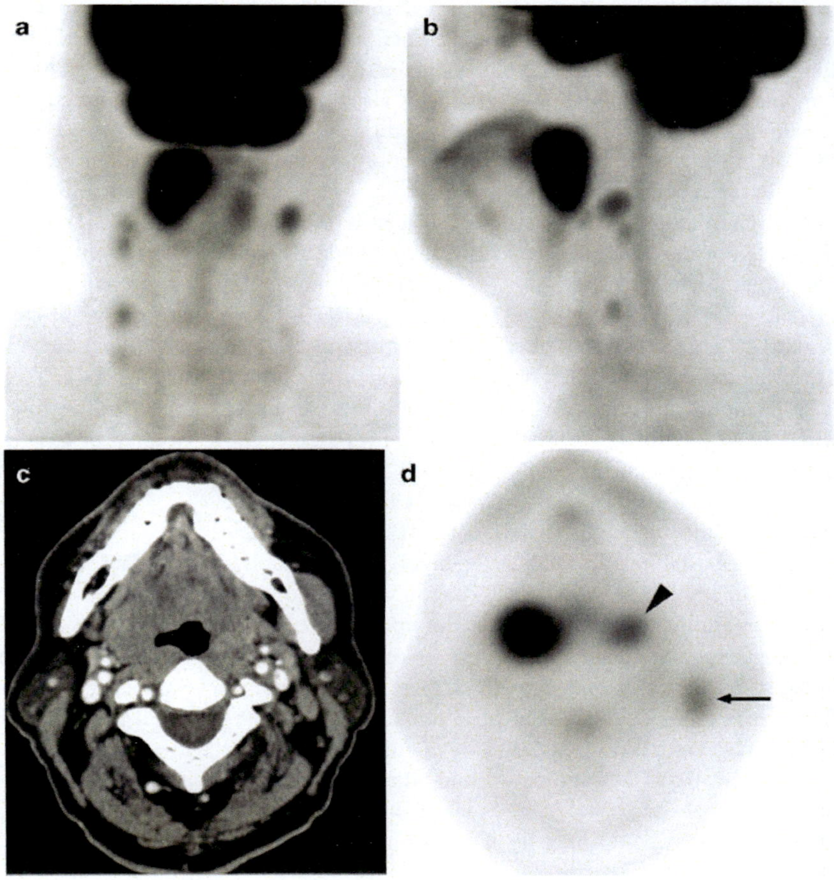

Fig. 22.8 Extranodal lymphoma involving Waldeyer's ring in the neck. Anterior (**a**) and lateral (**b**) FDG PET MIP images reveal intense FDG tracer uptake in the right parapharyngeal region with moderately low level physiologic FDG tracer activity seen elsewhere in Waldeyer's ring. Low level FDG tracer uptake is seen in cervical lymph nodes as well. On the transaxial contrast-enhanced CT image (**c**) the mass in the right palatine tonsil is discernable by nonenhancing asymmetric soft tissue which is intensely FDG avid on the corresponding FDG PET image (**d**) normal physiologic FDG tracer activity in the left palatine tonsil is seen (*arrowhead*), as well as low level tracer activity in a left level II cervical lymph node (*small arrow*) due to unrelated benign inflammatory response

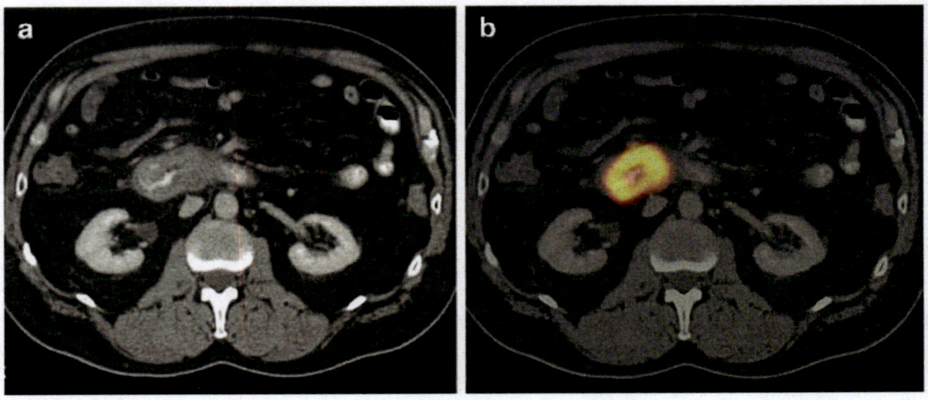

Fig. 22.9 High-grade diffuse B cell lymphoma involving small bowel. Transaxial contrast enhanced CT (**a**) and FDG PET-CT fusion (**b**) images demonstrate extensive soft tissue thickening of a segment of duodenum that is associated with intense abnormal FDG tracer uptake. Lymphomatous involvement of bowel typically is extensive before obstructive symptoms occur

stomach accounting for 50% of the gastrointestinal tract lymphoma presentations. Generally gastric lymphoma cannot be differentiated from gastric carcinoma, although luminal obstruction is uncommon with lymphoma due to lack of fibrous tissue response [56]. Low-grade primary gastric NHL of the MALT type is a common gastrointestinal tract lymphoma and there is a connection between this type of lymphoma with *Helicobacter pylori* infection [57]. In the small intestine, aneurysmal dilatation may be seen due to transmural extension of lymphoma, but differentiation from other malignant processes is not easy unless it is associated with bulky lymphadenopathy. The most common site for small intestinal lymphoma is the ileum; however, it may also involve the proximal jejunum particularly in association with celiac disease [58]. Colonic involvement is not common, but may occur in the cecum and rectum.

Lymphomatous involvement can be seen in the BM or the cortex of the bone. Bone and BM involvement is more common in NHL (especially in low-grade lymphoma) than in HD and confers stage IV disease. MRI is more sensitive than biopsy in detecting BM infiltration due to sampling errors associated with biopsy. It is becoming now feasible to routinely assess the entire marrow using MRI; however, in the follow-up period, persistent post-therapy MRI abnormalities may give rise to false positive results [59]. Cortical bone involvement can be primary or secondary, the former is usually of NHL type. Primary bone lymphoma has a tendency to involve the metaphyseal regions of the appendicular skeleton while secondary bone lymphoma usually involves the spine. In patients with bone involvement by direct extension from adjacent nodal disease, as it happens in HD, stage does not change. Bone involvement of HD is more often sclerotic (~50%) and NHL is osteolytic (~80%). This condition is denoted as "E." In patients with both BM and adjacent soft tissue involvement, MRI is preferred over CT; however, assessment of cortical bone integrity is performed with CT for better definition of disease.

Primary CNS lymphoma, which is exclusively of the NHL type (>80% B cell), is more frequently seen in immunocompromised patients, including patients with AIDS and those with prior organ transplantation; however, it can also occur in immunocompetent patients [60]. CT and MRI generally provide findings that are suggestive but not conclusive for CNS lymphoma [61]. The most frequent locations are supratentorial brain, including cerebral hemispheres, corpus callosum, basal ganglia, and rarely cerebellum and spinal cord [62]. Although MR perfusion imaging has been reported to distinguish between AIDS-associated CNS lymphoma and toxoplasmosis, imaging characteristics can be similar in both, and accurate differentiation between these two diseases still remains challenging.

The spleen is more frequently involved with lymphoma than is the liver. Approximately 30% of patients with either NHL or HD have splenic involvement while only up to 9% patients with HD and 14% patients with NHL have hepatic involvement [63]. The liver involvement is rare without the association of splenic lymphoma. In about one third of the time lymphoma involvement can be seen in normal size spleens [64]. CT can detect splenic lesions only when there are focal macroscopic lesions or substantial splenomegaly. Nodular disease is usually associated with aggressive NHL and diffuse disease with low-grade NHL [65].

FDG PET in Extranodal Lymphoma

A multitude of studies have reported that FDG PET may provide more information about the extent of disease in cases with extranodal lymphoma compared to CT alone [11, 15, 18, 66].

FDG PET can differentiate primary lymphomas of the CNS from infectious processes, with a reported accuracy of 89% [67, 68]. Distinguishing infectious etiology such as toxoplasmosis can be a challenge for morphologic imaging studies, including CT and MRI, particularly in patients with AIDS. Due to the low sensitivity and specificity of polymerase chain reaction test for toxoplasmosis and Epstein-Barr virus titers for lymphoma, patients with AIDS and CNS lesions are empirically treated with pyrimethamine and sulfadiazine for 2–4 weeks. Essentially, a lesion with an FDG uptake higher than the adjacent gray matter indicates a malignant process which should be biopsied for confirmation rather than empirically treated as infectious. T1-201 is also known as a valuable imaging tool in the differentiation of CNS lymphoma from infectious causes, especially toxoplasmosis [69]. There are no systematic prospective data comparing T1-201 findings with those of FDG PET in the evaluation of CNS lymphoma, however, in few anecdotal cases we have observed that the sensitivity of FDG PET appears to be better than T1-201 imaging in the detection of CNS lymphoma. Difficulty arises, however, when CNS lymphoma undergoes necrosis or is below the resolution limits of PET systems (<8 mm).

The detection of BM involvement identifies a group of high-risk patients and changes disease management; hence, this is particularly important in early stage patients given the trend toward less intensive treatment in this group of patients (Fig. 22.10). The incidence of BM involvement at diagnosis varies according to the type of lymphoma. In general, the

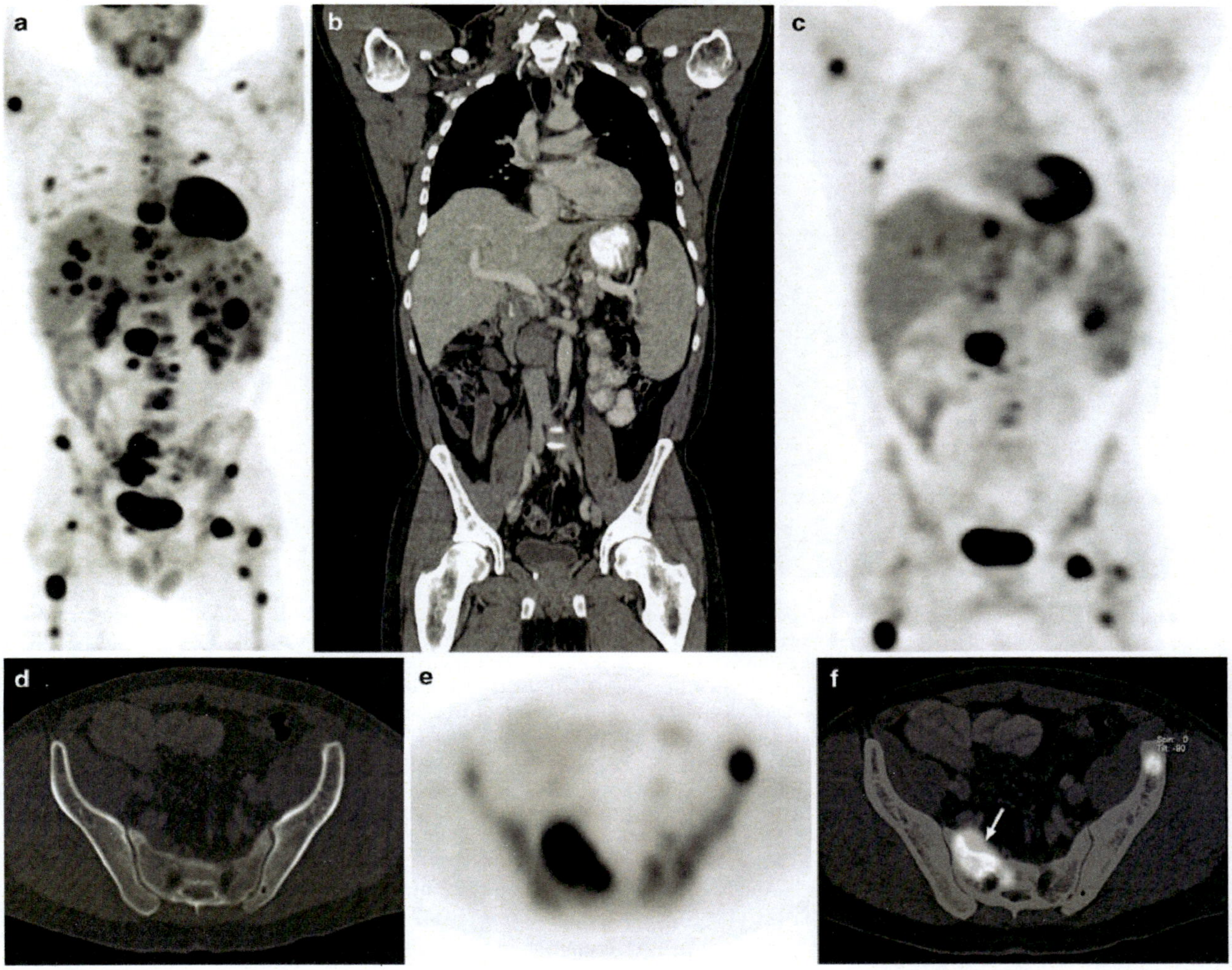

Fig. 22.10 Extranodal lymphoma. Anterior FDG PET MIP image (**a**) reveals abnormal FDG tracer uptake corresponding to a retroperitoneal nodal mass and extensive multiple foci of disease in the skeleton, liver, and spleen. Coronal contrast enhanced CT (**b**) and FDG PET (**c**) images show the 3-cm precaval lymph node mass which is intensely FDG avid, and multiple foci of abnormal FDG tracer uptake in the skeleton, and the liver and spleen with subtle corresponding findings on the portal venous–enhanced CT images of the liver and spleen, but no corresponding CT findings in the involved skeleton. Transaxial contrast-enhanced CT (**d**), FDG PET (**e**), and FDG PET-CT fusion images (**f**) reveal the osseous involvement in the right sacrum and left ileum are without discernable sclerotic or lytic abnormalities, including at the anterior cortex of the right sacrum where there is clear extension of soft tissue beyond the cortex (*arrow*). Osseous involvement of lymphoma is almost always marrow based and often without appreciable CT findings, despite extensive abnormal tracer uptake depicted on the FDG PET images. The disseminated involvement of extralymphatic organs renders the patient stage IV

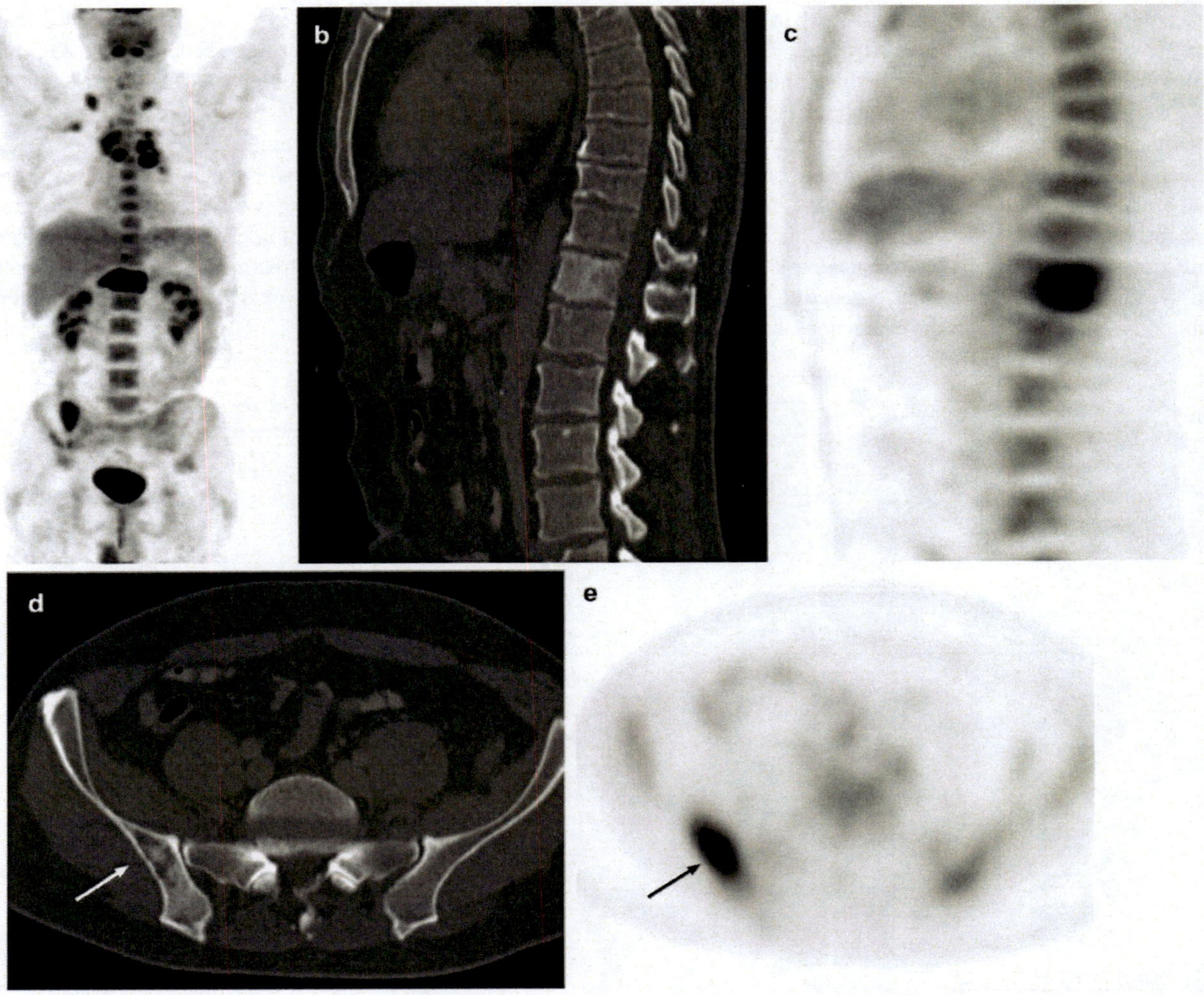

Fig. 22.11 Hodgkin's lymphoma with osseous involvement. Anterior FDG PET MIP image (**a**) demonstrates abnormal FDG tracer uptake corresponding to mediastinal lymphadenopathy and bilateral supraclavicular lymph nodes, and intense FDG tracer uptake at the T12 vertebral body and in the right ileum. Sagittal CT (**b**) and FDG PET (**c**) images reveal diffuse sclerosis in the T12 thoracic vertebral body and intense uniform FDG tracer uptake throughout the vertebral body. Transaxial CT (**d**) and FDG PET (**e**) images reveal mixed lytic and sclerotic changes in the region of intense FDG tracer uptake in the right ileum (*arrow*). Osseous involvement of Hodgkin's lymphoma more typically will have sclerotic changes on the CT images

incidence is very low in patients with HD (as low as 1–2%), while it is commonly observed in low-grade lymphoma (mainly follicular cell subtype) (60–70%), chronic lymphocytic leukemia, and mantle cell lymphoma (90–100%). In aggressive NHL (mainly diffuse large cell lymphoma), BM infiltration is seen in 25–40% of patients [70]. BM biopsy is the mainstay of BM evaluation despite its association with a high rate of false-negative findings due to sampling errors. MRI is especially useful in detecting BM involvement; however, its sensitivity is much higher than its specificity and thus benign entities such as hemangiomas and inflammatory processes can easily mimic lymphoma. Overall, focal FDG uptake suggests pathological BM activity, a pattern more commonly seen in HD patients (Fig. 22.11). In aggressive NHL, the degree of BM involvement may range from a few cells to complete marrow replacement. In cases with the latter condition, FDG uptake is usually diffuse and somewhat heterogeneous. Diffusely increased FDG uptake is also observed in patients with BM hyperplasia, particularly following administration of colony stimulating factors (e.g., G-CSF) (Fig. 22.12) [71, 72].

While several studies reported that FDG PET is an effective means for the detection of extranodal lymphoma, the sensitivity to detect BM infiltration is usually limited to about 80%, regardless of the subtype of lymphoma [41, 43, 73, 74]. In patients with negative BM biopsy, FDG PET may reveal

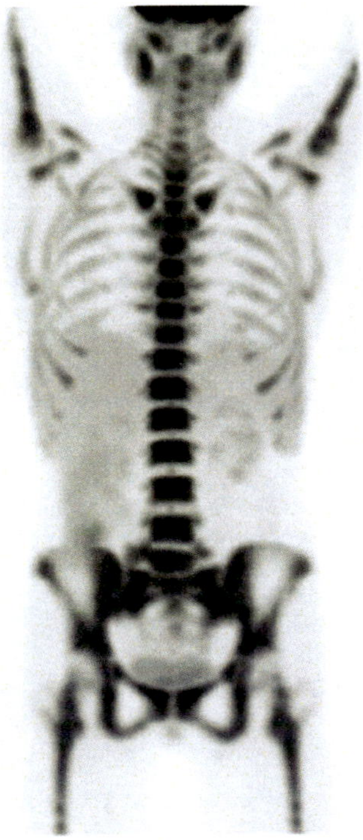

Fig. 22.12 Diffuse bone marrow hypermetabolism secondary to colony-stimulating factor on anterior FDG PET MIP image. Bone marrow stimulated by hematopoietic stimulation factors used in conjunction with chemotherapy can be very intense but uniform. Osseous lymphomatous involvement is usually heterogenous, but when extensive can be relatively uniform

focal BM infiltration is present remote to the biopsy site owing to the virtue of evaluating the entire body at one acquisition. Nevertheless, a minimal degree of BM involvement can result in false-negative findings on FDG PET due to the inherent resolution limits of FDG PET imaging [18, 73, 74].

Bone marrow involvement of lymphoma should not be confused with primary bone lymphoma which is a separate entity and accounts for less than 5% of all primary bone tumors. Although there is no series of cases performed using FDG PET, our experience is that FDG avidly accumulates in all primary bone lesions or osseous extension of lymphoma of advanced-stage disease unlike bone marrow involvement.

Splenic involvement by lymphoma is more sensitively detected on FDG PET images than CT [11, 15], or conventional Gallium-67 imaging [75]. Both focal and diffuse involvement can be seen on FDG PET images even when contrast-enhanced CT is normal (Fig. 22.13). Certain hemopoietic stimulants used in chemotherapy regimens, however, can cause diffuse splenic FDG uptake as well as diffuse bone marrow FDG activity. With the advent of combined PET-CT imaging, accuracy in the detection of extranodal lymphoma is advanced by the complementary strengths of the two modalities. In a small series involving 19 patients comparing PET-CT with non–contrast-enhanced CT to conventional fully optimized contrast-enhanced CT alone, the PET-CT detected extranodal disease (bone and splenic involvements) in three patients while separately acquired contrast-enhanced CT was false-negative at these sites. However, in one patient, contrast-enhanced CT revealed small bowel involvement while the non–contrast-enhanced PET-CT was false-negative [53]. Since PET-CT studies have now evolved to more widely include intravenous contrast administration, the fully complementary nature of combined PET-CT examination in the detection of extranodal involvement of lymphoma is realized.

FDG PET Versus Ga-67 Imaging

There is no comparative study using PET-CT and Ga-67 imaging in the same lymphoma population; however, and FDG PET has been shown to have superior sensitivity to Ga-67 scintigraphy and provide superior incremental value when combined with conventional diagnostic methods [76–80]. The discrepancy in the detection sensitivity between Ga-67 and FDG PET imaging has recently been shown to be independent of the disease volume, location, and histology in both nodal and extranodal disease. The discrepancy in the detection sensitivity between these two radiotracers can be explained not only by the superior counting statistics and spatial resolution of PET tomograph technology, but also by biologic differences considering the significant disparities in the mechanism of uptake of Ga-67 and FDG [80, 81]. Consequently, at present, FDG PET, particularly PET-CT, has largely downgraded Ga-67 imaging to an infection imaging agent from its past position as a staging or restaging modality in HD or aggressive NHL.

Influence of PET-CT on Patient Management at Initial Staging

As noted previously, accurate staging is more clinically relevant in aggressive NHL and HD than in indolent and mantle cell lymphoma, as the latter pair are associated with advanced-stage disease in a vast majority of patients. Even in the aggressive lymphomas, one should realize that not all stage changes as a result of PET-CT findings would translate into changes in therapeutic strategy. In routine practice, the stage category is usually altered within the same risk category (early stage vs advanced stage) and thus does not lead to management changes, but if additional information obtained from FDG PET, upstages early stage disease to advanced stage or vice versa, and therapy may be changed accordingly. Hence, the additional information provided by FDG PET is felt to be more useful in patients who are diagnosed with early stage

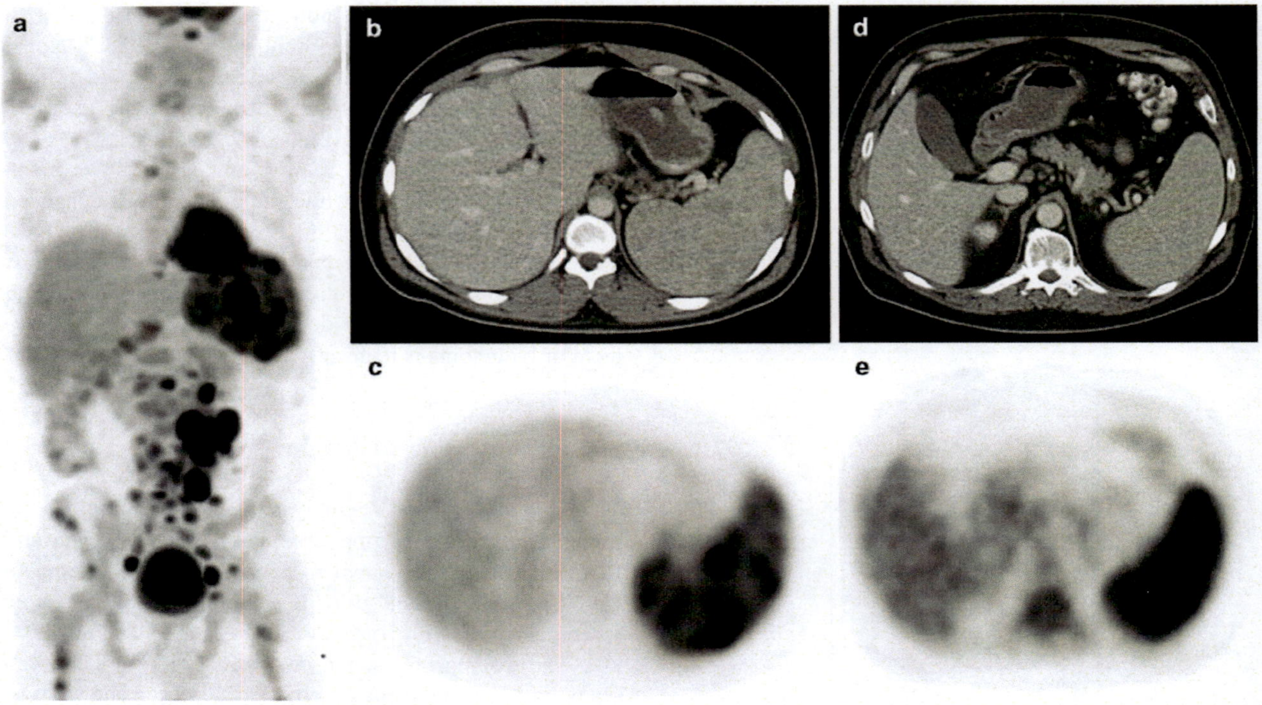

Fig. 22.13 Follicular B cell lymphoma with splenic involvement. Anterior FDG PET MIP image (**a**) reveals intense heterogenous FDG tracer uptake in the spleen as well as lymph node involvement above and below the diaphragm, including bulky retroperitoneal disease. Transaxial contrast-enhanced CT (**b**) and FDG PET (**c**) images demonstrate diffusely increased FDG tracer uptake throughout the spleen with additional multiple intense foci of abnormal FDG tracer uptake. Subtle corresponding regions of decreased attenuation are seen on the portal venous phase contrast-enhanced CT images. Lymphomatous involvement of the spleen can manifest as a spleen with no parenchymal abnormalities on the CT images, including contrast-enhanced CT images (**d**), but with uniform intense abnormal FDG tracer activity on the FDG PET images (**e**)

disease than in advanced stage disease as treatment strategy may be altered by detection of unexpected disease sites in the former patient population not in the latter [82].

The superior sensitivity of FDG PET has been reported to lead to a change in disease stage in 8–48% of patients with untreated NHL and HD by virtue of revealing additional disease sites not revealed on anatomic imaging that were confirmed by either biopsy or long-term clinical follow-up [9, 17, 48–50, 83–85]. Based on the significance of change in stage for therapeutic strategy, FDG PET findings may result in intra or intermodality treatment modifications in 8–25% of HD or aggressive NHL patients [17, 49, 50, 83–86].

The most important imaging data derived influence on therapy would be the accurate separation of patients into favorable and unfavorable risk categories, especially in the early-stage HD patient population. The relevant therapeutic changes in early-stage disease with favorable prognostic factors group include treatment reduction strategies, essentially shorter courses of chemotherapy rather than a longer course as exclusive treatment, as opposed to a shorter course of chemotherapy followed by radiation therapy.

PET-CT for Restaging and Evaluation of Therapy Response

Following therapy, evaluation of residual disease and the efficacy of therapy is crucial when alternative therapeutic strategies exist, so that intramodality or intermodality treatment changes can be made to increase progression-free or overall survival. In early stage lymphoma (aggressive NHL or HD) up to 90% of patients respond to therapy; however, advanced stage lymphoma confer poor prognosis with a cure rate of less than 50% in newly diagnosed patients [87, 88]. Assessment of therapy response is therefore, more important in patients with advanced stage disease than with early stage. Also one important issue is that the treatment strategy for aggressive NHL is determined based upon immunophenotype and molecular genetics of the tumor rather than the anatomic extent alone. Aggressive NHL is treated exclusively with chemotherapy except in some cases local therapy may be added. Thus in this patient population, the primary role for imaging is the assessment of therapy response.

CT in the Posttherapy Evaluation of Lymphoma

Evaluation of treatment response using CT can be quite challenging. Differences in slice thickness and inconsistencies in the use of intravenous contrast may render the comparisons difficult. Following therapy, the mass attenuation values of the lymph nodes decreases with or without overall reduction in lymph node size in responding patients; however, there is no established standard for an accurate categorization of responders and nonresponders based on CT criteria. Achieving a complete response, which is defined as complete disappearance of the tumor mass, is the goal of cytotoxic therapy. However, failure to completely eradicate tumor mass with chemotherapy does not always correlate with persistent tumor cells or unfavorable prognosis [89]. This dilemma on anatomic imaging has been recognized in the response criteria for both HD and NHL [90, 91]. Both systems designate residual masses of unclear etiology as CRu, or unconfirmed/uncertain complete responses due to inherent uncertainty associated with posttherapy residual CT masses. Naturally, further and aggressive treatment in patients with benign posttherapy masses only increases morbidity and risk of second malignancies [31]. The patients with HD are at a higher risk of developing solid tumors years after therapy as a long-term side effect of combination chemotherapy and radiotherapy. New masses discovered more than 10 years after therapy in the lung, thyroid, breast, and stomach should be considered as de novo primary tumors and must be verified by biopsy [92].

In patients with bulky lymphoma, chemotherapy followed by RT is the conventional treatment approach in those with residual posttherapy masses. Radiation related tissue changes usually appear within 3–6 months after completion of RT with a presentation of ground glass opacities confined to the mantle radiation ports. Acute changes eventually disappear after 6 months, usually replaced by chronic changes in the ensuing 18 months, presenting as retraction or traction bronchiectasis and mediastinal fibrosis which may resemble granulomatous disease but they are usually symmetrical and confined to the mantle port [93].

FDG PET in the Posttherapy Evaluation of Lymphoma

As many as 50–80% of patients with HD and 30% of those with NHL will have residual masses after treatment. However, only a small percentage (~15–20%) of these patients relapse. A multitude of studies have demonstrated that FDG PET is an effective imaging modality and more accurate than CT alone in the differentiation of posttherapy inert masses from active residual disease (Fig. 22.14), as well as monitoring response to therapy [13, 14, 86, 94–101].

FDG PET has been consistently reported to identify residual disease and/or preclinical relapse during the follow-up period (Fig. 22.15) [13, 14, 86, 94–101]. Despite reported high negative predictive values of greater than 90% obtained FDG PET by various investigators, false-negative findings are inevitable in cases with residual microscopic disease. Nevertheless, positive predictive value of FDG PET, also on the order of 90%, should be regarded more vital in the context of identifying patients who need immediate therapy changes or additional treatment after first-line therapy. In this group of patients, FDG PET could also avoid unnecessary further therapy in patients who achieve complete response to chemotherapy. One major concern that has not been addressed adequately, however, is the definition of patient population who would require further treatment with RT in the presence of false-negative findings associated with undetectable low-burden disease.

In summary, negative FDG PET findings in areas corresponding to persistent posttherapy masses usually indicate posttreatment fibrosis. Nevertheless, false-negative results can be obtained for small lesions that are below the detection limits of current PET tomographs (<5–6 mm) or diffusely distributed microscopic disease. False-positive FDG PET findings can occasionally be obtained in infectious or inflammatory processes, however, the pattern of FDG uptake in these situations is usually recognizable and can be differentiated in most cased, especially when CT findings are taken into account, with the notable exception of granulomatous disease coexisting with lymphoma. Posttherapy FDG tracer accumulation in the region of original disease should be recognized as a compelling evidence for further therapy, however, owing to the associated high positive predictive value (90%) for residual viable disease.

Prediction of Therapy Outcome After Completion of Therapy

Criteria based on clinical, imaging, and laboratory findings which allow for risk stratification have been developed and validated for HD, known as the international prognostic score (IPS), and for NHL, known as the international prognostic index (IPI) [90, 101]. The IPS for HD (Table 22.5) is based on seven adverse factors, while the IPI, the most widely used system for aggressive NHL (Table 22.6), predicts the risk of recurrence and overall survival by taking into account five adverse factors [102]. In this regard, sequential FDG PET imaging has a role in the determination of tumor

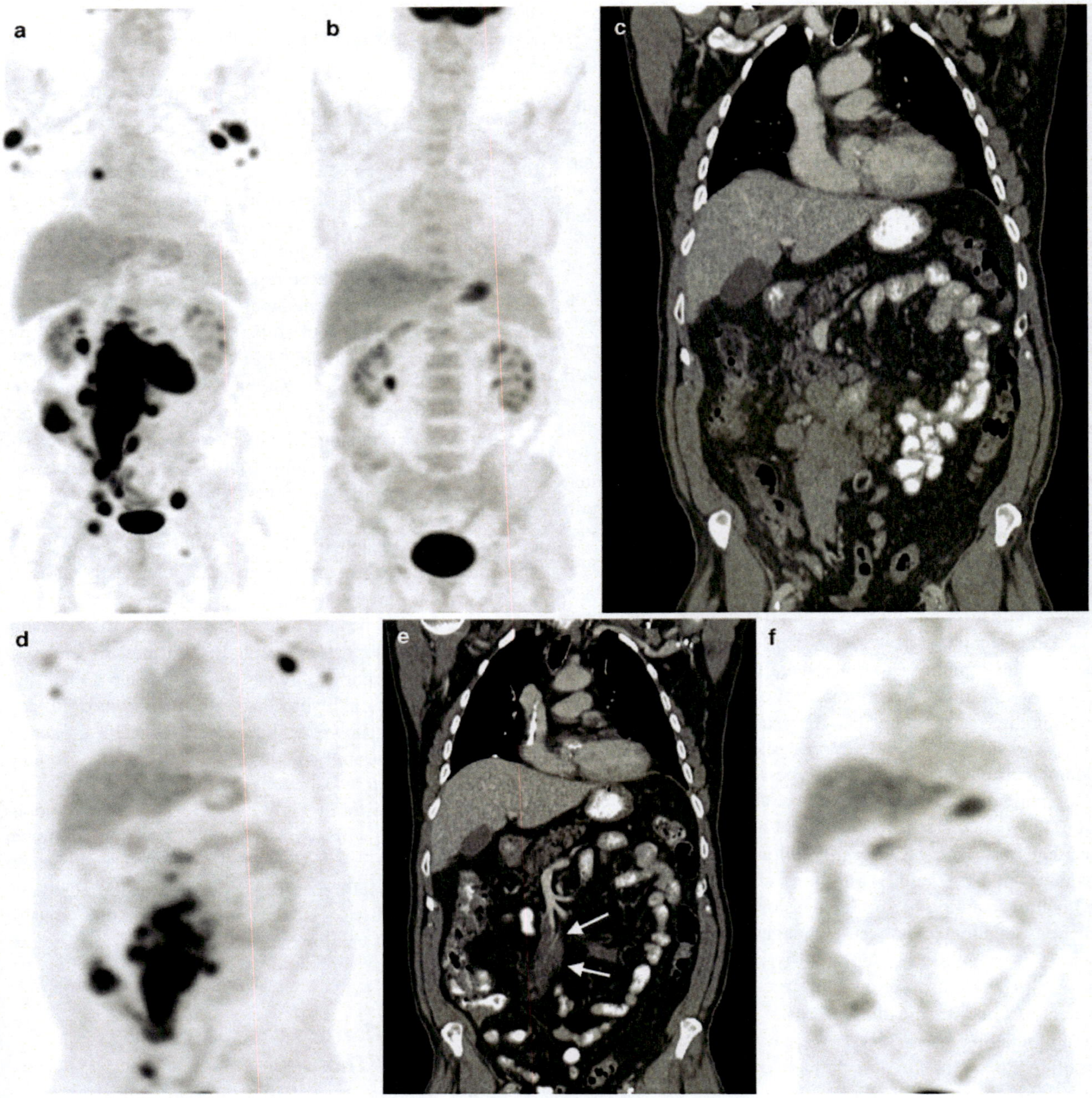

Fig. 22.14 Compete metabolic response of diffuse large B-cell non-Hodgkin's lymphoma to chemotherapy with ametabolic residual scarring. Anterior FDG PET MIP image (**a**) pre-chemotherapy demonstrates intense abnormal FDG tracer activity corresponding to extensive mesenteric lymphadenopathy as well as involvement of axillary and inguinal lymph nodes. The posttherapy anterior FDG PET MIP image (**b**) reveals complete resolution of all abnormal FDG tracer uptake, with normal physiologic tracer activity distribution. Coronal contrast-enhanced CT (**c**) and FDG PET images (**d**) performed prior to therapy reveal the extensive mesenteric lymph node involvement with a conglomerate mass as well as an involved left axillary lymph node. The posttherapy coronal contrast-enhanced CT (**e**) and FDG PET (**f**) images demonstrate the residual soft tissue (*arrows*) along the superior mesenteric vein is entirely without any abnormal FDG tracer activity, indicating this is residual scar tissue, without metabolically active macroscopic lymphoma

response rates [16, 95–99, 103, 104]. For example, in patients categorized as high risk for recurrence by IPI or IPS criteria, recurrent lymphoma should be anticipated in almost all patients with posttherapy residual abnormal FDG tracer uptake and in slightly under half of those with residual posttherapy CT masses [16, 97, 103].

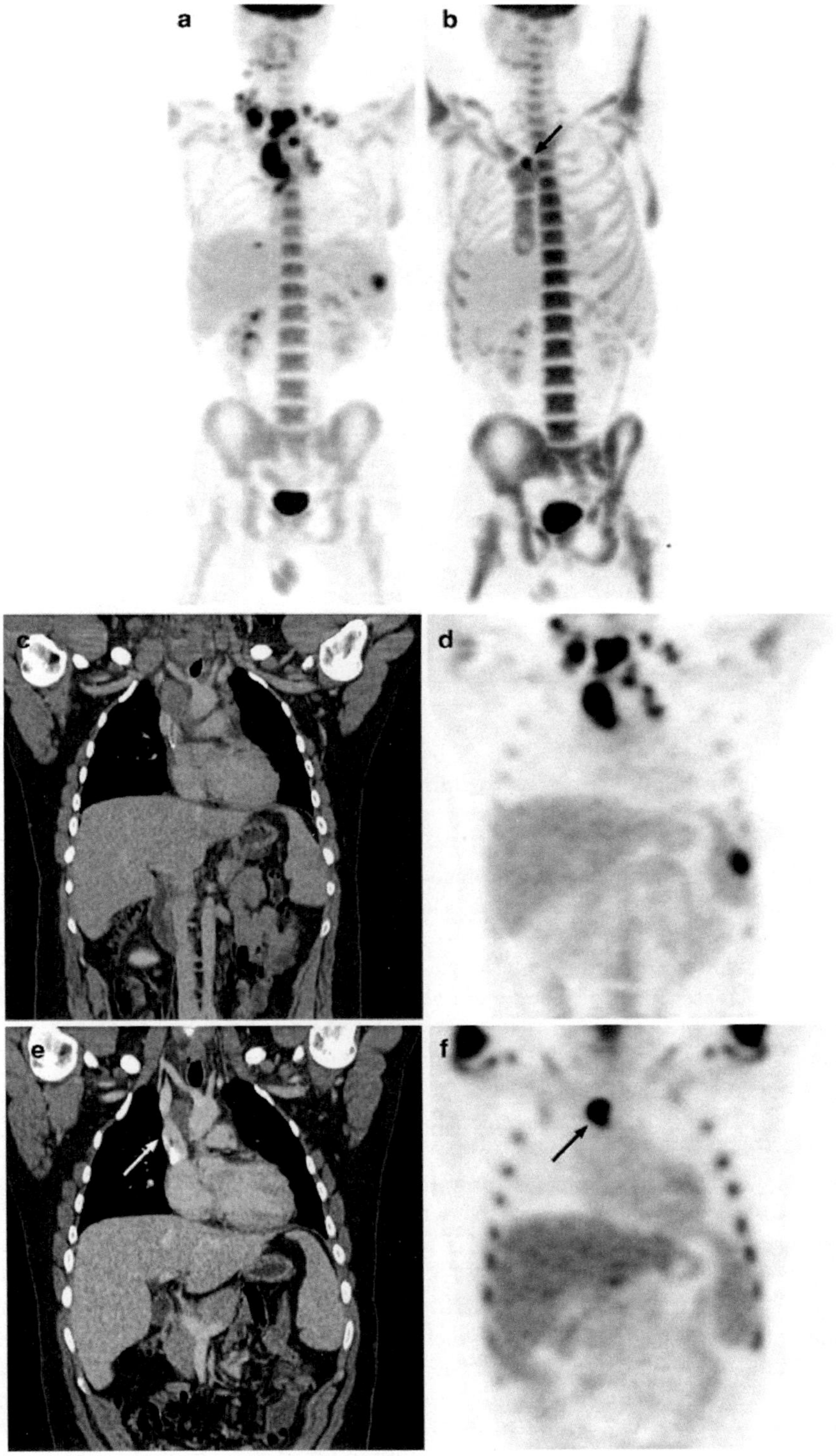

Fig. 22.15 Incomplete metabolic response of Hodgkin's lymphoma to chemotherapy. Anterior FDG PET MIP (**a**) prechemotherapy demonstrates intense abnormal FDG tracer activity corresponding to disease involving bulky mediastinal lymphadenopathy, bilateral lower cervical, and supraclavicular nodal involvement, an isolated right subdiaphragmatic lymph node, as well as focal involvement of the spleen. The posttherapy shallow left anterior oblique FDG PET MIP image (**b**) reveals complete resolution of all abnormal FDG tracer uptake, except a conspicuous single focus or abnormal FDG tracer uptake in the right mediastinum (*arrow*). There is additionally on the posttherapy FDG PET diffuse increased bone marrow FDG tracer uptake reflecting the use of hematopoietic stimulants in the chemotherapy regimen. Coronal contrast-enhanced CT (**c**) and FDG PET (**d**) images prechemotherapy reveal the intensely FDG avid mediastinal and supraclavicular lymphadenopathy and an intense focus of FDG tracer activity in the spleen The postchemotherapy coronal contrast-enhanced CT (**e**) and FDG PET (**f**) images show complete resolution of the lymphadenopathy and of the splenic lesion, with the exception of a 2-cm residual right mediastinal lymph node interposed (*arrow*) between the superior vena cava and ascending aorta, which maintains intense abnormal FDG tracer uptake, indicating the residual abnormal soft tissue is remaining viable lymphoma

Table 22.5 International prognostic score (IPS) for Hodgkin's lymphoma

Adverse factors	High risk	Low risk
Serum albumin	<4 g/dL	>4 g/dL
Hemoglobin	<10.5 g/dL	>10.5 g/dL
Patient gender	Male	Female
Age	>45 years	<45 years
Clinical stage	Stage IV	Stage I–III
WBC	>15,000/mm^3	<15,000/mm^3
Absolute lymphocytes	<600/mm^3	>600/mm^3

Table 22.6 International prognostic index (IPI) for non-Hodgkin's lymphoma

Adverse factors	High risk	Low risk
Age	>60 years	<60 years
Clinical stage	III/IV	I/II
Patient gender	Male	Female
Performance status	>2	<2
Extranodal sites of disease	>1	0 or 1
Serum lactate dehydrogenase	Elevated	Normal 15,000/mm^3

Combined Modality Therapy Including Radiation Therapy

The other important management issue is the avoidance of RT, especially in the HD population. The use of RT is associated with a short-term survival advantage; however, RT has an adverse effect on long-term survival due to significantly increased risk for many late complications such as development of a second malignancy or cardiovascular disease [31, 93]. Ongoing trials investigating treatment reduction, including reduction of radiation dose or radiation field size, and abbreviated chemotherapy, are intended to reduce RT treatment-related long-term complications [31]. PET-CT may well be a valuable imaging tool to risk stratify these patients and select the subgroups that will or not require RT followed by chemotherapy, based on the identification of residual viable disease on the FDG PET images.

In a mixed (HD and aggressive NHL) series of 44 patients presenting with bulky abdominal lymphoma, at the end of chemotherapy with or without RT, all those with positive FDG tracer uptake in residual masses eventually succumbed to disease relapse, while only 4% relapse occurred among those that had residual masses but no associated abnormal FDG tracer uptake [99].

Persistent FDG uptake after first-line chemotherapy was predictive of residual or recurrent disease after completion of first-line chemotherapy for aggressive NHL in a prospective study [103]. The negative predictive value of posttherapy FDG PET findings was 80% with a mean follow-up of approximately 24 months, while positive predictive value was 100% with a mean disease-free survival of only 3 months. This study highlights false-negative FDG PET findings can be as high as 20% probably due to microscopic residual disease. In the small number of studies evaluating exclusively patients with HD, after the first-line treatment, disease-free survival was significantly shorter for the PET positive group at 0–4% and longer for the PET negative group at 85–93% [105, 106]. These results provide grounds for future trials to evaluate the prognosis in patients who are administered abbreviated courses of chemotherapy with or without combined RT given at lower radiation doses in cases with negative FDG PET results.

High-dose Chemotherapy and Autologous Stem Cell Transplantation

For patients with relapsed lymphoma, high-dose chemotherapy (HDT) with autologous stem cell transplantation (SCT) is the treatment of choice resulting in 5-year event-free survival rates of up to 45% [107]. The outcomes after HDT/SCT, however, can be significantly different between chemosensitive and chemoresistant patients. Hence differentiation of these two patient populations is important for the identification of the optimal group that would benefit from HDT/SCT. Patients with less than 25% decrease in SUV measured FDG tracer uptake in the lymphoma after HDT had a progressive disease course while among those with more than 25% decrease in SUVs, 86% remained in complete remission [108]. Similarly, another study found none of the patients with complete resolution of FDG tracer uptake in response to the initial course of therapy before HDT/SCT relapsed subsequently [109], while seven or eight patients with a moderate or high FDG tracer uptake before HDT/SCT relapsed [109].

Early Prediction of Response During Therapy

The rapidity of response to therapy regimen has been suggested to be a good predictor of the ultimate response to that particular therapy regimen [110–112]. Patients with aggressive NHL who experience a partial response or who respond slowly to front-line chemotherapy have been reported to have a poor prognosis. In this group of patients, early introduction of dose-intensive salvage therapy before the development of progressive disease may be beneficial [111]. Since chemotherapy effect on tumor metabolic activity precedes the tumor size reduction, early evaluation of therapy response would be primarily based on the metabolic images.

Based on in vitro studies, FDG tracer uptake is proportional to the viable tumor cells, and viable tumor cells decrease early during effective chemotherapy. In a clinical study, 7 days after initiation of chemotherapy, tumor glucose metabolism as measured by FDG tracer uptake decreased by at least 74% in responding patients [113]. All lesions displayed a further decrease of FDG tracer uptake resulting in a total decrease of 83–96% from baseline to day 42 after initiation of therapy. There was no indication initial enhancement of FDG uptake as suggested by data from cell culture and animal studies. Further, the FDG tracer uptake values at day 42 were lower in patients with long-term remission compared to patients with early relapse [113]. Similarly, persistent FDG tracer uptake in the lymphoma after two to four cycles of chemotherapy was reported to predict poor progression-free survival in patients with aggressive NHL and HD [105, 106]. Persistent FDG uptake after a few cycles of chemotherapy was associated with relapse rates ranging from 70% to 100% while the relapse rate in patients with complete disappearance of FDG tracer uptake during therapy was as low as 8%. In one study, at midtreatment, none of the patients with persistent abnormal FDG tracer uptake achieved a durable complete remission, while 84% of patients with negative FDG PET results remained in complete remission after a median follow-up of approximately 3 years [106]. In this study, multivariate analysis revealed that FDG PET at midtreatment was a stronger prognostic factor for progression free survival compared with IPI criteria.

Could FDG PET predict as early as after one cycle of chemotherapy? It has been demonstrated that FDG PET after one cycle of chemotherapy was predictive of long-term outcome in aggressive NHL and HD [104, 114]. In one series by Kostakoglu et al., patients with persistent FDG uptake after one cycle of chemotherapy had a shorter progression free survival (median, 5 months) than those with negative FDG PET results (progression-free survival medians not reached) after a follow-up of 36 months [104]. The positive and negative predictive values for FDG PET after one cycle chemotherapy were 90% and 85%, respectively. However, these results were obtained on a dual-head camera system which lacks sensitivity and therefore may give rise false-negative results. Recently, in a study by the same investigators, using a dedicated full ring PET system, all patients (17 patients) with no appreciable FDG uptake after one cycle of chemotherapy remained in complete remission after a follow-up of 12 months, whereas 90% of patients with a positive FDG PET result had a relapse or persistent disease requiring further therapy, including bone marrow transplantation. These are promising results; nonetheless, these data should be interpreted with caution until larger, multi-institutional studies with a longer follow-up period are executed. Additionally, comparison of the predictive value of early FDG PET scanning to more conventional prognostic measures (such as the International Prognostic Index in aggressive lymphoma) as not yet been performed with sufficient patients to establish whether FDG PET derived early response criteria provides superior or complementary prognostic information.

If further studies confirm that persistent positive FDG PET results during therapy, preferably after one cycle, indicate a poor prognosis, one could consider an early change in therapy to a more aggressive approach (such as second-line chemotherapy and high-dose treatment with autologous stem cell transplant) early during the course of treatment (either before completion of a full course of initial chemotherapy or in first remission). However, the clinical benefit of such an approach, and whether this early change in therapy would improve upon a predicted outcome would require prospective testing in proper randomized clinical trials.

In conclusion, it appears that the superiority of FDG PET lies in its positive predictive value, especially early in the course of chemotherapy-based treatment of lymphoma, as to therapy resistance or failure. The negative predictive value of FDG PET, however, may not be as reliable as minimal residual disease, especially microscopic, that cannot be detected given the resolution limits of current PET tomographs. Thus, late relapses remain to be a possibility in patients with negative FDG PET results.

Comparison of FDG PET and Ga-67 Imaging in Posttherapy Evaluation

Ga-67 scintigraphy was the antecedent imaging modality to monitor response to chemotherapy in patients with lymphoma. However, with the proven advantages and strength of FDG PET imaging, Ga-67 scintigraphy is no longer widely used. There are only a few studies evaluating the potential of FDG and Ga-67 comparatively, in the posttherapy setting, but generally effective treatment sharply reduces tumor uptake of both Ga-67 and FDG activity within days and prior to volume response, whereas abnormal uptake of both Ga-67 and FDG persisted in treatment failure [115]. Nevertheless, the significantly higher sensitivity and specificity of FDG PET compared to Ga-67 scintigraphy for detection of nodal or extranodal lymphoma in both pretherapy and posttherapy setting has established FDG as the preferred metabolic tracer for lymphoma with Ga-67 scintigraphy in 93% versus 29%.

PET-CT systems provide important information particularly in the posttherapy setting; metabolic findings that are overlooked due to the subtlety of metabolic changes of FDG PET may result in the detection of residual disease after correlation with the simultaneously acquired and registered and aligned CT images. Furthermore, equivocal CT findings, which are suggestive of either recurrent tumor or posttherapy changes, can now be distinguished with the guidance of the additional information obtained from FDG PET images. In addition to diagnosis and staging and restaging of malignant disease, combined PET-CT is useful in planning radiation therapy and determining the optimum approach for CT-guided biopsy [21, 53]. Consequently, the addition of metabolic imaging can have a great effect on treatment in patients with a residual mass at the time of posttreatment evaluation.

Special Considerations with Lymphoma Imaging

Special considerations for imaging patients with lymphoma are summarized in Table 22.7.

Benign Lymphoproliferative Disorders

Benign lymphoproliferative disorders represent a spectrum of lymphoid abnormalities characterized by lymphocyte proliferation. LPD can be divided into two broad categories; benign and posttransplantation. The benign LPD most frequently manifest in the thorax, where the site can be the lymph nodes or in the bronchus associated lymphoid tissue of the lung [116]. Entities such as plasma cell granuloma, pseudolymphoma, posttransplant lymphoproliferative disorders, lymphoid interstitial pneumonia, and lymphomatoid granulomatosis involve the pulmonary parenchyma as a primary site of intrathoracic disease, while Castleman's disease, infectious mononucleosis and angioimmunoblastic

Table 22.7 Special consideration with FDG PET imaging in lymphoma

Entity	Pitfalls	Helpful features
Post Chemo	Varying degrees of FDG uptake in the region of original disease	• Residual uptake > surrounding background uptake suggests minimal residual disease Reduction in SUV >95% of initial SUV usually indicates complete resolution of disease
Post-RT	Diffuse, heterogeneous uptake in the portal region	• Uptake coinciding with exact location of original lesion indicates residual disease • Uptake outside the original disease suggests inflammatory changes • Optimal evaluation is usually performed at 3–4 months after RT
Post-GCSF	Diffuse, homogeneous, or heterogeneous uptake in the axial and appendicular BM	• In patients with known BM involvement, this is usually an equivocal finding
HIV + patients/LPD	FDG accumulation in multiple enlarged LNs Lesion confined to either LNs or organs, Multiple disease sites (LNs or organs)	• Low-grade uptake in multiple LNs (usually superficial LN stations) suggests benign LPD which can be due to infectious processes • High-grade FDG uptake in enlarged LNs (deep + superficial) indicates malignant LPD, i.e., lymphoma. Lymphoma in immunosuppressed patients is of aggressive NHL or HD • Low-grade uptake in intrathoracic LNs or lung parenchyma suggests benign etiology • High grade FDG uptake in multiple LNs or extranodal sites indicates lymphoma.
Sarcoidosis	Bilateral hilar uptake	• Hilar uptake is asymmetrical with HD or NHL, unlike sarcoidosis • Isolated hilar involvement without mediastinal disease does not occur • Pulmonary parenchymal lymphoma is considered as advanced HD or NHL
Renal transplant	Uptake in the pelvis	• Pelvic transplant kidney should not be confused with a pelvic mass; CT and clinical correlation is necessary if PET-CT is not available. Of note, the incidence of developing lymphoma is high in the posttransplant period.
Lung nodules	Isolated uptake in lung	• Focal lung nodule without mediastinal/hilar disease does not occur in lymphoma. • Primary pulmonary lymphoma (usually solitary nodule) is often of the MALT type. • Rapidly developing diffuse pulmonary opacities may be seen in cutaneous T-cell lymphoma, but these are usually in association with mediastinal and hilar disease.
Second malignancies Metachronous neoplasms)	Unusual lesion distribution pattern	• Distribution of FDG uptake outside patterns described in Tables 22.3A and B should raise a question about second malignancies, particularly in the breast, liver, lung, adrenals, pancreas, ovaries, and prostate.

BM Bone marrow, *chemo* chemotherapy, *GCSF* granulocyte colony stimulator factor, *HIV* human immunodeficiency virus, *LN* lymph nodes, *LPD* lymphoproliferative disorder, *RT* radiation therapy

lymphadenopathy involve intrathoracic lymph nodes. It is important to differentiate the "benign" forms of LPD from the more common, aggressive lymphomas. Overall, intrathoracic disease confined to one compartment, either lymph nodes or lung parenchyma, implies a more benign etiology whereas multiple sites of disease, a malignant neoplasm. There is considerable overlap between benign LPD and NHL, especially in the immunocompromised patients. One might assume that the FDG uptake would be lower in this benign form of LPD than that seen in aggressive NHL and HD. Only anecdotal case reports are available regarding the FDG uptake patterns in Castleman's disease in the literature [117, 118]. FDG accumulation in one of these case reports was modest (SUV: 6.2) in a hilar location and low in the other (SUV: 1.7–3.2) in a pelvic location. It is expected that in the indolent forms of NHL, the differentiation between benign LPD and lymphoma may not be possible. In the absence of a systematic study assessing FDG accumulation patterns, it is only speculative to discuss this topic; however, one must bear in mind that this category of diseases should be considered as a potential false-positive group among other granulomatous processes, especially in the posttherapy setting [119].

AIDS-Related Lymphoma

AIDS-related lymphomas, both NHL and HD, are characterized clinically by the presence of B symptoms (weight loss, night sweats, and fevers) at diagnosis in approximately 90%, advanced clinical stage with extranodal involvement in greater than 60% at presentation, and clinical aggressiveness with poor therapeutic outcomes. Extranodal involvement is a particularly distinctive feature, with the gastrointestinal tract being the most common location. Other sites of involvement include the central nervous system, the bone marrow, the oral cavity, the lungs, and the skin. Recently a primary effusion lymphoma (PEL) has been described in association with HIV. This rare lymphoma develops exclusively in serous body cavities (peritoneum, pleura, or pericardium) as a malignant effusion [120]. FDG PET findings follow the clinical presentation and CT findings with typically high levels of FDG tracer uptake due to the aggressive nature of these lymphomas.

Thymic Uptake

Following chemotherapy, thymic FDG uptake in young adults and pediatric patients is a known phenomenon and should not be mistaken with residual lymphoma, although at times differentiation between the two conditions may be challenging [121–123]. Thymic hyperplasia is a common phenomenon after treatment, especially in children, with an incidence of 16%. It has been proposed that this finding is due to an immunologic rebound phenomenon characterized by lymph follicles with large nuclear centers and infiltration of plasma cells following thymic aplasia secondary to steroid-induced apoptosis and inhibition of lymphocyte proliferation. Rebound thymic hyperplasia is associated with increased FDG tracer uptake and increased thymus volume. In children with a malignancy roughly 75% will have increased thymus FDG tracer uptake both prior to and following chemotherapy, although with a significant increase after therapy, while in young adults only about 5% will manifest increased thymic FDG uptake after chemotherapy [122, 123].

BM Uptake After Administration of Colony Stimulators

In patients with chemotherapy followed by bone marrow stimulants such as granulocyte colony-stimulating factor and granulocyte-macrophage colony-stimulating factor, the BM will have diffuse, intense increased FDG accumulation [71, 72]. Therefore, diffuse BM FDG uptake is commonly attributable to the effect of hematopoietic cytokines. Diffuse bone marrow FDG uptake can, however, also be caused by bone marrow involvement by lymphoma and at times this may be indistinguishable from hematopoietic cytokine-mediated FDG bone marrow uptake.

Posttransplantation Period

Bone marrow transplantation (BMT) and immunocompromised patients require special attention when interpreting images. Lymphoma patients after therapy, in particular after bone marrow transplantation, can develop cellular immunodeficiency until the transplanted marrow engrafts and creates new white blood cells. These patients are extremely susceptible to infections. Pulmonary infections are the most frequent complications in BMT recipients [124]. Idiopathic interstitial pneumonitis/ARDS, *pneumocystis carinii*, cytomegalovirus, *aspergillus*, and bacterial pneumonia are among the most common causes of infections [125]. Additionally, acute graft versus host disease (GVHD) often occurs during the first 3 months following an allogeneic BMT. To minimize the risk of graft rejection and GVHD, allogeneic BMT patients are given immunosuppressants to prevent GVHD before and after transplant. Use of these drugs, however, increases the risk of infection. Therefore, caution should be exercised when interpreting PET-CT images in immunocompromised patients as infectious/inflammatory lesions and granulomas can be falsely interpreted as persistent or recurrent tumor.

Conclusion

PET-CT is now the mainstay for imaging lymphoma patients. The complimentary nature of the metabolic and anatomic information provided by a PET-CT examination has become an essential component of patient management, complementing clinical and laboratory criteria used in staging, restaging, and therapy monitoring. As emphasized above, the nature of a particular lymphoma subtype and the patient's clinical presentation will determine the extent PET-CT imaging is best employed in a particular patient's management.

References

1. Canellos GP, Anderson JR, Propert KJ, et al. Chemotherapy of advanced Hodgkin's disease with MOPP, ABVD, or MOPP alternating with ABVD. NEJM 1992;327:1478–1484.
2. Fisher RI, Gaynor ER, Dahlberg S, Oken MM, et al. Comparison of a standard regimen (CHOP) with three intensive chemotherapy regimens for advanced non-Hodgkin's lymphoma. NEJM 1993;328:1002–1006.
3. Marshall WH Jr, Breiman RS, Harell GS, Glatstein E, Kaplan HS. Computed tomography of abdominal para-aortic lymph node disease: preliminary observation with a 6 second scanner. Am J Roentgenol 1977;128:759–764.
4. Bendini M, Zuiani C, Bazzocchi M, Dalpiaz G, Zaja F, Englaro E. Magnetic resonance imaging and 67Ga scan versus computed tomography in the staging and in the monitoring of mediastinal malignant lymphoma: a prospective pilot study. MAGMA 1996;4:213–224.
5. Nyman R, Forsgren G, Glimelius B. Long-term follow-up of residual mediastinal masses in treated Hodgkin's disease using MR imaging. Acta Radiol 1996;37:323–326.
6. Front D, Bar-Shalom R, Mor M, et al. Hodgkin's disease: prediction of outcome with ^{67}Ga scintigraphy after one cycle of chemotherapy. Radiology 1999;210:487–491.
7. Front D, Bar-Shalom R, Mor M, et al. Aggressive non-Hodgkin lymphoma: early prediction of outcome with ^{67}Ga scintigraphy. Radiology 2000;214:253–257.
8. Rodriguez M, Rehn S, Ahlstrom H, Sundstrom C, Glimelius B. Predicting malignancy grade with PET in non-Hodgkin's lymphoma. J Nucl Med 1995,36:1790–1796.
9. Jerusalem G, Warland V, Najjar F, Paulus P, Fassotte MF, Fillet G, Rigo P. Whole-body 18F-FDG PET for the evaluation of patients with Hodgkin's disease and non-Hodgkin's lymphoma. Nucl Med Commun 1999;20:13–20.
10. Hoh CK, Glaspy J, Rosen P, et al. Whole-body FDG PET imaging for staging of Hodgkin's disease and lymphoma. J Nucl Med 1997;38:343–348.
11. Thill R, Neuerburg J, Fabry U, et al. Comparison of findings with 18-FDG PET and CT in pretherapeutic staging of malignant lymphoma. Nuklearmedizin 1997;36:234–239.
12. Mainolfi C, Maurea S, Varrella P, Alaia C, Imparato C, Alfano B, Aate G, Bazzicalupo L. Positron emission tomography with fluorine-18-deoxyglucose in the staging and control of patients with lymphoma. Comparison with clinico-radiologic assessment. Radiol Med 1998;95:98–104.
13. Cremerius U, Fabry U, Neuerburg J, Zimny M, Osieka R, Buell. Positron emission tomography with 18F-FDG to detect residual disease after therapy for malignant lymphoma. Nucl Med Commun 1998;19:1055–1063.
14. Stumpe KD, Urbinelli M, Steinert HC, Glanzmann C, Buck A, von Schulthess GK. Whole-body positron emission tomography using fluorodeoxyglucose for staging of lymphoma: effectiveness and comparison with computed tomography. Eur J Nucl Med 1998;25:721–728.
15. Moog F, Bangerter M, Diederichs CG, Guhlmann A, Merkle E, Frickhofen N, Reske SN. Extranodal malignant lymphoma: detection with FDG PET versus CT. Radiology 1998;206:475–481.
16. Jerusalem G, Beguin Y, Fassotte MF, Najjar F, Paulus P, Rigo P, Fillet G. Whole-body positron emission tomography using 18F-fluorodeoxyglucose for post-treatment evaluation in Hodgkin's disease and non-Hodgkin's lymphoma has higher diagnostic and prognostic value than classical computed tomography scan imaging. Blood 1999;94:429–433.
17. Bangerter M, Kotzerke J, Griesshammer M, Elsner K, Reske SN, Bergmann L. Positron emission tomography with 18-fluorodeoxyglucose in the staging and follow-up of lymphoma in the chest. Acta Oncol 1999;38:799–804.
18. Wiedmann E, Baican B, Hertel A, et al. Positron emission tomography (PET) for staging and evaluation of response to treatment in patients with Hodgkin's disease. Leuk Lymphoma 1999;34:545–551.
19. Hany TF, Steinert HC, Goerres GW, Buck A, von Schulthess GK. PET diagnostic accuracy: improvement with in-line PET-CT system: initial results. Radiology 2002;225:575–581.
20. Kostakoglu L, Leonard JP, Kuji I, et al. Comparison of fluorine-18 fluorodeoxyglucose positron emission tomography and Ga-67 scintigraphy in evaluation of lymphoma. Cancer 2002;94:879–888.
21. Townsend DW, Beyer T. A combined PET/CT scanner: the path to true image fusion. Br J Radiol 2002;75:S24–30.
22. National Cancer Institute–sponsored study of classifications of non-Hodgkin's lymphomas: summary and description of a working formulation for clinical usage. The Non-Hodgkin's Lymphoma Pathologic Classification Project. Cancer 1982;49:2112–2135.
23. Jaffe E, Harris N, Diebold J, Muller-Hermelink H-K. World Health Organization classification of neoplastic diseases of the hematopoietic and lymphoid tissues. A progress report. Am J Clin Pathol 1999;111(Suppl 1):S8–S12.
24. Harris N, Jaffe E, Diebold J, et al. The World Health Organization classification of hematological malignancies. Report of the Clinical Advisory Committee Meeting. Mod Pathol 2000;13:193–207.
25. Armitage JO. Treatment of non-Hodgkin's lymphoma. NEJM 1993;328:1023–1030.
26. Orlandi E, Lazzarino M, Brusamolino E, Paulli M, Astori C, Magrini U, Bernasconi C. Nodular lymphocyte predominance Hodgkin's disease: long-term observation reveals a continuous pattern of recurrence. Leuk Lymphoma 1997;26:359–368.
27. Lister TA, Crowther D, Sutcliffe SB, et al. Report of a committee convened to discuss the evaluation and staging of patients with Hodgkin's disease: Cotswold meeting. J Clin Oncol 1989;7:1630–1636
28. Rosenberg S. Validity of the Ann Arbor staging system classification from the non-Hodgkin's lymphomas. Cancer Treat Rep 1977;61:1023–1027.
29. Leibenhaut MH, Hoppe RT, Efron B, Halpern J, Nelsen T, Rosenberg SA. Prognostic indicators of laparotomy findings in

clinical stage I-II supradiaphragmatic Hodgkin's disease. J Clin Oncol 1989;7:81–91.
30. Josting A, Diehl V. Current treatment strategies in early stage Hodgkin's disease. Curr Treat Options Oncol 2003;4:297–305.
31. Ng AK, Bernardo MV, Weller E, et al. Second malignancy after Hodgkin disease treated with radiation therapy with or without chemotherapy: long-term risks and risk factors. Blood 2002;100: 1989–1996.
32. Cheson BD. Radioimmunotherapy of non-Hodgkin lymphomas. Blood 2003;101:391–398.
33. Winter JN, Gascoyne RD, Van Besien K. Low-grade lymphoma. Hematology 2004;1:203.
34. Hoane BR, Shields AF, Porter BA, et al. Comparison of initial lymphoma staging using computed tomography (CT) and magnetic resonance (MR) imaging. Am J Hematol 1994;47:100–105.
35. Jung G, Heindel W, von Bergwelt-Baildon M, et al. Abdominal lymphoma staging: is MR imaging with T2-weighted turbo-spin-echo sequence: a diagnostic alternative to contrast-enhanced spiral CT? J Comput Assist Tomogr 2000;24:783–787.
36. Ferrucci JT. Advances in abdominal MR imaging. RadioGraphics 1998;18:1569–1586.
37. North LB, Libshitz HI, Lorigan JG. Thoracic lymphoma. Radiol Clin North Am 1990;28:745–762.
38. Tateishi U, Muller NL, Johkoh T, Onishi Y, Arai Y, Satake M, Matsuno Y, Tobinai K. Primary mediastinal lymphoma: characteristic features of the various histological subtypes on CT. J Comput Assist Tomogr 2004;28:782–789.
39. Cazals-Hatem D, Lepage E, Brice P, et al. Primary mediastinal large B-cell lymphoma: a clinicopathologic study of 141 cases compared with 916 nonmediastinal large B-cell lymphomas – a GELA ("Groupe d'Etude des Lymphomas de l'Adulte") study. Am J Surg Pathol 1996;20:877–888.
40. Lee JKT, Stanley RJ, Sagel SS, et al. Accuracy of computed tomography in detecting intra-abdominal and pelvic adenopathy in lymphoma. Am J Roentgenol 1978;131:675–679.
41. Elstrom R, Guan L, Baker G, et al. Utility of FDG PET scanning in lymphoma by WHO classification. Blood 2003;101:3875–3876.
42. Jerusalem G, Beguin Y, Najjar F, Hustinx R, Fassotte MF, Rigo P, Fillet G. Positron emission tomography (PET) with 18F-fluorodeoxyglucose (18F-FDG) for the staging of low-grade non-Hodgkin's lymphoma (NHL). Ann Oncol 2001;12:825–830.
43. Hoffmann M, Kletter K, Becherer A, et al. 18F-fluorodeoxyglucose positron emission tomography (18F-FDG PET) for staging and follow-up of marginal zone B-cell lymphoma. Oncology 2003;64: 336–340.
44. Yeung HW, Young KS, Schoder H, Beal K, Larson SM. Extranodal marginal zone lymphoma (LAT) is frequently positive on FDG PET scan. J Nucl Med 2004;45:93P.
45. Nathwani B, Anderson JR, Armitage JO, et al. Marginal zone B-cell lymphoma: A clinical comparison of nodal and mucosa-associated lymphoid tissue types. J Clin Oncol 1999;17:2486–2492.
46. Ben-Haim S, Bar-Shalom R, Israel O, et al. Utility of gallium-67 scintigraphy in low-grade non-Hodgkin's lymphoma. J Clin Oncol 1996;14:1936–1942.
47. Shrikanthan S, Zhuang HM, Schuster S, Alavi A. FDG PET imaging in diagnosis of mantle cell lymphoma. J Nucl Med 2004;45:93P.
48. Moog F, Bangerter M, Diederichs CG, Guhlmann A, Kotzerke J, Merkle E. Lymphoma: role of FDG PET in nodal staging. Radiology 1997;203:795–800.
49. Menzel C, Dobert N, Mitrou P, Mose S, Diehl M, Berner U. Positron emission tomography for the staging of Hodgkin's lymphoma. Acta Oncol 2002;41:430–436.
50. Weihrauch MR, Re D, Bischoff S, Dietlein M, Scheidhauer K, Krug B. Whole-body positron emission tomography using 18F-fluorodeoxyglucose for initial staging of patients with Hodgkin's disease. Ann Hematol 2002;81:20–25.
51. Naumann R, Beuthien-Baumann B, Reiss A, Schulze J, Hanel A, Bredow J. Substantial impact of FDG PET imaging on the therapy decision in patients with early-stage Hodgkin's lymphoma. Br J Cancer 2004;90:620–625.
52. Bangerter M, Moog F, Buchmann I, et al. Whole-body 2-[18F]-fluoro-2-deoxy-D-glucose positron emission tomography (FDG PET) for accurate staging of Hodgkin's disease. Ann Oncol 1998;9:1117–1122.
53. Schaefer NG, Hany TF, Taverna C, Seifert B, Stumpe KD, von Schulthess GK, Goerres GW. Non-Hodgkin lymphoma and Hodgkin disease: coregistered FDG PET and CT at staging and restaging – do we need contrast-enhanced CT? Radiology 2004;232:823–829.
54. Sohaib SA, Turner B, Hanson JA, Farquharson M, Oliver RT, Reznek RH. CT assessment of tumour response to treatment: comparison of linear, cross-sectional and volumetric measures of tumour size. Br J Radiol 2000;73:1178–1184.
55. Economopoulos T, Asprou N, Stathakis N, et al. Primary extranodal non-Hodgkin's lymphoma of the head and neck. Oncology 1992;49:484–488.
56. Dodd GD. Lymphoma of the hollow abdominal viscera. Radiol Clin North Am 1990;28:771–783.
57. Yoo CC, Levine MS, Furth EE, Salhany KE, Rubesin SE, Laufer I, Herlinger H. Gastric mucosa-associated lymphoid tissue lymphoma: radiographic findings in six patients. Radiology 1998;208:239–243.
58. Levine MS, Rubesin SE, Pantongrag-Brown L, Buck JL, Herlinger H. Non-Hodgkin's lymphoma of the gastrointestinal tract: radiographic findings. AJR Am J Roentgenol 1997;168(1):165–172.
59. Yuki M, Narabayashi I, Yamamoto K, Shimizu T, Tanaka Y, Tatsumi T, Komori T. Multifocal primary lymphoma of bone: scintigraphy and MR findings before and after treatment. Radiat Med 2000;18:305–310.
60. Lanfermann H, Heindel W, Schaper J, Schroeder R, Hansmann ML, Lehrke R, Ernestus RI, Lackner K. CT and MR imaging in primary cerebral non-Hodgkin's lymphoma. Acta Radiol 1997;38:259–267.
61. Herrlinger U, Schabet M, Clemens M, Kortmann RD, Petersen D, Will BE, Meyermann R, Dichgans J. Clinical presentation and therapeutic outcome in 26 patients with primary CNS lymphoma. Acta Neurol Scand 1998;97:257–264.
62. Buhring U, Herrlinger U, Krings T, Thiex R, Weller M, Kuker W. MRI features of primary central nervous system lymphomas at presentation. Neurology 2001;57:393–396.
63. Buckley JA, Fishman EK.CT evaluation of small bowel neoplasms: spectrum of disease. Radiographics 1998;18:379–392.
64. Gospodarowicz MK, Ferry JA, Cavalli F. Unique aspects of primary extranodal lymphomas. In: Mauch PM, Armitage JO, Coiffier B, Dalla-Favera R, Harris NL (eds.). Non-Hodgkin's lymphomas. Philadelphia: Lippincott Williams & Wilkins, 2004:685–707.
65. Gorg C, Weide R, Schwerk WB. Malignant splenic lymphoma: sonographic patterns, diagnosis and follow-up. Clin Radiol 1997;52:535–540.
66. Rodriguez M, Ahlstrom H, Sundin A, Rehn S, Sundstrom C, Hagberg H, Glimelius B. 18F FDG PET in gastric non-Hodgkin's lymphoma. Acta Oncol 1997;36:577–584.
67. Hoffman JM, Waskin HA, Schifter T, et al. FDG PET in differentiating lymphoma from non-malignant central nervous system lesions in patients with AIDS. J Nucl Med 1993;34:567–575.
68. Heald AE, Hoffman JM, Bartlett JA, Waskin HA. Differentiation of central nervous system lesions in AIDS patients using positron emission tomography (PET). Int J STD AIDS 1996;7:337–346.
69. Skiest DJ, Erdman W, Chang WE, Oz OK, Ware A, Fleckenstein J. SPECT thallium-201 combined with Toxoplasma serology for the presumptive diagnosis of focal central nervous system mass lesions in patients with AIDS. J Infect 2000;40:274–281.

70. Shipp M, Mauch PM, Harris NL. Non-Hodgkin's lymphomas. In: Devita VT, Hellman S, Rosenberg SA (eds.). Cancer Principles and Practice of Oncology. Philadelphia: Lippincott, 1997, pp. 2165–2220.
71. Abdel-Dayem HM, Rosen G, El-Zeftawy H, Naddaf S, Kumar M, Atay S, Cacavio A. Fluorine-18 fluorodeoxyglucose splenic uptake from extramedullary hematopoiesis after granulocyte colony-stimulating factor stimulation. Clin Nucl Med 1999;24:319–322.
72. Gundlapalli S, Ojha B, Mountz JM. Granulocyte colony-stimulating factor: confounding F-18 FDG uptake in outpatient positron emission tomographic facilities for patients receiving ongoing treatment of lymphoma. Clin Nucl Med 2002;27:140–141.
73. Carr R, Barrington SF, Madan B, ÓDoherty MJ, Saunders CA, van der Walt J, Timothy AR. Detection of lymphoma in bone marrow by whole-body positron emission tomography. Blood 1998;91: 3340–3346.
74. Moog F, Bangerter M, Kotzerke J, Guhlman A, Frickhofen N, Reske SN. 18-F-fluorodeoxyglucose-positron emission tomography as a new approach to detect lymphomatous bone marrow. J Clin Oncol 1998;16:603–609.
75. Rini JN, Manalili EY, Hoffman MA, Karayalcin G, Mehrotra B, Tomas MB, Palestro CJ. F-18 FDG versus Ga-67 for detecting splenic involvement in Hodgkin's disease. Clin Nucl Med 2002;27:572–577.
76. Bar-Shalom R, Yefremov N, Haim N, et al. Camera-based FDG PET and ^{67}Ga SPECT in evaluation of lymphoma: comparative study. Radiology 2003;227:353–360.
77. Wirth A, Seymour JF, Hicks RJ, et al. Fluorine-18 fluorodeoxyglucose positron emission tomography, gallium-67 scintigraphy, and conventional staging for Hodgkin's disease and non-Hodgkin's lymphoma. Am J Med 2002;112:262–268.
78. Hong SP, Hahn JS, Lee JD, Bae SW, Youn MJ. 18F-fluorodeoxyglucose-positron emission tomography in the staging of malignant lymphoma compared with CT and 67Ga scan. Yonsei Med J 2003;44:779–786.
79. Sasaki M, Kuwabara Y, Koga H, Clinical impact of whole body FDG PET on the staging and therapeutic decision making for malignant lymphoma. Ann Nucl Med 2002;16:337–345.
80. Larson SM, Rasey JS, Allen DR, Nelson NJ, Grunbaum Z, Harp GD, Williams DL. Common pathway for tumor cell uptake of gallium-67 and iron-59 via a transferrin receptor. J Natl Cancer Inst 1980;64:41–53.
81. Nejmeddine F, Caillat-Vigneron N, Escaig F, Moretti JL, Raphael M, Galle P. Mechanism involved in gallium-67 (Ga-67) uptake by human lymphoid cell lines. Cell Mol Biol (Noisy-le-grand) 1998;44:1215–1220.
82. Diehl V, Stein H, Hummel M, Zollinger R, Connors JM. Hodgkin's lymphoma: biology and treatment strategies for primary, refractory, and relapsed disease. Hematology 2003;225–247.
83. Buchmann I, Reinhardt M, Elsner K, et al. 2-(Fluorine-18)fluoro-2-deoxy-D-glucose positron emission tomography in the detection and staging of malignant lymphoma. A bicenter trial. Cancer 2001;91:889–999.
84. Partridge S, Timothy A, ÓDoherty MJ, et al. 2-fluorine-18-fluoro-2-deoxy-D glucose positron emission tomography in the pretreatment staging of Hodgkin's disease: Influence on patients management in a single institution. Ann Oncol 2000;11:1273–1279.
85. Schoder H, Meta J, Yap C, et al. Effect of whole-body (18)F-FDG PET imaging on clinical staging and management of patients with malignant lymphoma. J Nucl Med 2001;42:1139–1143.
86. Hueltenschmidt B, Sautter-Bihl ML, Lang O, et al. Whole body positron emission tomography in the treatment of Hodgkin disease. Cancer 2001;91:302–310.
87. Brandt L, Kimby E, Nygren P, Glimelius B. A systematic overview of chemotherapy effects in Hodgkin's disease. Acta Oncol 2001;40:185–197.
88. Coiffier B, Gisselbrecht C, Vose JM, et al. Prognostic factors in aggressive malignant lymphomas. Description and validation of prognostic index that could identify patients requiring a more intensive therapy. J Clin Oncol 1991;9:211–219.
89. Lewis E, Bernardino ME, Salvador PG, Cabanillas FF, Barnes PA, Thomas JL. Post-therapy CT-detected mass in lymphoma patients: is it viable tissue? J Comput Assist Tomogr 1982;6:792–795.
90. Cheson BD, Horning SJ, Coiffier B, et al. Report of an international workshop to standardize response criteria for non-Hodgkin's lymphomas. NCI Sponsored International Working Group. J Clin Oncol 1999;17:1244–1253.
91. Hasenclever D, Diehl V. International Prognostic Factors Project on Advanced Hodgkin's Disease. A prognostic score for advanced Hodgkin's disease. NEJM 1998;339:1506–1514.
92. Rodriguez MA, Fuller LM, Zimmerman SO, et al. Hodgkin's disease: study of treatment intensities and incidences of second malignancies. Ann Oncol 1993;4:125–131.
93. Theuws JC, Seppenwoolde Y, Kwa SL, Boersma LJ, Damen EM, Baas P, Muller SH, Lebesque JV. Changes in local pulmonary injury up to 48 months after irradiation for lymphoma and breast cancer. Int J Radiat Oncol Biol Phys 2000;47:1201–1208.
94. Cremerius U, Fabry U, Kroll U, Zimny M, Neuerburg J, Osieka R, Bull U. Clinical value of FDG PET for therapy monitoring of malignant lymphoma. Results of a retrospective study in 72 patients. Nuklearmedizin 1999;38:24–30.
95. Weihrauch MR, Re D, Scheidhauer K, et al. Thoracic positron emission tomography using 18F-fluorodeoxyglucose for the evaluation of residual mediastinal Hodgkin's disease. Blood 2001;98:2930–2934.
96. Naumann R, Vaic A, Beuthien-Baumann B, et al. Prognostic value of positron emission tomography in the evaluation of post-treatment residual mass in patients with Hodgkin's disease and non-Hodgkin's lymphoma. Br J Haematol 2001;115:793–800.
97. Mikhaeel NG, Timothy AR, ÓDoherty MJ, Hain S, Maisey MN. 18-FDG PET as a prognostic indicator in the treatment of aggressive Non-Hodgkin's lymphoma: comparison with CT. Leuk Lymphoma 2000;39:543–553.
98. de Wit M, Bohuslavizki KH, Buchert, Bumann D, Clausen M, Hossfeld DK. ^{18}FDG PET following treatment as valid predictor for disease-free survival in Hodgkin's lymphoma. Ann Oncol 2001;12:29–37.
99. Zinzani PL, Magagnoli M, Chierichetti F, et al. The role of positron emission tomography (PET) in the management of lymphoma patients. Ann Oncol 1999;10:1181–1184.
100. Jerusalem G, Beguin Y, Fassotte MF, et al. Early detection of relapse by whole-body positron emission tomography in the follow-up of patients with Hodgkin's disease. Ann Oncol 2003;14: 123–130.
101. Dittmann H, Sokler M, Kollmannsberger C, et al. Comparison of 18FDG PET with CT scans in the evaluation of patients with residual and recurrent Hodgkin's lymphoma. Oncol Rep 2001;8:1393–1399.
102. Shipp MA. Prognostic factors in aggressive non-Hodgkin's lymphoma: who has "high-risk" disease? Blood 1994;83:1165–1173.
103. Spaepen K, Stroobants S, Dupont P, et al. Prognostic value of positron emission tomography (PET) with fluorine-18 fluorodeoxyglucose ([^{18}F]FDG after first line chemotherapy in non-Hodgkins lymphoma: is ([^{18}F]FDG PET a valid alternative to conventional diagnostic methods? J Clin Oncol 2001;19:414–419.
104. Kostakoglu L, Coleman M, Leonard JP, Kuji I, Zoe H, Goldsmith SJ. Positron emission tomography predicts prognosis after one cycle of chemotherapy in aggressive lymphoma and Hodgkin's disease. J Nucl Med 2002;43:1018–1027.
105. Mikhaeel NG, Mainwaring P, Nunan T, Timothy AR. Prognostic value of interim and post treatment FDG PET scanning in Hodgkin lymphoma [abstract]. Ann Oncol 2002;13(Suppl 2):21.

106. Spaepen K, Stroobants S, Dupont P, et al. Early restaging positron emission tomography with 18F-fluorodeoxyglucose predicts outcome in patients with aggressive non-Hodgkin's lymphoma. Ann Oncol 2002;13:1356–1363.
107. Philip T, Guglielmi C, Hagenbeek A, et al. Autologous bone marrow transplantation as compared with salvage chemotherapy in relapses of chemotherapy-sensitive non-Hodgkin's lymphoma. NEJM 1995;333:1540–1545.
108. Cremerius U, Fabry U, Wildberger JE, et al. Pre-transplant positron emission tomography using fluorine-18-fluoro-deoxyglucose predicts outcome in patients treated with high-dose chemotherapy and autologous stem cell transplantation for non-Hodgkin's lymphoma. Bone Marrow Transplant 2002;30:103–111.
109. Becherer A, Mitterbauer M, Jaeger U, et al. Positron emission tomography with [18F]2-fluoro-D-2-deoxyglucose (FDG PET) predicts relapse of malignant lymphoma after high-dose therapy with stem cell transplantation. Leukemia 2002;16:260–267.
110. Armitage JO, Weisenburger DD, Hutchins M, et al. Chemotherapy for diffuse large-cell lymphoma – rapidly responding patients have more durable remissions. J Clin Oncol 1986;4:160–164.
111. Haw R, Sawka CA, Franssen E, Berinstein HL. Significance of a partial or slow response to front-line chemotherapy in the management of intermediate-grade or high-grade non-Hodgkin's lymphoma: a literature review. J Clin Oncol 1994;12:1074–1084.
112. Verdonck LF, van Putten WL, Hagenbeek A, Schouten HC, et al. NEJM 1995;20(332):1045–1051.
113. Romer W, Hanauske A-R, Ziegler S, et al. Positron emission tomography in non-Hodgkin's lymphoma: assessment of chemotherapy with fluorodeoxyglucose. Blood 1998;91:4464–4471.
114. Kostakoglu L, Coleman M, Somrov S, Leonard JP, Verma S, Sherman CH,. Goldsmith SJ. FDG PET after one cycle of chemotherapy accurately predicts response to therapy in large cell (aggressive) non-Hodgkin's lymphoma (NHL) and Hodgkin's disease (HD). J Nucl Med 2004;45:316P.
115. Hoekstra O, Ossenkoppele GJ, Golding R, et al. Early treatment response in malignant lymphoma, as determined by planar fluorine-18-fluorodeoxyglucose scintigraphy. J Nucl Med 1993;34: 1706–1710.
116. Koss MN. Pulmonary lymphoid disorders. Semin Diagn Pathol 1995;12:158–171.
117. Reddy MP, Graham MM. FDG positron emission tomographic imaging of thoracic Castleman's disease. Clin Nucl Med 2003;28:325–326.
118. Murphy SP, Nathan MA, Karwal MW. FDG PET appearance of pelvic Castleman's disease. J Nucl Med 1997;38:1211–1212.
119. Bragg DG, Chor PJ, Murray KA, et al. Lymphoproliferative disorders of the lung: histopathology, clinical manifestations, and imaging features. Am J Roentgenol 1994;163:273–281.
120. Tirelli U, Spina M, Gaidano G, Vaccher E, Franceschi S, Carbone A. Epidemiological, biological and clinical features of HIV-related lymphomas in the era of highly active antiretroviral therapy. AIDS 2000;14:1675–1688.
121. Weinblatt ME, Zanzi I, Belakhlef A, Babchyck B, Kochen J. False-positive FDG PET imaging of the thymus of a child with Hodgkin's disease. J Nucl Med 1997;38:888–890.
122. Ferdinand B, Gupta P, Kramer EL. Spectrum of thymic uptake at 18F-FDG PET. Radiographics 2004;24:1611–1616.
123. Kawano T, Suzuki A, Ishida A, et al. The clinical relevance of thymic fluorodeoxyglucose uptake in pediatric patients after chemotherapy. Eur J Nucl Med Mol Imag 2004;31:31–36.
124. Armitage JO. Bone marrow transplantation. NEJM 1994;330: 827–838.
125. Sandherr M, von Schilling C, Link T, Stock K, von Bubnoff N, Peschel C, Avril N. Pitfalls in imaging Hodgkin's disease with computed tomography and positron emission tomography using fluorine-18-fluorodeoxyglucose. Ann Oncol 2001;12: 719–722.

Chapter 23
PET-CT Imaging in Multiple Myeloma, Solitary Plasmacytoma, and Related Plasma Cell Dyscrasias

Ronald C. Walker, Marisa H. Miceli, and Laurie Jones-Jackson

Multiple myeloma (MM), also called plasma cell myeloma, comprises about 1% of all malignancies and 10% of hematologic malignancies. It is the second most common hematologic malignancy in the USA. It is a malignancy of terminally differentiated B cells (plasma cells), typically associated with secretion by these plasma cells of a complete and/or partial (light chain) monoclonal immunoglobulin protein (M protein) [1, 2].

About 50,000 people live with MM. There are approximately 15,000 new cases diagnosed and 11,000 patients dying annually. It is typically a disease of the late middle-aged to elderly people, with the median age at diagnosis being 65 years, although MM even occurs in teenagers. MM occurs more commonly in men than women and, in the USA, in African-American men than in the general population. Although the etiology of MM is unknown, several cytogenetic abnormalities associated with the disease define biologically and prognostically distinct entities. Chromosome 13 deletions, in particular, confer a poor prognosis. Most cases of MM evolve from a premalignant condition known as monoclonal gammopathy of undetermined significance (MGUS), which converts to MM at 1% annually, though some cases of MM probably develop de novo [2, 3].

Tumor Biology

MGUS, solitary plasmacytoma, and MM all belong to a spectrum of disorders known as *plasma cell dyscrasias*. The tumor growth is typically restricted to the bone marrow until late in tumor evolution, with the exception of solitary extramedullary plasmacytoma. The myeloma plasma cells induce changes in the bone marrow microenvironment that are critical for tumor cell survival, growth, and microenvironment-mediated drug resistance, as well as osteolysis. These signals eventually contribute to disease manifestations (e.g., bone disease). Investigators are increasingly recognizing the MM/microenvironment-associated signals as fundamental to the disease development, evolution, and ultimately development of treatment resistance. Thus, investigators are increasing interested in exploring these fundamental MM–microenvironmental interactions for disease control and, ultimately, cure. Genetic expression profiling (GEP) of these myeloma associated genes (MAG) is entering widespread use to guide treatment selection for these patients as well as to give upfront long-term risk assessment.

Clinical symptoms occur through a variety of mechanisms. These include direct tumor mass effect, such as cord compression, cytokine production (leading to secondary anemia, systemic osteoporosis, and compression fractures), and immune system dysfunction (with resultant immunosuppression causing increased infections, secondary malignancies, and autoimmune disorders). The clinical course depends on the individual biologic behavior of the specific clonal cell line, and can vary from a relatively indolent course to highly aggressive disease.

Solitary plasmacytoma exists in two varieties, solitary extramedullary plasmacytoma (SEP) and solitary bone plasmacytoma (SBP). SEP occurs exclusively in the soft tissues and has a high potential for cure. SBP is the more common of the two entities, and occurs in association with a focal tumor of bone. SBP is the more ominous of these two diseases, frequently a harbinger for future development of MM. Indeed, 3% of SBP patients convert annually to MM. If more than one focal lesion is detected in a patient with suspected solitary disease, then the diagnosis is almost always MM, with the exception being the uncommonly recognized condition "multiple solitary plasmacytomas." MM and multiple solitary plasmacytomas are distinguished by the presence of 10% or more diffuse plasma cell infiltrate on random marrow biopsy in MM.

Other plasma cell dyscrasias include rare conditions such as Castleman's disease (recently classified as a non-Hodgkin's lymphoma), alpha-heavy-chain disease, and Waldenström's macroglobulinemia [4–11].

R.C. Walker (✉)
Department of Clinical Radiology & Radiological Sciences, Vanderbilt University Medical Center, 1121 21st Avenue South CCC-1121, Nashville, 37232-2675 TN, USA
e-mail: ronald.walker@vanderbilt.edu;

P. Shreve and D.W. Townsend (eds.), *Clinical PET-CT in Radiology: Integrated Imaging in Oncology*,
DOI 10.1007/978-0-387-48902-5_23,

Diagnosis and Conventional Staging

Radiographic and laboratory findings form the basis of classical diagnosis using the canonical Durie-Salmon (DS) staging system. The most common clinical presentations are fatigue and bone pain (typically of the back or ribs, with or without associated fractures) or unexplained recurrent infections due to immunosuppression. About 15–30% of patients present with hypercalcemia and renal insufficiency from precipitation of M protein in the collecting tubules. Another 10% present with miscellaneous symptoms, such as hyperviscosity syndrome, compression of the spinal cord, radicular pain, soft-tissue tumors/plasmacytomas, or abnormal bleeding. In patients with asymptomatic disease, incidental laboratory findings of anemia or hyperproteinemia lead to the diagnosis.

The hallmark of MM is the detection in blood and/or urine of a monoclonal protein, called M protein, produced by the malignant plasma cells. Serum protein electrophoresis reveals a monoclonal peak in 80% of patients. The remaining 20% of patients will have either hypogammaglobulinemia or a normal-appearing (nonsecretory) electrophoresis profile. By using more sensitive techniques, such as the free-light chain analysis, M protein (in serum and/or urine) will be detected in 99% of patients. Additional parts of the diagnostic evaluation include a radiographic skeletal survey and a random bone marrow aspiration and biopsy to permit histologic examination, cytogenetic analyses, and determination of plasma cell labeling index (PCLI). Minimal criteria for establishing a diagnosis of MM is the detection of 10% or more abnormal plasma cells in a random bone marrow biopsy and M protein in either the serum (typically >3 g/dL) and/or urine (typically >1 g/24-h collection). Osteolytic lesions are the classic findings on skeletal survey in greater than or equal to 80% of patients [3].

Most plasma cell dyscrasias result from the expansion of a single clone of cells that secrete the hallmark monoclonal protein. A small fraction (3% at diagnosis) will be hyposecretory or nonsecretory, either with very low levels or without the secretion of the M protein. Serial M protein levels can be very useful to determine response to treatment. Thus, the hyposecretory or nonsecretory state, occurring in 3% at diagnosis but developing more frequently during treatment, is problematic for clinical management and reflects dedifferentiation of the tumor. This dedifferentiation is typically associated with a more aggressive form of the disease. Sensitive assays for serum free light chain protein allow quantifiable detection of free kappa/lambda proteins in approximately 70% of patients with nonsecretory disease and/or minimally secretory disease. Positron emission tomography (PET) scanning, using ^{18}F-fluorodeoxyglucose (FDG) as the radiotracer is useful in this clinical setting since the secretory status of the tumor does not alter the uptake of FDG [3–11].

Staging at diagnosis is still often based on the classic Durie-Salmon staging (D-S staging) (Table 23.1). In order to incorporate advances in medical technology (especially in imaging) in the interval since the DS staging system was initially adopted in 1975, Durie and others have recently proposed the Durie-Salmon Plus Imaging Staging (D-S–Plus Imaging) system. New protocols are increasingly making use of this modified and updated staging system.

The D-S–Plus Imaging staging system incorporates the number of either magnetic resonance imaging (MRI) or FDG PET defined focal lesions into staging. Specifically, increasing numbers of focal lesions on either MRI and/or FDG PET result in upstaging of the patient since an increasing number of MRI or FDG PET defined focal lesions is inversely related to prognosis, both independently and, in a multivariate analysis, with or without the presence of significant cytogenetic abnormalities (CA). Indeed, the statistical significance of this increasing number of focal lesions as defined by MRI or FDG PET was second only to CA in prognostic significance, superior to standard prognostic factors in either a univariate or multivariate analysis in terms of both event free survival (EFS) and overall survival (OS), independent of standard prognostic factors (i.e., elevated LDH, M protein, C-reactive protein, creatinine, or β-2 microglobulin, or abnormally depressed levels of hemoglobin or platelets) (Fig. 23.1a, b and Table 23.2) [4, 8, 12].

Table 23.1 Durie-Salmon PLUS staging system (DS+) (From Ref. [4]. With permission)

Classification	PLUS	New imaging: MRI and/or FDG PET
MGUS		All negative
Stage IA* (smoldering or indolent)		Can have single plasmacytoma and/or limited disease on imaging
Multiple myeloma stage IB*		<5 Focal lesions; mild diffuse disease
Multiple myeloma stage IIA/B*		5–20 Focal lesions; moderate diffuse disease
Stage III A/B*		>20 Focal lesions; severe diffuse disease
	*A Serum creatinine <2.0 mg/dL and No extramedullary disease	
	*B Serum creatinine >2.0 mg/dL or extramedullary disease	

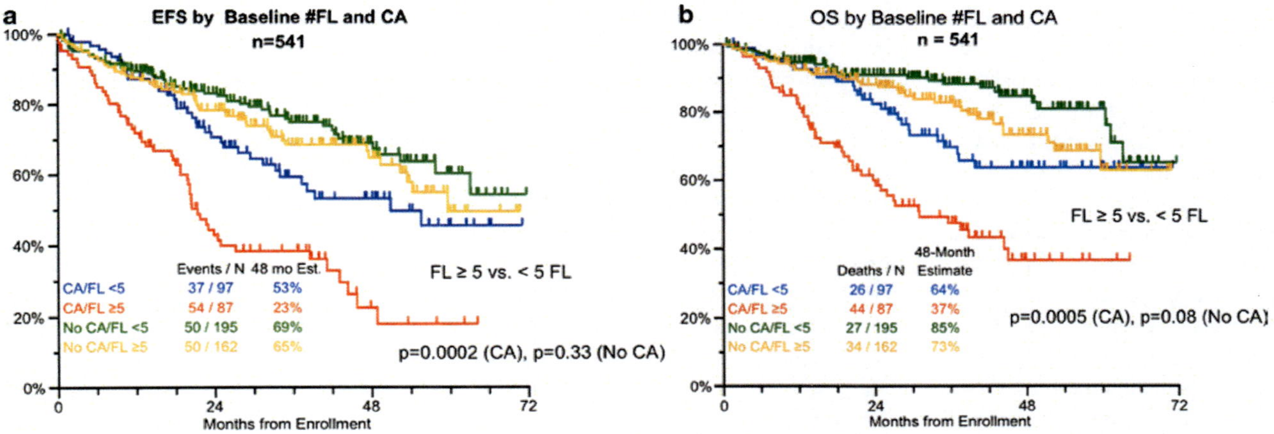

Fig. 23.1 Impact of the presence of cytogenetic abnormalities and number of focal lesions at diagnosis on event free survival (*EFS*) and overall survival (*OS*). (**a**) Kaplan-Meier (*KM*) curves for event free survival (*EFS*). (**b**) Overall survival (*OS*) correlating significance of number of focal lesions of bone at baseline with or without cytogenetic abnormalities with outcome (From Ref. [7]. With permission)

Table 23.2 Criteria for diagnosis of multiple myeloma[a] (From Ref. [1]. With permission)

Major criteria
Plasmacytomas on tissue biopsy
Marrow plasmacytosis with >30% plasma cells
Monoclonal globulin spike on serum electrophoresis >3.5 g/dL for IgG or >2.0 g/dL for IgA; 1.0 g/24 h of κ or λ light-chain excretion on urine electrophoresis in the absence of amyloidosis
Minor criteria
Marrow plasmacytosis 10–30%
Monoclonal globulin spike present, but less than the levels defined above
Lytic bone lesions
Normal IgM <0.05 g/dL, IgA <0.1 g/dL, or IgG <0.6 g/dL

[a] The diagnosis of plasma cell myeloma is confirmed when at least one major and one minor criterion or at least *three minor criteria* are documented in *symptomatic* patients with *progressive* disease. The presence of features not specific for the disease supports the diagnosis, particularly if of recent onset: anemia, hypercalcemia, azotemia, bone demineralization, or hypoalbuminemia

Current Treatment

Autologous peripheral blood stem cell transplant supported by high-dose melphalan is now considered standard therapy for symptomatic patients with MM up to 70 years of age, with tandem autotransplants achieving an almost 50% complete remission rate, and with median survival extending beyond 6–7 years. "Mini-allotransplants" are less toxic than standard therapy, exploiting a graft-versus-myeloma effect, and are used in the very old or very frail patient. New active drugs include immunomodulatory agents, such as thalidomide and CC-5013 (Revlimid, lenalidomide, Celgene, Warren, NJ), and the proteasome inhibitor, Velcade (bortezomib, Millennium, Cambridge, MA), all of which not only target MM cells directly but which also modulate the MM–microenvironmental interactions which support the tumor growth and ultimate development of drug resistance [13].

Role of PET-CT Imaging in Multiple Myeloma

Historically, x-ray metastatic surveys were a mainstay of the classic Durie-Salmon staging established in 1975, with the number of osteolytic lesions used to stage the patient. However, x-ray has less importance in the new Durie-Salmon Plus Imaging staging system since plain x-rays will often under represent the tumor burden. Indeed, accurate determination of the number of focal lesions at diagnosis and on follow-up is of great prognostic significance, secondly only to the presence of significant CA. There are two components of MM in the skeletal system imaged with PET-CT, the diffuse infiltration component and the focal lesion (FL) component. *A FL is defined as a well-circumscribed area of abnormal uptake in the skeletal system that is thought to represent tumor with at least one dimension measuring 5 mm or more.* These FL may or may not be associated with areas of x-ray osteolysis, and indeed, with effective treatment the FL will resolve before osteolysis occurs. Unlike many malignancies associated with osteolytic bone disease, the osteolytic lesions from MM often do not heal, even after years of remission.

Thus, functional imaging at baseline, such as with FDG PET-CT, is of prime importance for determining both upfront prognosis and subsequent tumor response. FDG PET-CT is superior to other imaging modalities for detection of progression on treatment or relapse since other modalities, including MRI, may require months to years to occur. MRI is probably best, however, to document completeness of response since patients who ultimately achieve a normal MRI scan have superior outcome to those who do not.

PET-CT is superior to other imaging modalities, including MRI, for detection of extramedullary tumor (MM that has become independent of the bone marrow microenvironment), because of its wider field of view. This is important since the presence of EMD defines a tumor population independent of the bone marrow microenvironment, resistant to the many treatments for MM that exploit this dependency. EMD confers a poor prognosis, with patients needing close followup and aggressive treatment.

PET-CT is also superior for detection of occult infection, a frequent and life-threatening occurrence in these immune-compromised patients. FDG PET-CT is useful for detection of occult infection even in the neutropenic patient on high-dose glucocorticoid medications, such as dexamethasone, a mainstay in MM treatment. This ability of FDG PET-CT to detect and localize infection in such a clinical setting is very useful since the utility of other methods for detection of occult infection, such as radiolabeled white cells, gallium scans, etc., will be adversely affected. Because infection is a significant source of morbidity and mortality in patients with hematologic malignancies, detection of suspected infection in not only useful but important to communicate in a rapid fashion to the clinical caregivers (Fig. 23.2) [3, 4, 15].

MRI is an important staging tool to distinguish truly solitary bone plasmacytoma from MM by identifying additional focal lesions of bone that are occult on standard radiographs, an ability shared with PET-CT. Both MRI and PET-CT can document the extent and pattern of marrow involvement. This overall pattern can range from diffuse involvement to microfocal (speckled appearance due to innumerable focal lesions of between 1 and 4 mm in maximum dimension) and/or to macrofocal disease (5 mm or more in at least on dimension, hereafter referred to as focal lesions), often occurring in various combinations. Both PET-CT and MRI can demonstrate "breakout" lesions, focal areas of disease that break through the cortex of bone into the soft tissues (including epidural spread which is seen with both modalities but best seen with MRI), yet which still occur in the context of and dependency upon the bone marrow microenvironment.

Both PET-CT and MRI can reveal exclusively soft tissue myeloma, called extramedullary disease (EMD). EMD represents a tumor population that is no longer dependent on the bone marrow microenvironment for growth and survival. Since therapy targets both the myeloma cells and the synergistic tumor–bone marrow interaction, loss of bone marrow microenvironment dependency identifies high-risk disease in need of aggressive monitoring and treatment. It is essential for the imaging physicians to communicate the presence, size, location, and number of sites of EMD in the report, including in the summary or impression, so the presence of EMD is not overlooked.

There are several relative disadvantages of MRI compared to PET-CT in this setting. Extensive imaging of the marrow space with MRI requires greater time and expense for a thorough examination compared to PET-CT, about 2–3 h versus 45 min of scan time, respectively. The much greater time and expense of MRI versus PET-CT are due to the need for separate studies of the brain and meninges, calvarium, vertebral column, pelvis, shoulder girdles, and sternum by MRI with multiple sequences (Whole body MRI may obviate some of these issues, but is if limited availability at this time and not yet established in this context.). MRIs has a field-of-view limited to the region under examination, resulting in failure to detect tumor (especially EMD) that is outside the region of study, which also limits detection of occult infection to regions being imaged.

It is neither safe nor permissible to image some patients by MRI, such as patients with pacemakers, certain aneurysm clips, cochlear implants, etc., all frequent occurrences in patients in the highest risk age group for MM; PET-CT can still safely image such patients. Regional artifacts, such as occurring in the sternum or mid-thoracic spine from cardiac motion or sternal wires, or in the pelvis from a hip replacement, also limit MRI relatively more than PET-CT.

The relative advantages of MRI compared to PET-CT imaging are the superior spatial and contrast resolution of MRI (with spatial resolution typically 2 mm for a high-field system versus about 1 and 4 mm for the CT and PET portions of the PET-CT imaging study, respectively) and its more widespread availability at this time. The high spatial/contrast resolution of MRI is important in the high-detail delineation of common problems in myeloma such as cord compression, infections of the spine, epidural and/or calvarial disease, and spinal fractures, though such conditions are often detected with PET-CT as well.

MRI easily depicts avascular necrosis (AVN) of the femoral or humeral heads resulting from glucocorticoid treatment, a common complication of treatment for MM. PET-CT does not detect AVN until late in the course of this condition when femoral or humeral head collapse occurs.

MRI easily depicts leptomeningeal spread of MM, an uncommon but important complication of MM, which is not well seen on PET-CT imaging due to the nearby normal intense brain uptake. The superior soft tissue contrast (compared to CT) and spatial resolution (compared to FDG PET) of MRI are particularly helpful to demonstrate involvement of the skull, including skull base and upper face, areas relatively difficult to evaluate on PET-CT examinations due to the high normal FDG uptake in the brain (Fig. 23.3).

If severe diffuse marrow infiltration with tumor is present, focal lesions (FL) from MM can be masked on both FDG PET-CT and MRI, but especially so on MRI. This diffuse

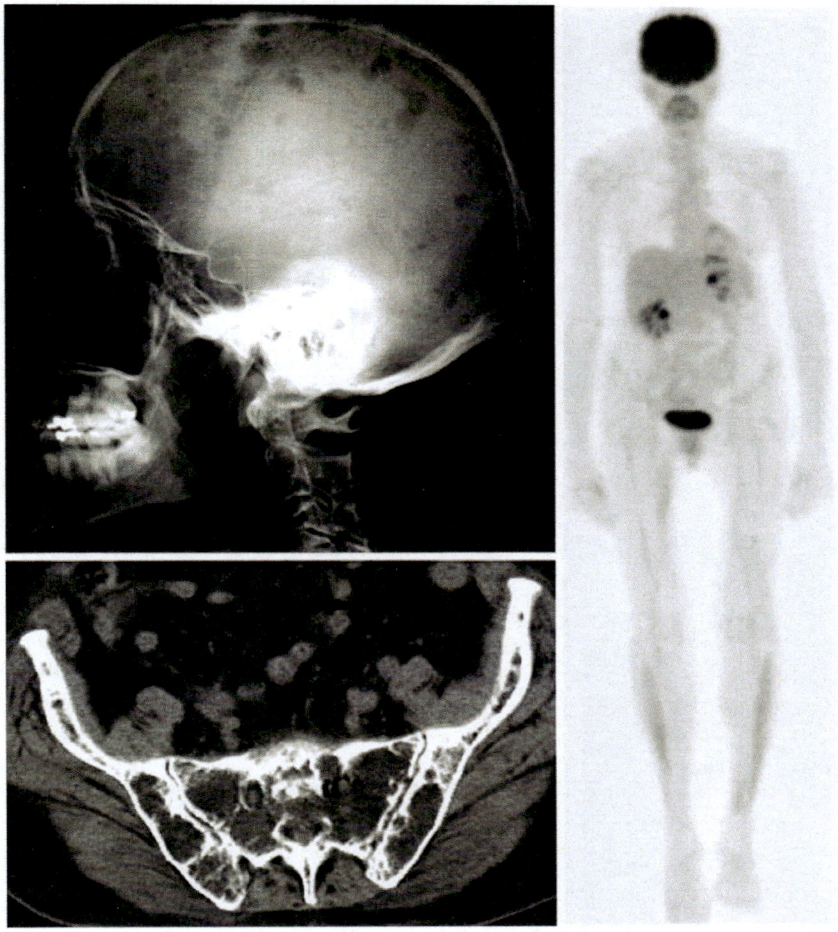

Fig. 23.2 Classic x-ray osteolytic lesions from MM. Lateral skull (*upper left*) and transaxial CT of the pelvis (*lower left*) demonstrate the focal osteolytic lesions from MM which will never heal. A concurrent FDG PET scan (*right*) of the same patient is normal in this patient who has been in remission for more than 2 years (From Ref. [14]. With permission)

tumor infiltration of the marrow will have the same signal characteristics on MRI as focal disease, specifically high signal on short-T1 inversion recovery weighted (STIR-wt) and low signal on T1-weighted (T1-wt) imaging sequences. Additionally, the severe diffuse marrow infiltration from MM will enhance diffusely after gadolinium injection similar to the underlying FL. Thus, severe diffuse tumor infiltration can obscure the presence of FL on MRI on all sequences. FDG PET or integrated PET-CT, however, can still visualize these FL against the diffuse infiltration because of the typically greater metabolic rate of the FL (Fig. 23.4).

MRI and PET-CT both track response to treatment of the diffuse infiltration from MM in real time demonstrating rapid return to normal appearance on both imaging modalities in close temporal relation to the M protein, appearance of random marrow aspirate, etc. However, the FL seen on MRI typically require months or even years to resolve, and indeed may never resolve despite prolonged complete remission. MRI can detect relapse if these FL increase in size or number or by the presence of FL gadolinium enhancement. These MRI-defined FL can still harbor viable tumor cells detected by biopsy on a microscopic level, and thus may represent sanctuaries or sources for relapse months to years after remission.

PET-CT tracks treatment response of both the diffuse and focal lesions in near real-time, in both secretory or, importantly, nonsecretory disease. Also importantly, PET-CT will demonstrate relapse during treatment as areas of persisting, new, and/or recurrent metabolic uptake on treatment. Indeed, the PET-CT can provide high-yield targets for biopsy of the areas of relapse, with gene expression profiling of such tissue samples of possible usefulness in selection for changes in treatment.

Thus, MRI and PET-CT have complementary roles in diagnosis, staging, and restaging of MM and related plasma cell dyscrasias. MRI is ideal to document the ultimate

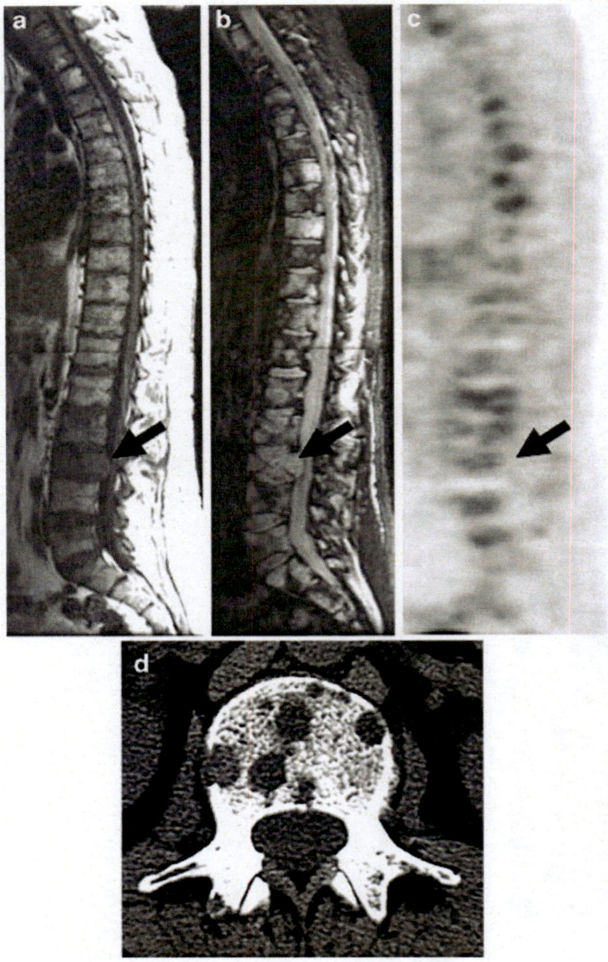

Fig. 23.3 (**a–d**) Severe diffuse and focal disease demonstrated on MRI T1 (**a**) and STIR-weighted (**b**) and FDG PET imaging (**c**) of the vertebral column with an axial CT (**d**) demonstrating classic osteolytic disease of advanced MM. The compression fracture with neural arch compromise at L3 (*arrow*) is not seen by FDG PET (From Ref. [14]. With permission)

completeness of response to treatment, though a normal MRI may take years to achieve. Nonetheless, obtaining a normal MRI examination is a favorable prognostic finding (*p* value with table). PET-CT is ideal for monitoring short-term treatment response, detection of sites of relapse on treatment, and/or detection of EMD or occult infection (Fig. 23.5) [7].

Clinical PET and PET-CT Imaging Protocols

The FDG PET-CT imaging protocol for MM and related plasma cell dyscrasias is designed to image the entire marrow space and the soft tissues from the vertex to the feet, similar to protocols for melanoma. The day before the PET-CT is to be done the patient begins a high-protein, low-carbohydrate diet and limits physical activity. Because excessive muscular uptake will significantly obscure imaging of the marrow space (diversion of isotope from the target to the muscles and direct obscuration of the regions of high interest from nearby soft-tissue activity), the patient is instructed to avoid any unnecessary physical activity for 24 h as well, including what the patient may think is trivial (yard work, grocery shopping, house work, etc.). Insulin-dependent diabetics are instructed to withhold insulin for a minimum of 6 h before administration of FDG if possible. The serum glucose level at time of injection of the FDG is measured and documented in the report.

Because of the frequent use of high-dose glucocorticoids in MM and related diseases, high serum glucose levels are common, frequently ranging between 100 and 200 mg/dL. This hyperglycemia interferes to some degree with the quality of the PET images. The degree of uptake by tumors is reduced due to competitive inhibition, decreasing measured standard uptake values (SUVs). These SUV values are also affected by the volume of distribution of the isotope in the patients, with fatty tissue adding to the weight of the patient but not significantly to the volume of distribution of the isotope. Since glucocorticoid medications can cause wide swings in both the weight of the patient and the level of glucose, normalization for these factors is important to provide meaningful comparison of SUVs between studies. Thus, reporting SUV values normalized to lean body mass, rather than body weight, is essential for meaningful comparisons between studies.

Due to the devastating effect of the MM on the immune system, compounded by the frequent use of high-dose glucocorticoid medications, occult infection is very common in these patients and is a frequent source of morbidity and mortality. Some simple steps in performance of the PET-CT scan can provide important information in detection of occult infection. For instance, if possible, it is very important to administer the radiopharmaceutical via a peripheral vein rather than a central line. Thrombi typically occur at the tips of central catheters and may become secondarily infected. Avoiding the use of the central catheter for FDG injection allows detection of infected thrombi that may form at the tip of these catheters as focal areas of uptake on the PET-CT image. If direct venous access is not technically feasible, flushing the central catheter with 200 mL of sterile normal saline helps diminish residual activity in the central catheter and improves the image appearance in general, though detection of infection associated with the central catheter will be less reliable [16–19].

A dose of FDG 555 MBq (15 mCi) of FDG is typically administered intravenously 60 min prior to beginning image acquisition. During the distribution time, the patient rests quietly in a semirecumbent position, and avoids talking. The patient voids immediately prior to imaging.

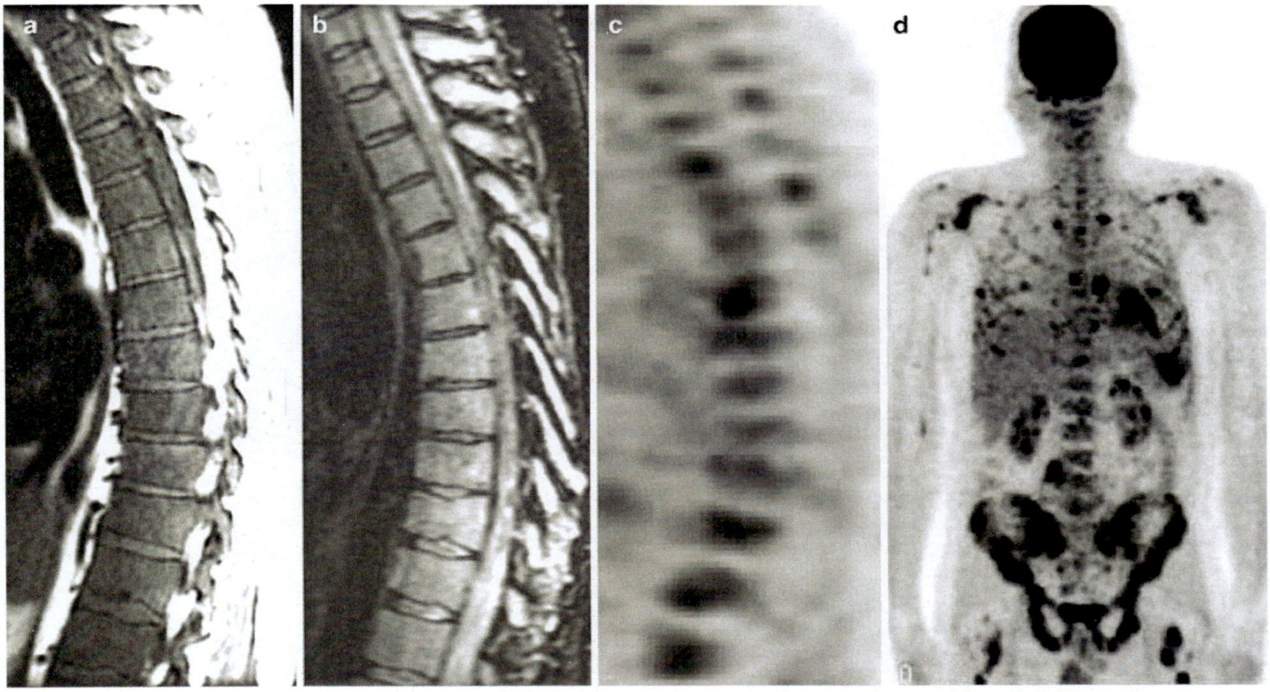

Fig. 23.4 (**a–d**) Masking of focal lesions on MRI from the signal produced by diffuse, intense tumor infiltration on T1 (**a**) and STIR (**b**) weighted sagittal thoracic spine MRI images. The many focal lesions as well as areas of diffuse infiltration are shown clearly on sagittal (**c**) and anterior 3D maximum intensity projection (*MIP*) (**d**) FDG PET images (From Ref. [14]. With permission)

Protocols for PET image acquisition and processing are identical to the technical settings used for other malignancies, such as melanoma, though specific settings vary from manufacturer to manufacturer. The whole-body protocol for MM is similar to that for melanoma, imaging from vertex to feet.

At the University of Arkansas Medical Center, PET-CT imaging is performed using one of two integrated PET-CT systems. One system is a CTI Reveal 16 "Hi Res" system from CTI Medical Systems, Knoxville, TN, with the CT portion being a Siemens Sensation 16 helical CT scanner and with the PET portion having 4-mm LSO detectors. The other is the similar Siemens PET-CT, with an identical "Hi Rez" PET imaging portion made by CTI Medical Systems (Knoxville, TN), and a 6-slice Siemens helical CT. These are 3D only systems. PET-CT imaging is performed from vertex to feet in a continuous manner, with whole-body CT attenuation correction, beginning at the vertex. Patients are imaged in one continuous examination, unless too tall (in which case they are imaged from the vertex to the knees, turned on the table, and then imaged from the knees to the feet). The use of identical PET gantries permits, as much as possible, similar results in terms of image resolution and SUV values for comparison between studies.

For the typical patient, a 1-mm helical CT topogram is performed with 120 kV and 50 mA for the full length of the body. If the patient exceeds the single pass length capability of the system (about 76 in. or 196 cm), the knees to feet region is imaged separately. The protocol for CT image acquisition includes a kV of 120 with effective mAs of 190, with 1.5 mm "fast" slice with 18 mm feed/rotation. A general whole-body kernel filter is used, B.31f, with medium smoothing with a 500 mm field of view, with reconstruction increments of 3.4 mm.

For the PET acquisition of the PET-CT examination, 4-min bed position emission images are acquired, though this time is increased on a floating scale if the patient is obese in order to obtain sufficient count statistics for adequate image quality and SUV measurement.

With both systems, the raw data are transferred to Wizard workstations (CTI Medical Systems) for reconstruction to permit scanning of the next patient. The PET images are reconstructed with a 6-mm FWHM filter, with FORE sinogram rebinning, using iterative reconstruction (two iterations on eight subsets), and scatter correction. The processed images are transferred to PACS and multiple PET-CT reading workstations.

With these types of PET-CT systems, it is not necessary to reconstruct separately the CT data with a bone filter since the resolution of the CT scanners using the whole-body filtering mentioned above demonstrates excellent bone detail using the appropriate window and level settings.

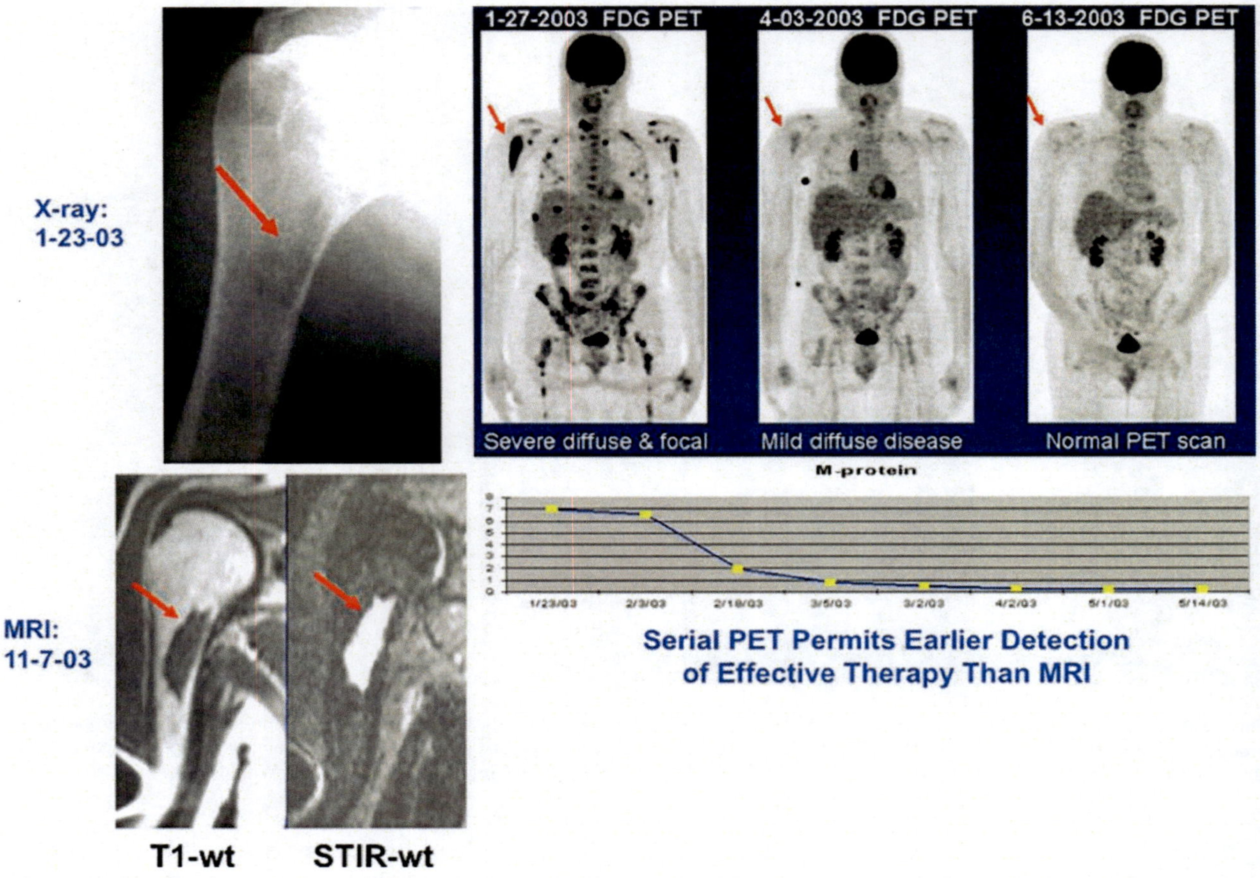

Fig. 23.5 PET normalization of diffuse and focal disease components tracks clinical response. X-ray is abnormal permanently. MRI-focal lesion normalization lags behind M protein and FDG PET for months to years. Patient in complete remission since April 2003 (From Ref. [14]. With permission)

Therefore, both the skeletal system and the soft tissues are evaluated with one image set. The CT images are processed in a 512×512 pixel matrix. The PET images, acquired with 4-mm high-resolution LSO detectors, are reconstructed in a 168×168 pixel matrix and interpolated to a 512×512 matrix to match the CT.

The images are interpreted on dedicated Mirada MVS workstations (CTI Medical Systems), using proprietary FDA-approved software provided by the manufacturer that includes deformable fusion. Raw data are archived on disc for long-term storage in addition to transfer of processed images to the university PACS system. When the patient returns for followup PET or PET-CT imaging, the raw data from the most recent study (or more, if needed) are reconstructed for direct comparison on the workstations between new and old studies. PACS image comparison of older studies is also available, though without the SUV information.

Role of FDG PET and PET-CT in MM and Related Plasma Cell Dyscrasias

The findings of great importance in PET imaging of MM are:

1. Detecting and quantifying the size, number and SUV (normalized to lean body mass) of skeletal focal lesions.
2. Detecting and quantifying location, size, and SUV of extramedullary disease sites.
3. Detecting and rapidly communicating the presence of occult infection.
4. Detection and quantifying the number of focal CT osteolytic lesions (CT metastatic bone survey) with documentation of maximum size of an osteolytic lesion and rapid communication of any at-risk lesions for pathologic fracture. Not infrequently, the number of focal CT osteolytic

lesions is too many to practically quantify, in which case a range, such as 25–50, or 100+, is given, with a comment as to whether or not this has changed from prior examinations, given in the report. In general, most CT osteolytic lesions are not FDG-avid, and thus do not represent sites of active tumor.

Comparison with baseline examinations for change in number of active focal lesions is very important since FDG PET imaging demonstrates tumor response as decreasing size, number, and uptake of FDG-avid focal lesions. Similarly, relapse and/or progression of disease appear on FDG PET imaging as increasing values of these parameters. The presence of persistent, metabolically active focal lesions after treatment correlates with early relapse. A high number of focal lesions (five or more) on baseline examination is associated with poor long-term prognosis, especially in the presence of cytogenetic abnormalities, but does not correlate with short-term response. The presence of extramedullary disease (tumor occurring completely independent of bone), confers a very poor prognosis in the relapsing/refractory patient, especially if present at baseline, with overall survival of 42% versus 70% ($p=0.005$) and event free survival of 20% versus 47% ($p = 0.002$) at 12 months after relapse ($n=48$) [7, 11].

Tumor involvement with MM, as seen with FDG PET and PET-CT imaging, occurs as a diffuse infiltration of the marrow, focal bone lesions, and/or soft tissue lesions (extramedullary disease). About 20% of newly diagnosed patients have normal baseline PET or PET-CT images. The skeletal lesions can achieve a sufficient mass to break through the cortex of the involved bone, producing breakout lesions, but these lesions do not have the same ominous prognostic significance as true extramedullary disease, which grows entirely independently of the bone marrow microenvironment (Fig. 23.6a–c) [6–8, 11].

Focal Lesions

Focal lesions are defined as *well-circumscribed areas of increased uptake relative to the marrow background that are thought to represent areas of tumor involvement, measuring at least 5 mm in one dimension.* This definition specifically excludes focal areas of uptake that are not thought to be due to tumor, such as rib fractures not associated with focal bone lesions (common in MM and other osteoporotic patients), acute or subacute compression fractures (also common), arthritis, and sites of infection. The use of PET-CT rather than PET only imaging is very helpful in deciding if focal uptake is due to tumor or not.

Active focal lesions seen on FDG PET resolve very quickly with effective treatment, similar to the time course of M protein normalization in secretory disease and to the time course of abnormal diffuse uptake. Most patients (85%) will develop focal lesions during the course of their disease. The number of focal lesions at baseline is inversely related to prognosis for both event-free survival (EFS) and overall survival (OS). The adverse impact of the number of focal lesions at baseline is second only to the presence of cytogenetic abnormalities (CA). The presence of CA in MM defines a condition in which the tumor cells proliferate outside the bone marrow microenvironment, a condition both very aggressive and refractory to treatment. The physician interpreting PET or PET-CT imaging for MM should report the

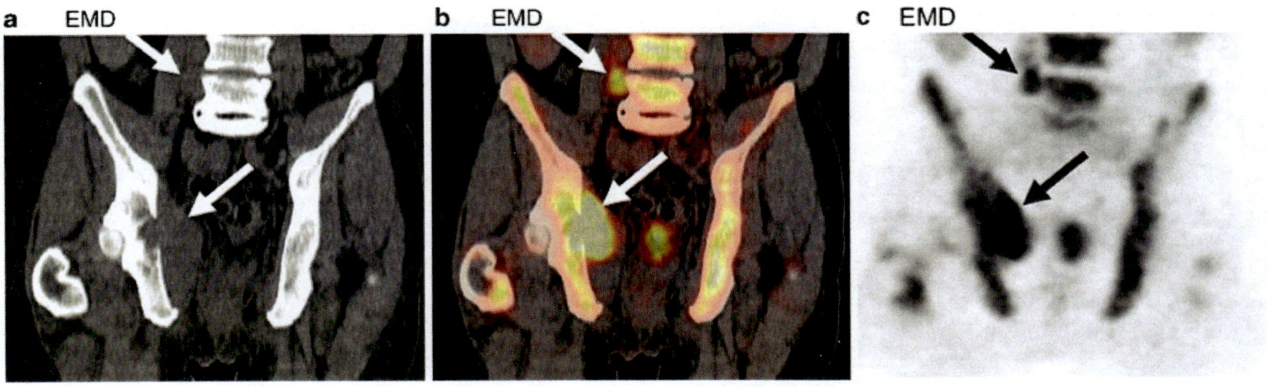

Fig. 23.6 Classic breakout lesion seen on coronal pelvic views, CT (**a**), fused PET-CT (**b**), and FDG PET (**c**, *unlabeled arrows*), and extramedullary disease (*EMD*, *labeled arrows*). A large focal plasmacytoma from MM has penetrated the cortex of the periacetabular pelvis on the right with a soft tissue component extending medially (breakout, *unlabeled arrows*). These breakout lesions are still dependent on the bone marrow microenvironment, unlike exclusively soft tissue or extramedullary disease (*EMD*) such as seen in the right rectus muscle, which has ominous prognostic significance (From Ref. [14]. With permission)

number of PET defined focal lesions to the referring physician since this information helps define the risk category of the patient. On follow-up examination, decreasing size, uptake, and/or number of focal lesions is seen with response to treatment. Conversely, new focal lesions and/or increasing number or size of preexisting active focal lesions indicate lack of response, progression of disease or relapse. Reporting specific, quantitative changes between scans is necessary to determine effectiveness of treatment and to detect progression or relapse [4–8].

It is clinically important to obtain cytogenetic information on patients with MM. Random marrow biopsy of the iliac crest or sternum is generally sufficient. However, the PET-interpreting physician can aid in selection of biopsy sites by describing in the report areas of focal uptake that are accessible to biopsy (for example, large breakout lesions, locations of large lesions within the pelvis, or expansile lesions elsewhere). Since MM is a genetically heterogeneous tumor, focal lesions with the greatest metabolic activity (SUV) should also be identified in the report as possible biopsy sites as these regions can demonstrate a higher percentage of abnormal cytogenetics than random biopsy [20].

The presence of one or more focal lesions of bone constitutes the diagnosis of MM in the presence of abnormal diffuse marrow infiltration with greater than or equal to 10% abnormal plasma cells. If only one focal lesion is present in the skeletal system and the patient does not have diffuse marrow tumor infiltration, the patient may have solitary bone plasmacytoma. Progression of solitary bone plasmacytoma to MM occurs at about 3% annually. FDG PET imaging can often find additional lesions not detected on skeletal survey or on MRI, properly upstaging the patient. FDG PET imaging is thus useful for periodic screening of patients with solitary bone plasmacytoma to assess response of the solitary tumor to treatment and screen for progression to MM.

If a focal area of uptake is present exclusively in the soft tissues, with no diffuse marrow infiltration, the patient may have solitary extramedullary plasmacytoma. This condition does not have the ominous progression rate to MM as seen in solitary bone plasmacytoma and is often curable. However, FDG PET imaging may detect the presence of additional lesions elsewhere in this condition, because of the whole-body nature of the procedure. FDG PET imaging can also assess effectiveness of treatment for this condition.

Multiple focal lesions of bone without diffuse marrow infiltration occurs in a condition known as multiple solitary plasmacytomas. This is a relatively uncommon condition that has only been recognized recently and that cannot be reliably distinguished from MM by MRI, FDG PET, or PET-CT imaging (a marrow biopsy is required) [12, 21, 22].

Extramedullary Disease

It is of great importance that the PET or PET-CT interpreting physician distinguishes between intramedullary and extramedullary disease. The presence of extramedullary disease defines a high-risk population with poor survival in need of close monitoring and aggressive treatment. Breakout lesions (focal areas of tumor that expand beyond the confines of the bone from which they originate, via erosion/permeation through the cortex) do not have the same biologic significance as true extramedullary disease since the breakout lesions are still growing in association with (and presumed dependency upon) the bone marrow microenvironment. Extramedullary disease represents a clinical entity that is less differentiated, often nonsecretory, and more aggressive, capable of growing without dependency on the marrow microenvironment. Since much of the treatment of MM is directed not only at the tumor but also at the tumor/bone marrow interaction and dependency, development of extramedullary disease indicates development of resistance to many therapeutic agents. Median survival for relapsing or refractory patients with extramedullary disease is less than 1 year (Fig. 23.7) [7].

Diffuse Uptake

Attention to diffuse FDG uptake in the hematopoietic marrow is essential. Diffuse increased uptake can be due to tumor infiltration, especially if the pattern is irregular or heterogeneous or in the untreated condition. Other situations can simulate the diffuse uptake from tumor, such as bone marrow stimulating medication or bone marrow hyperplasia following chemotherapy. Similarly, MRI will also demonstrate increased diffuse signal in the same conditions, and therefore cannot help to distinguish between these etiologies (Fig. 23.8).

Severe diffuse increased uptake can hide or "mask" the presence of underlying focal lesions that have a similar metabolic rate. Since treatment results in rapid suppression of the diffuse component, on subsequent PET imaging the focal lesions may become visible against the now less active diffuse background activity, producing the spurious appearance of interval development of new focal lesions (unmasking). In truth, the focal lesions were present earlier but obscured by the diffuse uptake (or on MRI, signal component) of the diffuse cellular infiltration of the marrow space. Thus, it is important to document in the report for each examination the SUV of a representative region of the hematopoietic marrow that is not involved with focal uptake. If, on follow-up PET examination, the diffuse component SUV has dramatically decreased, whereas the number of focal lesions appears to have increased, unmasking of focal lesions may be present, representing tumor responding to treatment.

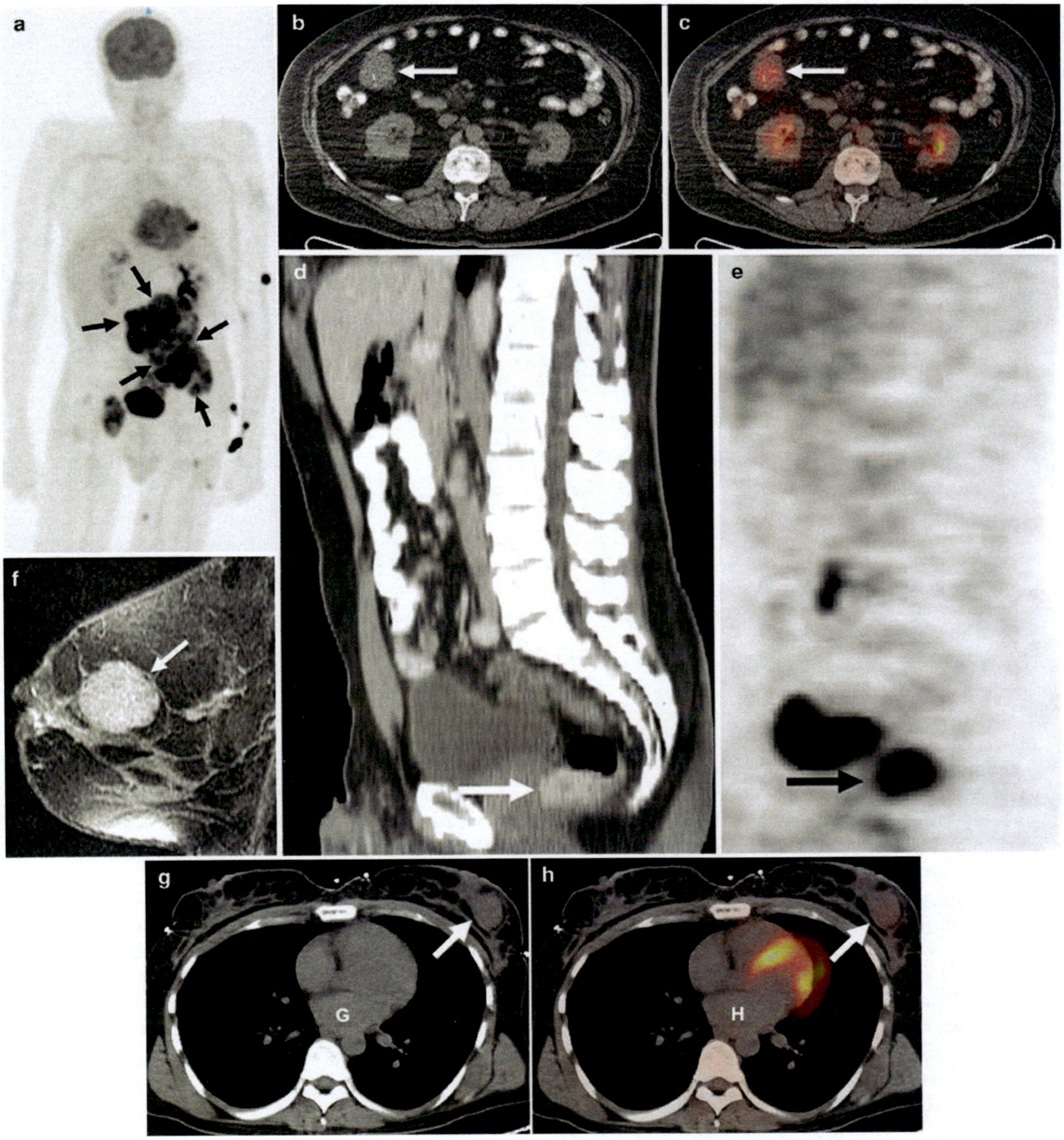

Fig. 23.7 (**a**) 3D MIP FDG PET image of a patient with newly diagnosed multiple myeloma with severe extramedullary disease (*EMD*, *arrows*) of the retroperitoneum. Smaller foci of EMD are in the soft tissues of the left lower extremities. Injection artifact is in the left arm. (**b, c**) Occult extramedullary disease (*EMD*) from MM discovered with PET-CT (*arrows*): Transaxial CT (*left*) and fused FDG PET-CT (*right*) demonstrate an occult focus of extramedullary MM (*arrows*). This region of disease was asymptomatic and outside the field of view of MRI, discovered only with FDG PET-CT. (**d–e**) Extramedullary MM of the rectum (*arrows*). Sagittal CT (*left*) and FDG PET (*right*). (**f–h**) Extramedullary MM of the breast (*arrows*). RODEO MRI sequence (**f**, *above left*), verifies the focal mass of the left breast previously seen on CT (**g**, *upper right*) and fused PET-CT (**h**, *lower right*) with slight FDG uptake, is a lobulated mass. Biopsy revealed MM (From Ref. [14]. With permission)

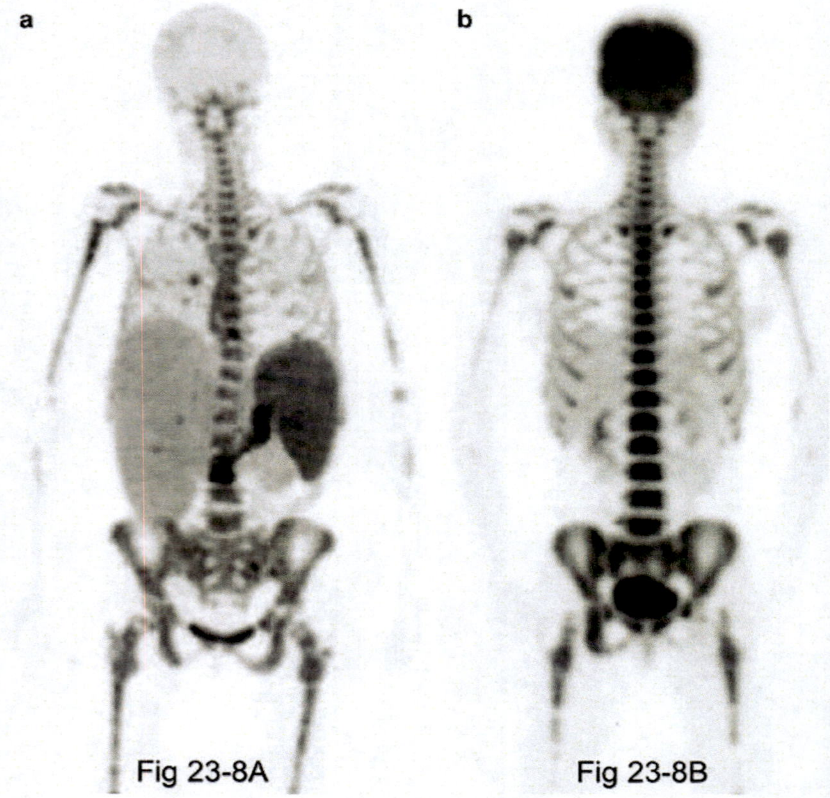

Fig. 23.8 (**a**) Superscan appearance from severe, intramedullary and extramedullary (stomach, liver, and spleen) multiple myeloma. Notice the brain see-through effect from the massive tumor steal of the FDG. Anterior 3D MIP FDG PET. (**b**) Superscan appearance from bone marrow stimulating medication (*G-CSF*, granulocyte colony stimulating factor). Anterior 3D MIP FDG PET (From Ref. [14]. With permission)

At the University of Arkansas, the maximum SUV of the L5 or L4 vertebral body is typically reported, assuming there are no compression fractures, vertebroplasty, focal lesion, or other abnormality present. If an abnormality is present at these levels, the SUV of the next normal appearing more cephalad vertebral body is reported. All SUV values are measured from the transaxial images. While nonspecific, comparison between SUV values of diffuse uptake between examinations can thus provide suggestive information, with careful correlation with clinical information, as to possible unmasking versus progression of disease on treatment, with the latter indicating a need for rapid intervention.

Skeletal disease in MM typically mirrors the distribution of hematopoietic marrow. The hematopoietic marrow in the typical late middle-aged to elderly patient with MM typically extends from the calvarium to the pelvis and includes the sternum, the ribs, portions of the scapulae (the glenoid and coracoid regions and inferior scapular tips), and the proximal portions of the humeri and femora. In more aggressive or later stages of the disease, spread to more peripheral locations occurs.

After bone marrow transplantation, alteration of the normal hematopoietic distribution can be significant, with FDG uptake extending to the peripheral skeleton, sometimes with an irregular or patchy appearance of the more central marrow (This irregular pattern can be due to repopulation of a scarred marrow space from antecedent large, focal lesions with or without associated focal osteolysis.). Thus, active marrow in the distal femurs or proximal tibias is sometimes seen without active tumor.

Since MM does rarely occur as young as the teenage years, the age of the patient must be considered when evaluating the extent and intensity of diffuse skeletal uptake. In the adolescent to young adult, the hematopoietic marrow normally extends further into the extremities than in the older adult, and is more metabolically active than in the typical, otherwise healthy older adult [3].

Detection of Infection

Infection continues to represent a diagnostic and therapeutic challenge in the management of immunosuppressed patients, including those with MM, in whom timely diagnosis and treatment is often delayed because of the absence of the typical signs and symptoms [23, 24].

Because FDG accumulates nonspecifically in cells with increased glucose metabolism, including both neoplastic and inflammatory cells, it represents a potentially important tool for the diagnosis of infection in this patient population [25–29].

Recent studies have demonstrated the ability of FDG PET scan to identify a wide range of infections caused by various pathogens (bacteria, fungi, and/or viruses) at a variety of sites, including pneumonia, sinusitis, discitis, osteomyelitis, septic arthritis, cellulitis, colitis, diverticulitis, esophagitis, abdominal abscess, and periodontal abscess, even in the presence of severe neutropenia [16–18].

Additionally, FDG PET imaging was particularly useful for the diagnosis of vascular infections such as septic thrombophlebitis, either spontaneous or in association with implantable catheters. FDG PET imaging also contributed to the management of patients with infection, particularly those involving the vascular system, skeleton, and joints, including detection of infectious foci that were silent clinically and not identified by conventional diagnostic methods. FDG PET imaging was also useful in this clinical context for determination of the extent of infection, modification of the diagnostic workup, and both determining and directing the therapeutic strategy [16, 18].

Other nuclear imaging techniques have a significant role in the diagnosis of infection, for example, using tracers such as ^{111}In- or ^{99m}Tc-labeled white blood cell scans or ^{67}Ga citrate. Compared to these tracers, FDG PET is less labor intense, allows earlier diagnosis because of earlier imaging time (about 1 h after injection vs 4–24 h or longer), and provides less radiation dose to the patient than ^{67}Ga citrate. In addition, FDG PET imaging can be diagnostic in the setting of severe neutropenia and the use of high-dose glucocorticoid medications, not to mention being useful for staging the underlying cancer. With PET-CT imaging, the foci of abnormal FDG uptake can be precisely localized anatomically [16–18, 23–31].

A potential limitation of FDG PET imaging for diagnosing infection is the inability to discriminate between malignancy and infection simply by uptake alone. This potential difficulty is largely circumvented by discriminative interpretation of the imaging findings by experienced imaging physicians in the context of the typical anatomic distribution of the underlying malignancy versus the findings on the study under review. For instance, foci of FDG uptake in certain locations would be extremely unlikely to represent metastatic spread, such as foci in the vascular system, dentition, sinuses, discs, and joints.

The interpreter must be familiar with the usual pattern of spread of the malignancy affecting the patient. For example, MM rarely involves the lung tissue (though pleural involvement is not uncommon). MM can involve the gut, but typically in focal masses; thus, diffuse gut involvement, especially seen on PET-CT to have concomitant wall thickening and peri-bowel inflammatory change, may well be due to mucositis (a frequent complication of the use of melphalan, commonly used in MM). Thus, abnormal FDG uptake in sites unusual for tumor, but not for infection, strongly suggests infection.

Evaluation of response of the underlying malignancy by standard clinical or laboratory parameters (for example, clinical examination, serum markers such as C-reactive protein, M-protein, and LDH, or bone marrow aspirate and biopsy) can also assist in the discrimination between infection and tumor. Specifically, if lab values indicate the tumor is likely under control, whereas the C-reactive protein is elevated, infection is favored, whereas if serum LDH, M protein, etc., are climbing and the C-reactive protein is not, tumor is favored.

The radiopharmaceutical should be administered in a peripheral vein rather than through a central catheter. Such administration will prevent retention of isotope in the central catheter. While such retention will introduce some degree of error in SUV measurements, more importantly focal uptake seen at the catheter tip following peripheral venous injection of the radiopharmaceutical strongly suggests infection of the thrombus at the catheter tip due to hematogenous microorganism seeding (typically from GU or GI sources). Similarly, FDG uptake along the catheter tract or associated with the reservoir of an indwelling catheter strongly suggests infection. However, if injection of the isotope was via the central catheter, discrimination of uptake due to infection versus injection is problematic, even if the catheter is flushed liberally with saline after injection. Uptake associated with a central line can also be due to recent placement, especially within the first 2 weeks.

FDG PET imaging should be considered in immunosuppressed patients with suspected infection that have a negative diagnostic workup to detect and localize a source of infection. FDG PET imaging should similarly be considered to evaluate the significance of persistent findings of infection by conventional radiologic tests following a recently treated infection, such as a persistent lung infiltrate on chest x-ray or chest CT scan. A negative FDG PET study, in the absence of other clinical or laboratory markers for infection, suggests resolution of the infection, hence allowing safe resumption of antineoplastic chemotherapy. FDG PET imaging should also be obtained when an intravascular infection is suspected, including spontaneous septic thrombophlebitis and infections of implantable catheters.

Finally, abnormal areas of FDG uptake at extramedullary sites should prompt an evaluation for infection, particularly when the location of the abnormal uptake is not typical of organ system involvement by the underlying malignancy. Detecting and properly treating such infections prior to immunosuppressive therapy may avoid serious clinical consequences [16–18].

Since detection of infection in MM and related malignancies frequently results in significant changes in patient management, rapid communication of the presence of suspected infection to the referring physician is essential (Fig. 23.9).

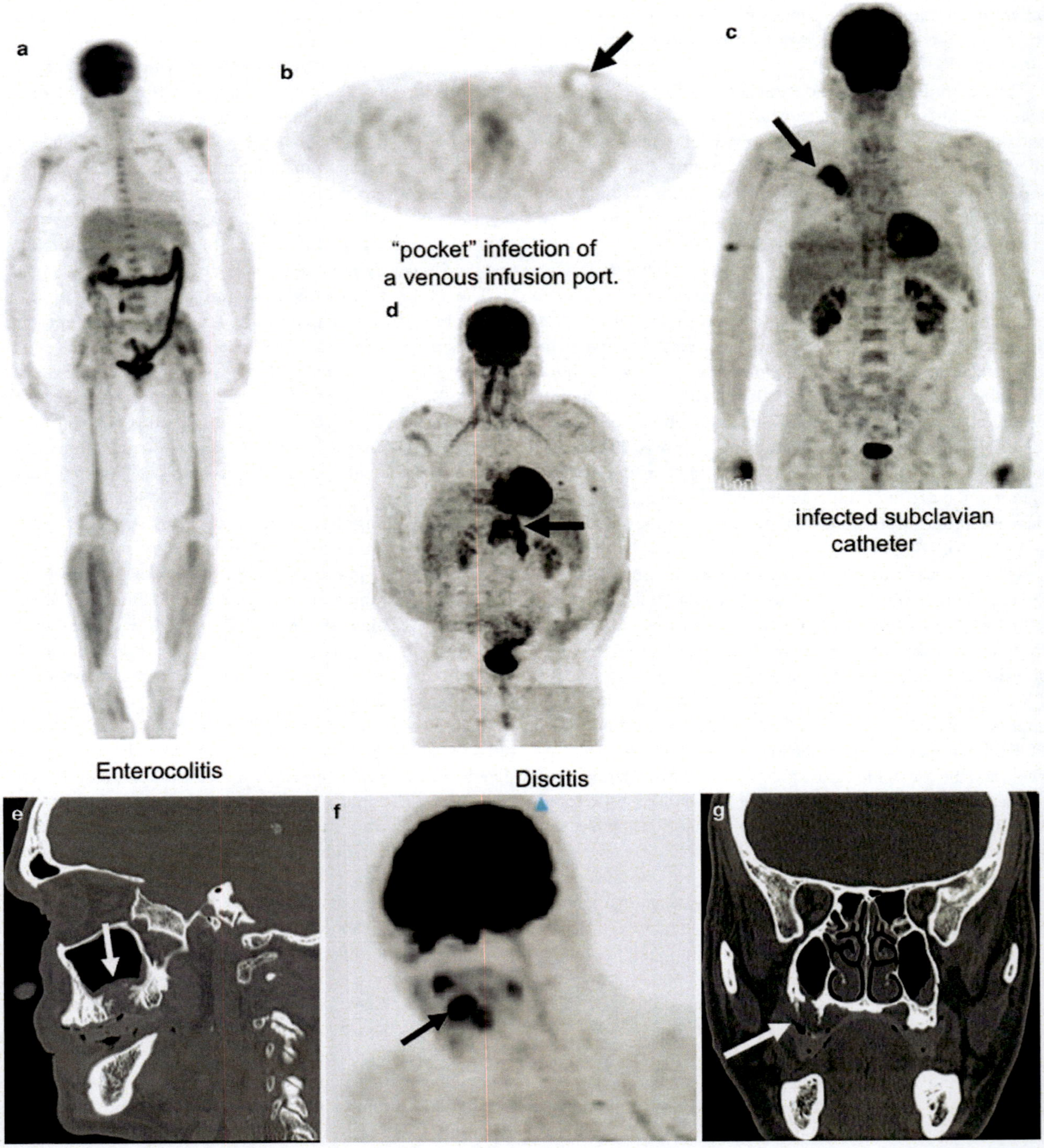

Fig. 23.9 **(a–d)** Proven examples of infections discovered with FDG PET in patients with hematologic malignancies. Sagittal **(e)** and coronal **(g)** images demonstrate osteomyelitis of the maxilla (*arrows*) in a patient with multiple myeloma, with a severe periodontal abscess. Maxillary or mandibular infections in this population can be bacterial or fungal (e.g., actinomycosis) and their incidence may be increased by the use of bisphosphonate medications, which may also predispose to osteonecrosis of the mandible (From Ref. [14]. With permission) **(f)** CT and oblique 3D MIP FDG PET

Pitfalls, Pearls, and Caveats

Vertebroplasty

Much of the morbidity of MM comes from the bone disease resulting from inhibition of osteoblasts (termed *osteoblastic anergy*) and stimulation of osteoclasts from various cytokines (notably RANKL, also called NF-κ B) released from the tumor/marrow microenvironmental interactions. Systemic osteoporosis, with or without coexisting focal osteolytic lesions, is a frequent cause of compression and other insufficiency fractures of the vertebral bodies and pelvis.

Vertebroplasty is now a common procedure performed for acute to subacute compression fractures, often with dramatic and rapid relief of pain. The vertebroplasty cement is radiopaque. Depending on the PET or PET-CT manufacturer's imaging algorithm and method of attenuation correction, the levels of vertebroplasty can appear as areas of increased or decreased uptake on the attenuation corrected PET or PET-CT images. Additionally, since compression fractures often occur at levels with concurrent osteolytic focal lesions, careful attention, and comparison to prior examinations is needed to determine if uptake is from the compression fracture alone, from attenuation correction artifact (by reviewing the nonattenuation corrected images) and/or is also associated with focal tumor uptake (Fig. 23.10) [19].

Biopsies

Bone marrow biopsy is a mainstay for diagnosis and restaging of MM. This is typically done in the posterior iliac crest but can be performed in the sternum and occasionally elsewhere (for example, the anterior, superior iliac spine, a specific focal bone lesion or area of extramedullary disease, etc.). As with other surgical interventions, biopsies can produce FDG uptake from the induced inflammatory response in the acute to subacute time frame. The interpreting physician should recognize focal uptake in these typical locations as possible biopsy sequelae, especially for new areas of uptake. PET-CT imaging is particularly helpful in this regard, often showing the needle tracks. On PET-only images, extension of uptake from the area of suspected biopsy to the skin is often visible, particularly in the region of the iliac wing (Fig. 23.11a–e) [19].

False-Negative (Chemotherapy Effect)

Any partially effective treatment, such as dexamethasone for MM, can produce false-negative FDG images despite the presence of extensive disease in the bone marrow on a diffuse and/or a focal basis. As in other malignancies, it is important to coordinate the timing of the treatment and performance of PET imaging following treatment to avoid false negative examinations (Fig. 23.12) [5].

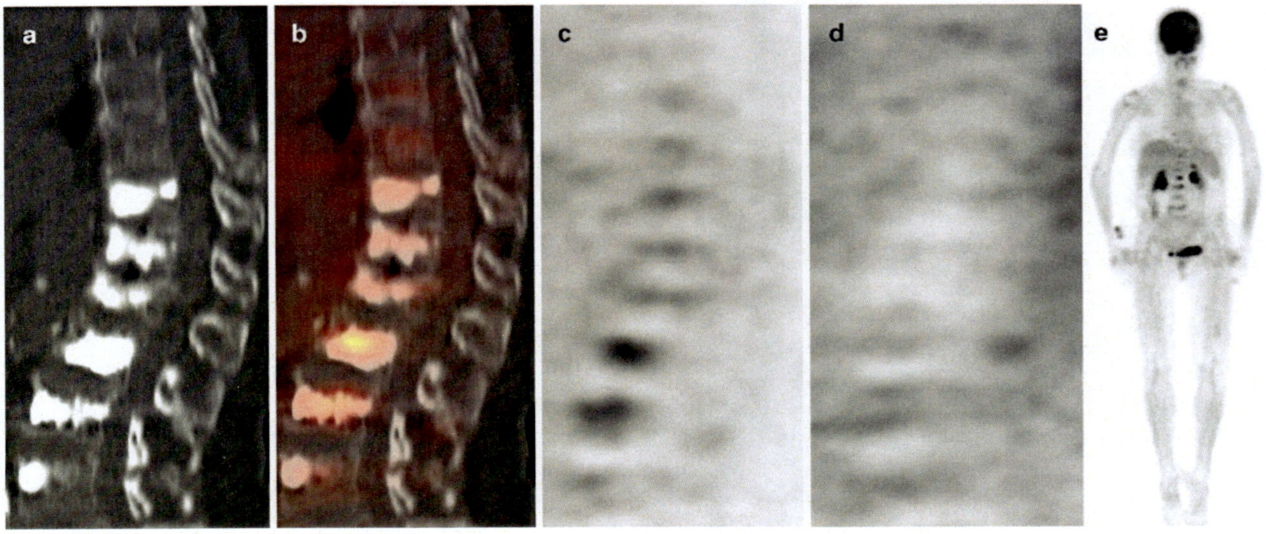

Fig. 23.10 (a–e) Attenuation correction (*AC*) artifact producing spurious appearance of focal lesions of the lumbar spine. These images are from a MM patient in remission with multilevel vertebroplasty. Attention to the sagittal non-AC image demonstrates no focal lesions (From Ref. [14]. With permission)

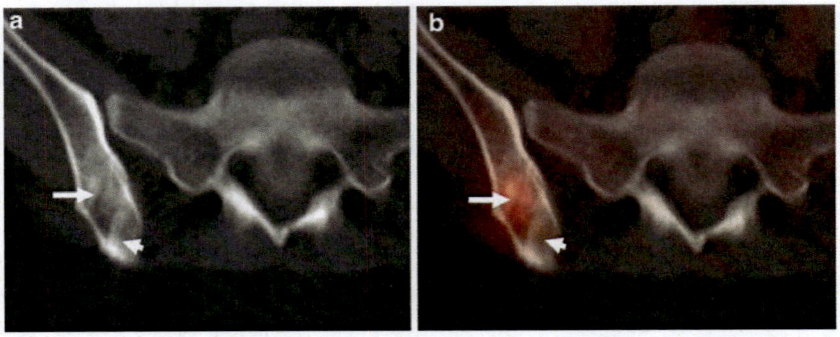

Fig. 23.11 **(a, b)** Focal uptake from a bone marrow biopsy the previous day, not to be mistaken for a focal lesion from MM (*long arrow*). The linear needle tract is seen on the CT image. An old, healed biopsy site with sclerotic margins is also visible (*short arrow*) (From Ref. [14]. With permission)

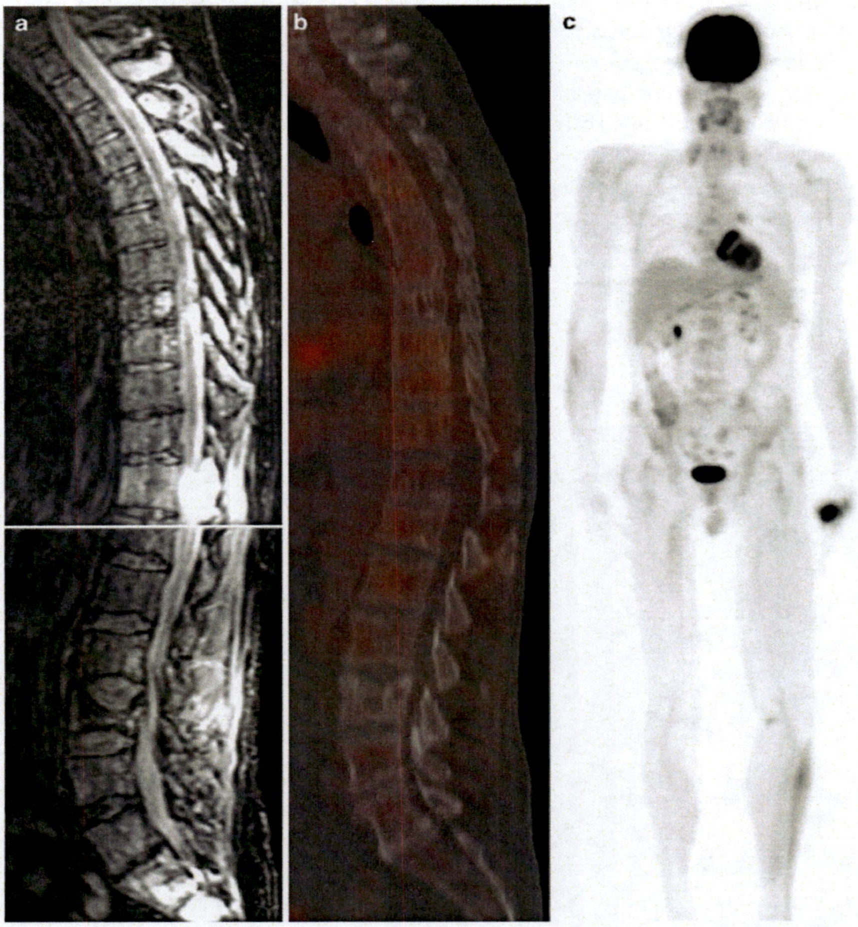

Fig. 23.12 **(a–c)** False-negative PET-CT in a newly diagnosed patient with active MM. The MRI examination **(a)** STIR-weighted sagittal images obtained one day before the FDG PET-CT (corresponding sagittal fused PET-CT images of the vertebral column **(b)** with anterior 3D MIP **(c)** image). The MRI demonstrates severe diffuse and focal disease with T12 level epidural disease. Administration of dexamethasone to the patient resulted in a rapid but transient suppression of FDG uptake (From Ref. [14]. With permission)

Other Plasma Cell Dyscrasias

Monoclonal Gammopathy of Undetermined Significance (MGUS)

Most authorities consider monoclonal gammopathy of undetermined significance (MGUS) the usual precursor of MM, being indistinguishable from MM based on gene expression profiling and having the same genomic instability. There is progression to MM in approximately 1% of patients annually. PET imaging in MGUS is usually normal. Since focal lesions or extramedullary disease are not seen in MGUS, PET, or PET-CT scans revealing such findings demonstrate progression to MM. Because of the whole body nature of FDG PET imaging, this procedure is an excellent means to screen for progression (Fig. 23.13a, b) [11].

Solitary Plasmacytoma

Solitary plasmacytoma occurs in two varieties, solitary extramedullary plasmacytoma (occurring exclusively in the soft tissues) and solitary bone plasmacytoma (involving the skeletal system). Solitary extramedullary plasmacytoma has a high likelihood of cure with radiation treatment and is unlikely to progress to MM. Solitary extramedullary plasmacytoma appears as a nonspecific FDG-avid soft tissue mass involving bone, shown on biopsy to be a plasmacytoma. Solitary bone plasmacytoma is more likely to progress to MM, with a conversion rate of about 3% annually. Solitary bone plasmacytoma has the same osteolytic appearance on x-ray as a plasmacytoma associated with MM. FDG PET and PET-CT imaging can demonstrate unsuspected multiple lesions, upgrading the diagnosis to MM. FDG PET and PET-CT can also demonstrate response of either solitary extramedullary plasmacytoma or solitary bone plasmacytoma to treatment (Fig. 23.14) [11, 21].

Castleman's Disease

Benjamin Castleman first described Castleman's disease in 1956. It was later divided into two subtypes, unicentric (with a relatively favorable prognosis and often diagnosed incidentally) and multicentric. The multicentric variant has a relatively poor prognosis, representing a polyclonal lymphoproliferative disorder characterized by recurrent fevers, lymphadenopathy, hepatosplenomegaly, and autoimmune phenomena, sometimes progressing to malignant lymphoma. The plasma cell variant of multicentric Castleman's disease frequently occurs in the setting of underlying HIV infection, and appears to be associated with HHV-8 infection.

FDG PET imaging can demonstrate active areas of tumor in Castleman's disease in an analogous manner to lymphoma,

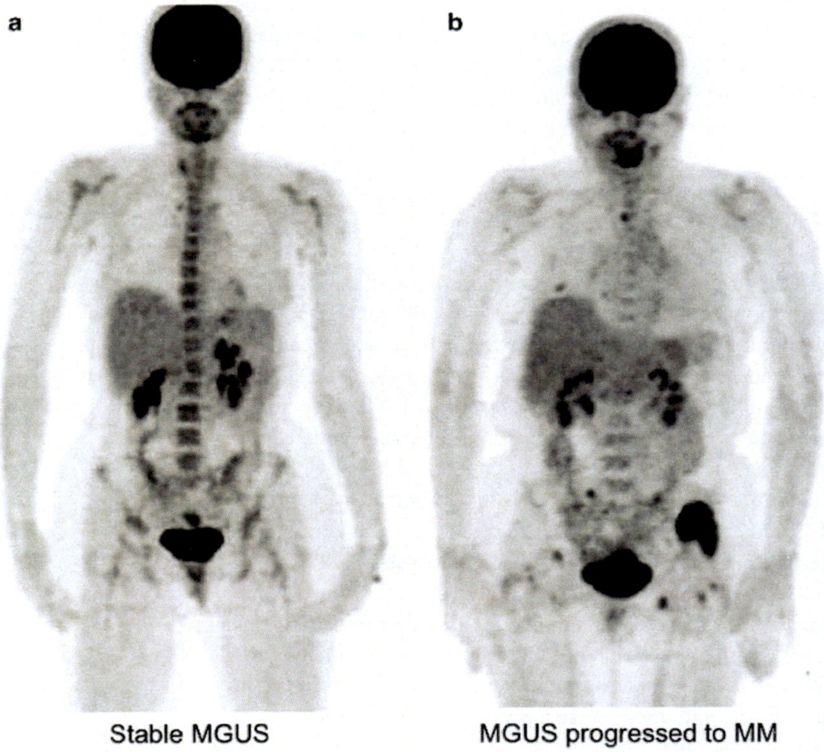

Fig. 23.13 (**a, b**) Anterior 3D MIP FDG PET images of patients with monoclonal gammopathy of undetermined significance (*MGUS*). The patient in stable MGUS (**a**) demonstrates no focal lesions. The patient progressing to MM (**b**) has focal lesions on FDG PET (From Ref. [7]. With permission)

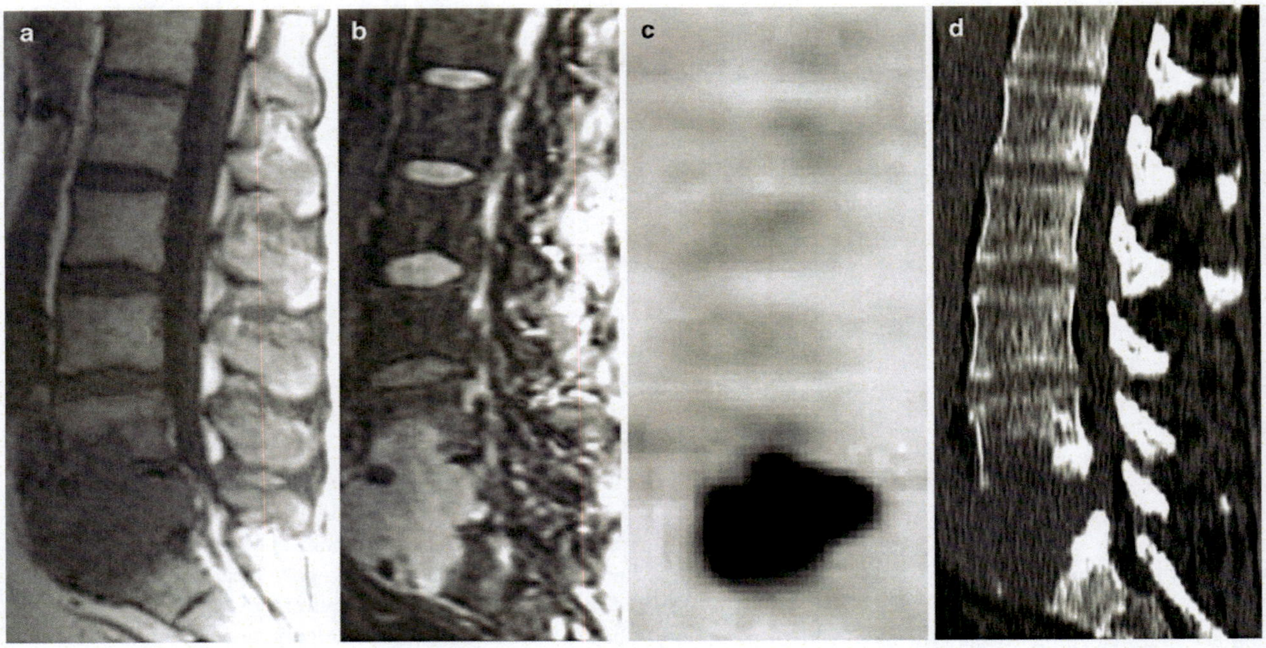

Fig. 23.14 (**a–d**) Solitary bone plasmacytoma (*SBP*) at the lumbosacral junction. The tumor is extending from L5 to the upper end plate of S1, with direct extension anterior and posterior to the vertebral column, invading the neural arch with epidural involvement. T1- (**a**) and (**b**) STIR-weighted MRI, FDG PET (**c**), and CT (**d**) sagittal lumbar spine images are shown. Note the normal appearance of all regions away from the solitary lesion (From Ref. [14]. With permission)

demonstrating FDG uptake in active regions of disease, as well as response to treatment. FDG PET-CT imaging is particularly helpful because, as in lymphoma, the CT imaging allows demonstration of lymphadenopathy that may not be FDG-avid, allowing comparison on follow-up examinations for both anatomic and physiologic changes (Fig. 23.15) [32, 33].

Waldenström's Macroglobulinemia

Waldenström's macroglobulinemia is a variant of non-Hodgkin's lymphoma, a lymphoid neoplasm characterized by a monoclonal lymphoplasmacytic expansion accompanied by secretion of a serum monoclonal immunoglobulin M (IgM). Jan G. Waldenström originally described the disease in 1944, reporting two patients with epistaxis, anemia, lymphadenopathy, and hypergammaglobulinemia. The monoclonal protein often results in a characteristic hyperviscosity syndrome. Current therapeutic modalities include alkylator agents, purine nucleoside analogues, and rituximab.

Waldenström's macroglobulinemia is uncommon disorder, comprising 6% of all B-cell lymphoproliferative diseases, with about one tenth the estimated prevalence of MM. Waldenström's macroglobulinemia has an overall better prognosis and median survival than MM. Waldenström's macroglobulinemia is believed to be more common in white

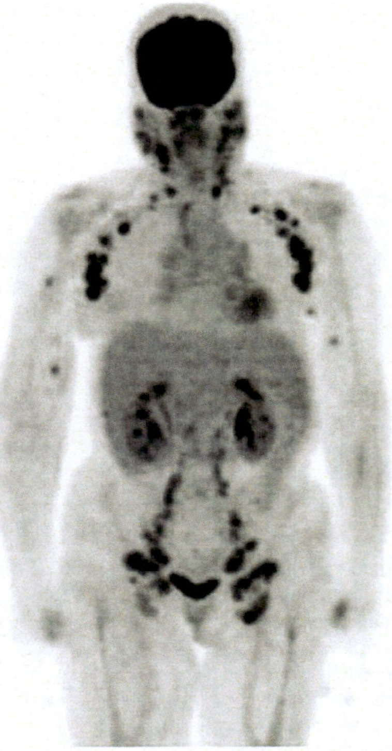

Fig. 23.15 Anterior 3D MIP image of a patient with active Castleman's disease. Note the extensive nodal pattern of uptake indistinguishable from lymphoma (From Ref. [14]. With permission)

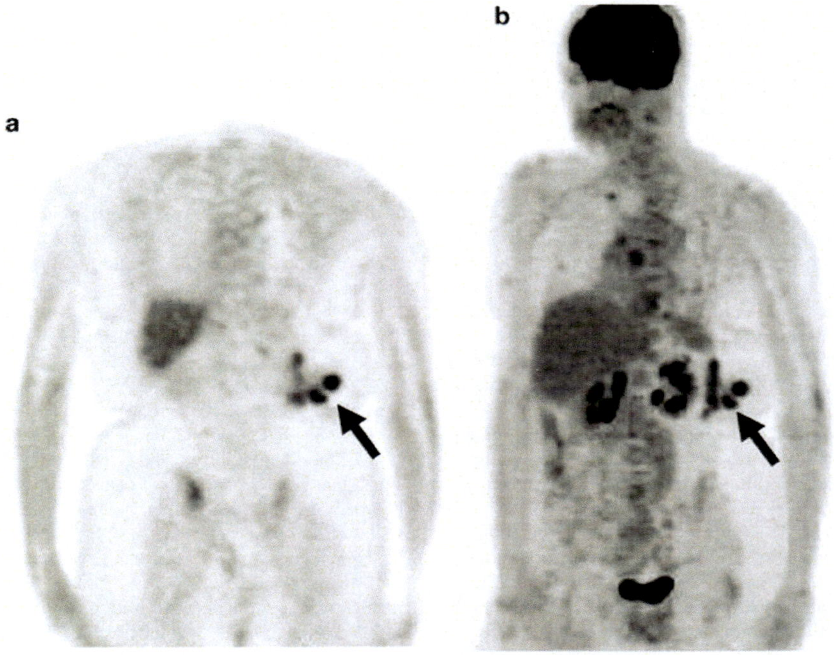

Fig. 23.16 (**a, b**) FDG PET scan in a patient with Waldenström's macroglobulinemia with a lobulated left flank mass (*arrows*) as seen on coronal (**a**) and LAO 3D MIP (**b**) images (From Ref. [14]. With permission indistinguishable from lymphoma)

populations and in men. The median age at presentation is 63 years. Analogous to MM, the predominant risk factor for development of the disease is the presence of IgM-MGUS [34, 35].

The typical findings of Waldenström's macroglobulinemia on FDG PET and PET-CT imaging are those of lymphoma, with hepatosplenomegaly (especially with splenic enlargement), lymphadenopathy with increased nodal uptake, and rarely focal lytic lesions of skeleton similar to MM. Increased diffuse uptake in the marrow may also be present (Fig. 23.16) [19].

Summary

In MM and related plasma cell dyscrasias, either FDG PET or PET-CT imaging is useful and reliable techniques for assistance in the diagnosis by identifying optimal sites for biopsy, staging and restaging the tumor, detecting extramedullary disease, and monitoring response to treatment, though PET-CT is superior for precise localization of regions of involvement, discrimination between infection and tumor, and detection of important additional findings, such as epidural disease, spinal cord compression, lytic bone disease (including areas at risk for fracture), etc. FDG PET and PET-CT are equally effective in either secretory or nonsecretory disease, with the latter developing with an increasing frequency during the course of the disease, causing difficulty in monitoring disease response or progression via laboratory means.

FDG PET or PET-CT imaging is also a useful technique for detecting occult infection in patients with hematologic malignancies, finding the source of infection, and documenting response to treatment of infection, even in the setting of severe neutropenia/immunosuppression. The information gained by FDG PET or PET-CT related to infectious disease often contributes to changes in patient management. The presence of a suspected infection should be rapidly communicated to the referring physician since the patient is often at significant risk from immune compromise and because such infections are often clinically occult.

The presence of a high number of focal lesions, especially with cytogenetic abnormalities and/or chromosome 13 deletions, and/or the presence of extramedullary tumor, defines patients at high risk with poor long-term prognosis who will need aggressive monitoring and treatment.

Failure to achieve normalization of FDG PET or PET-CT images after treatment identifies patients at high risk for early relapse.

Progression of disease on treatment is a poor prognostic sign identifying patients in need of immediate intervention.

References

1. Barlogie B, Shaughnessy J, Epstein J, Sanderson R, Anaissie R, Walker R, Tricot G. Plasma cell myeloma. Williams' Hematology, 7th edn. New York: McGraw-Hill, 2005.
2. Shaughnessy J, Barlogie B. Interpreting the molecular biology and clinical behavior of MM in the context of global gene expression profiling. Immunol Rev 2003;194:140–163.
3. Angtuaco EJC, Fassas AB, Walker RC, et al. Multiple myeloma: clinical review and diagnostic imaging. Radiology 2004;231:11–23.
4. Durie B, Kyle R, Belch A, et al. Myeloma management guidelines: a consensus report from the Scientific Advisors of the International Myeloma Foundation. Hematol J 2003;4:379–398.
5. Walker R, Jones-Jackson L, Miceli M, et al. FDG PET functional imaging in multiple myeloma clinically important caveats, pitfalls, and pearls. Blood 2004;104:11.
6. Walker R, Jones-Jackson L, Rasmussen E, et al. Rapid response to treatment of multiple myeloma detected with FDG PET scanning in multiple myeloma—early results from total therapy III. Blood 2004;104:11.
7. Walker R, Jones-Jackson L, Rasmussen E, et al. Diagnostic imaging of multiple myeloma—FDG PET and MRI complementary for tracking short vs. long term tumor response. Blood 2004;104(11):217a.
8. Walker R, Jones-Jackson L, Rasmussen E, et al. MRI-detectable focal lesions (FL) in multiple myeloma (MM) at relapse frequently involve novel sites not involved at diagnosis. Blood 2004;104(11):364b.
9. Orchard K, Barrington S, Buscombe et al. A. Fluoro-deoxyglucose positron emission tomography imaging for the detection of occult disease in MM. Br J Haematol 2002;117:133–135.
10. Schirrmeister H, Bommer M, Buck AK, et al. Initial results in assessment of MM using ^{18}F-FDG PET. Eur J Nucl Med 2002;29:361–366.
11. Durie B, Waxman A, D'Agnolo A, et al. Whole-body ^{18}F-FDG PET identifies high-risk myeloma. J Nucl Med 2002;43:1457–1463.
12. Durie BG, Salmon SE. A clinical staging system for MM: correlation of measured myeloma cell mass with presenting clinical features, response to treatment and survival. Cancer 1975;36:842–854.
13. Barlogie B, Shaughnessy J, Tricot G, et al. Treatment of multiple myeloma. Blood 2004;103:20–32.
14. Walker RC, Jones-Jackson LB, Rasmussen E, et al. PET and PET-CT imaging in multiple myeloma, solitary plasmacytoma, MGUS and other plasma cell dyscrasias. In: Valk PE, Delbeke D, Bailey DL, et al. (eds.). Positron Emission Tomography Clinical Practice. London: Springer, 2006.
15. Roodman GD. Pathogenesis of myeloma bone disease. Blood Cells Mol Dis 2004;32:290–292.
16. Miceli MH, Atoui R, Walker R, et al. Diagnosis of deep septic thrombophlebitis in cancer patients by Fluorine-18 fluorodeoxyglucose positron emission tomography scanning: a preliminary report. J Clin Oncol 2004;22:1949–1956.
17. Miceli MH, Jones-Jackson LB, Walker RC, et al. Diagnosis of infection of implantable central venous catheters by Fluorine-18 fluorodeoxyglucose positron emission tomography Nucl Med Commun 2004;25:813–818.
18. Anaissie E, Miceli M, Stroud S, et al. ^{18}F-Fluorodeoxyglucose (FDG) positron emission tomography (pet): an important tool in the management of infection in patients with hematological cancer. Blood 2004;104:11.
19. Walker RC. Personal communication, unpublished data. Little Rock, AR: University of Arkansas for Medical Sciences, 2005.
20. Avva R, Vanhemert R, Barlogie B, et al. CT-guided biopsy of focal lesions in patients with multiple myeloma may reveal new and more aggressive cytogenetic abnormalities. Am J Neuroradiol 2001;22(4):781–785.
21. Kyle R, Child JA, Anderson K, et al. Criteria for the classification of monoclonal gammopathies, MM and related disorders: a report of the International Myeloma Working Group. Br J Haematol 2003;121:749–757.
22. Migliorati CA. Bisphosphonates and oral cavity avascular bone necrosis. J Clin Oncol 2003;21:4253–4254.
23. O'Brien SN, Blijlevens NM, Mahfouz TH, et al. Infections in patients with hematological cancer: recent developments. Am Soc Hematol Educ Program 2003; 438–472.
24. Crawford J, Dale DC, Lyman GH. Chemotherapy-induced neutropenia: risks, consequences, and new directions for its management. Cancer 2004;100:228–237.
25. Sugawara Y. Infection and inflammation. In: Wahl R, Buchanam J (eds.). Principles and Practice of Positron Emission Tomography, 1st edn. Philadelphia: Lippincott Williams & Wilkins, 2002:381–394.
26. Stumpe KD, Dazzi H, Schaffner A, et al. Infection imaging using whole-body FDG-PET. Eur J Nucl Med 2000;27:822–832.
27. Zhuang H, Alavi A. 18-Fluorodeoxyglucose positron emission tomographic imaging in the detection and monitoring of infection and inflammation. Semin Nucl Med 2002;32:47–59.
28. Rennen H, Boerman O, Oyen W, et al. Imaging infection/inflammation in the new millennium. Eur J Nucl Med 2001;28:241–252.
29. De Winter F, Vogelaers D, Gemmel F, et al. Promising role of 18-F-fluoro-D-deoxyglucose positron emission tomography in clinical infectious diseases. Eur J Clin Microbiol Infect Dis 2002;21:247–257.
30. Gibel LJ, Hartshorne MF, Tzamaloukas AH. Indium-111 oxime leukocyte scan in the diagnosis of peritoneal catheter tunnel infections. Perit Dial Int 1998;18:234–235.
31. Mettler F, Guiberteau M. Inflammation and infection imaging. In: Mettler F (ed.). Essentials of Nuclear Medicine Imaging, 4th edn. Philadelphia: Saunders, 1998:387–403.
32. van Rhee F, Alikhan M, Munshi N, et al. Anti-IL6 antibody (ab) based strategies improve the management of HIV negative castleman's disease. Blood 2004;104:11.
33. Volberding P, Baker K, Levine A. Human immunodeficiency virus hematology. Hematology 2003;294–313. (www.hematology.org).
34. Brown J, Skarkin A. Clinical mimics of lymphoma. Oncologist 2004;9:406–416.
35. Ghobrial IM, Gertz MA, Fonseca R. Waldenström macroglobulinaemia. Lancet Oncol 2003;4:679–685.

Chapter 24
PET-CT of Melanoma

Chuong Bui and Paul Shreve

Cutaneous melanoma is the most aggressive form of skin cancer and accounts for 4.5% of all cancer cases and 1.4% of cancer deaths. In the USA, there are over 60,000 new cases of melanoma each year and nearly 8,000 melanoma related deaths [1]. Most cutaneous melanomas are diagnosed at a localized stage throughout the adult years with slight male predominance [2]. The incidence of cutaneous melanoma has increased substantially in the last several decades in persons with light-colored skin throughout the world. Recent data suggest that the rates of increase in melanoma incidence have begun to slow down in Western Europe and North America [3]. A major modifiable risk factor is exposure to solar ultraviolet radiation. Host risk factors include light-colored skin, a tendency to sunburn, numerous common or atypical nevi, immunosuppression, and personal or family history of melanoma. Of the four major histopathologic subtypes of melanoma, nodular melanoma demonstrates pure vertical growth phase with the potential to metastasize early, whereas the other three subtypes (superficial spreading, lentigo maligna, and acral lentiginous melanomas) show variable horizontal or radial growth phase first before entering the vertical or invasive phase. Superficial spreading is the most common subtype, comprising 70% of melanomas, with nodular accounting for approximately 15%, and lentigo maligna and acral lentiginous comprising the balance. Other variants (such as desmoplastic, mucosal, and ocular melanomas) are rare.

Melanoma is well known for the propensity to metastasize unpredictably to a wide variety of locations, including unusual sites such as cutaneous sites, the spleen, bowel, and leptomeninges. Recurrent disease can occur around the melanoma scar, in the regional nodal basins, or in remote locations, most commonly the lungs, liver, brain, bone, and gastrointestinal tract. Most recurrences occur within 3 years of treatment of the primary melanoma. The risk of recurrence is lifelong, however, and delayed locoregional and distant recurrences after 5, 10, or 15 years, although uncommon, are well documented [4].

P. Shreve (✉)
Advanced Radiology Services, Michigan State University College of Human Medicine, 3264 North Evergreen Drive North East, Spectrum Health Lemmen-Holten Cancer Center, Grand Rapids, MI 49525
e-mail: pshreve@earthlink.net

Overview of Contemporary Management

Surgical excision with adequate margins remains the standard and most successful therapy for primary melanoma that has not metastasized. For patients with proven regional nodal metastases (whether at macroscopic or microscopic level; with or without identifiable primary tumor; and at diagnosis or at the time of regional relapse), therapeutic lymphadenectomy is effective for regional control of disease and may improve survival [2]. Adjuvant therapy with high-dose interferon improves relapse free survival and overall survival in patients with high-risk primary melanoma without lymph node metastases (stage IIB or IIC) or with proven regional nodal involvement (stage III) rendered disease free by surgery [5]. Isolated limb perfusion or infusion therapy is useful for locoregional control in patients with unresectable tumor (at diagnosis or recurrent disease) confined to an extremity. For patients with distant metastases, there are currently no reliable and effective therapeutic options that have significantly improved survival, which is usually measured in months. Selected patients may benefit from the resection of isolated distant metastases. The numerous systemic therapeutic regimens described in the literature generally provide benefits to only a low percentage of patients with advanced melanoma. Durable response can occur however, but this is rare. Biologic response modifiers such as alfa interferonand interleukin-2 (IL-2) are the two agents that have been used in clinical trials for the treatment of advanced melanoma. Melanoma vaccines are being actively evaluated [6].

Radiation therapy is most commonly used in the palliative setting for cutaneous, nodal, visceral, skeletal, and brain metastases [7]. Elective/adjuvant radiation therapy may be of value to improve regional control in situations where complete surgical resection is difficult or when pathologic

P. Shreve and D.W. Townsend (eds.), *Clinical PET-CT in Radiology: Integrated Imaging in Oncology*,
DOI 10.1007/978-0-387-48902-5_24, © Springer Science+Business Media, LLC 2011

findings are suggestive of high risk for relapse (such as extracapsular lymph node extension). Superficial radiation therapy is a valid alternative to surgery for facial lentigo maligna melanoma in elderly patients who decline surgery or in whom the risks of surgical morbidities are considered unacceptable.

Staging of Melanoma

Staging System

Conventional staging of cutaneous melanoma may require some or all of surgical, histopathologic, imaging, and biochemical modalities. The recently revised and validated staging system endorsed by the American Joint Society on Cancer (AJCC) and International Union Against Cancer (UICC) for cutaneous melanoma is summarized in Table 24.1 [8, 9]. The four overall stages are grouped according to local (stage I and II), regional (stage III), and distant (stage IV) disease, and strongly correlate with prognosis (Table 24.2).

Full-thickness biopsy should be performed to confirm melanoma in any suspicious skin lesion for accurate microstaging. In localized cutaneous melanoma, the most important prognostic factor is the thickness or vertical height of the primary tumor. The level of invasion (Clark's level) adds prognostic information only in thin melanoma (≤1 mm thickness). Histologic ulceration of the primary tumor denotes poor prognostic feature in stage I–III disease. For patients with intermediate-risk primary tumors (thickness 1–4 mm) and clinically negative regional lymph nodes, lymphatic mapping and sentinel lymph node (SLN) biopsy assist in the selection of patients who may benefit from regional lymphadenectomy (those with involved SLNs) and who can be spared of this procedure (those with negative SLNs). Sentinel lymph node biopsy alone has a very low complication rate of 5%, whereas the complication rate of completion lymph node dissection is 23% [10]. The number of positive regional lymph nodes (instead of the dimensions of the lymph nodes involved) is used to stratify regional nodal disease. Satellite and in-transit metastases are now grouped together with regional nodal metastases. There is considerable overlap in the expected survival rates between stage II and stage III disease (see Table 24.2). The sites of distant metastases and elevation of serum lactate dehydrogenase (LDH) are used to stratify stage IV disease. Patients with distant cutaneous, subcutaneous, distant nodal metastases; or with lung metastases in the presence of normal LDH carry slightly more favorable prognosis at 1 year than those with other visceral metastases.

Clinical Staging and Restaging of Melanoma

There is no universal agreement among clinicians regarding the laboratory and imaging tests required to search for metastases in patients with melanoma. Asymptomatic patients with stage 1A melanoma do not appear to benefit from any additional diagnostic tests. Patients with intermediate risk primary cutaneous melanoma (between 1 and 4 mm, and Clark's level IV or V or ulceration) and clinically negative lymph nodes (nonpalpable), sentinel lymph node mapping and biopsy are performed to determine the presence or absence of regional lymph node metastases. Clinically abnormal lymph nodes often undergo percutaneous or excision biopsy straight away when lymphatic drainage from the primary lesion is unambiguous (for example palpable axillary and supraclavicular lymph nodes ipsilateral to an arm melanoma), whereas in the setting of ambiguous lymphatic drainage such as a truncal cutaneous melanoma, lymphatic mapping may be required to confirm the draining nodal basins of the primary lesion. The sentinel lymph node status is the most important staging procedure for prediction of recurrence and survival. The likelihood of sentinel lymph node metastases is strongly correlated with the thickness of the primary cutaneous melanoma, rising from 7% with primary lesions less than 1 mm, to 20% for lesions 1.01–2.0 mm, to 33% for lesions2.01–4 mm, and to 40% for lesions greater than 4 mm [11].

Patients with intermediate risk primary lesions (1–4 mm) and negative sentinel lymph node status typically require no further workup, but commonly have laboratory tests, including serum alkaline phosphatase and lactate dehydrogenase (LDH), and a chest radiograph to serve as a baseline for future comparison. Patients with positive sentinel lymph nodes or clinically positive lymph nodes commonly undergo comprehensive imaging studies to determine distant metastatic disease status. Likewise, due to the increased propensity for hematogenous spread, patients with high risk primary lesions (thickness >4 mm with or without ulceration; or 2–4 mm with ulceration) may also undergo comprehensive imaging studies in search of distant metastatic disease. These patients (stage IIB and IIC) have similar guarded prognosis as stage IIIA and IIIB, respectively.

In the setting of recurrent disease, either at the site of the primary melanoma, within regional draining lymph node basins, or distant visceral, lymph node, or cutaneous sites, comprehensive imaging studies are often performed to determine the nature of the local recurrence as well as the status of distant metastatic disease. Such comprehensive imaging is typically performed following biopsy proof of the recurrent or metastatic disease, but may also be pursued when there are clinical or laboratory findings highly suspicious for recurrence or metastases in patients at high risk of

Table 24.1 AJCC TNM staging for melanoma (Used with the permission of the American Joint Committee on Cancer (AJCC), Chicago, IL. The original source for this material is the *AJCC Cancer Staging Manual,* Seventh Edition (2010) published by Springer Science and Business Media LLC. www.springer.com)

Definitions of TNM		
Primary tumor (T)		
TX	Primary tumor cannot be assessed (e.g., curettaged or severely regressed melanoma)	
T0	No evidence of primary tumor	
Tis	Melanoma in situ	
T1	Melanomas 1.0 mm or less in thickness	
T2	Melanomas 1.01–2.0 mm	
T3	Melanomas 2.01–4.0 mm	
T4	Melanomas >4.0 mm	
T classification	**Thickness**	**Ulceration status/mitoses**
T1	≤1.0 mm	a: w/o ulceration and mitosis $<1/\text{mm}^2$
		b: with ulceration or mitoses $\geq 1/\text{mm}^2$
T2	1.01–2.0 mm	a: w/o ulceration
		b: with ulceration
T3	2.01–4.0 mm	a: w/o ulceration
		b: with ulceration
T4	>4.0 mm	a: w/o ulceration
		b: with ulceration
Note: a and b subcategories of T are assigned based on ulceration as shown below:		
Regional lymph nodes (N)		
N0	No regional metastases detected	
NX	Patients in whom the regional nodes cannot be assessed (e.g., previously removed for another reason)	
N classification	**No. of metastatic nodes**	**Nodal metastatic mass**
N1	1 node	a: micrometastasis[a]
		b: macrometastasis[b]
N2	2–3 nodes	a: micrometastasis[a]
		b: macrometastasis[b]
		c: in transit met(s)/satellite(s) *without* metastatic nodes
N3	4 or more metastatic nodes, or matted nodes, or in transit met(s)/ satellite(s) *with* metastatic node(s)	
N1–3 Regional metastases based upon the number of metastatic nodes and presence or absence of intralymphatic metastases (in transit or satellite metastases)		
Note: N1–3 and a–c subcategories assigned as shown below:		
Distant metastasis (M)		
M0	No detectable evidence of distant metastases	
M1a	Metastases to skin, subcutaneous or distant lymph nodes	
M1b	Metastases to lung	
M1c	Metastases to all other visceral sites or distant metastases to any site combined with an elevated serum LDH	
Note: Serum LDH is incorporated into the M category shown below:		
M classification	**Site**	**Serum LDH**
M1a	Distant skin, subcutaneous, or nodal mets	Normal
M1b	Lung metastases	Normal
M1c	All other visceral metastases	Normal
	Any distant metastasis	Elevated

[a]Micrometastases are diagnosed after sentinel lymph node biopsy and completion lymphadenectomy (if performed)

[b]Macrometastases are defined as clinically detectable nodal metastases confirmed by therapeutic lymphadenectomy or when nodal metastasis exhibits gross extracapsular extension

Table 24.2 Simplified AJCC/UICC staging system and prognosis for melanoma

Stage	Brief criteria	5-Year survival
Localized cutaneous melanoma		
IA	≤1 mm, no ulceration	95%
IB(T1b)	≤1 mm, with ulceration or Clark's level IV/V;	89–91%
(T2a)	1.01–2.0 mm, no ulceration	
IIA(T2b)	1.01–2.0 mm, with ulceration;	77–79%
(T3a)	2.01–4.0 mm, no ulceration	
IIB(T3b)	2.01–4.0 mm, with ulceration;	63–67%
(T4a)	>4.0 mm, no ulceration	
IIC	>4.0 mm, with ulceration	45%
Cutaneous melanoma with regional nodal metastases		
IIIA	Any T, no ulceration, 1–3microscopic node metastases	63–70%
IIIB	Any T, with ulceration and1–3 microscopic node metastases	46–59%
	Any T, no ulceration and1–3 macroscopic node metastases	
	Any T, ulcerated or not, with satellite/in-transit mets and without N	
IIIC	Any T, with ulceration and1–3 macroscopic node metastases	24–29%
	Any T, ulcerated or not and≥4 microscopic or macroscopic node metastases or matted lymph node metastases or satellite/in-transit lymph node metastases	
Cutaneous melanoma with distant metastases		
IV	Any T, any N, with distant metastases	10–19%

Clark's level IV/IV, invasion to the reticular dermis/subcutaneous fat, respectively; *in-transit mets,* skin or subcutaneous deposits greater than 2 cm from the primary tumor but not beyond the regional lymph nodes; *mets*, metastases; *N*, regional nodal metastasis; *satellite mets*, tumor nests or nodules within 2 cm of the primary tumor; *T* primary tumor

relapse, such as those with high risk primary lesions (stage IIb and IIc) or regional lymph node metastases at initial diagnosis (stage III).

Morphologic cross-sectional imaging modalities such as CT, MRI, and ultrasound have been useful for the precise delineation of anatomic details associated with recurrent disease and have been the mainstay for evaluation of patients with advanced staged melanomas (stage III and IV disease) and symptomatic patients. Contrast-enhanced MRI is particularly well suited for detecting metastatic melanoma in the brain and leptomeninges, and contrast-enhanced CT or MRI is well suited for detecting liver and splenic metastatic deposits. With careful attention to technique and interpretation, contrast enhanced CT can detect small (<1 cm)metastases to the bowel. Morphologic imaging modalities are generally associated with limited accuracy for the detection of lymph node metastases due to the nonspecific nature of nodal size criteria, although specific MRI contrasts agents for lymph node metastases are in development [12]. In addition, melanoma is well known for the random and unpredictable nature of distant lymph node and cutaneous metastases, requiring extensive anatomic coverage (head and neck and entire torso, and often extremities). Such whole body scans are now possible with CT and increasingly MRI, but the interpretive task can be formidable, amounting to a search for a "needle in a haystack."

Bone scintigraphy is a sensitive and widely available screening tool for metastases to the whole skeleton, although melanoma osseous metastases tend to be lytic, and hence more difficult to detect on bone scintigraphy. Also, abnormalities in bone scintigraphy are frequently nonspecific and may require additional imaging studies to differentiate metastases from fractures and degenerative disease.

PET-CT and Melanoma

Melanoma is among the most FDG-avid malignancies known [13]. Hence FDG PET is particularly well suited for detecting small deposits of melanoma anywhere in the body. The detectability of malignancy by FDG PET is dependent on tumor volumes, the extent of tumor necrosis, and the extent of background activity. FDG PET is reliable in the detection of melanoma metastases in normal sized lymph nodes of volumes equal to or greater than 80 mm^3 (about 5.4 mm in diameter or greater) [14]. The utility of FDG PET in the detection of cerebral metastases is limited because of prominent physiologic FDG activity in the brain, although melanoma metastases are not uncommonly detected in the brain on FDG PET due to the very high FDG uptake in melanoma metastases. Elsewhere, the very high tumor to background uptake ratio of melanoma on FDG PET permits the detection of small metastases in visceral organs, bones, bowel, and mesentery. Likewise, small lymph node, subcutaneous nodules, and cutaneous deposits of melanoma are readily detected on FDG PET imaging. Maximum intensity projection(MIP) images of the attenuation corrected PET emission image reconstructions affords a very efficient and convenient assessment of the whole body for focal abnormal

FDG tracer accumulation, and is especially well suited for delineating the presence and extent of metastatic melanoma.

Focal FDG uptake is not specific for melanoma, however, and may be seen in a wide variety of unrelated malignant and nonmalignant tumors, and benign states, including normal variants, inflammation, infection, and postsurgical repair. Benign nonspecific inflammation in lymph nodes, particularly lymph nodes in the neck, mediastinum, axilla, and inguinal nodal basins is common and can result in false-positive findings on FDG PET. Even cutaneous carbuncles can be detected on FDG PET and be potentially mistaken for cutaneous melanoma metastases. In general, histopathologic verification of the presence or absence of melanoma in FDG-avid foci is required if this would alter patient management or prognosis.

With the complementary merging of metabolic and anatomic information, PET-CT enables the precise localization of abnormalities on FDG PET, which may assist the clinicians in the selection of the appropriate management approach such as further imaging, biopsy or therapy [15]. Evidence is accumulating that PET-CT is more accurate that PET or CT alone in the detection of distant metastases from melanoma [16]. The morphologic features demonstrated on CT corresponding to a site of focal abnormal FDG uptake can be invaluable in specifying the nature of the nonspecific FDG PET finding. On the other hand, FDG PET can assist in the metabolic characterization of nonspecific anatomic abnormalities on CT that may result in downstaging of melanoma.

Role of PET-CT in the Initial Diagnosis of Melanoma

PET-CT has no established role in the diagnosis of melanoma. Most primary melanomas are cutaneous lesions that are readily accessible for diagnostic biopsy.

Role of PET-CT in the Staging of Melanoma

FDG PET has no established role in the staging of the primary cutaneous melanoma (T staging). This is best achieved by histopathologic examination of a full-thickness biopsy of a suspicious lesion.

Because melanoma is typically a cutaneous lesion, metastatic spread to lymph nodes follows the lymphatic drainage pattern of the regional lymph node basin(s) draining the skin of the site of the primary melanoma. These drainage patterns are largely predictable for the extremities, but head and especially torso lesions can have multiple possible draining lymph node basins due to the superficial drainage routes of cutaneous melanoma. The expected location of locoregional lymph node metastases, and in-transit lymph node metastases are predictable if this lymphatic drainage pattern of a given primary lesion is known, such as can be demonstrated on lymphoscintigraphic mapping. The greater depth a primary melanoma lesion, and the presence of ulceration, increase the likelihood of hematogenous route of metastatic spread. Hematogenous metastatic spread of melanoma is unpredictable, with a remarkably wide variety of potential sites, including in order of decreasing likelihood, lymph nodes (74%), lung (71%), skin and muscles (68%), liver (58%), brain (49%), bone (49%), heart (47%), peritoneum (43%), and spleen (31%) [17]. Small bowel involvement includes, in addition to serosal implants (Fig. 24.1), carcinomatosis, intraluminal masses, ulcerating lesions, and diffuse infiltration [18]. Osseous metastases tend to be lytic and expansile, and favor the spine. Rare noncutaneous melanomas similarly follow the unpredictable hematogenous routes of metastatic spread, with exception of ocular (uveal) melanoma, which most commonly metastasizes tothe liver (87%) [19]. In contrast to the extremely common pattern of multiple organ involvement in advanced melanoma of cutaneous origin (95%), single organ involvement is seen in almost one third of patients with metastatic ocular melanoma [17].

The role of FDG PET, and hence PET-CT, is not well established in the staging of regional lymph nodes (N staging). In patients with higher risk primary melanoma (thickness >1 mm or with ulceration) and clinically negative regional lymph nodes, lymphatic mapping and SLN biopsy procedures are highly accurate and are the procedures of choice in the detection of metastases to regional nodal basins. The value PET-CT in this situation is to exclude distant metastases because FDG PET is unreliable for microscopic or small volumes of tumor deposits [20]. In patients with prior resection of primary cutaneous melanoma and with palpable or enlarged regional lymph nodes on CT and ultrasound, a negative FDG PET study (negative predictive value at 89%) [21] is helpful but not completely reliable in ruling out regional nodal disease. Although a positive FDG PET has high positive predictive value (92%) [21], this may not be diagnostic of regional nodal spread because of the potentially false-positive PET findings, especially in lymph nodes in locations subject to inflammatory response such as inguinal, axillary, and cervical (Fig. 24.2). These patients should be evaluated with PET-CT directed fine needle aspiration biopsy, followed by excisional biopsy or imaging follow-up if the results of the fine needle aspiration are inconclusive.

Due to the very high avidity of melanoma for FDG, FDG PET is a sensitive imaging technique in the detection of metastatic melanoma (M-staging) and is superior to CT for small lesions in locations other than the brain and the lungs [22, 23], particularly small metastases to lymph nodes, soft tissue,

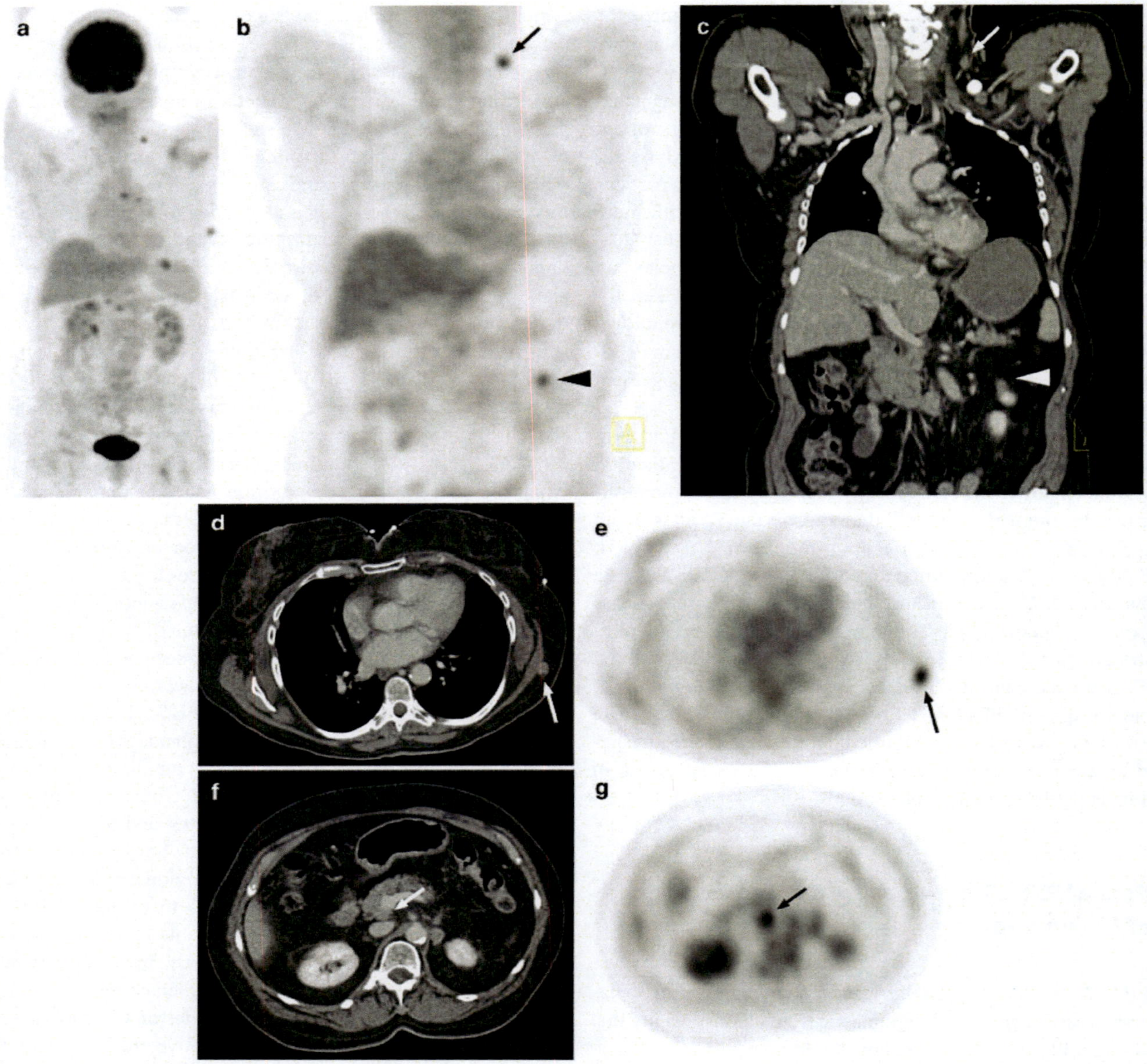

Fig. 24.1 Widespread distribution of metastatic melanoma. Multiple small foci of metastatic melanoma seen on anterior FDG PET maximum intensity projection image (**a**) coronal CT (**b**) and FDG PET (**c**) images show a left cervical level IV FDG avid node (*arrow*) and a small metastatic implant on small bowel (*arrowhead*). Transaxial CT (**d**) and FDG PET (**e**) images demonstrate a subcutaneous soft tissue FDG avid nodule at the left chest wall (*arrow*) and additional transaxial CT (**f**) and FDG PET (**g**) images show a FDG avid portocaval lymph node (*arrow*)

and small bowel(see Fig. 24.1) [24]. Very small pulmonary metastases (<4 mm) may be too small for detection on FDG PET images, but such are detected on CT images of contemporary helical CT. As noted, the normal high gray matter glucose metabolism obscures brain metastases on FDG PET, although it is not uncommon to identify brain metastases of melanoma on FDG PET images as melanoma commonly has greater FDG uptake than brain. FDG PET appears most useful for patients at high risk for harboring distant spread who are under consideration for further surgical therapy. This generally applies to patients with more advanced disease (stage III and IV with isolated distant metastases). These patients may benefit from the identification of unsuspected or additional distant metastases with subsequent change in management by means of additional surgical resection or avoidance of unnecessary procedures [22]. In patients with clinical stage III melanoma, abnormal PET findings from unsuspected distant metastases were reported to result in a change in of

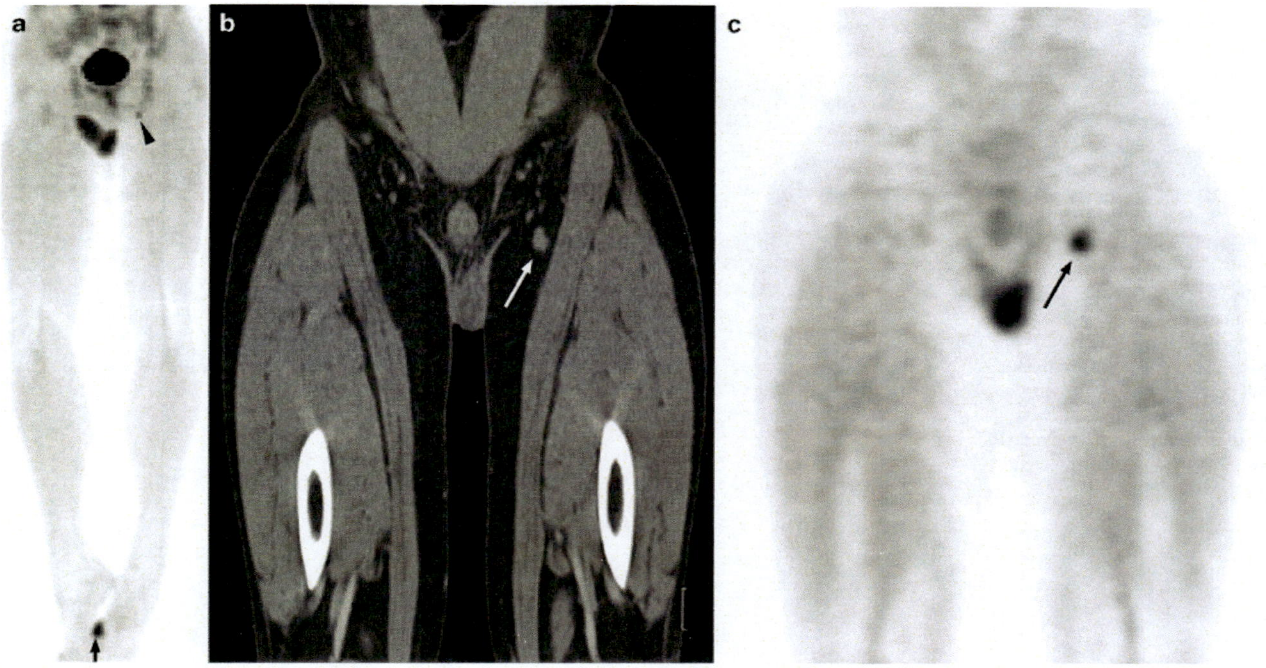

Fig. 24.2 FDG avid left inguinal lymph node in patient 10 days post left foot cutaneous melanoma resection. On the anterior FDG PET MIP image (**a**) FDG tracer uptake is present in the left foot (*arrow*) due to normal postoperative inflammatory changes at the site of resection and there is a very small focus of FDG tracer uptake at the left inguinal nodal basin is seen (*arrowhead*). Coronal CT (**b**) and FDG PET (**c**) images show an 8 × 10 mm left inguinal lymph node with associated abnormal FDG tracer uptake (*arrow*). The lymph node was negative on needle biopsy and resolved on subsequent scan, consistent with a reactive inflammatory lymph node

management in 15% of cases [25]. The most common indications for PET-CT in the initial staging of melanoma, then, would include patients with locoregional disease at high risk for distant metastases including patients with in-transit and regional lymph node metastases based on clinical findings, biopsy, or sentinel node biopsy (stage III). The routine use of FDG PET and hence PET-CT is not well defined in asymptomatic patients with clinically early staged melanoma (stage I and II). FDG PET is not indicated for thinner primary melanoma (<1.5 mm depth) because of low probability of disseminated disease at diagnosis [26].

The role of FDG PET and PET-CT in clinically localized, higher-risk melanomas with thickness greater than 1.5 mm is controversial. FDG PET and hence PET-CT have the potential to upstage and influence management of these patients by detecting occult distant metastases[27]. There are also consensus guidelines supporting a probably useful role of FDG PET in these patients [26], particularly for primary tumors greater than or equal to 4 mm in thickness [28]. Limitations of FDG PET in the M-staging of early staged melanomas include low yield due to low tumor burden at diagnosis and problems with false positive findings due to the nonspecific nature of FDG uptake [29, 30].

Role of PET-CT in Surveillance and Restaging of Melanoma

There is no universal consensus on the optimal protocol in the follow-up and surveillance of patients with previously treated melanoma. Because there is a lack of clearly effective systemic therapy for advanced recurrent melanoma, the major goal in the followup of these patients is the early detection of locoregional relapses and limited distant metastatic recurrences that may be amendable to complete resection by salvage surgical therapy. There is a wide spectrum of possible clinical presentations at relapse of melanoma ranging from isolated local recurrence (Fig. 24.3) to widespread distant metastases (Fig. 24.4). The local lymph node metastatic burden at the time of initial diagnosis, as typically determined by sentinel lymph node mapping and biopsy, most strongly influences the likelihood of relapse, with the increasing number of positive nodes and the presence of extranodal invasion increasing the likelihood of subsequent relapse [31, 32]. Most cases of relapses from cutaneous melanoma are actually discovery by history, physical examination, and laboratory tests (LDH in particular) alone, and confirmed with

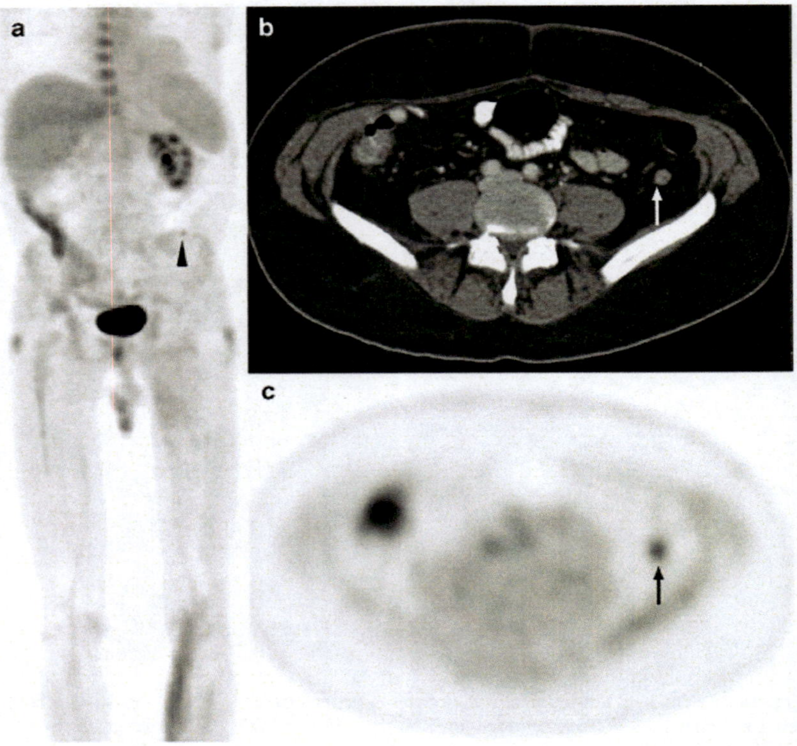

Fig. 24.3 Left leg malignant melanoma with popliteal and inguinal metastases treated with chemoradiation therapy 1 year prior. There is no evidence of recurrence of malignant melanoma in the left leg or inguinal region on the FDG PET anterior MIP image (**a**), although there is a subtle focus of FDG uptake projecting over the left iliac crest (*arrowhead*). Transaxial CT (**b**) and FDG PET (**c**) images reveal the subtle abnormality seen on the MIP image corresponds to an isolated left pelvic 10 mm FDG avid mesenteric lymph node (*arrow*). This was the only new metastasis and was subsequently resected

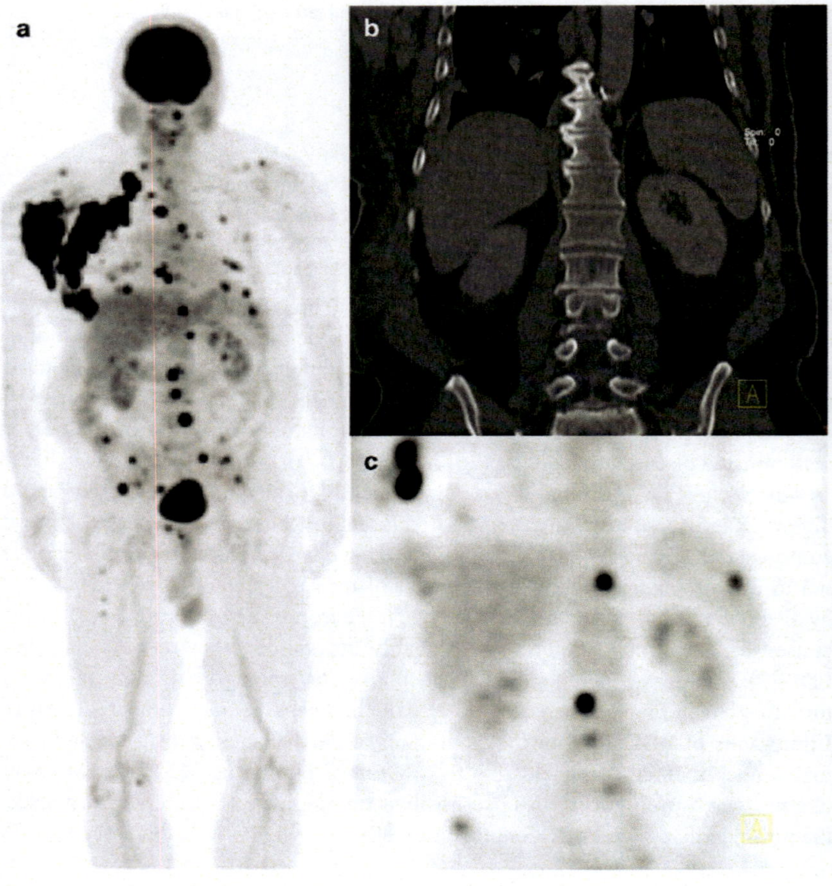

Fig. 24.4 Right upper back recurrent malignant melanoma with bulky right axillary and supraclavicular lymph node metastases, as well as numerous osseous metastasesinvolving spine, ribs, pelvis and right femur demonstrated on anterior FDG PET MIPimage (**a**). On coronal CT (**b**) and FDG PET (**c**) images the osseous metastases are clearly depicted on the FDG PET image, but no lytic or sclerotic changes evident on CT (Only unrelated discogenic sclerosis is seen). The right axillary nodal metastases are seen and an isolated splenic metastasis is also present

biopsy of physical findings or directed limited morphologic imaging of such as chest CT or brain MRI, for example.

For those patients with a known malignant melanoma recurrence, PET-CT can play a useful role in the accurate restaging in patients with apparently limited burden of suspected or proven melanoma recurrence. This is primarily attributed to the greater sensitivity of FDG PET over conventional imaging (such as CT and bone scan) in the detection of distant melanoma metastases other than small lesions in the brain and lungs [27]. In a retrospective study, the addition of FDG PET to conventional imaging resulted in a change of management in 24% of patients with proven locoregional recurrence by upstaging (identification of unsuspected or additional metastases) or downstaging (negative PET findings at suspicious lesions on morphologic imaging); however, in patients with known distant metastases management was changed in only 6% [31]. For example, locoregional recurrent disease (lesions at the primary melanoma site, satellite lesions less than 2 cm from the primary melanoma site, in-transit metastases, and involved regional lymph nodes) is often the harbinger of further systemic metastases from hematogenous spread with poorer outcome; hence, in these patients a PET-CT is helpful to determine the presence or absence of distant metastatic disease and fully characterize the locoregional recurrence (Fig. 24.5). For patients with known extensive distant metastatic disease, PET-CT would add little to patient management, except perhaps as baseline inventory for the metastatic burden prior to systemic therapy. In patients with known distant metastatic disease that appears limited, and resection of the metastasis is considered, PET-CT is useful to exclude additional unsuspected metastases.

Pitfalls and Selected Issues in Performing and Reporting PET-CT of Melanoma

As discussed, the combination of FDG PET and CT images is especially well suited for delineating the presence and extent of metastatic melanoma. FDG PET images depict potential sites of metastatic melanoma in the entire body (except for the brain to some extent), even relatively small deposits of macroscopic neoplasm, while the registered and aligned CT images permit precise anatomic localization of the FDG PET abnormality and probably improved specificity (benign cause of FDG tracer uptake vs metastasis) based on morphologic features. Inflammatory responses can result in false-positive FDG PET findings, and as with any PET-CT examination, regions of recent surgery or intervention, when abnormal on the FDG PET images, must be carefully evaluated on the CT images for specific signs of abscess, fistula, or soft tissue inflammatory changes. The propensity of melanoma to metastasize to unusual sites requires careful attention to all aspects of the FDG PET images, including the skin and immediate subcutaneous fat. Cutaneous abnormalities also require caution, however. A simple carbuncle can cause focal abnormal FDG tracer uptake at the skin and with a corresponding very small soft tissue nodule identified on the CT images, and be indistinguishable from a cutaneous melanomametastasis. Physical examination of the site can be a simple and inexpensive means of differentiation.

Inflammatory changes in lymph nodes can be entirely indistinguishable from macroscopic metastatic melanoma on both the FDG PET and CT images. On initial staging of melanoma, the PET-CT scan will typically be performed after excisional biopsy of the primary lesion. Both draining basin and in-transit lymph nodes of the primary lesion are the potential sites of local lymph node metastases, but also the sites of potential inflammatory reaction to postoperative changes at the site of excisional biopsy. Hence it is important to know the extent of excision and postoperative inflammatory changes at the primary site and the interval between biopsy and the PET-CT scan, as false-positive lymph node FDG PET findings will be increased in the setting of inflammatory changes at the site of primary cutaneous melanoma resection (see Fig. 24.2). Melanoma can also metastasize to distant lymph nodes, in an unpredictable pattern, and such metastases carry a poor prognosis as stage IV disease. There is an elevated false-positive rate in lymph nodal basins draining the extremities, the head and neck, and the lungs due to nonspecific inflammatory reaction. Hence abnormally increased FDG uptake in lymph nodes in the neck, mediastinum, pulmonary hila, axillae, and inguinal nodal basins must be approached with caution, as normal false-positive rates in these lymph node groups is elevated, and can be as high as 20% in the neck, mediastinum, and pulmonary hila. CT findings can be helpful, for example, preservation of a fatty hilus generally favors benign lymph nodes. Nevertheless, loss of ovoid shape and fatty hilus, anatomic enlargement, and increased contrast enhancement all can occur with inflammation as well as metastatic melanoma (Fig. 24.6). Biopsy or follow-up imaging will be sometimes be required for isolated and limited lymph nodes positive on FDG PET, although such may be in practice be resected in any case both as a diagnostic and potentially therapeutic procedure.

Malignant melanoma is among the most FDG tracer avid cancers known, and hence typically is depicted on FDG PET images as foci of remarkably intense tracer uptake. Malignant melanoma can also demonstrate rapid growth, and central necrosis can occur in masses and lymph node metastases, resulting in much reduced overall intensity of FDG tracer uptake on the FDG PET images (Fig. 24.7). Careful review of CT findings, particularly those corresponding to any PET abnormality, must be maintained despite the usual ease of detection of malignant melanoma on the FDG PET images. Additionally, since extranodal invasion is an important

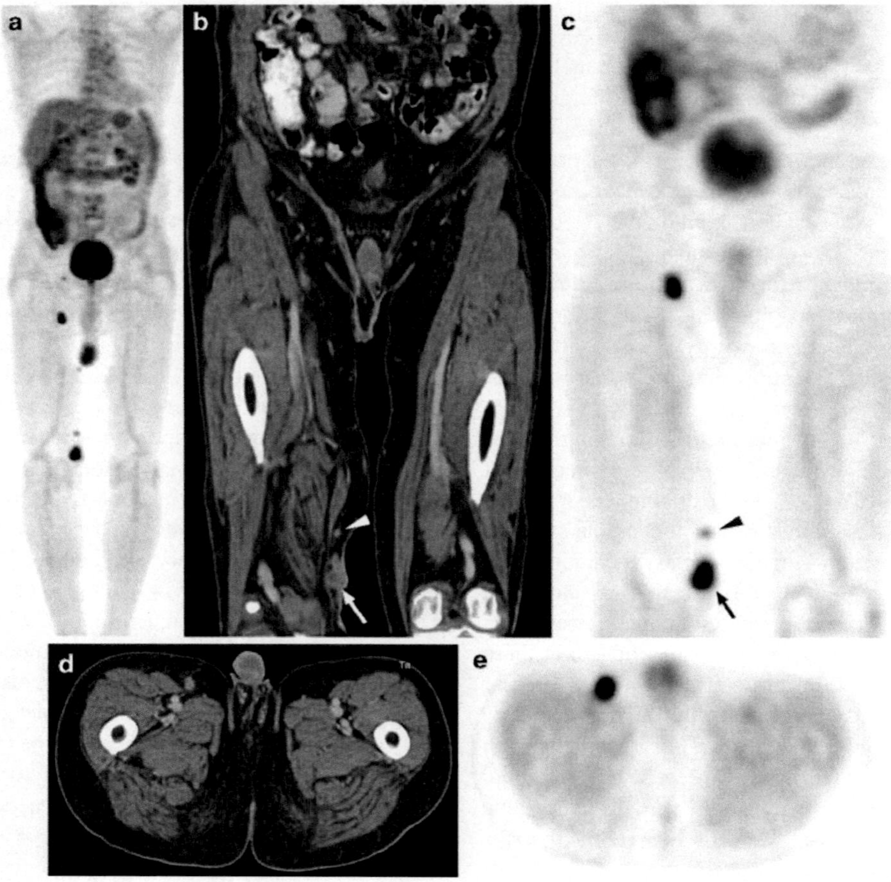

Fig. 24.5 Locally recurrent melanoma in right distal thigh with an associated nearby in-transit lymph node metastasis as well as right inguinal and external iliac lymph node metastases seen on the anterior FDG PET MIP image (**a**), but no distant metastatic disease otherwise. Coronal CT (**b**) and FDG PET (**c**)images reveal the local recurrence is a nearly 2 cm subcutaneous fat mass (*arrow*) which does not invade the fascia, and there is an associate 3 mm in-transit nodal metastasis (*arrowhead*). A 12 × 10 mm enhancing right inguinal lymph node which is intensely FDG avid is depicted on the transaxial CT (**d**) and FDG PET images (**e**)

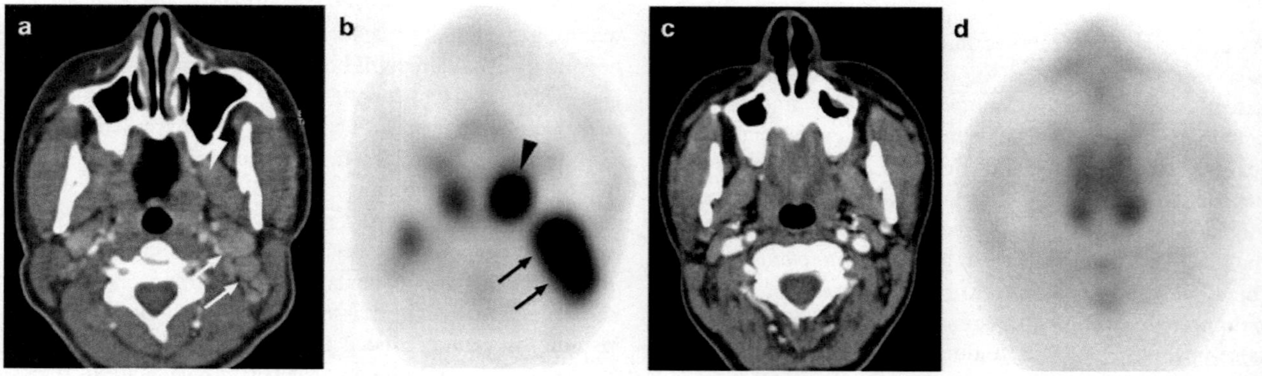

Fig. 24.6 False-positive findings du to inflammation in a patient with face melanoma. Transaxial CT (**a**) and FDG PET (**b**) images reveal left level II cervical lymph nodes up to 2 cm short axis diameter with increased contrast enhancement and intense abnormal FDG tracer uptake (*arrow*) as well as left tonsillar abnormal FDG tracer uptake and tonsillar soft tissue asymmetry (*arrowhead*). The cervical lymph node and tonsillar abnormal FDG tracer uptake, and the cervical lymphadenopathy and tonsillar asymmetry, completely resolved without treatment (**c**, **d**), reflecting locoregional inflammatory changes of tonsillitis

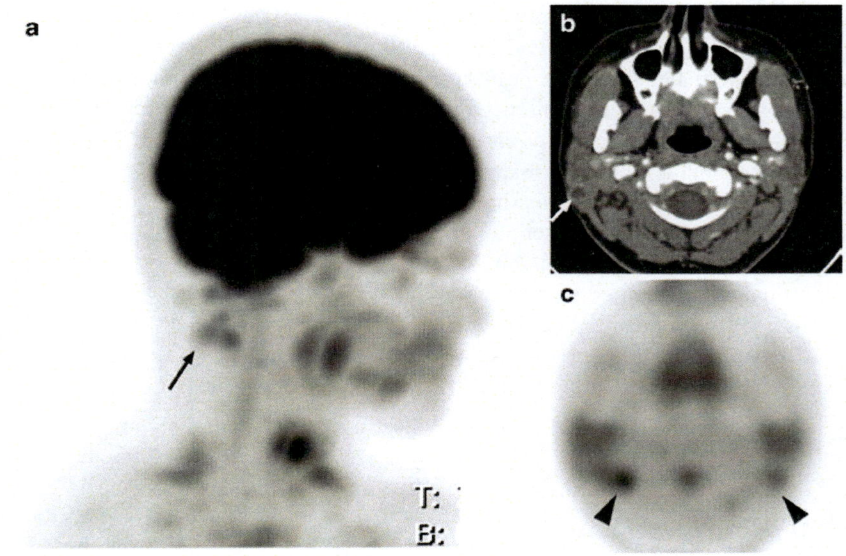

Fig. 24.7 Necrotic lymph node metastases. Patient with right scalp melanoma and palpable right posterior auricular lymph nodes. Lateral FDG PET MIP image (**a**) reveals mild FDG tracer uptake in posterior auricular lymph nodes (*arrow*), projecting just posterior to the cervical spinal cord. There is modest physiologic brown fat FDG tracer uptake at the base of the neck. On transaxial CT (**b**) a necrotic lymph node adjacent to the parotid gland (*arrow*) is seen that shows central low attenuation with peripheral contrast enhancement. On the corresponding FDG PET images (**c**), however, no appreciable FDG tracer uptake is seen due to the extent of necrosis. Brown fat FDG uptake is also seen. On resection the lymph node was positive for metastatic melanoma (*arrowhead*)

criterion in the N staging of melanoma (see Table 24.1), lymph nodes positive on FDG PET images require careful review on the CT images for findings of extranodal soft tissue extension or contiguous soft tissue matting amongst the lymph nodes. Careful review of CT findings is also important when there are recent postoperative changes in a nodal basin, as postoperative inflammation can result in increased FDG tracer uptake mimicking residual malignancy. Osseous metastasesare typically depicted on the FDG PET images well before corresponding CT abnormalities are seen due to their lytic nature and the typically intense FDG tracer uptake by melanoma. It is not unusual for extensive osseous metastases clearly seen on the FDG PET images to have little or no CT correlative abnormalities (see Fig. 24.4).

Due to the propensity of malignant melanoma to metastasize in widespread and unpredictable patterns, the PET-CT imaging protocols for staging and restaging melanoma require extensive axial coverage, usually the entire body, or nearly so (see PET-CT Protocols in Body Oncology Imaging). Since lung is one of the most common sites for melanoma metastases, and very small pulmonary metastases (<4 mm) may be detected primarily on the CT images, optimized CT technique for imaging the lungs is thus important, and may include both breath-hold and dedicated lung algorithm image reconstruction. Normal physiologic FDG tracer activity in bowel can confound detection of small metastatic deposits of melanoma to bowel. Optimized CT diagnostic technique, including the use of oral and intravenous contrast material, can improve ease and certainty of the diagnosis of bowel metastases. Brain and leptomeninges metastases can be obscured on FDG PET images due to the high physiologic uptake of FDG in brain gray matter, but detected on the CT images, especially if intravenous contrast enhancement is used. The use of CT contrast agents in PET-CT may provide additional benefits in the precise anatomic localization of PET abnormality by distinguishing the lesion from its surrounding structures. This is of particular value in the head and neck as well as in the abdomen and pelvis where the accurate differentiation of focal pathology from surrounding normal tissues (muscles, vessels, intestines, etc.) is crucial[33].

In a hybrid PET-CT system, the additional radiation exposure from the CT portion is obligatory, and commonly in the order of 10 mSv over the usual radiation dose of 5–10 mSv from the PET emission scan [34]. Younger patients who have received curative therapy for melanoma may undergo repeated whole body PET-CT scans over their lifetime for surveillance for early recurrence. Efforts to reduce overall ionizing radiation exposure in these patients on follow-up surveillance scans include reducing the dose of FDG for the PET portion of the examination and the total mAs employed in the CT portion of the examination.

As with any PET-CT report, the history should contain a concise summary relevant to the particular cancer. Since the thickness of the primary lesion (T stage) strongly influences survival and the anticipated pattern of metastases (lymphatic vs hematogenous), the pathologic diagnosis of the primary lesion, including vertical height and presence or absence of ulceration in the primary lesion, should be included in the report history. Results of the sentinel lymph node mapping and biopsy, including the precise N stage, if available, should also be included in the history, as well as subsequent treatments and surgeries. Relevant historical information for interpretation includes locations and time intervals from previous surgery or open biopsy, the injection sites of interferon or melanoma vaccine, the time intervals from previous radiation or chemotherapy, and the sites of intercurrent infection and inflammation.

Therapy Monitoring with PET-CT During Treatment

Currently little is known regarding the utility of routine FDG PET or PET-CT in the evaluation of response (or lack of response) to therapy in patients with melanoma. As with other cancers, indications of response include both metabolic response (reduction or complete resolution of abnormal FDG tracer uptake) and anatomic response (decrease in size or complete resolution of the abnormal soft tissue). Such responses are observed in systemically treated melanoma (Fig. 24.8), but the relative significance of metabolic vs anatomic response in predicting progression-free survival has yet to be systematically evaluated. Preliminary data do suggest the potential of FDG PET in the assessment of response of melanoma lesions 1 month after isolated limb perfusion therapy [35]. Further studies are required before any definitive conclusions can be made regarding the ability of FDG PET or PET-CT to predict patient outcomes during therapy. It should be noted that at present the predicative value of a complete metabolic response for melanoma is unknown, and complete resolution of abnormal FDG tracer uptake in treated melanoma may not predict a fully sterilized tumor. Also, immunomodulatory therapies used to treat malignant melanoma may by virtue of the intended inflammatory response result in residual FDG tracer uptake in successfully treated tumors.

Radiation Therapy Planning for Melanoma with PET-CT

For patients with melanoma, radiation therapy is mostly utilized in the palliative setting of metastatic disease which generally carries very poor prognosis. The value of adjuvant radiation therapy following surgical therapy for locoregional disease remains controversial. Consequently, little specific data exist about the role of FDG PET or PET-CT in the planning of radiation therapy for patients with melanoma.

Conclusion

At present, most patients with melanoma are diagnosed at an early stage and have a favorable prognosis after initial treatment. Melanoma is well known for the propensity to metastasize to any part of the body with unpredictable natural history. Lifelong surveillance is required, as some thin melanomas can relapse locoregionally or systemically after many years of an apparent disease-free period. The best treatment for melanoma is complete surgical resection of all tumor burdens when feasible. This applies to patients with resectable locoregional disease with or without isolated distant metastases. Patients with extensive metastatic disease are candidates for palliative or experimental systemic therapies. PET-CT combines the advantages of the high sensitivity of PET with the excellent spatial resolution of CT in one session without moving the patient and without time lag, thus overcoming the individual limitations of each modality (Table 24.3). PET-CT with its inherent whole body capability is arguably the best imaging option to search for metastases from melanoma with the potential to change treatment plan in as high as 48% [16]. More studies are required to determine the optimal surveillance schedules of PET-CT in patients with high-risk melanomas to maximize the chance to detect early relapse, whereas minimizing the radiation exposure from the procedure, particularly in younger patients. Hopefully with future advances in treatment options, the role of PET-CT would become more defined in the assessment of response to melanoma therapy. Until further definitive studies become available, at present, when the clinicians are faced with the question of whether or not to proceed with an FDG PET-CT examination, the following indications appear justified (Table 24.4): (1) Patients at high risk for distant metastases based on the extent of locoregional disease at diagnosis; (2) patients with known isolated distant metastatic disease under consideration for surgical resection with curative intent; (3) patients with nonspecific morphologic abnormalities suspicious for distant metastases; (4) patients with locoregional relapse and/or isolated distant metastatic recurrence under consideration for surgical resection; and (5) patients with high risk locoregional disease undergoing surveillance after initial treatment.

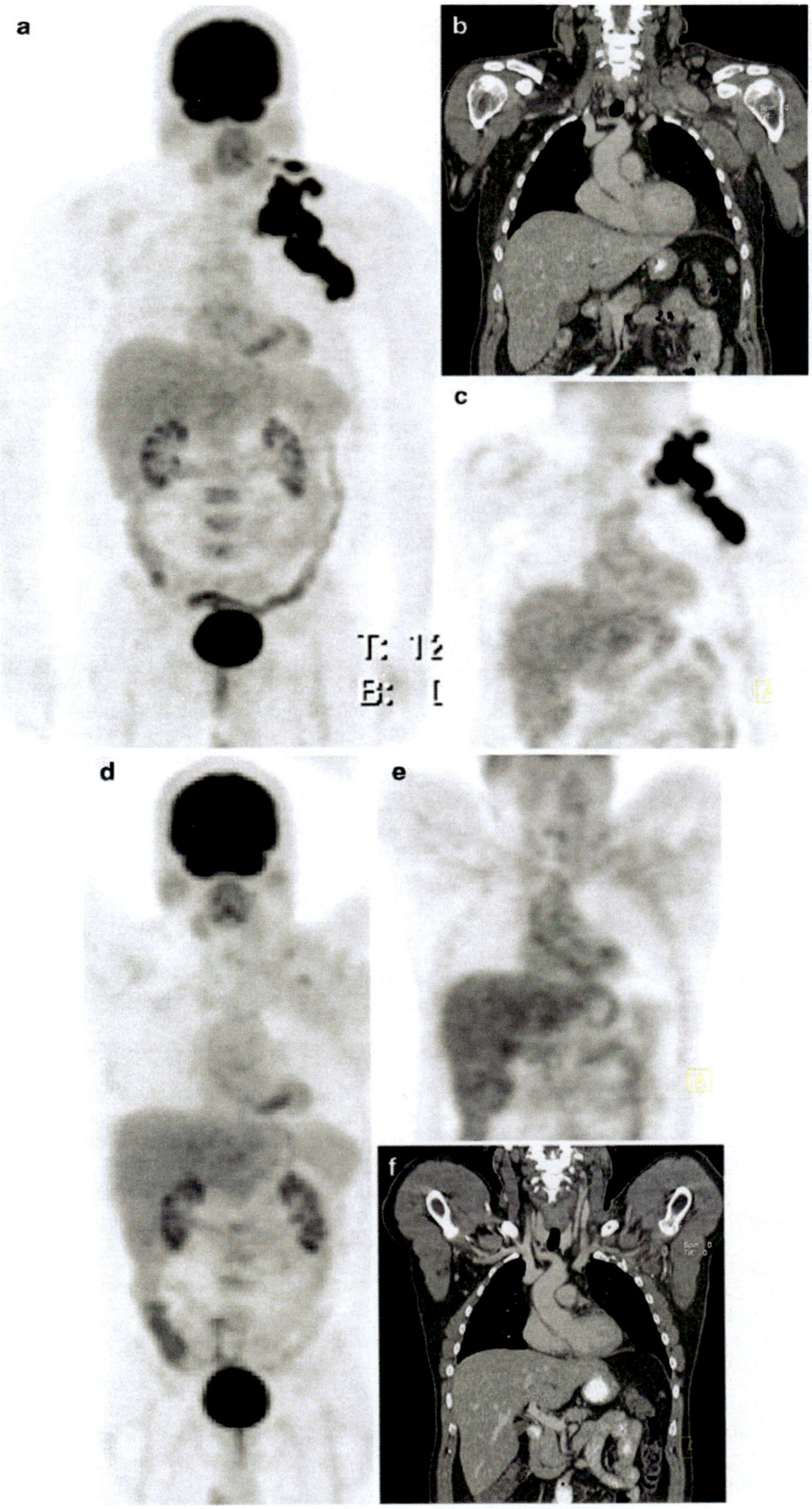

Fig. 24.8 Melanoma response to therapy. Left upper back melanoma with recurrence 9 years later as bulky left axillary and supraclavicular adenopathy seen an onterior FDG PET MIP image (**a**) and coronal CT (**b**) and FDG PET image (**c**). Following interferon therapy, the anteriorFDG PET MIP image (**d**) shows complete resolution of all the abnormal FDG tracer activity. Residual necrotic left axillary and supraclavicular lymph nodes are seen on the posttherapy CT (**e**), but these are without any abnormal FDG tracer uptake (**f**)

Table 24.3 Pitfalls and pearls

Natural history
- Melanoma can metastasize widely to unpredictable sites.
- Delayed recurrence beyond 10 years after initial treatment is uncommon but well described.

Treatment options
- Complete surgical resection of tumor burdens at diagnosis or at relapse is the most effective therapy when feasible.
- Currently, there is no routinely reliable and successful systemic therapy for extensive metastatic melanoma.

PET-CT
- Whole body PET-CT for melanoma frequently covers from vertex to toes and takes longer to acquire than other common cancers.
- Melanoma is among the most FDG avid tumors known.
- PET detectability depends on tumor volumes (>80 mm^3 or >5–6 mm in diameter), surrounding background activity and degree of tumor necrosis.
- Common distant metastatic sites include lymph nodes (including mesenteric lymph nodes), lung, skin, and subcutaneous tissues, liver, brain, and leptomeninges, bone, adrenal gland, bowel, and spleen.
- The use of CT contrast with PET-CT can provide additional localization value of lesions and specificity of PET findings.
- FDG avid foci are not necessarily diagnostic of metastases and should, when feasible, have histologic verification if this would alter management.

Table 24.4 Potential indications for PET-CT for melanoma

1. Locoregional disease at high risk for distant metastases at diagnosis (satellite, in-transit, or regional nodal metastases and probably for primary tumor thickness >1.5 mm, particularly with ulceration)
2. Known isolated distant metastatic disease under consideration for surgical resection with curative intent
3. Characterization of nonspecific morphologic abnormalities suspicious for distant metastases
4. Locoregional relapse and/or isolated distant metastatic recurrence under consideration for surgical resection
5. Surveillance of high-risk locoregional disease after initial treatment

References

1. Jemal A, Seigel R, Ward E, et al. Cancer statistics, 2006. CA Cancer J Clin 2006;56:106–130.
2. Chang AE, Karnell LH, Menck HR. The national cancer data base report on cutaneous and noncutaneous melanoma: a summary of 84,836 cases from the past decade. Cancer 1998;83:1664–1678.
3. Lens MB, Dawes M. Global perspectives of contemporary epidemiological trends of cutaneous malignant melanoma. Br J Dermatol 2004;150:179–185.
4. Christianson DF, Anderson CM. Close monitoring and lifetime follow-up is optimal for patients with a history of melanoma. Semin Oncol 2003;30:369–374.
5. Kirkwood JM, Ibrahim JG, Sosman JA, et al. High dose interferon alfa-2b significantly prolongs relapse-free and overall survival compared with the GM2-KLH/QS-21 vaccine in patients with resected stage IIB-III melanoma: results of intergroup trial E1694/S9512/C509801. J Clin Oncol 2001;19:2370–2380.
6. Lange JR, Sharfman WH, Alani RM, et al. Melanoma. In: Abeloff MD, Armitage JO, Niederhuber JE, et al.(eds.). Abeloff: Clinical Oncology, 3rd edn. New York: Elsevier-Churchill Livingstone, 2004, pp. 1561–1588.
7. Ballo MT, Ang KK. Radiation therapy for malignant melanoma. Surg Clin North Am 2003;83:323–342.
8. Balch CM, Buzaid AC, Soong SJ, et al. Final version of the American Joint Society on Cancer staging system for cutaneous melanoma. J Clin Oncol 2001;19:3635–3648.
9. Malignant melanoma of skin. In: Sobin LH, Wittekind Ch (eds.). TNM Classification of Malignant Tumours, 6th edn. New York: Wiley-Liss, 2002, pp. 126–130.
10. Wrightson WR, Wong SL, Edwards MJ, et al. Complications associated with sentinel lymph node biopsy for melanoma. Ann Surg Oncol 2003;10:676–680.
11. Morton DL, Hoon DSB, Cochran AJ, et al. Lymphatic mapping and sentinel lymphadenectomy for early-stage melanoma. Ann Surg 2003;238:538–550.
12. Will O, Purkayastha S, Chan S, et al. Diagnostic precision of nanoparticle-enhanced MRI for lymph-node metastases: a meta-analysis. Lancet Oncol 2006;7:52–60.
13. Wahl RL, Hutchins GD, Buchsbaum DJ, et al. 18F-2-deoxy-2 fluoro-D-glucose uptake into human xenografts. Cancer 1991;67:1544–1550.
14. Wagner JD, Schauwecker D, Davidson D, et al. FDG PET sensitivity for melanoma lymph node metastases is dependent on tumor volume. J Surg Oncol 2001;77:237–242.
15. Schöder H, Larson SM, Yeung WD. PET/CT in oncology: integration into clinical management of lymphoma, melanoma and gastrointestinal malignancies. J Nucl Med 2004;45:72S–81S.
16. Reinhardt MJ, Joe AY, Jaeger U, et al. Diagnostic performance of whole body dual modality 18F-FDG PET/CT imaging for N- and M-staging of malignant melanoma: experience with 250 consecutive patients. J Clin Oncol 2006;24:1178–1187.
17. Patel JK, Didolkar MS, Pickren JW, et al. Metastatic pattern of malignant melanoma: a study of 216 autopsy cases. Am J Surg 1978;135:807–810.
18. Kawashima A, Fishman EK, Kuhnlman JE, et al. CT of malignant melanoma: pattern of small bowel and mesenteric involvement. J Comput Assist Tomogr 1991;15:570–574.
19. Kath R, Hayungs J, Bornfeld N, et al. Prognosis and treatment of disseminated uveal melanoma. Cancer 1993;72:2219–2223.
20. Wagner JD, Schauwecker D, Davidson D, et al. Prospective study of fluorodeoxyglucose-positron emission tomography of lymph node basins in melanoma patients undergoing sentinel node biopsy. J Clin Oncol 1999;17:1508–1515.
21. Crippa F, Leutner M, Belli F, et al. Which kind of lymph node metastases can FDG PET detect? A clinical study in melanoma. J Nucl Med 2000;41:1491–1494.
22. Friedman KP, Wahl RL. Clinical use of positron emission tomography in the management of cutaneous melanoma. Semin Nucl Med 2004;34:242–253.
23. Segall GM, Swetter SM. PET imaging in melanoma. In: Valk PE, Bailey DL, Townsend DW, Maisey MN (eds.). Positron Emission Tomography. Basic Science and Clinical Practice. London: Springer-Verlag, 2003:625–636
24. Swetter SM, Carroll LA, Johnson DL, et al. Positron emission tomography is superior to computed tomography for metastatic detection in melanoma patients. Ann Surg Oncol 2002;9:646–653.
25. Tyler DS, Onaitis M, Kherani A, et al. Positron emission tomography scanning in malignant melanoma, Clinical utility in paitenst with stage III disease. Cancer 2000;89:1019–1025.
26. Reske SN, Kotzerke J. FDG PET for clinical use: results of the 3rd German interdisciplinary consensus conference, "Onko-PET III," 21 July and 19 September 2000. Eur J Nucl Med 2001;28:1707–1723.

27. Rinne D, Baum RP, Hör G, et al. Primary staging and follow-up of highriskmelanomapatientswithwholebody18F-Fluorodeoxyglucose positron emission tomography, results of a prospective study of 100 patients. Cancer 1998;82:1664–1671.
28. Dummer R, Panizzon R, Bloch PH, et al. Updated Swiss guidelines for the treatment and follow-up of cutaneous melanoma. Dermatology 2005;210:39–44.
29. Wagner JD, Schauwecker D, Davidson D, et al. Inefficacy of F-18 fluorodeoxy-d-glucose-positron emission tomography scans for initial evaluation in early-stage cutaneous melanoma. Cancer 2005;104:570–579.
30. Acland KM, O'Doherty MJ, Russell-Jones R. The value of positron emission tomography scanning in the detection of subclinical metastatic melanoma. J Am Acad Dermatol 2000;42:606–611.
31. Calabro A, Singletary SE, Balch CM. Pattern of relapse in 1001 consecutive patients with melanoma nodal metastases. Arch Surg 1989;124:1051–1055.
32. Stas M, Stroobants S, Dupont P, et al. 18-FDG PET scan in the staging of recurrent melanoma: additional value and therapeutic impact. Melanoma Res 2002;12:479–490.
33. Antoch G, Freudenberg LS, Beyer T, et al. To enhance or not to enhance? 18F-FDG and CT contrast agents in dual-modality 18F-FDG PET/CT. J Nucl Med 2004;45:56S–65S.
34. Vogel WV, Oyen WJG, Barentsz JO, et al. PET/CT: panacea, redundancy, or something in between. J Nucl Med 2004;45:15S–24S.
35. Mercier GA, Alavi A, Fraker DL. FDG positron emission tomography in isolated limb perfusion therapy in patients with locally advanced melanoma: preliminary results. Clin Nucl Med 2001;26:832–836.

Further Reading

1. Antoch G, Saoudi N, Kuehl H, et al. Accuracy of whole-body dual-modality fluorine-18-2-fluoro-2-deoxy-D-glucose positron emission tomography and computed tomography (FDG PET/CT) for tumor staging in solid tumors: comparison with CT and PET. J Clin Oncol 2004;22:4357–4368.
2. Essner R. Surgical treatment of malignant melanoma. Surg Clin North Am 2003;83:109–156.
3. Mack LA, McKinnon JG. Controversies in the management of metastatic melanoma to regional lymphatic basins. J Surg Oncol 2004;86:189–199.
4. Reinartz P, Wieres FJ, Schneider W, et al. Side-by-side of PET and CT scans in oncology: which patients might profit from integrated PET/CT. Eur J Nucl Med Mol Imaging 2004;31:1456–1461.
5. Tsao H, Atkins MB, Sober AJ. Management of cutaneous melanoma. N Engl J Med 2004;351:998–1012.

Chapter 25
PET-CT of Ovarian Cancer

Carlos A. Buchpiguel

Ovarian cancer represents one of the most deadly cancers in women. More than 23,000 new cases will be diagnosed causing 13,900 deaths in USA [1]. Initial diagnosis of ovarian cancer occurs after the disease has spread in up to 75% of patients, limiting effective treatment and resulting in the high mortality rate. Ovarian cancer originates from epithelial, stromal, or germ cell elements, and this chapter focuses on management of celomic epithelial carcinoma since it accounts for more than 90% of all subtypes of ovarian cancers. These cancers actually may arise in any part of the peritoneal cavity; however, they nearly always arise from the ovarian epithelium. Ovarian cancer spreads by direct invasion and dissemination throughout peritoneal space, lymphatic spread, and/or more rarely hematogenous routes. Risk factors for ovarian cancer include age, nulliparity, and personal or family history of ovarian, endometrial, or breast cancer. Management is primarily surgical, and is directly dependent on clinical stage based largely on surgical findings. As very few symptoms appear on the initial onset of the ovarian cancer, the majority of patients present with advanced disease at the time of clinical staging. An accurate staging is mandatory to classify the disease as limited or advanced as well as to define the proper management and prognosis.

Patients may present with abdominal pain, bowel obstruction, or ascites related to advanced disease, or a mass may be found on bimanual pelvic exam or incidentally on imaging studies. Diagnosis and staging is almost always on laparotomy with exploration, usually involving total abdominal hysterectomy, bilateral salpingo-oophorectomy, omentectomy, and peritoneal cavity exploration. Further management is based on the clinical stage (Table 25.1), either limited disease (stage I–II) or advanced disease (stage III–IV).

Ovarian tumors are relatively common, and overall only 15–20% of ovarian masses removed are found to be malignant. Epithelial ovarian neoplasm includes serous and mucinous, endometrioid, clear cell, and Brenner tumors. Patients with disease limited to the pelvis that is completely removed on surgical exploration can be considered low risk and kept on observation. In selected young women who desire to maintain fertility, stage 1A disease can be managed by unilateral oophorectomy. Those patients with limited disease but elevated risk of recurrence due to tumor histology (poorly differentiated and clear cell tumors, positive peritoneal washings, ascites, or involvement of pelvic structures other than uterus and adnexa) may undergo additional adjuvant platinum-based chemotherapy (high-risk).

Patients found to have advanced disease on surgical exploration, including those with peritoneal implants outside the pelvis and/or retroperitoneal or inguinal lymph node metastases (stage III) or distant metastases (stage IV), undergo maximum cytoreduction (resection of as much metastatic disease as possible) at the time of surgery followed by systemic combined chemotherapy. Debulking should achieve absence of visible disease or at least residual disease less than 1 cm diameter at each site of involvement. Patients with nonresectable lesions might benefit from neoadjuvant chemotherapy with interval debulking surgery, although controversies still exist regarding its therapeutic impact. Radiation therapy has limited roles including selected patients after optimal debulking and palliation in patients with localized recurrent disease.

Role of PET-CT on Initial Diagnosis of Ovarian Cancer

PET-CT has no current role in the initial diagnosis of ovarian cancer. Since stage on initial presentation is one the major prognostic factors, and early stage disease is largely curable with surgical resection, there has been an interest in identifying early stage ovarian cancer in high-risk patients [3]. Physical examination, endovaginal ultrasound with duplex Doppler and serum CA-125 assay have not proven sufficiently sensitive, specific or of sufficient positive predictive value for the early detection of ovarian cancer, although in patients of high

C.A. Buchpiguel (✉)
Department of Radiology, São Paulo University School of Medicine, São Paulo, Brazil PET-CT Laboratory, Hospital do Coração, São Paulo, Brazil
e-mail: buch@usp.br

P. Shreve and D.W. Townsend (eds.), *Clinical PET-CT in Radiology: Integrated Imaging in Oncology*,
DOI 10.1007/978-0-387-48902-5_25,

risk such as those with a strong family history of ovarian cancer may routinely undergo such tests. Serum CA-125 levels are elevated in most patients with epithelial ovarian cancer, but not generally in patients with early disease (stage I) or mucinous ovarian carcinoma. Further, there are several conditions which also raise serum CA-125 levels, including endometriosis, uterine fibroids, pelvic inflammatory disease, cirrhosis, and tumors of the cervix, endometrium, pancreas, liver, lung, breast, and colon.

Regarding FDG PET detection of primary ovarian cancer, even with large-sized primary lesions, sensitivity and specificity is limited for detecting primary ovarian cancer [4]. Benign ovarian masses such as cystadenomas, endometriomas, follicular or corpus luteum cysts, granuloma, abscess, thecoma, and even hydrosalpinx have been reported to concentrate FDG tracer and appear to be indistinguishable on FDG PET [5]. Physiologic ovarian FDG tracer uptake can also be seen in premenopausal [6]. Moreover, very early ovarian carcinomas (small volume) or mucinous, cystic, or well-differentiated ovarian tumors may lack sufficient FDG tracer uptake on FDG PET for detection. The false-negative rate of FDG PET can be as high as 71% for stage IA or mucinous or cystic ovarian cancer [7]. The addition of the diagnostic CT images to FDG PET may reduce the false-negative rate for larger tumors that are without detectable FDG tracer uptake; however, not enough data are available in the literature yet regarding combined PET-CT technology for the detection of primary ovarian cancers. Preliminary studies evaluating the value of PET-CT in 97 patients with pelvic masses and with high risk of malignancy index (RMI) showed very high sensitivity (100%) and high specificity (92.5%) for PET-CT in identifying primary ovarian cancer, despite some limitations on patient selection bias [8].

Staging of Ovarian Cancer with PET-CT

Staging of ovarian cancer is based on findings at laparotomy in accordance with the recommendations of the International Federation of Gynecology and Obstetrics (FIGO) [2]. Surgical findings and pathological diagnosis of surgical specimens and biopsies determine the diagnosis the extent of disease (Table 25.1). While imaging studies are not the basis of staging, imaging studies are often performed preoperatively (usually CT or MRI of the abdomen and pelvis) on patients suspected of advanced disease. Ovarian masses are also frequently disclosed as incidental findings on CT or ultrasound examinations performed for other indications. Correct staging of ovarian cancer is crucial for proper therapeutic planning and for prognostic estimation. Survival is strongly affected by stage of ovarian cancer at initial presentation. Although the survival rate can be as high as 93% when the disease is restricted to ovaries, it decreases to 25% in more advanced stages. For all stages, the 5-year survival rate is only 46%, reflecting the advanced stage at diagnosis for a majority of patients [9].

Table 25.1 FIGO staging system for ovarian cancer (Data from Ref. [2])

Stage	Description
I	Growth limited to the ovaries
IA	One ovary; no ascites; capsule intact, no tumor on external surface
IB	Two ovaries; no ascites; capsule intact, no tumor on external surface
IC	One or both ovaries with either: surface tumor; ruptured capsule; ascites or peritoneal washings with malignant cells
II	Pelvic extension
IIA	Involvement of uterus and/or tubes
IIB	Involvement of other pelvic structures
IIC	Stage IIA or IIB with factors as in stage IC
III	Peritoneal implants outside pelvis and/or positive retroperitoneal or inguinal nodes
IIIA	Grossly limited to pelvis; negative nodes; microscopic seeding of abdominal peritoneum
IIIB	Implants of abdominal peritoneum <2 cm; nodes negative
IIIC	Abdominal implants >2 cm and/or positive retroperitoneal or inguinal nodes
IV	Distant metastases

As mentioned, surgery is the gold standard for staging patients with ovarian cancer and at the same time allows for cytoreduction in those patients with advanced disease. Accurate preoperative identification of malignant sites, however, can be important for surgical planning and to define sites at which biopsy should be performed at surgery. This is also of value since complete removal of tumor tissue is not possible in approximately 60% of patients with ovarian cancer [10]. Patients found to have bulky nonresectable disease on imaging studies may be referred to neoadjuvant chemotherapy before undergoing primary debulking at surgery.

It is important to recognize the pathways for tumor spread in ovarian cancer to understand the considerations of surgical exploration for staging. Ovarian cancer spreads from confinement to the ovary (stage I) to local extension involving adjacent pelvic structures (stage II) and then beyond the pelvis as peritoneal implants or extrapelvic lymph node metastases (stage III), and finally as distant metastases (stage IV). Peritoneal spread is the most common route of dissemination of disease beyond the pelvis. Peritoneal implants typically are found in the pelvis, on the liver, along the right paracolic gutter, under the right hemidiaphragm and on bowel and omentum. Therefore, in order to stage ovarian cancer on imaging studies such as PET-CT, it is important to evaluate all major anatomic areas within the pelvis and abdomen according to the FIGO staging system (see Figs. 25.1, 25.2, 25.3, and 25.4).

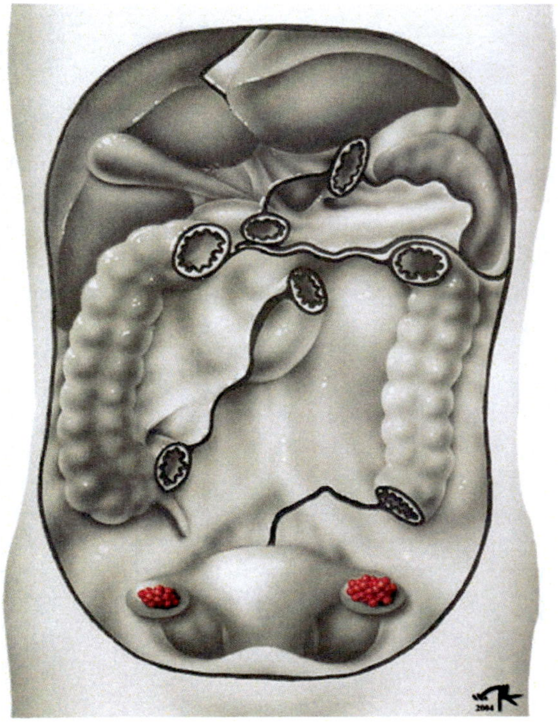

Fig. 25.1 Stage I ovarian cancer. Tumor involvement is restricted to one or both ovaries (*pink*) (Courtesy of Walther Yoshiharu Ishikawa)

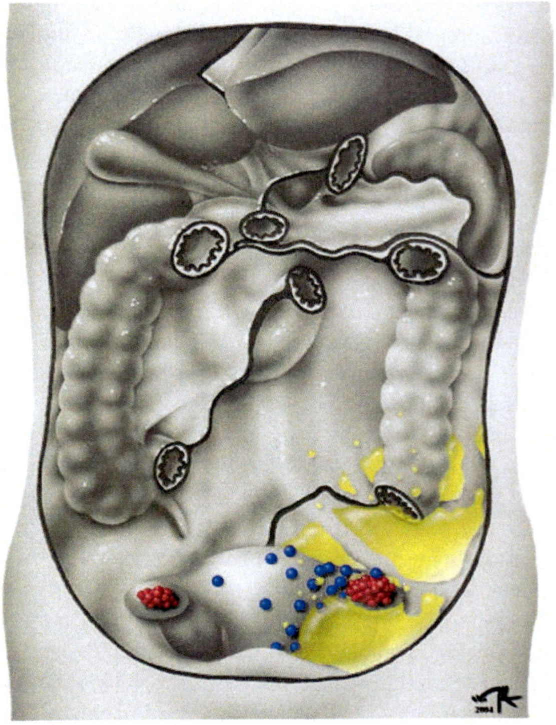

Fig. 25.2 Stage II ovarian cancer. Tumor involvement extends beyond ovary to include adjacent pelvic structures. *Pink* illustrates ovarian involvement; *blue* the uterus and tube involvement; and *yellow* the presence of ascitic fluid (Courtesy of Walther Yoshiharu Ishikawa)

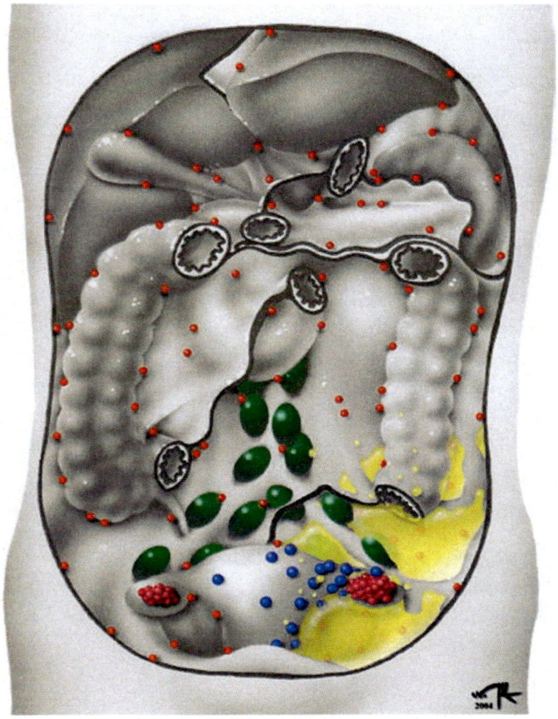

Fig. 25.3 Stage III ovarian cancer. Tumor has spread via peritoneal implants (*red*) and/or retroperitoneal lymph nodes (*green*) (Courtesy of Walther Yoshiharu Ishikawa)

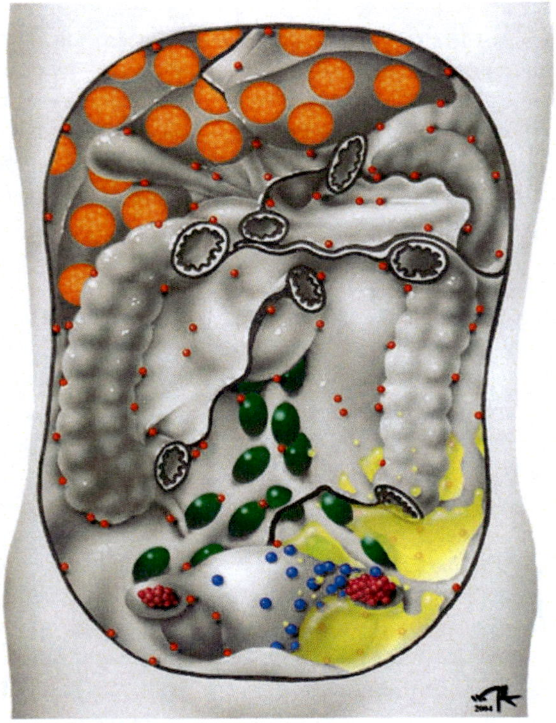

Fig. 25.4 Stage IV ovarian cancer. Presence of metastatic disease, in this example intraparenchymal liver metastasis (*orange*) defines systemic advanced disease (Courtesy of Walther Yoshiharu Ishikawa)

In the pelvic space it is important to detect structural and/or metabolic evidence for involvement of uterus, pelvic sidewall, sigmoid colon, urinary bladder, and cul-de-sac. This will allow characterizing as local (stage I) or regionally advanced (stage II) disease. Optimized CT technique, including use of oral and intravenous contrast agents as part of the PET-CT examination is helpful to identify local extension into the fallopian tube, uterus, and adjacent structures including bowel wall invasion. For abdominal staging, the potential targets can be separated in three main groups: peritoneum, lymph nodes, and liver-spleen. According to a previous radiologic standardized form [11], the peritoneum can be divided into the following, which should be specifically addressed with regard to involvement in the imaging evaluation:

- The anterior part of the abdomen
- The paracolic gutters
- The subdiaphragmatic spaces
- The mesentery
- The liver surface
- The omenta
- Lymph node staging includes porta hepatis, splenic hilum, and paraaortic and iliac (common, external, and internal) chain nodal groups.
- Distant metastatic disease includes hepatic metastases, in distinction from liver surface implants.

A major advantage of PET-CT is the registered and aligned nature of the detailed anatomic images generated by the multidetector CT technology with the images of tissue metabolism possible by the PET technology. This allows for staging based on anatomical classification such as determining local extension of tumor into adjacent structures. Moreover, subtle metabolic abnormalities on FDG PET can be missed or misinterpreted as physiologic concentration of tracer, and the coregistration of the PET images with CT helps to further identify the lesion based on morphologic criteria. This is particularly important in assessing for peritoneal implants of ovarian cancer. FDG PET, on the other hand, can detect metastatic involvement of nonenlarged lymph nodes and greatly aids in the search throughout the peritoneal cavity for small implants of tumor, which may be easily overlooked on CT. Hence the combination of PET and CT is particularly well suited for staging of ovarian cancer.

Very limited data are currently available in the literature regarding the value of PET-CT in staging ovarian cancer. The majority of data in the literature presently is based on FDG PET alone, in comparison with structural imaging modalities. A very interesting work done by Yoshida et al. showed significant increase of accuracy in staging abdominal disease by adding PET data into CT staging information [12]. In the pelvis, only mild improvement was observed by including FDG PET findings in the analysis. However, for abdominal staging the addition of FDG PET improved the sensitivity from 24% (only CT) to 63% (CT + PET), the specificity from 95% to 98%, the positive predictive value from 45% to 88%, and the negative predictive value from 88% to 93%. Diagnostic accuracy in comparison with surgical findings changed from 53% (only CT) to 87% (CT + PET). A recent prospective study evaluating 50 patients with pelvic lesions and rising serum Ca-125 levels already scheduled for surgery showed that PET-CT was concordant with final pathological staging in 69% of patients while CT results alone were concordant in 53%. Moreover, CT incorrectly downstaged four out of six which were correctly detected by PET-CT [13]. Thus, despite a limited number of prospective studies using PET-CT for staging ovarian cancer, particularly in patients suspected of having advanced disease based on clinical, laboratory and available imaging studies preoperatively, PET-CT may be of values in more completely determining the full extent of disease for surgical planning and consideration of preoperative adjunctive chemotherapy.

Restaging of the Ovarian Cancer with PET-CT

Even though ovarian cancer is considered one of the most chemo sensitive solid tumors, with more than 80% of response after first-line chemotherapy, the majority of patients will present with tumor recurrence after primary therapy. Recurrence can be found on pelvis, abdomen, or as distant metastases. The most common clinical presentations for recurrent disease are peritoneal implants (Fig. 25.5) and lymph node metastases (Fig. 25.6). The pattern of recurrent disease is not quite different from that seen on primary staging of ovarian cancer. A significant proportion of patients with persistent or recurrent tumor remain clinically silent. The value of an elevated serum CA-125 measurement has been established in the follow up of patients with ovarian cancer. When elevated, serum CA-125 is a strong indication of recurrence in patients with ovarian cancer, however, a normal serum CA-125 cannot rule out the presence of tumor. Residual or recurrent disease was found in 62% of patients with ovarian cancer in whom CA-125 levels were normal [14]. Even if positive, serum CA-125 does not provide site localization, nature and extent of recurrence, all of which influence decisions on salvage therapy.

Conventional morphologic imaging has also been investigated for restaging patients with ovarian cancer. Sensitivities for CT and MR have ranged from 46% to 84% [15]. A principal limitation of conventional morphologic imaging is detection of small peritoneal implants and metastatic disease in normal or borderline enlarged lymph nodes. Few reports are available in the literature evaluating the role of FDG-PET in restaging ovarian cancer patients. Early studies reported

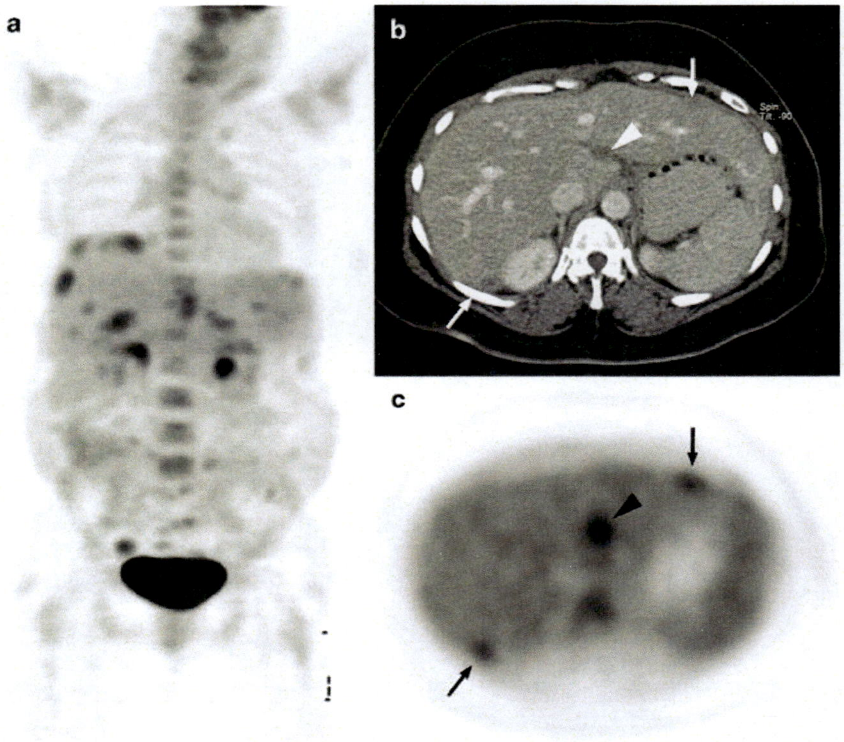

Fig. 25.5 Recurrent ovarian cancer as peritoneal implants. Anterior FDG PET MIP image (**a**) shows multiple small foci of abnormal FDG tracer distributed throughout the peritoneal cavity including over the surface of the liver and under the right hemidiaphragm. Transaxial CT (**b**) and FDG PET image (**c**) demonstrate liver surface implants at the posterior right lobe and anterior aspect of the left lobe of the liver (*arrows*) as well as within an intrahepatic fissure (*arrowhead*)

higher sensitivities (83–91%) for FDG PET in comparison with conventional imaging in detecting recurrent ovarian cancer. More recent papers of using modern PET-CT scanners have reported limitations in the detection of microscopic and low volume disease detection [15], reflecting the difficulty in detecting very small peritoneal implants on either FDG PET or CT images. The inability to accurately define extent of small peritoneal implants on noninvasive imaging studies has been a reason for second-look laparotomies for restaging patients with ovarian cancer. In a prospective study of patients undergoing second-look exploration following treated with primary cytoreductive surgery and platinum based chemotherapy, PET-CT was found to have positive and negative predictive values of 89% and 57%, respectively [16]. A recent study performed by Sebastian et al. showed that PET-CT accuracy exceeded CT for abdomen (91% vs 79%) and total body recurrence (92% vs 83%), and the interobserver agreement was better for PET-CT than for CT alone [17].

The registered and aligned images of PET-CT technology provide a few advantages in comparison to PET- or CT-alone interpretation. Subtle abnormalities on FDG PET can be confirmed as disease on careful review of the CT images. This is specially observed when small implants or small volume disease show mild FDG uptake, either because of partial volume effect on small sized lesions (Fig. 25.7) or due to biologic properties of the tumor itself. Even when the exact nature of a mild abnormality seen on PET cannot be precisely determined, it is believed that PET can at least guide surgeons toward a more optimal cytoreductive second-look surgery. However, there are no prospective data in the literature yet to prove that PET-CT might have prognostic impact in promoting more effective cytoreductive surgeries. It is important to fully interpret both the CT and FDG PET images, as ovarian cancer is not always highly FDG avid and thus peritoneal implants and masses may not be strikingly abnormal on FDG PET (Fig. 25.8). In addition, important distinctions in local extend of disease and the nature of metastases requires careful review of fully optimized CT images (Fig. 25.9).

On the other hand, lymph node metastases clearly demonstrated on FDG PET images may not be easily confirmed as corresponding to a lymph node identified on CT when the lymph node is small or in a region of postoperative changes (see Fig. 25.6c).

Reports should be done according to the FIGO staging system, since gynecologic oncologists and gynecologic surgeons usually follow these standards. Providing detailed description of lesions with information regarding the size,

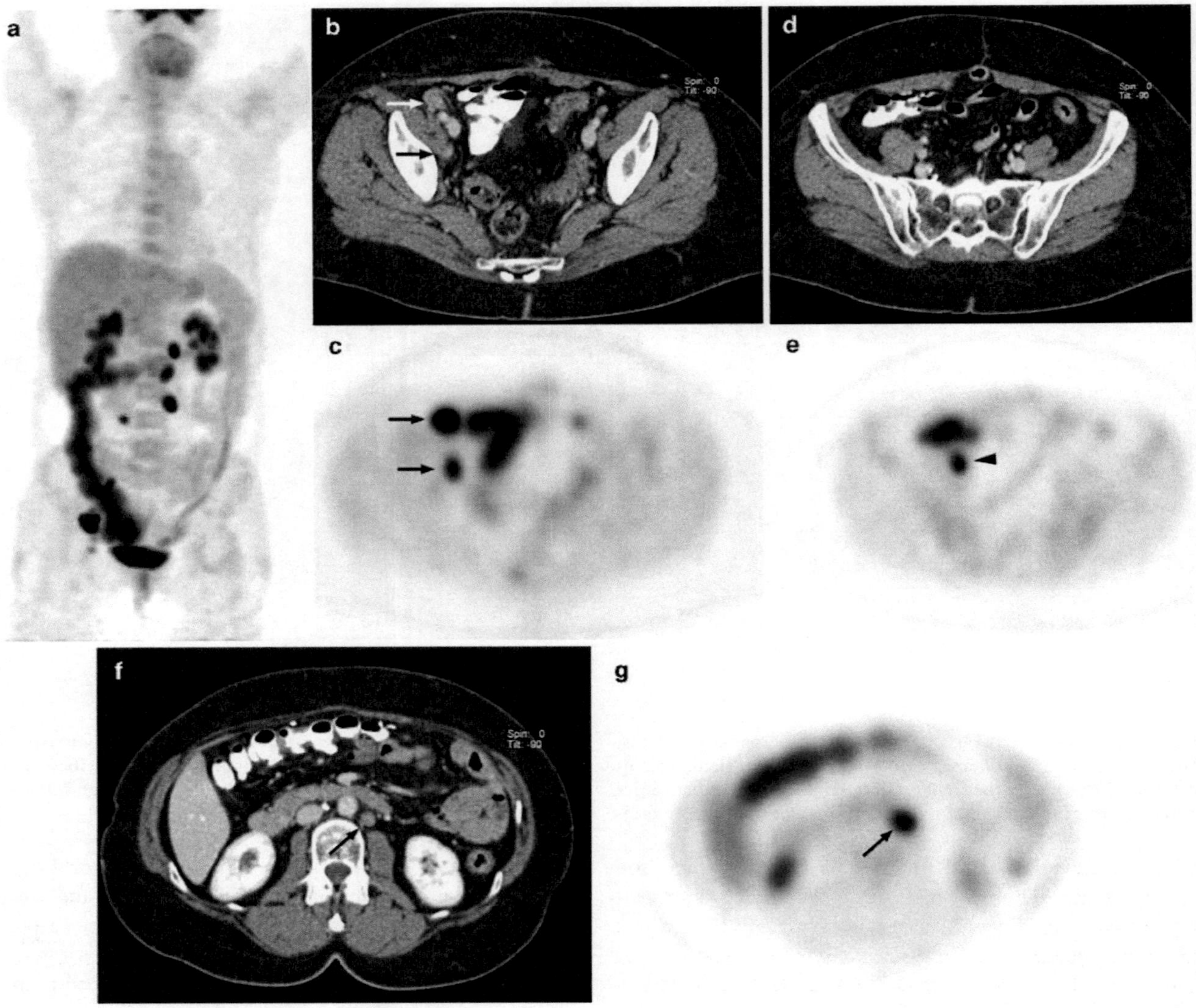

Fig. 25.6 Recurrent ovarian cancer as lymph node metastases. Anterior FDG PET MIP image (**a**) demonstrates intense foci of abnormal FDG tracer uptake following right iliac and left paraaortic lymph node chains. Physiologic tracer activity is seen in the right colon. Transaxial CT arrows (**b**) and FDG PET (**c**) images show a 1.4-cm right external iliac lymph node and 6-mm right obturator lymph node metastases (*arrows*), a 5-mm right iliac lymph node metastasis (*arrowhead*) adjacent to the right psoas muscle (**d, e**), and a 1.2 cm left paraaortic lymph node (*arrow*) metastasis (**f, g**)

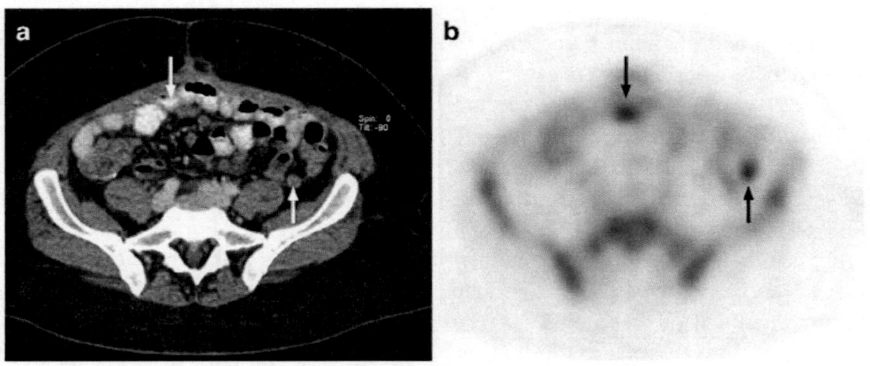

Fig. 25.7 Peritoneal implants of ovarian cancer. (**a, b**) On CT and FDG PET transaxial images there are two isolated foci of FDG tracer activity that correspond to subcentimeter soft tissue nodules depicted on the registered and aligned CT image (*arrows*)

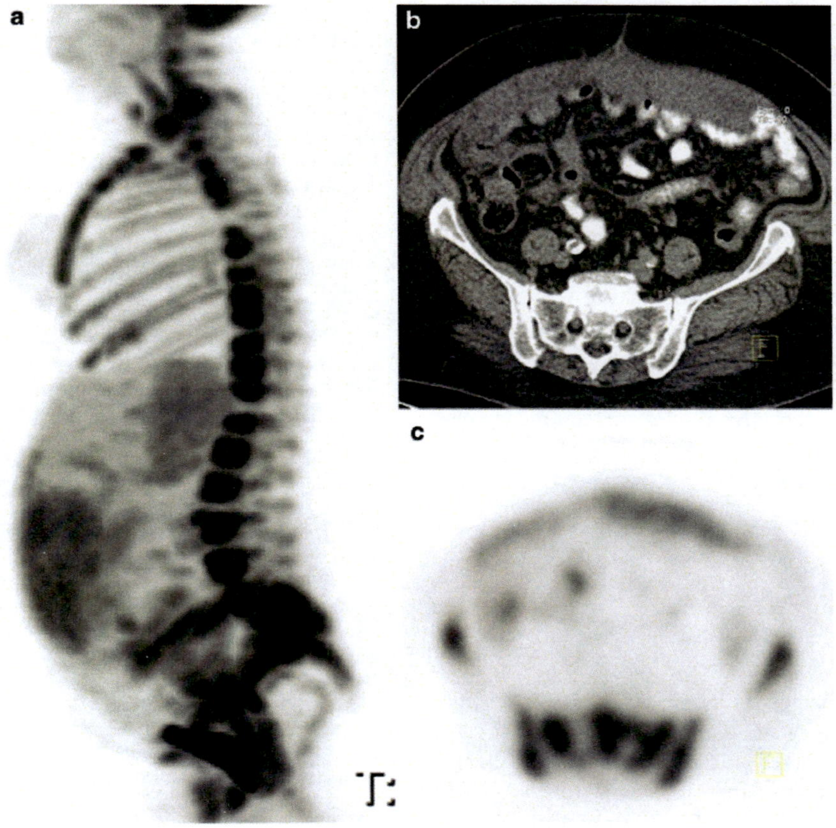

Fig. 25.8 Extensive omental implants (omental cake) of ovarian cancer. Lateral FDG PET MIP image (**a**) reveals diffuse modestly abnormal FDG tracer activity in the anterior abdomen. Increased tracer activity in bone marrow reflects recent use of hemopoietic stimulate as part of chemotherapy regimen. CT (**b**) and FDG PET (**c**) transaxial images reveal extensive abnormal soft tissue contiguous with the anterior abdominal wall displacing bowel loops posteriorly associated with only modest FDG tracer uptake in a patient 6 weeks following completion of chemotherapy

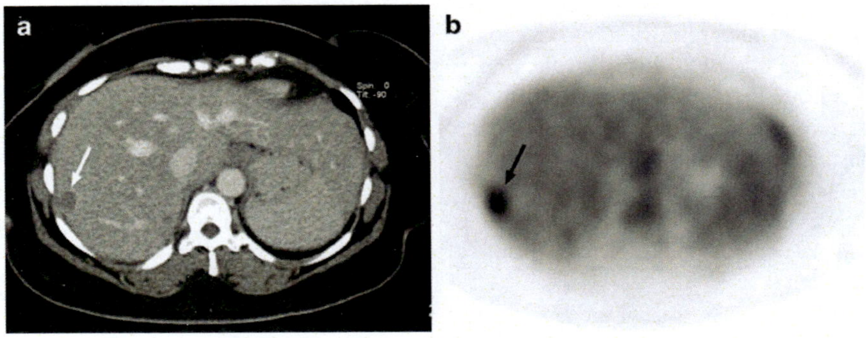

Fig. 25.9 Metastatic (stage IV) ovarian cancer. On CT (**a**) and FDG PET (**b**) transaxial images the focal FDG tracer activity corresponds to a lesion which is shown on the contrast enhanced CT to be within the liver parenchymal rather than a surface implant (*arrow*)

location, extension, and relation with neighborhood structures are important for guiding precise cytoreduction surgery that may be employed for treatment of relapse. The reports should follow the same scheme for primary staging of ovarian cancer noted previously which must describe detailed evaluation of pelvic and extrapelvic structures, including nodal and peritoneal staging.

PET-CT would be more commonly employed, then, in patients needing restaging for clinical or laboratory (rising serum CA-125) findings suggesting disease recurrence.

Identifying the site(s) and extent of recurrent disease can be particularly helpful in planning further systemic therapy vs. cytoreduction surgery. Uncertainties remain exist concerning the economic impact of PET-CT on management of patients with ovarian cancer. Again, very few relevant data are available in the literature, but some authors have shown that management can be changed in 76% of high-risk patients. Another recent study evaluating PET-CT impact on patient management in ovarian cancer recurrence showed that on 34% of patients the clinical decision making was changed based on PET-CT findings [18]. However, no effect on survival rate or disease-free survival has been clearly demonstrated by adding FDG PET to the clinical algorithm. Therefore, additional prospective studies are required to confirm the clinical and prognostic impact of PET-CT on restaging ovarian cancer patients.

Therapy Monitoring with PET-CT During Treatment

Even though ovarian cancer is very sensitive to front-line therapy, including surgery and platinum chemotherapy, second-line or salvage therapies after relapses can be challenging with response rates ranging from 14% to 34% [19]. Conventional imaging, especially CT, has not proven to be effective on monitoring treatment of ovarian cancer [20]. A study of FDG PET imaging alone of patients undergoing adjuvant chemotherapy prior to cytoreductive surgery found a significant correlation between the reduction in FDG tracer uptake in tumor after first and third cycles of chemotherapy and overall patient survival [21]. The FDG PET findings were more accurate than clinical or histopathologic response criteria or changes in serum CA-125, suggesting there may be an important role for using PET-CT in therapy monitoring of ovarian cancer. A recent study evaluating 179 patients with advanced ovarian cancers showed that large bowel mesentery implant was the only independent predictor of incomplete response by multivariate analysis ($p = 0.004$); However, it should not be used to withhold patients from primary cytoreductive surgery [22].

References

1. Jemal A, Thomas A, Murray T, Thun M. Cancer statistics, 2002. CA Cancer J Clin 2002;52:23–47.
2. FIGO Cancer Committee. The new FIGO stage grouping for primary carcinoma of the ovary (1985). Gynecol Oncol 1986;25:383.
3. Piver MS, Baker TR, Jishi MF, Sandecki AM, Tsukada Y, Natarajan N, Mettlin CJ, Blake CA. Familial ovarian cancer: a report of 658 families from the Gilda Radner Familial Ovarian Cancer Registry (1981–1991). Cancer 1993;71:582–588.
4. Casey MJ, Gupta NC, Muths CK. Experience with positron emission tomography (PET) scans in patients with ovarian cancer. Gynecol Oncol 1994;53:331–338.
5. Rieber A, Nussle K, Stohr I, Grab D, Fenchel S, Kreienberg R, Reske SN, Brambs HJ. Preoperative diagnosis of ovarian tumors with MR imaging: comparison with transvaginal sonography, positron emission tomography, and histologic findings. Am J Roentgenol 2001;177:123–129.
6. Lerman H, Metser U, Grisaru D, Fishman A, Lievshitz G, Even-Sapir E. Normal and abnormal 18F-FDG endometrial and ovarian uptake in pre- and postmenopausal patients: assessment by PET/CT. J Nucl Med 2004;45:266–271.
7. Fenchel S, Grab D, Nussle K, Kotzerke J, Rieber A, Kreienberg R, Brambs HJ, Reske SN. Asymptomatic adnexal masses: correlation of FDG PET and histopathologic findings. Radiology 2002;223:780–788.
8. Risum S, Hogdall C, Loft A, et al. The diagnostic value of PET/CT for primary ovarian cancer – a prospective study. Gynecol Oncol 2007;105(1):145–149.
9. American Cancer Society. Cancer facts and figures: 1998. Atlanta: American Cancer Society, 1998;13.
10. Kuhn W, Rutke S, Spathe K. Neoadjuvant chemotherapy followed by tumor debulking prolongs survival for patients with poor prognosis in International Federation of Gynecology and Obstetrics stage IIIC ovarian carcinoma. Cancer 2001;92:2585–2591.
11. Tempany CMC, Zou KH, Silverman SG, Brown DL, Kurtz AB, McNeil BJ. Staging of advanced ovarian cancer: comparison of imaging modalities. Report from the Radiological Diagnostic Oncology Group. Radiology 2000;215:761–767.
12. Yoshida Y, Kurokawa T, Kawahara K, Tsuchida T, Okazawa H, Fujibayashi Y, Yonekura Y, Kotsuji F. Incremental benefits of FDG positron emission tomography over CT alone for the preoperative staging of ovarian cancer. Am J Roentgenol 2004;182:227–233.
13. Gadducci A, Cosio S. Surveillance of patients after initial treatment of ovarian cancer. Crit Rev Oncol Hematol 2009;71(1):43–52.
14. Rubin SC, Hoskins WJ, Hakes TB, Markman M, Reichman BS, Chapman D, Lewis JL Jr. Serum CA125 levels and surgical findings in patients undergoing secondary operations for epithelial ovarian cancer. Am J Obstet Gynecol 1989;160:667–671.
15. Kim EE. Whole-body positron emission tomography and positron emission tomography/computed tomography in gynecologic oncology. Int J Gynecol Cancer 2004;14:12–22.
16. Sironi S, Messa C, Mangili G, et al. Integrated FDG PET/CT in patients with persistent ovarian cancer: correlation with histologic findings. Radiology 2004;233:433–440.
17. Sebastian S, Lee SI, Horowitz NS, et al. PET-CT vs. CT alone in ovarian cancer recurrence. Abdom Imaging 2008;33:112–118.
18. Poveda A. Ovarian cancer treatment: what is new? Int J Gynecol Cancer 2003;13:241–250.
19. Simcock B, Neesham D, Quinn M, et al. The impact of PET/CT in the management of recurrent ovarian cancer. Gynecol Oncol 2006;103(1):271–276.
20. Patsner B. Is there a role for CT scanning to monitor therapy of optimally debulked patients with advanced ovarian epithelial cancer? Int J Gynecol Cancer 1994;4:19–21.
21. Avril N, Sassen S, Schmalfeldt B, et al. Prediction of response to neoadjuvant chemotherapy by sequential F-18 fluorodeoxyglucose positron emission tomography in patients with advanced-stage ovarian cancer. J Clin Oncol 2005;23:7445–7453.
22. Risum S, Høgdall C, Loft A, et al. Prediction of suboptimal primary cytoreduction in primary ovarian cancer with combined positron emission tomography/computed tomography – a prospective study. Gynecol Oncol 2008;108(2):265–270.

Chapter 26
PET-CT of Cervical and Uterine Cancer

Yat Yin Yau

Uterine cancers can be considered in two separate entities: carcinoma of the cervix and carcinoma of the uterine corpus. They behave clinically and biologically dissimilar to each other and are staged and treated differently. Cancer of the corpus in essence is represented by endometrial carcinoma and is the most common gynecologic cancer [1]. Endometrial cancer occurs most commonly in postmenopausal women, with the risk increasing with age. The mode of spread of endometrial cancer is local (myometrial) and later hematogenous. Cervical malignancy usually occurs in the premenopausal women and spreads locally (parametrial) and through lymphatics in a relatively predictable pattern. Overall, cervical cancer is the third most common gynecologic cancer and ranks after ovarian and uterine carcinoma as the third leading cause of death by gynecologic malignancy [1].

The pathogenesis of these uterine and cervical cancers is also different. Carcinoma of the cervix is associated with human papillomavirus, while carcinoma of the uterine corpus is either developed de novo or is hormonally induced by estrogens. A subtype of uterine cancer, clear cell carcinoma of the cervix is linked to in utero exposure to diethylstilbestrol [2]. Early detection with Papanicolaou (Pap) smear and advances in treatment have improved the mortality rate of early stage cervical carcinoma, but the mortality rate of invasive or advanced cervical cancer has not changed substantially. Management for both tumors relies heavily on staging. Staging carcinoma of the cervix is clinically based while endometrial carcinoma staging is primarily surgical.

Y.Y. Yau (✉)
Department of Radiology, University of Hong Kong, Hong Kong, China
and
Diagnostic Imaging, Nuclear Medicine and PET-CT, Hong Kong Adventist Hospital, 1/F, 40 Stubbs Rd, Hong Kong, China
e-mail: yatyin@gmail.com

Cervical Carcinoma

Cervical carcinoma is most commonly diagnosed in the women during their fifth and sixth decades of life. Cervical carcinoma is thought to progress from a preexisting dysplastic lesion over many years. The progenitor lesion, known as cervical intraepithelial neoplasm (CIN), is commonly associated with Type II human papillomavirus (HPV) infection. In particular, certain subtypes (16, 18, 51, 52) of HPV are known to have the highest risk in inducing invasive squamous cell carcinoma [3]. Other less common etiologic factors include immunosuppression, cigarette smoking, and history of sexually transmitted disease. CIN is potentially reversible and the period of transition to invasive carcinoma is unknown and may take up to 20 years [1]. This time window permits early detection and allows for curative therapy. The majority (roughly 80%) of cervical cancer is squamous cell carcinoma originating at the squamocolumnar junction. Adenocarcinoma, which accounts for 10–20% of the cell types, arises from the endocervix and tends to grow endophytically, resulting in relatively late detection. Adenocarcinoma of the cervix is associated with poorer prognosis than squamous cell carcinoma at every stage. The remaining cell types include adenosquamous, mixed epithelial, neuroendocrine, and various sarcomatous subtypes. Small cell carcinoma of the neuroendocrine group disseminates rapidly and has the worst prognosis.

Prognosis and mode of treatment for cervical cancer are strongly dependent on the clinical stage. The 5-year survival for patients with cervical cancer is 90–95% for stage I, 50–70% for stage II, 30% for stage III, and <20% with stage IV [4]. Stage I disease, which is microscopic and diagnosed on cytology or colposcopy (IA), is treated by cone biopsy or simple hysterectomy. Stage I disease that is clinically detectable (IA) is treated by radical hysterectomy with pelvic lymph node dissection or external beam and intracavitary radiotherapy. For stage IIA disease, the patient is treated with external and intracavitary radiation therapy later followed by simple hysterectomy. Cervical cancer with locoregional extension (Stage III and IVA) is typically treated by combination radiotherapy and chemotherapy. Pelvic irradiation with or without extended

P. Shreve and D.W. Townsend (eds.), *Clinical PET-CT in Radiology: Integrated Imaging in Oncology*,
DOI 10.1007/978-0-387-48902-5_26,

field or neoadjuvant chemotherapy is reserved for advanced disease of the cervix (stage II and greater). Extended field irradiation including the paraaortic nodes has been found to improve survival by 31–50% [5]. No optimal therapeutic option has been agreed upon for adenocarcinoma. In cases of node positive and high-risk node-negative patients (e.g., large tumor volume), chemoradiation may replace combine radical surgery and post operative radiotherapy [6].

Role of PET-CT in Initial Diagnosis of Cervical Cancer

There is little place for imaging in establishing the diagnosis of cervical cancer. The diagnosis is based on histology on colposcopic biopsy. Cancer of the cervix is characterized by a long asymptomatic period before the disease becomes clinically evident, and is now often detected in its earliest stage on screening cytologic Pap smear followed by colposcopic biopsy.

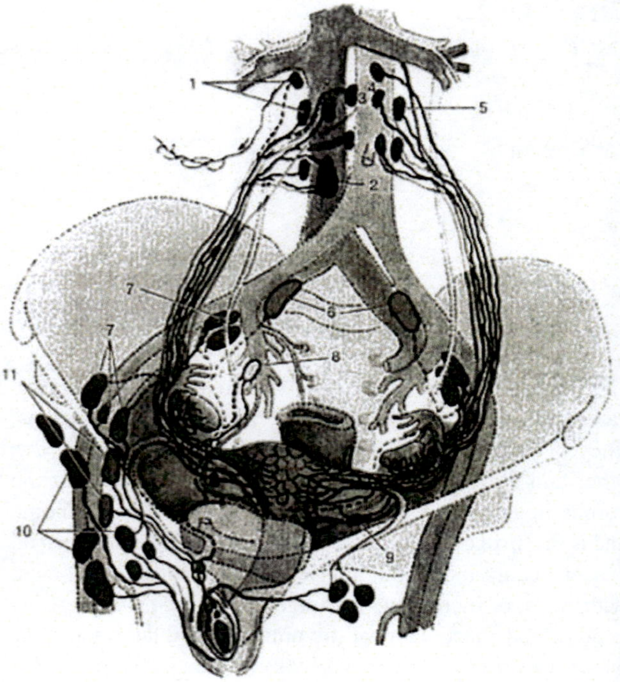

Fig. 26.1 Patterns of lymphatic spread of cervical cancer (From [7]. With permission). 1-5 paracaval, aortocaval and paraoortic nodes, 6 common iliac nodes, 7 eternal iliac nodes, 8 internal iliac nodes, 9 parauterine nodes, 10 superficial iliac nodes, 11 deep inguinal nodes

Staging of Cervical Cancer with PET-CT

Cervical cancer metastasizes in a predictable fashion. Direct extension occurs first laterally to the parametrium followed by anteroposterior extension and then later extension into the vagina and uterus. Lymphatic spread (Fig. 26.1) begins early in the disease in the following order: parametrial, obturator, internal iliac, external iliac, common iliac, lateral sacral, paraaortic, and finally mediastinal and supraclavicular nodes [8, 9]. It is uncommon to have extrapelvic disease without pelvic nodal metastases. The order of frequency for hematogenous dissemination, which is uncommon at initial diagnosis of cervical cancer, is lung, bones, brain, and liver. Peritoneal seeding is rare. The essence of staging is to be able to differentiate surgically treated disease (Stage I and IIA) from nonsurgical types (advanced lesion Stage IIB or greater).

Staging Method

The currently accepted staging method is that of the International Federation of Gynecology and Obstetrics (FIGO) rather than the TNM system. It comprises 4 stages (Table 26.1) based on clinical findings and historically used standard radiologic imaging. This has significant shortfalls, as inaccuracy occurs with clinical determination of tumor volume and localized pelvic involvement. Nodal status (the presence of lymph node metastases) is also not considered in the FIGO staging [1, 10]. Reported underestimation compared with surgical

Table 26.1 FIGO Staging of cervical carcinoma (From [1]. With permission of Elsevier)

Stage 0	Carcinoma in situ
Stage I	Carcinoma confines to the cervix. Extension into uterine corpus should be disregarded
Stage IA	Preclinical invasive carcinoma
Stage IA1	Stromal invasion not greater than 3mm deep and 7mm wide
Stage IA2	Stromal invasion 3-5mm deep and 7mm wide
Stage IB	Clinically detectable lesions confined to the cervix
Stage IB1	Tumor not greater than 4cm
Stage IB2	Tumor greater than 4cm
Stage II	Carcinoma extends beyond uterus. Excludes involvement of pelvic wall and lower third of the vagina
Stage IIA	No parametrial invasion
Stage IIB	Parametrial invasion
Stage III	Pelvic wall invasion and/or involvement of the lower third of the vagina and/or hydronephrosis or nonfunctioning kidney
Stage IIIA	Involvement of the lower third of the vagina
Stage IIIB	Pelvic wall extension and/or hydronephrosis or nonfunctioning kidney
Stage IV	Extension beyond the true pelvis and/or bladder or rectum invasion
Stage IVA	Bladder or rectal involvement
Stage IVB	Distant organs (extension beyond the true pelvis)

FIGO International Federation of Gynecology and Obstetrics

staging was 25% in stage I-IIA disease and increased to 65–90% in stages thereafter [11]. Surgical staging, while more accurate, could not be a routine replacement of purely clinical staging due to its invasiveness and high comorbidity, especially in those patients who subsequently receive radiotherapy. Surgical staging is also not cost-effective in early-stage cervical cancer patients in which only a small number of patients (10–20%) will have paraaortic disease requiring extended field of irradiation [1]. Modern imaging is becoming an effective tool providing the missing data between these two staging methods, and has become crucial to treatment planning as well as predicting response and disease-free interval.

Stage of Cervical Cancer and Prognosis

As noted above, the 5 year survival for patients with cervical cancer based on clinical staging is 90–95% for stage I, 50–70% for stage II, 30% for stage III and <20% with stage IV [4]. Some prognostic factors depicted on imaging that predict progression-free interval include primary tumor size and the presence and extent of lymph node metastases. Nodal involvement and location at the time of diagnosis, rather than nodal size or treatment related issues, are the most important variables determining the recurrence of the disease and death from cervical cancer [1, 12]. The 5-year disease-free survivals were 74–75% for those with negative nodes, 43–58% for those with microscopic nodal involvement, and 39–50% for those with macroscopic disease [13, 14]. However, those with common iliac nodal involvement did poorer than those with external or internal iliac nodes [1]. The survival rate with paraaortic nodal metastases is further reduced to about 30%, irrespective of the clinical stage and dismal with supraclavicular involvement [9]. The prevalence of paraaortic nodal spread at the time of diagnosis in Stage IIB-IVA patients can be as high as 24% [15]. Presence of inguinal or paraaortic nodal metastases although not classified by the FIGO system, is equivalent to a stage IVB [16]. The number of nodes involved was another outcome predictor and is inversely related to prognosis [1].

Another important prognosticator is tumor volume. Patients with larger primary tumor fare poorer than those with a smaller primary cervical mass both in terms of progression-free survival and overall survival [17]. However, tumor volume has no direct relationship to the presence of disease in lymph nodes, but extension of the primary cervical cancer into the uterine body is correlated with increased risk of lymph node metastases [6]. Stage IB of the FIGO staging system further subdivides a clinically-detected cancer confined to the cervix into IB1 for tumors <4 cm and IB2 for tumors >4 cm, reflecting the increased risk of more advanced disease and recurrence associated with large primary tumors. Approximately 35% of the invasive cervical carcinoma will have recurrent and persistent disease after treatment. This is associated with a 1-year survival rate of 10–15% and a 5 year survival rate of <5% [18].

PET-CT Findings in Staging of Cervical Cancer

In clinically stage I disease or tumor <2 cm, contribution from imaging (CT, PET, or MRI) to staging is of little value as the prevalence of extra-cervical spread is low [1, 19, 20]. For tumor >2 cm or when the lesion is endocervical in origin, MRI is the imaging modality of choice, although even MRI cannot reliably detect superficial stromal invasion (Stage IA).

Due to the low soft tissue contrast resolution of CT, small cervical cancer (<2 cm) cannot be detected, and accurate tumor volume cannot be obtained even in larger lesion. Primary cervical tumor visualization, when it is possible, appears merely either as cervical enlargement without any apparent lesion or just as a hypodense mass in noncontrast scans (Fig. 26.2a, b). Intravenous contrast enhancement improves delineation of cervical cancer (Fig. 26.2c), but the true size and extent of the neoplasm relative to normal uterine tissue is not truly depicted. Up to 50% of the stage IB primary cervical cancer mass can be isodense on CT and thus cannot be differentiated from the normal cervix or corpus [21]. Larger primary cervical cancer may appear as an irregular mass protruding into and/or obstructing the endocervical canal, producing endometrial cavity distension and fluid collection (Fig. 26.2d).

Since cervical cancer is typically associated with high levels of FDG tracer uptake (SUV values ranging from 4 to 15), the primary cervical cancer is more sensitively detected on the PET images than the CT images. The reported detection rate of Stage IB cervical cancer is 76% improving to 91–100% after reducing the spillover effect of urinary activity with postvoiding scan or bladder catheterization, in comparison to 58–88% with CT alone [22]. Primary cervical cancer lesions less than 1 cm in size are not sensitively detected by FDG PET [19]. Primary cervical cancer tumors with higher proliferative behavior tend to have higher levels of FDG tracer uptake, but this has not been shown to change the tumor staging [22]. Tumor volume itself does have predictive value for disease-free interval and has been estimated by either visual assessment [10] or with the help of special computer software [17].

The hallmark of stage II disease is parametrial invasion from the primary cervical mass. Parametrial invasion is depicted on CT images as an irregular or blurred cervical margin, parametrial soft tissue stranding, obliterated periureteral fat planes, or as an eccentric parametrial mass (Fig. 26.3). Parametrial stranding is a nonspecific CT sign, as it is more

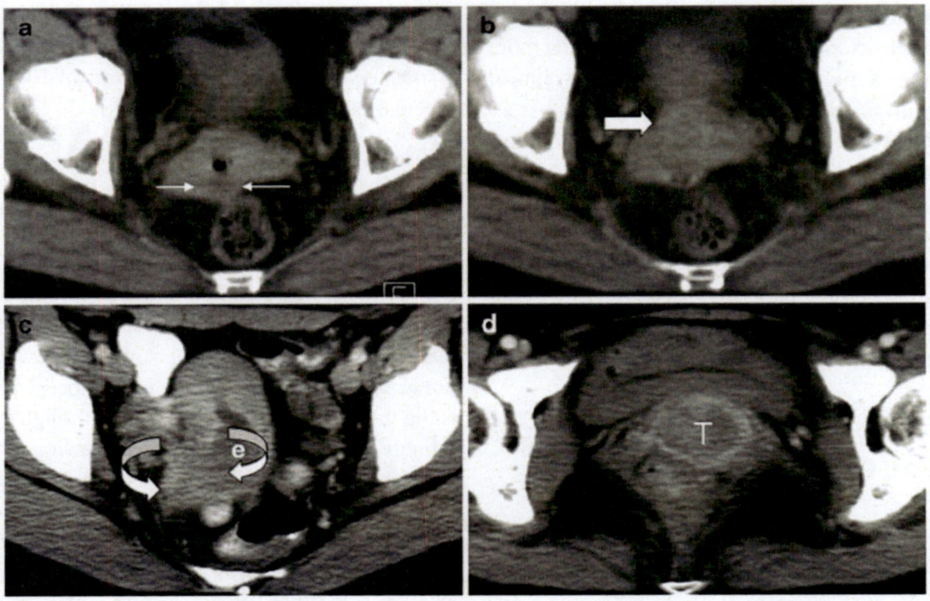

Fig. 26.2 Different appearances of cervical carcinoma on computed tomography. On the noncontrast images, it can appear as a small faint low density mass (*white arrows* in **a**) or as isodense focal enlargement (*white block* arrow in **b**). In the post contrast images, it is either hypodense relative to the enhancing myometrium (*curved arrows* in **c**) or as a ring enhancing hypodense larger mass (*T* in **d**). In **c**, the tumor is producing endometrial canal obstruction (*e*)

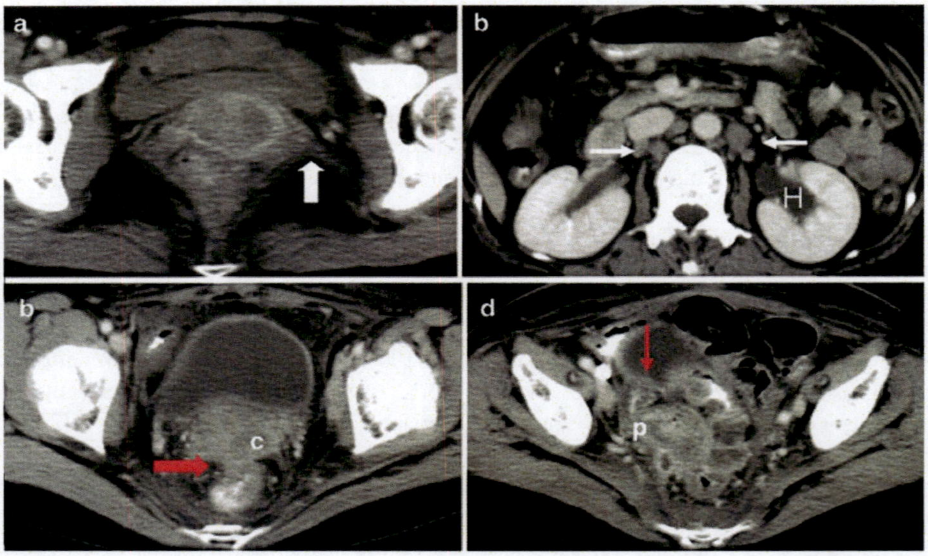

Fig. 26.3 Cervical carcinoma Stage II, IIIB & IV. Contrast-enhanced computed tomography image (**a**) shows large heterogeneous cervical mass with left cervical margin blurring indicative of parametrial extension (*white block arrow*). Image (**b**) demonstrates left sided hydronephrosis (*H*) and retroperitoneal nodes (*white arrows*). Image (**c**) shows hypodense cervical carcinoma (*c*) invading rectum (*red block arrow*) and (**d**) bladder (*red arrow*). There is right pelvic side wall (*p*) extension (**d**)

often due to parametritis. The FDG PET images have little role in the imaging diagnosis of parametrial invasion, although the more extensive the primary cervical cancer mass as delineated by the FDG PET images, the greater the concern for parametrial invasion.

Stage III disease is defined by pelvic side wall extension or involvement of the lower third of the vagina. Pelvic side wall invasion is evident on CT images by tumor extension within 3 mm of the pelvic sidewalls, enlargement of the obturator or piriformis muscles, and encasement of the iliac vessels. The

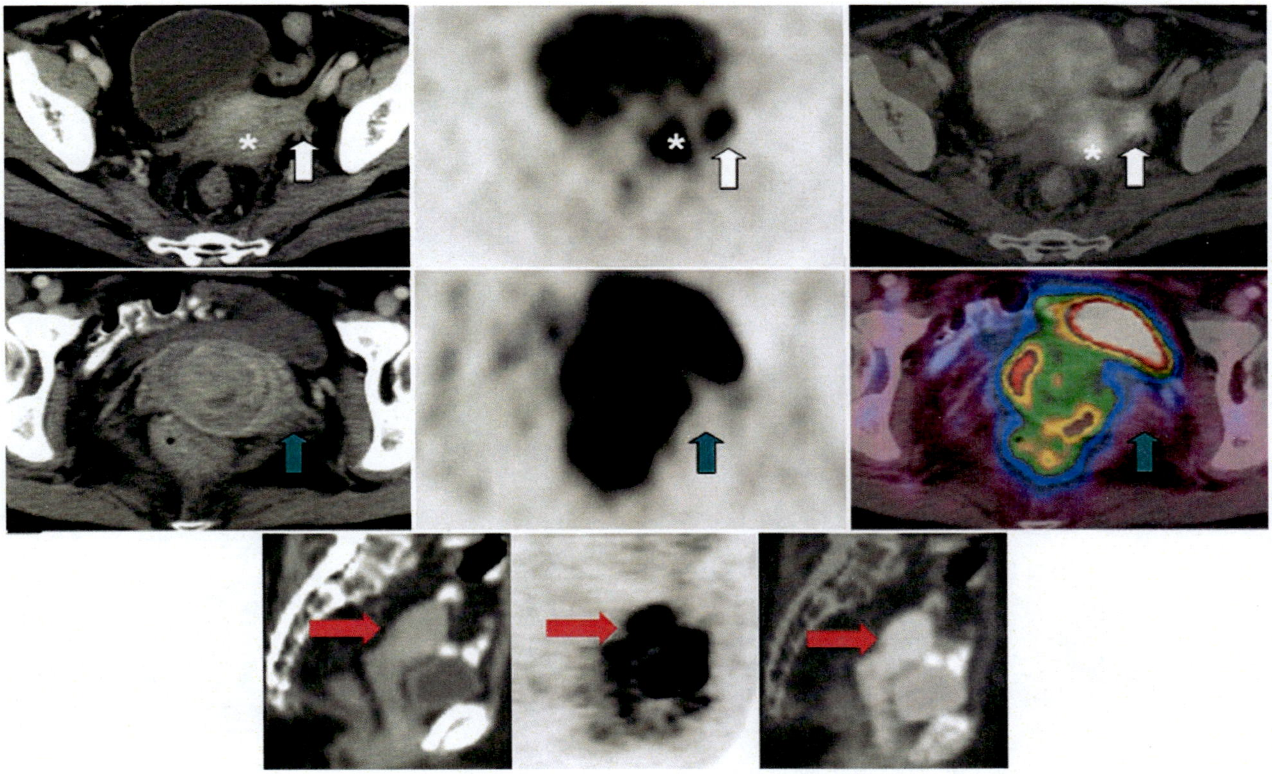

Fig. 26.4 Value of PET-CT in staging of cervical cancer. The cervical carcinoma (*) is not well seen on the CT but visualized on the PET and fusion images (*top row*), enabling PET-CT to obtain reliable multiplanar tumor volume assessment. Presence of an eccentric hypermetabolic left parametrial mass (*white block arrows*) indicates parametrial invasion. The middle row of images shows blurring of left parametrial soft tissue plane on CT but not on PET or fusion images (*green block arrows*), which was confirmed in surgery to be due to parametritis and not neoplastic spread. Uterine extension by the cervical tumor is best appreciated on the sagittal PET-CT images (*pink block arrow in bottom row*)

FDG PET images are valuable in identifying the soft tissue that is truly neoplasm, particularly cancer invasion of the muscles, and confirming subtle soft tissue encasement of iliac vessels (Fig. 26.4). Ureteric obstruction secondary to local tumor extension producing hydroureter and hydronephrosis can be reliably identified on the CT images (and by persistent tracer in the upper urinary tract on PET images), and the site of tumor ureteral encasement localized by the presence of abnormal FDG tracer uptake on the PET images (see Fig. 26.3b).

Stage IV disease involves bladder or rectal invasion (IVA) and distant metastatic disease (IVB). Rectal and bladder invasion are depicted on the CT images either as loss of fat planes, irregular wall thickening, or tumor replacement (see Fig. 26.3c). Early or minimal involvement of the bladder or rectal walls by cervical cancer is difficult to determine on CT due to limitations of contrast resolution and not seen on FDG PET images due to spatial resolution limitations of PET. MRI is consequently superior to PET-CT in detecting very early contiguous invasion of the bladder wall and rectal wall.

PET-CT is particularly well suited for the detection of distant metastatic disease of cervical cancer, including to the lung where CT will be more sensitive for very small pulmonary nodules, and to the visceral organs and bone where FDG PET will generally be more sensitive for small metastatic deposits (Figs. 26.5 and 26.6). Another recognized strength is in localizing distant metastases. On reviewing the literature [21–27], the whole body imaging allows identification of extrapelvic disease, including distant sites such as the supraclavicular fossa, bone, lung, or liver. PET-CT has achieved a sensitivity, specificity, positive predictive value (PPV), and negative predictive value (NPV) of 100%, 94%, 63%, and 100%, respectively, for uncovering distant secondaries [15]. Histologic verification should be obtained with PET-CT-positive extrauterine site especially if it is a solitary focus, as a second unrelated pathology may coexist. This is particularly important in lung and liver, irrespective of the SUV level, as tuberculosis and hepatocellular carcinoma in endemic areas may simulate metastases. PET-CT in this setting can give an accurate anatomic and metabolic road mapping to the biopsy site as well as for radiotherapy planning.

As noted above, lymph node metastasis status has important prognostic significance, but nodal status is not included in the FIGO staging. A major usefulness of PET-CT in the staging of cervical cancer lies in determining noninvasively

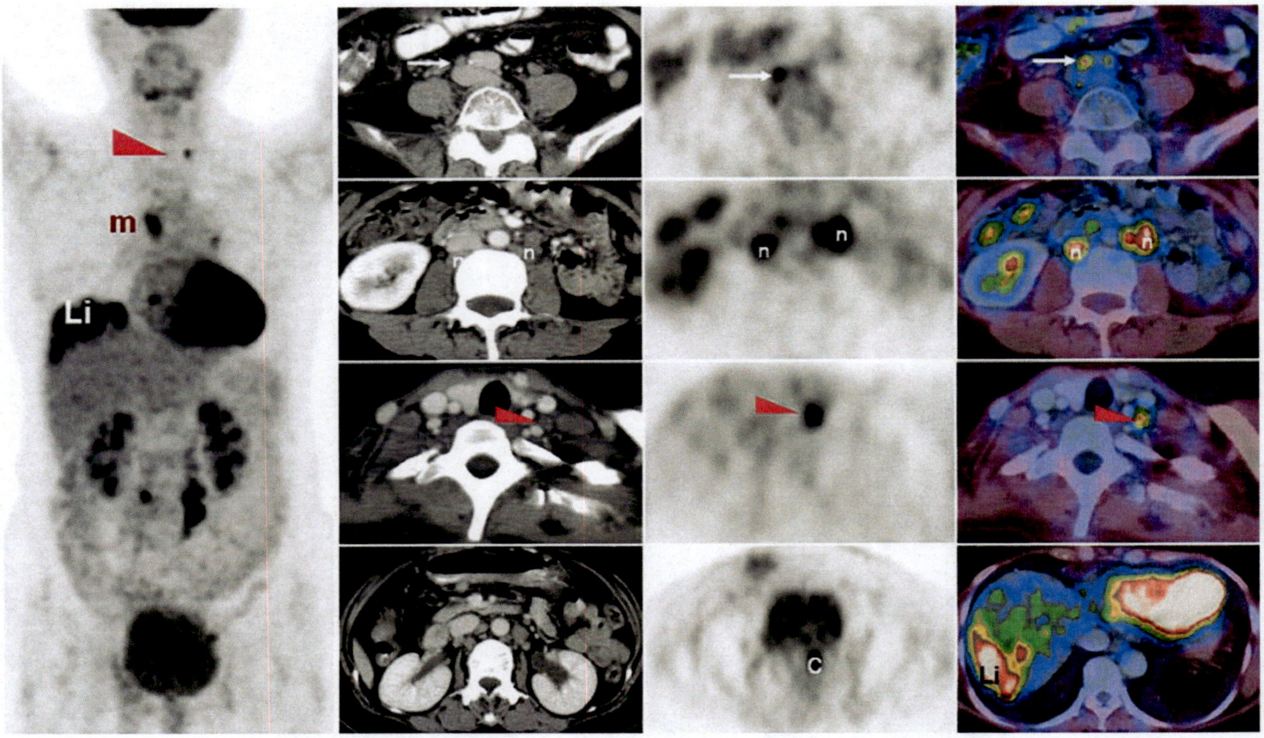

Fig. 26.5 Stage IV carcinoma of cervix (*c*). There are hypermetabolic metastases to retroperitoneal (*n*), mediastinal (*m*), common iliac (*white arrow*) and left supraclavicular fossa lymph nodes and liver secondaries (*Li*). The left supraclavicular node (*red arrowhead*) is 8 mm in size, which is not pathologic by CT criteria but hypermetabolic on PET confirming metastatic involvement (*third row of axial images*). Similarly the PET-CT image revealed an abnormal right common iliac node (*white arrow*), which is 6mm size and would not have been regarded as a true pathology by CT alone

the lymph node metastasis status in patients clinically diagnosed with cervical cancer (stage Ib and higher). The CT criteria for pathologic nodes are lymph node >1 cm or nodes with central low density necrosis. The latter finding has higher specificity for neoplastic involvement [1]. Metastatic nodal detection on CT has a reported sensitivity of 44%, specificity of 93% and an accuracy of 70–80% [1]. FDG PET alone is significantly superior to CT alone for nodal staging of cervical cancer, with an average sensitivity of 89%, specificity of 95% and accuracy of 93% (21–26). The much greater sensitivity of FDG PET reflects the detection of macroscopic metastases in nonenlarged lymph nodes. Failed nodal metastatic detection in FDG PET occurs with microscopic disease and macroscopic tumor volume less than 5 mm [19]. Current literatures have shown comparable superior results of PET-CT in nodal evaluation over conventional imaging. PET-CT achieved better detection rate for metastatic paraaortic node than pelvic nodes. The sensitivity, specificity, PPV, and NPV for pelvic nodes involvement were 75%, 96%, 75% and 96%, respectively. They were 100%, 99%, 94%, and 100% for paraaortic nodes [15]. The high detection rate of neoplastic paraaortic node appeared to be consistent and well supported [15, 28–30]. This has great clinical importance, as presence of paraaortic nodal metastases affects the extent of the radiation field as well as prognosis. Such treatment strategy modification was noted in 25% of patient in one series [31]. Compared with PET, PET-CT appeared to be even more sensitive as it could locate metastatic nodes with tumor volume under 5 mm [32].

Due to the greater sensitivity of FDG PET in detection of lymph node metastases over the size criteria of CT, the size criteria on CT need not be strictly adhered to; lymph nodes in the expected distribution of cervical cancer metastases associated with abnormal FDG tracer uptake should be considered suspicious for metastatic involvement. Since central low density is a specific finding for lymph node metastases of cervical cancer, careful review of the CT images, especially with attention to lymph nodes in the obturator, internal iliac, external iliac, common iliac, lateral sacral, paraaortic, and mediastinal and supraclavicular node basins and chains is important, as necrotic lymph nodes may not be highly FDG avid due to the relative volume of the necrotic tumor within the lymph node.

Abnormal FDG tracer uptake in lymph nodes can be due to inflammation or benign tumor (i.e., histiocytosis), and in certain lymph node groups, specifically neck, mediastinum and hila, axillary and inguinal, there is a significant false positive rate on FDG PET associated with lymph nodes in these locations [15, 33]. With the exception of mediastinum,

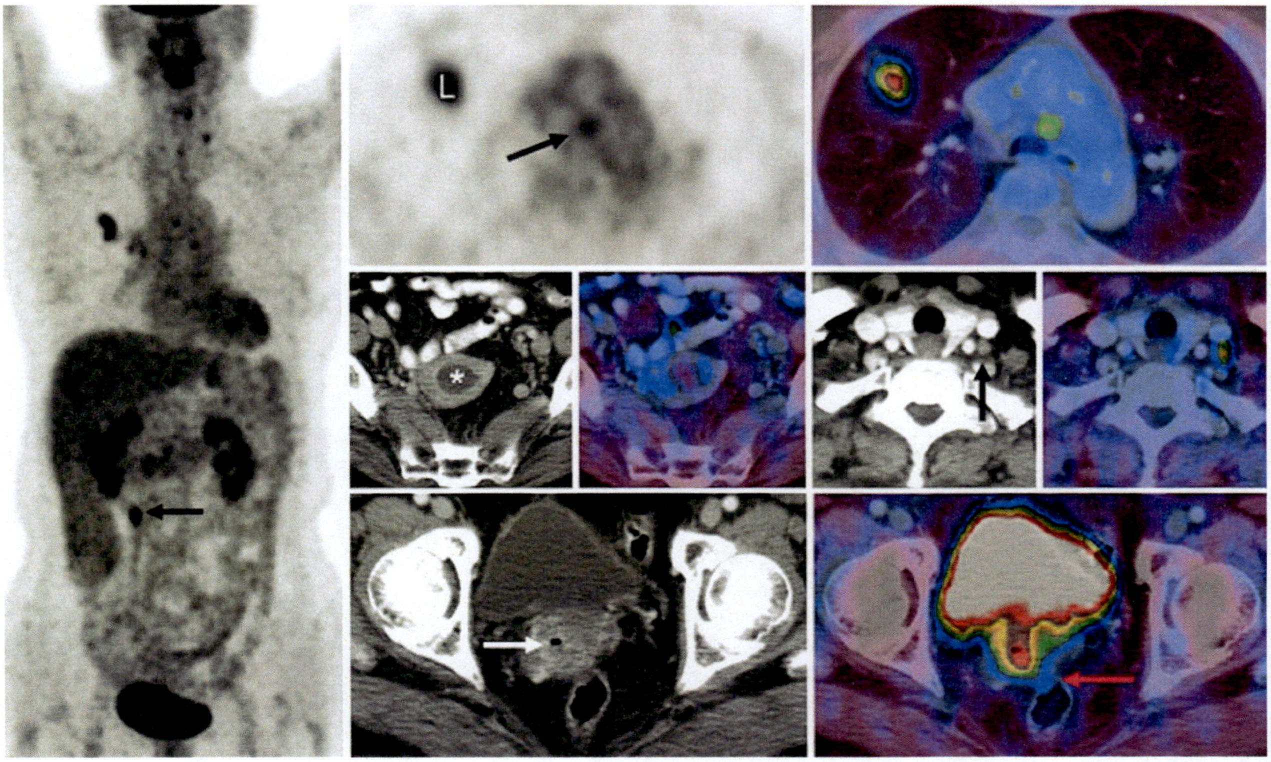

Fig. 26.6 Small cell carcinoma of the cervix stage IV. This is a highly malignant tumor, which disseminates early and does not conform to the normal metastatic pathways. The cervical cancer is infected as evident by the air bubble (*white arrow*). It is obstructing the endometrial canal, producing cavity distension (* in). There is an invasion into the rectum (*red arrow*), despite small size of the tumor and no pelvic side wall extension. Nodal metastases occur at para-aortic area, mediastinum and supraclavicular fossa (*black arrows*). Right lung secondary is also present (*L*)

these nodal groups are not in the expected and typical pattern of metastases of cervical cancer, and hence positive findings on FDG PET and/or enlargement on CT should be approached with caution. Mediastinal lymph node metastases in the absence of pelvic lymph node metastases are rare in cervical cancer. Isolated paraaortic lymph nodes positive on PET-CT imaging may warrant fine needle aspiration biopsy when there is borderline abnormal FDG tracer uptake or enlargement with equivocal or absent FDG tracer uptake if the lymph node metastasis would change the extent of radiation field. Addition of a 3 hour delayed PET scan has been reported to be helpful in differentiating inflammatory from metastatic para-aortic nodes when staging cervical cancer [34].

Pitfalls and Selected Issues in Performing and Reporting PET-CT In Patients with Cervical Carcinoma

The registered and aligned CT and PET images routinely generated by PET-CT scanners greatly facilitates interpretation of the PET findings in general and specifically in the pelvis, where physiologic tracer activity in bowel, the urinary tract and uterus and ovaries can be confounding if not properly identified with the corresponding anatomic structures. Since local staging of cervical cancer involves delineating the local extension of the cervical cancer and is largely defined by CT findings, CT technique should be fully optimized for imaging of pelvic structures. Use of both oral and intravenous contrast material improves delineation of pelvic structures and facilitates interpretation of local invasion. Thin section technique with slice thickness of 5 mm or less is preferred. On the PET images, urinary tracer activity in the bladder results in image degradation due to increased scatter from the intense bladder tracer activity, and methods to reduce urinary tracer activity can improved overall quality of the reconstructed PET images of the pelvis. Since cervical cancer frequently occurs in premenopausal women, physiologic FDG tracer uptake in ovaries and endometrium can be seen, and menstrual status of patients at the time of scanning should be known.

Necrosis in lymph nodes is highly suggestive of metastatic cervical cancer but may result in reduced FDG uptake in the PET images (Fig. 26.7a). When there is a large tumor mass obstructing the endometrial canal, infection is common and may produce FDG avid endometritis simulating parametrial invasion (Fig. 26.7c). Small lung metastases (<6 mm) of cervical cancer may not be detected on FDG PET images,

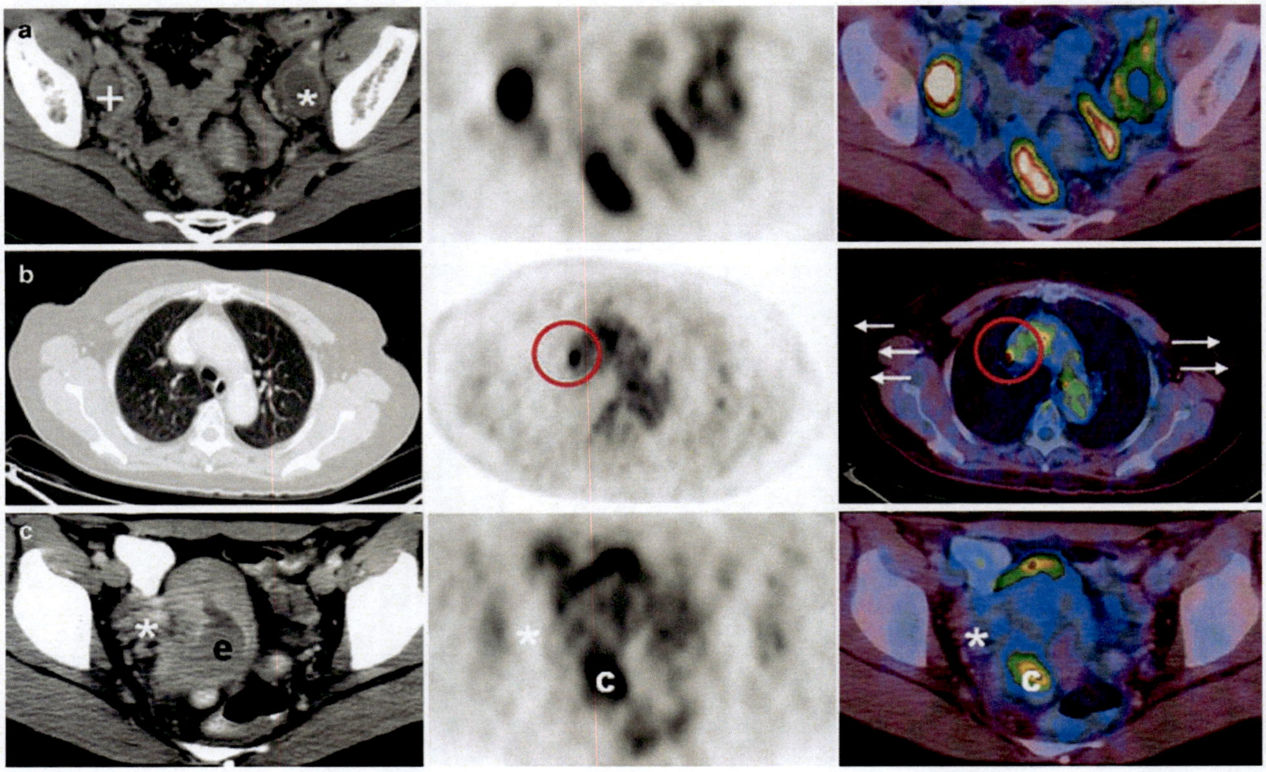

Fig. 26.7 Pitfalls in PET-CT. The left external iliac node (* in **a**) shows central necrosis, which is highly specific for malignant involvement but it can decrease the overall FDG uptake of the node. The left external iliac node has a SUV max of 3, while the nonnecrotic node (+) has a SUV max of 12. The lung secondary (*pink circle*) on CT (**a**) appears on PET (**b**) and fusion PET-CT (**c**) to resemble a mediastinal node. The clue to this is due to the patient's movement to the side during the PET acquisition. This is demonstrated by the *white arrows* along the skin lines of this patient. They do not superimpose exactly between the PET and CT images (**c**). Contrast enhanced CT demonstrated a hypometabolic right parametrial mass (*white * in bottom row*) associated with endometrial canal obstruction by the tumor (**c**).This is subsequently confirmed to be an inflammatory mass in surgery

but a pulmonary nodule evident on the CT images will be seen (Fig. 26.7b). Small cell carcinoma of the cervix is highly malignant and disseminates more rapidly and in a less predictable pattern than other cervical cancer on presentation (Fig. 26.6). It is unusual to have skipped nodal or atypical site involvement during first presentation e.g., axillary or supraclavicular lymph node without paraaortic disease. The chance of a reactive node is higher in these cases, except in the case of small cell.

The PET-CT report of a patient with new diagnosis of cervical cancer should include the following:

- Primary tumor morphology including sizes of the tumor or in the case of nonvisualization, the functional size and a qualitative or semiquantitative assessment of FDG tracer uptake. This is important as a baseline value for follow-up study posttreatment
- Presence of endometrial or ureteric obstruction
- Local extension of the primary tumor: parametrial, uterine, pelvic sidewall, rectal, or bladder
- Lymph node status: location of FDG PET positive lymph nodes, size of enlarged and FDG PET positive nodes, and presence of central necrosis in lymph nodes. Specific level of positive or suspicious paraaortic lymph nodes is important for management decision to include radiation field to the paraaortic region
- Presence and location of any distant metastases

Restaging Cervical Cancer with PET-CT

Treatment failure occurs commonly within the first 2 years for carcinoma of the cervix [1]. Relapse of cervical cancer can develop locally or distantly, or both, with no predictable pattern. Failed local control by the above mentioned management equates poor salvage rate and reduced long-term survival. This tends to occur in patients with larger tumor volume and nodal metastases at the time of diagnosis. Studies have shown that aggressive initial therapy with combined modalities produced a survival advantage in these groups with cervical cancer [35].

In cervical cancer, FDG PET is a reliable restaging tool with an average sensitivity and specificity of 89% and an accuracy of 93% in detecting recurrence (10, 24, 25, 35). It had already been shown to have impact on survival, altering management decisions in nearly two thirds of cases with relapses [36]. FDG PET-CT through better anatomical localization and metabolic characterization of the PET findings had displayed similar result with a sensitivity of 90%, a specificity of 81%, and accuracy of 86.5% [37]. Similarly, the therapeutic choice between curative intent and palliation (i.e., from surgery + radiation to chemotherapy + radiation) can be made more effectively by precisely localizing the sites of dissemination to above or below the diaphragm on the PET-CT. This had lead to treatment modification in 23% of patients in one series [37]. This lower clinical influence compared with PET was attributed to the small numbers in the study.

In asymptomatic patients with raised SCC-Ag level, PET can detect relapse with a sensitivity of 97.5% and an accuracy of 94%. This ability had been incorporated into a proposed prognostic scoring system to determine which groups of patient would benefit from follow up FDG PET. It is found that the presence of clinical symptoms; elevated SCC-Ag (>4 ng/mL) and primary radiation treatment correlate with poorer survival and earlier surveillance with FDG PET, and hence PET-CT may help in this high-risk group of patients with cervical cancer to reduce mortality rate and to avoid unnecessary salvage therapy [36].

Despite such knowledge and general agreement that vigilant screening is necessary for high risk patients during those periods, no standardized follow-up protocol has been currently formed. Serum tumor marker such as squamous cell carcinoma antigen (SCC-Ag) for cervical cancer is a sensitive and specific indicator for recurrence, which may be positive up to 6 months preceding clinical and radiologic evidence of recurrence of the cervical cancer. SCC-Ag can also be elevated in benign gynecologic or non- gynecologic diseases, which reduces the specificity of this tumor marker [38]. Physical examination, CT, or MRI cannot differentiate pelvic soft tissue thickening as a result of surgery or radiation therapy form recurrent neoplasm.

Pitfalls and Selected Issues in Performing and Reporting PET-CT in Restaging Patients with Uterine Cancer

With the advent of PET-CT, the above-noted limitations of physical exam and purely morphologic imaging can be overcome, since recurrent or metastatic cervical FDG avid PET can reliably distinguish posttreatment scarring from recurrence (Fig. 26.8), in addition to localizing extrapelvic metastases. Since the relapse of cervical cancer does not conform to the initial pattern of spread, with recurrence occurring at distant or atypical sites or combination of local and distant involvement, PET-CT is particularly helpful in assessing the overall disease status. Unlike the pattern of spread of primary cervical cancer where hematogenous route metastases to the lungs, skeleton, brain, and liver are uncommon, in the setting of recurrent cervical cancer these routes of metastatic spread are important

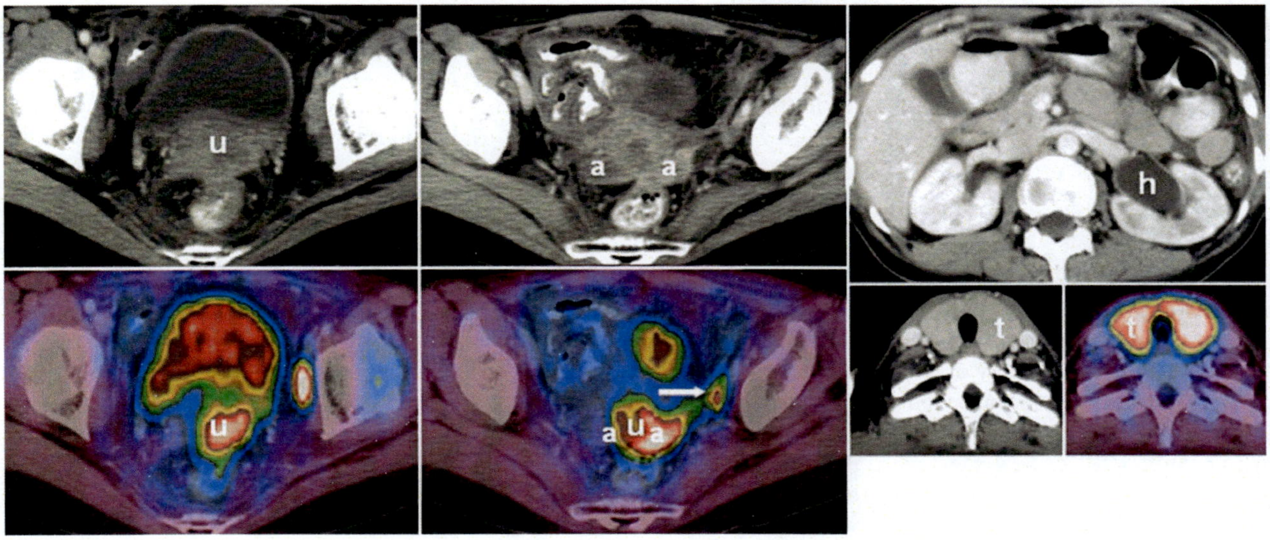

Fig. 26.8 Patient had been treated with chemoradiation for carcinoma of cervix with pelvic nodal metastases 12 months ago. There is evidence of local relapse with involvement of the uterus (*u*), both adnexae (*a*), left obturator node (*white arrow*), and left ureter resulting in hydronephrosis (*h*). Incidental finding of metabolically active goiter most likely thyroiditis (*t*)

and can be key findings on PET-CT. Brain metastases are best assessed on contrast enhanced MRI or CT.

The ovaries are often not removed for treatment of cervical cancer. They are frequently transposed outside the pelvis to avoid damage from radiotherapy. Physiologic FDG tracer uptake due to abscess, fistula, or complication of radiation therapy such as proctitis, enteritis, cystitis, and osteonecrosis may simulate tumor recurrence. In order to assess treatment response or recurrence more reliably, a baseline staging PET-CT should be carried out prior to surgery or radiotherapy. Although the optimal time to perform imaging as a followup has not been established, persistent disease at 3 months is associated with a poorer long-term survival, and hence the PET-CT may be appropriate at this time. Similar uptake time and dosage of FDG should be given between the initial and follow-up scans to ensure a fair comparison between the two series of PET-CT if SUV level is used as a guide. It is also important to use the same type of PET image acquisition and reconstruction parameters between the 2 scans [37].

PET-CT Reports for restaging cervical cancer should include the following:

- Surgical site evaluation should include the description of the presence of residual mass or abnormal FDG tracer uptake, anatomical sizes of the residual tumor (in the case of nonvisualization on CT), the functional size and degree of FDG tracer uptake, and comparison of the size and degree of FDG tracer uptake with the prior scan
- Any resolution of hydronephrosis or hydroureter
- Lymph node status: abnormal tracer uptake and comparison of the size and degree of FDG tracer uptake with the prior PET-CT scan(s)
- Status of distant metastases, change in comparison to prior scan

Cervical Cancer Therapy Monitoring with PET-CT

Currently there is no study demonstrating the value of PET-CT in assessing cervical cancer treatment response. Anatomic imaging alone had not been accurate enough since morphologic change often lags behind metabolic ones and distinction between fibrosis and persistent/residual disease is difficult. FDG PET not only overcomes these issues, it also allows survival prediction in the following manner. Persistent FDG tracer uptake in the primary tumor or metastatic sites (particularly SCF) or new sites after radiotherapy indicate poor outcome [39]. Persistent cervical disease at 3 months posttreatment is another bad sign [40]. Patients with no metabolically active tumor detected post treatment had a 5 year progression-free survival rate of 92%. This drops to 46% for those with partial response (residual abnormal uptake at one or more sites). No patients with persistent disease in SCF nodes lived beyond 3.5 months. Those who developed new disease did not live to 2 years [40]. With FDG PET-CT, patients with a negative follow-up study had been found to have a better 2 year disease-free interval than those with positive findings [37]. Example of usage of PET-CT in evaluating treatment response is shown in Fig. 26.9.

Potential erroneous interpretation and survival prediction by PET can occur as FDG uptake increases in both dying and treated tumors and radiation induced inflammatory process might last up to 6 months [41]. The complimentary information offered by CT acquired as part of PET-CT might help in this dilemma. The useful clues to determine if the increased FDG uptake is spurious are increasing necrosis and decreasing sizes of the treated area.

The optimal time to perform a post treatment surveillance PET-CT scan had not been defined. Also, there is no currently published literature using PET or PET-CT to assess therapy response post chemotherapy in cervical cancers as chemotherapy is rarely used alone.

Role of PET-CT in Radiotherpy Planning

No large series has been reported for RT planning for cervical cancer using PET-CT. The extent of pelvic and retroperitoneal lymph node metastases detected on PET-CT noninvasively may be of considerable value for planning the extent of radiation therapy in patients both on initial diagnosis and at relapse for salvage. It has been demonstrated that tumor volume of primary cervical cancer and 3D functional information can be reliably obtained from FDG PET [10, 17]. This allows accurate spatial orientation of the tumor as well as better delineation of the degree of spread between of spread between the tumor and bladder as well as the rectum. Such information had been used to guide placement of the tandem and ovoid applicators in brachytherapy for cervical carcinoma [42]. This may be useful for subsequent brachytherapy planning as tumor size is expected to be smaller. A boost dose can be adjusted accordingly with the information provided by PET-CT. PET-guided IMRT has been tried in extrapelvic involvement in cervical cancer which allows dose escalation to the para-aortic bed permitting minimal dose to the surrounding critical structures [37].

Cancer of the Uterine Corpus

Cancer of the uterine corpus is essentially endometrial carcinoma and is the most common gynecologic cancer [1]. Endometrial cancer occurs later in life, with 75% of the cases developed in the postmenopausal period [44]. There are

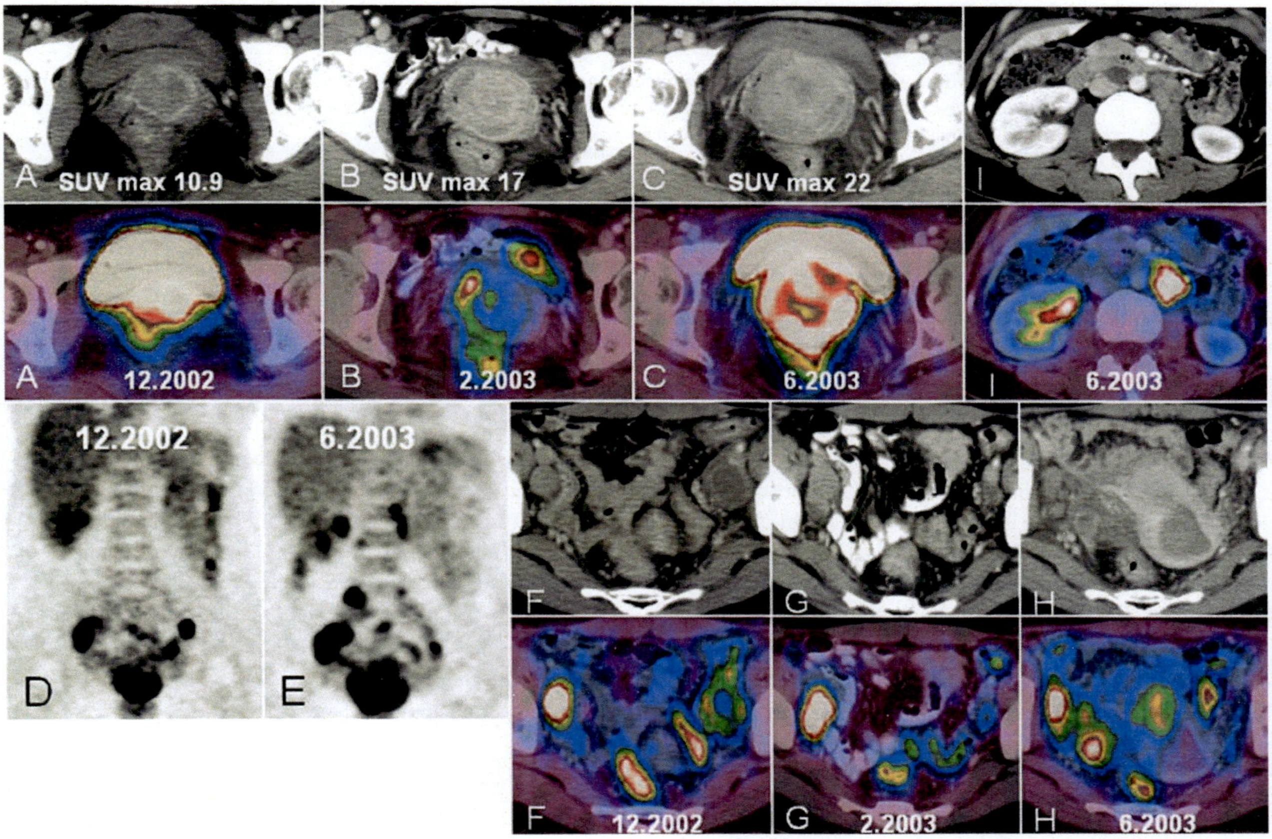

Fig. 26.9 Carcinoma of cervix pre- and post-treatment PET-CT (**d-e**). The primary tumor has shown both size and metabolic activity increases over 6 months (**a–c**) in keeping with disease progression. The pelvic nodes are showing mixed response (**f–h**) with left side nodes showing decreasing size and glycolysis. The right pelvic nodes are getting more numerous. Paraaortic nodes developed in the last scan (**e, i**)

many etiologic factors but the etiology of endometrial cancer is broadly divided into 2 groups. Type I endometrial cancer is more common, and occurs in middle age women between 40 to 60. The precursor is atypical hyperplasia, which is related to unopposed estrogen stimulation. It tends to be a low grade and nonmyoinvasive carrying a favorable response after curative surgery. Most of these tumors are additionally estrogen or progesterone receptor (ER/PR) positive allowing opportunity for anti-hormonal therapy. Type II endometrial develops de novo in the context of endometrial atrophy and tends to be high grade with poorer outcome. It affects older women and is associated with diabetes, hypertension, obesity, infertility, low parity, Stein-Leventhal syndrome, gonadal dysgenesis, tamoxifen exposure, and pelvic radiation [3].

Nearly 90% of uterine cancer is adenocarcinoma with the endometrioid type predominates. The clear cell and papillary serous type are the most aggressive and with the worst prognosis [1]. Sarcoma, primary uterine lymphoma, and metastases account for a minor portion of the corpus cancers.

The majority of endometrial carcinoma (74%) remains confined to the uterine corpus and is consequently more amendable to surgical treatment than cervical cancer. The prognosis for endometrial carcinoma depends on the FIGO staging (see below and Table 26.2), depth of myometrial invasion and histologic grade (in order of importance). Peritoneal involvement is associated with higher recurrence rate [44]. The 5 year survival for uterine cancer is 89% for stage I disease, 80% for stage II, 30% for stage III and 9% in stage IV [3]. These figures deteriorated further with increasing tumor histologic grade. Uterine sarcoma, with the majority being leiomyosarcoma, has poorer prognosis with a 5 year survival rate of 15–25% [3]. The size in leiomyosarcoma has prognostic value with >5 cm associated with poorer survival [44].

Hysterectomy is the mainstay of management of uterine cancer as this provides both the means of staging and initial treatment. Additional therapy or option employed would depend on extent of disease, risk of recurrence and medical status of the patient. For stage IA disease, patient receives total hysterectomy and bilateral salpingo-oophorectomy (TAHBSO). Hormonal therapy is an alternative if there is a higher risk of perioperative morbidity. Radical surgery carrying more serious complication is reserved for advanced cancer and in those with

Table 26.2 FIGO Staging of endometrial carcinoma (From [1]. With permission of Elsevier)

Stage 0	Carcinoma in situ
Stage IA	Confined to uterine corpus and limited to the endometrium
Stage IB	Confined to uterine corpus with invasion to less than one half of myometrium
Stage IC	Confined to uterine corpus with invasion to more than one half of myometrium
Stage IIA	Involves corpus and endocervical gland
Stage IIB	Involves corpus with cervical stroma invasion
Stage IIIA	Tumor extension beyond the uterus but confines to the true pelvis; has invasion of the uterine serosa, adnexa, and/or positive peritoneal cytology
Stage IIIB	Extends outside the uterus but confined to the true pelvis with invasion of the vagina (direct or metastasis)
Stage IIIC	Extends outside the uterus but confined to the true pelvis; regional lymph node metastases
Stage IVA	Extension beyond the true pelvis and/or bladder or rectal involvement
Stage IVB	Distant metastases including abdominal or inguinal lymph nodes

FIGO International Federation of Gynecology and Obstetrics

high risk of relapse. Thus in stage IB, additional pelvic nodal sampling is required and in stage IC radical lymph nodal resection [16]. Stage II disease is treated with radical hysterectomy, pelvic lymphadenectomy, and aortic nodal dissection followed by radiotherapy (external or intravaginal), except when the cervix is involved. In such case, radiotherapy is carried out prior to surgery. Patients with stage III and IV endometrial carcinoma receive primary pelvic radiation followed by residual tumor removal if resectable. Additional extended-field radiation therapy and/or concurrent chemotherapy or antiestrogen therapy are used to treat extrapelvic metastases. Imaging plays an important role in striking a balance between undertreating resulting in relapse and over treatment causing significant morbidity and mortality.

Role of PET-CT in the Diagnosis of Uterine Cancer

The majority of the endometrial carcinoma is symptomatic on presentation (bleeding) and easily confirmed with endometrial biopsy, rendering imaging for diagnosis unnecessary. In asymptomatic and marginally symptomatic patients, endovaginal ultrasound has led to earlier diagnosis, although abnormal sonographic findings are followed by endometrial biopsy. Uterine cancer can, however, present atypically as a widespread malignancy from tumor of unknown origin. PET-CT may be useful to identify the culprit, gynecologic cancer (Fig. 26.10).

Staging Uterine Cancer with PET-CT

Carcinoma of the endometrium tends to arise from the upper uterine body and spreads by direct extension. It first extends into the endometrial cavity and later the myometrium. In a more advanced stage, it spreads to the cervix, vagina, parametrium, and other pelvic organs. Unlike carcinoma of the cervix, lymphatic spread is variable due to multiple drainage routes. Uterine cancer can spread to inguinal, internal iliac, or high paraaortic areas without any order of preference [1]. Hematogenous spread occurs to lung, liver, brain, and bone.

Staging Method

Since initial treatment of uterine caner almost always involves hysterectomy, staging of uterine cancer is based on surgical and histologic findings (see Table 26.2), as developed by the International Federation of Gynecology and Obstetrics (FIGO), rather than TNM staging method. The FIGO system relies on evaluation of the hysterectomy specimen and interoperative findings and biopsies to assess the extent of uterine and pelvic spread. The extent of myometrial invasion is an important prognostic factor. Locoregional and or paraaortic nodal spread increases from 3% in superficial myometrial invasion to 46% with deeper myometrium involved. Conventional macroscopic inspection of surgical specimen and frozen section analysis intraoperatively are found to be inaccurate in a significant proportion of patients [16].

The degree of nuclear atypia and tissue growth pattern give an additional three grades of stratification, with the lower score representing the most well differentiated and best prognosis [3]. Extension of tumor beyond the uterus (stage III) is determined at time of surgical exploration. Lymph node status is likewise determined at time of surgery for both pelvic nodes (stage IIIC), and as required for retroperitoneal lymph nodes (stage IVB).

As noted above, prognosis for endometrial carcinoma is related to, in addition to stage, the depth of myometrial invasion and the histologic grade (in order of importance). The 5-year survival for uterine cancer is 89% for stage I disease, 80% for stage II, 30% for stage III, and 9% in stage IV [3]. These survival rates are further deteriorated with increasing tumor histologic grade.

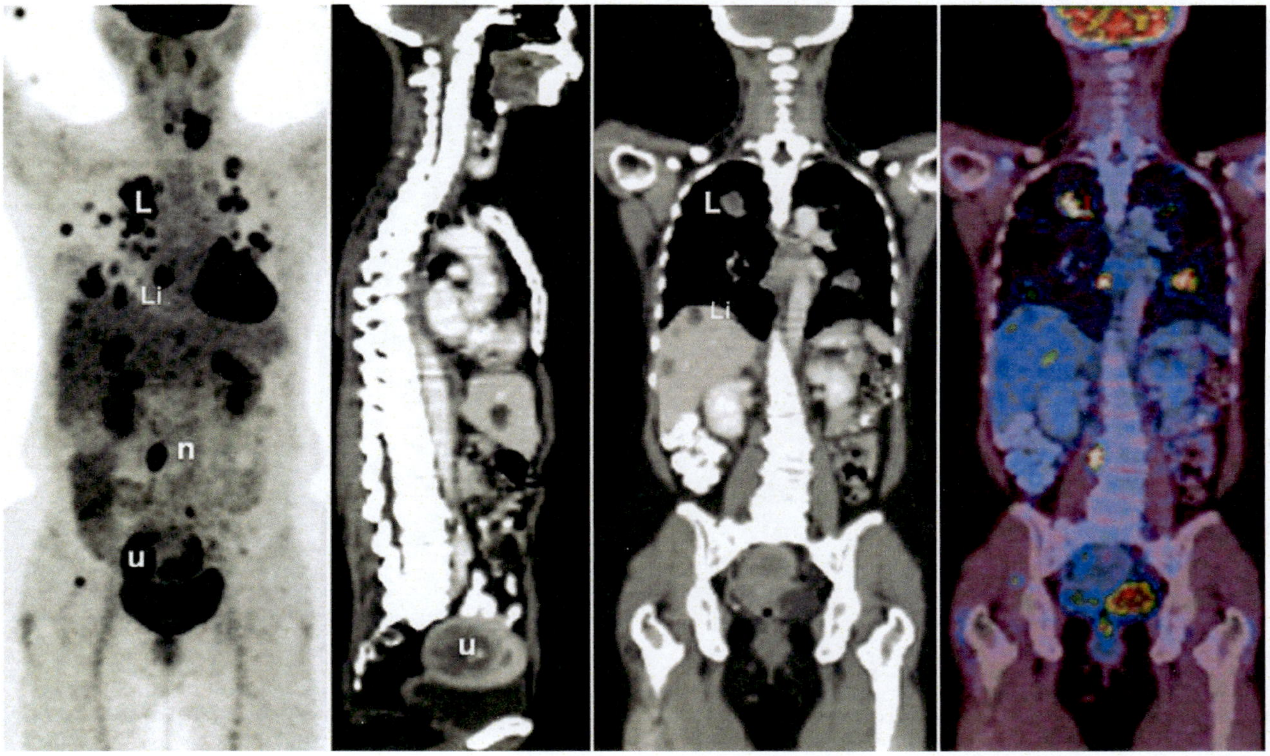

Fig. 26.10 Uterine sarcoma (*u*) presented with widespread dissemination to node (*n*), lung (*L*) and liver (*Li*) as cancer of unknown origin

PET-CT Findings in Staging Uterine Cancer

The role of PET-CT in the staging of endometrial carcinoma is primarily in the identification of metastasis to lymph node, peritoneum, and distant organs (stage III and IV).

Stage I and II

It is noteworthy that 75% of the endometrial carcinoma presents as stage I, which has a good outcome, and consequently there is typically little imaging workup prior to hysterectomy. This is supported in a study by Kim [45] when 53 patients with corpus cancer underwent MRI and PET-CT for staging prior to surgery. Both modalities showed similar results of moderate success for primary lesion detection. PET-CT only had a sensitivity of 89%, specificity of 50%, PPV of 93%, NPV of 37%, and accuracy of 85%. If imaging evaluation of tumor size, cervical and myometrial invasion is required prior to hysterectomy, this is better assessed with MRI than by PET-CT [16].

The primary tumor of the uterine corpus manifests either as diffuse or focal endometrial enlargement on the CT images and can be delineated by the abnormal contrast enhancement (Fig. 26.11). Depth of myometrial invasion may be appreciated when there is sufficient distinction between the normal myometrium and the contrast enhancement of the primary neoplasm when intravenous contrast is employed. Cervical involvement is suspected when there is heterogeneous cervical enlargement. When the tumor is located in a low position, it may obstruct the endometrial canal producing cavity distension secondary to retention of blood, debris or fluid. Signs of parametrial extension are as those described in cervical cancer with the addition of irregular uterine margin. The increased FDG uptake in the primary tumor on the PET images is helpful in roughly delineating the extent of the primary tumor, and excluding malignancy in CT abnormalities such as incidental uterine fibroids.

Stage III and IV

There are very few published FDG PET or PET-CT data in staging or survival prediction of cancer of corpus. This is understandable, as most of these patients tend to have undergone hysterectomy both for curative intent and staging prior

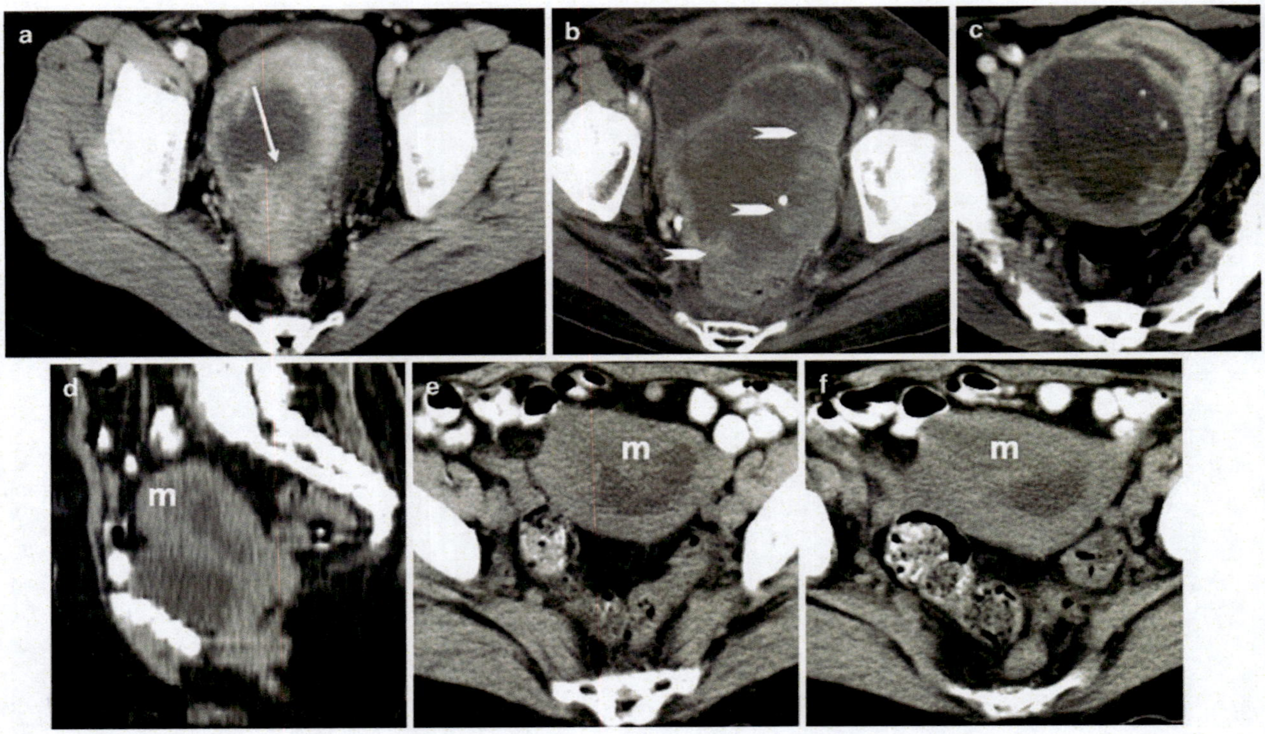

Fig. 26.11 CT appearances of corpus cancer. It can occur as focal endometrial enlargement (*white arrow* in **a**) or as irregular diffuse thickening (*white arrowheads* in **b**). Mixed solid and low density uterine mass is seen in uterine sarcoma (**c**). Myometrial involvement can occasionally be visualized (*m* in **d–f**)

to any imaging investigation. The capability of recognizing abnormality in a normal-sized node with anatomical precision gives PET-CT an edge over other modalities for whole body assessments of extrauterine sites of metastases. This includes nodal station beyond the extent of interoperative nodal dissection and if necessary it also serves as a roadmapping for biopsy (Fig. 26.12). In a study by Grisaru [30], PET-CT picked up all metastatic nodes while standard imaging (MRI, CT, US) failed to do in 28% of the cohort. Another study showed PET-CT being more sensitive than MRI (69% vs. 46%) in nodal staging and outperformed MRI in depicting distant metastasis [45].

Pitfalls and Selected Issues in Performing and Reporting PET-CT in Patients with Uterine Cancer

As with cervical cancer, optimization of both CT and PET technique for imaging the pelvis is important to minimize errors of interpretation of pathologic vs. physiologic FDG tracer uptake in pelvis structures. Use of both oral and intravenous contrast material improves delineation of pelvic structures and facilitates interpretation of local invasion in patients who have not yet undergone hysterectomy. Thin section technique with slice thickness of 5 mm or less is preferred. On the PET images, urinary tracer activity in the bladder results in image degradation due to increased scatter from the intense bladder tracer activity, and methods to reduce urinary tracer activity can improved overall quality of the reconstructed PET images of the pelvis. Special attention should also be given to the ovaries as an occasional endometrioid carcinoma can develop simultaneously in uterus and ovary. In this regard, PET-CT would help to differentiate physiologic ovarian uptake from ovarian neoplasm. CT images of the lungs should be reviewed carefully for small lung nodules, as very small pulmonary metastases (<6 mm) may be below the threshold of FDG PET detection. Benign parametritis may simulate parametrial extension on the CT images or even be associated with mild FDG tracer uptake on the PET images, as with cervical cancer. Miliary peritoneal implants do occur with endometrial cancer and will have minimal, if any associated abnormal FDG tracer activity on the FDG PET images, but will be seen on CT. They often deposit on bowel and are confused with normal bowel uptake on the FDG PET images. The presence of ascites is an important clue for the possibility of peritoneal implants and warrants careful review of the CT images. The mucinous type of endometrioid cancer may have very low FDG activity both in the primary tumor and metastases (Fig. 26.13). Cervicitis may take up FDG and simulate cervical extension.

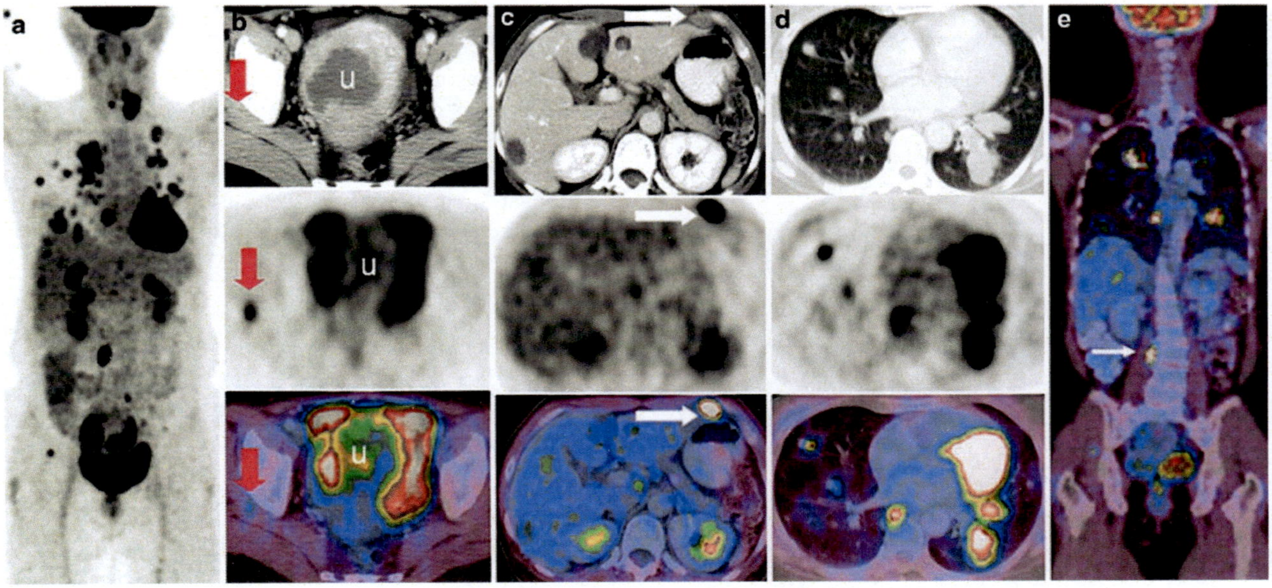

Fig. 26.12 PET-CT in staging of uterine sarcoma (**a–e**). The sarcoma (*u*) involves the entire uterus with central necrosis (**b**). The whole body evaluation shows metastases to liver (**c**), lungs (**d**), right gluteus medius muscles (*pink block arrows* in **b**), left intercostal muscle (*white block arrows* in **c**) and right psoas muscle (*white arrow* in **e**). PET-CT provides roadmap for site of muscle biopsy (in this case the left intercostal muscle) confirming uterine sarcoma. Subsequent hysterectomy also supported this diagnosis

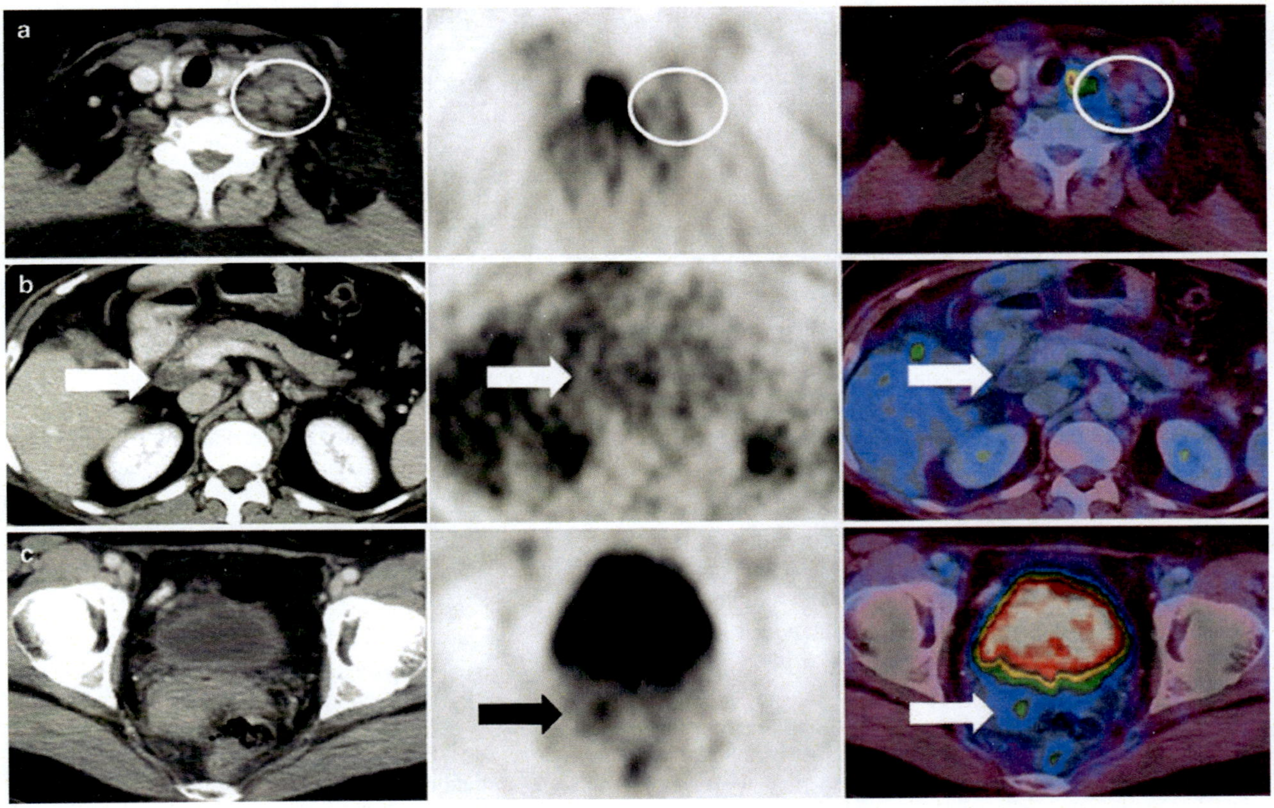

Fig. 26.13 PET-CT pitfalls in corpus cancer. Mucinous endometrioid carcinoma and secondary tends to have low glycolytic activity. PET-CT images in **a** show multiple hypometabolic nodal metastases >1cm at the left lower cervical region (*white circle*) and peripancreatic area (*white block arrow* in **b**) from mucinous carcinoma relapse. Note the absence of FDG tracer uptake in the low density lymph nodes containing mucinous carcinoma. PET-CT images in **c** show a focus of cervical uptake in a case of endometrial carcinoma suspicious of cervical spread. This was confirmed to be due to cervicitis in surgery

When initial staging of endometrial cancer is required by PET-CT, it should include the following:

- Primary tumor- anatomical or functional size, degree and distribution of abnormal FDG tracer uptake, and any protrusion into endometrial cavity
- Presence of ascites or peritoneal implants
- Any local invasion from the primary tumor: myometrial, cervical, parametrial, pelvic sidewall, rectal or bladder
- Co-existing ovarian lesion suspicious for endometrioid ovarian neoplasm
- Lymph node status: distribution and size of FDG avid lymph nodes and location of any enlarged lymph nodes
- Sites of distant metastases

Restaging of Uterine Cancer with PET-CT

Treatment failure occurs commonly within the first 3 years for endometrial cancer [1]. Endometrial carcinoma, if treated solely by surgery, has local recurrence in 53% of the cases and tends to be at the vaginal cuff, which is easily identified clinically [1]. If uterine cancer was treated with combined modality therapy, development of distant metastases rather than local disease is more likely [1]. Tumor marker such as CA 125 antigen for endometrial cancer is a sensitive and specific indicator for recurrence and may be positive for recurrent neoplasm up to 6 months preceding clinical and radiologic. Physical examination and anatomic imaging modalities such as CT or MRI cannot differentiate pelvic soft tissue thickening as a result of surgery or radiation from relapse [46]. Also, tumor relapse may not conform to the initial pattern of spread, with recurrence occurring at distant or atypical sites or combination of local and distant.

Since recurrent or metastatic endometrial cancer is FDG avid, the FDG PET images can reliably distinguish posttreatment scarring from recurrence [46] in addition to localizing extrapelvic metastases. The poor spatial resolution of PET is now compensated by the registered and aligned CT images [46], allowing differentiation between physiologic/nonmalignant uptakes from true pathologies (as discussed in staging). The registered and aligned PET and CT images also give precise anatomic information for biopsy guidance and radiotherapy planning. Occasionally, the PET-CT examination may pick up other pathologies or second tumor (Fig. 26.14).

Little had been written on the identification of endometrial carcinoma recurrences. From those reported, it seems that PET has good potential in detecting most of the recurrences, including unsuspected sites and asymptomatic patients, leading to change of management in 35% of cases [11]. For PET-CT, results so far seemed to confirm its superiority in disclosing local and/or distant recurrence. In one study, it localized disease in all tumor sites that were missed by standard imaging [30]. A sensitivity of 100%, specificity of 94%, accuracy of 92%, PPV of 100%, and NPV of 97% were obtained for posttreatment surveillance, resulting in a change of management in 22%. It also allowed for progression-free-survival prediction whereby those with a negative PET-CT fared significantly better than those with a positive scan [37].

Pitfalls and Selected Issues in Performing and Reporting PET-CT in Restaging Patients with Uterine Cancer

Radiation- induced ureteric stricture, proctitis, enteritis, cystitis, and osteonecrosis can be symptomatic and become the indication for a PET-CT exam, but these inflammatory lesions will simulate tumor recurrence due to FDG tracer uptake. If there is disagreement between the anatomic and functional images after treatment, either perform a biopsy or perform a follow-up imaging study in 1 month. In cases of enlarging pulmonary nodules despite low to no metabolic uptake, there is a higher probability to be due to metastases than benign disease. The time to perform imaging as a follow up has not been established. Since persistent disease at 3 months is associated with a poorer long-term survival, a 3-month follow up after initial surgical staging and treatment may be indicated.

PET-CT Reports for restaging or follow up surveillance of uterine cancer should include the following:

- Surgical site evaluation should include the description of the presence of residual mass or abnormal FDG tracer uptake, anatomical size of the residual tumor (in the case of nonvisualization on CT, the functional size and degree of FDG tracer uptake), and comparison of the size and degree of FDG tracer uptake with the prior scan
- Any resolution of hydronephrosis or hydroureter
- Lymph node status: abnormal tracer uptake and comparison of the size and degree of FDG tracer uptake with the prior PET-CT scan(s)
- Status of distant metastases, change in comparison to prior scan

Uterine Cancer Therapy Monitoring with PET-CT

There are no data available on monitoring therapy response of uterine cancer using PET-CT. The basic principle and application would be similar to cervical cancer. Both the morphologic as well as functional change should be used together to guide management decision or modification of therapy.

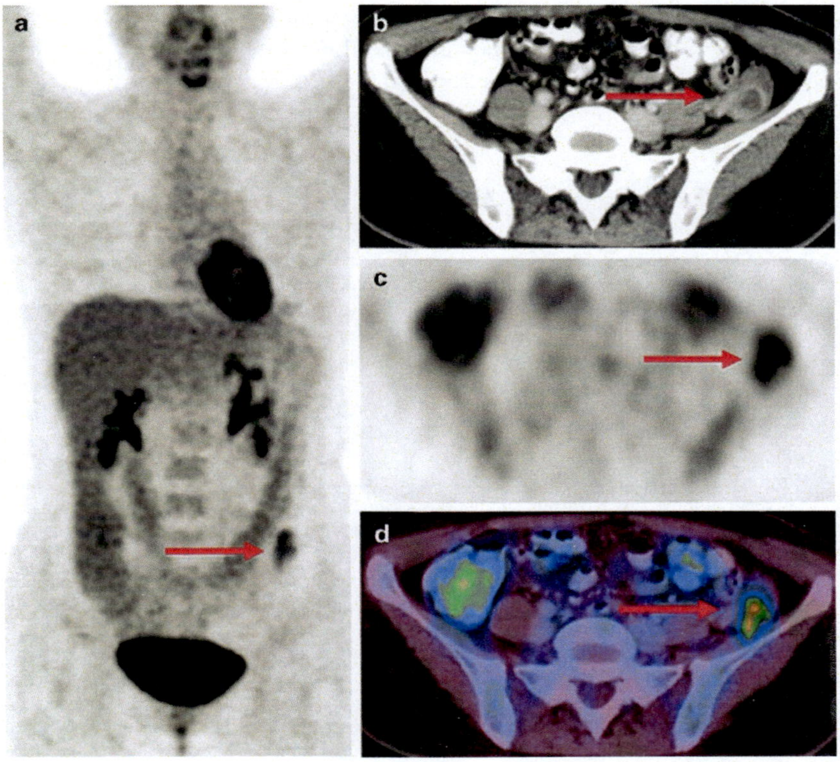

Fig. 26.14 Ectopic ovary simulates recurrence. Patient had hysterectomy for cervix cancer without ovarian transportation 1 year ago. PET-CT performed for follow up showed uptake in the left lower quadrant (**a**, **c**) which was confirmed on the contrast CT image and fusion PET-CT to be due to a soft tissue mass with central lucency (**b, d** *red arrows*). Recurrence was suspected but biopsy found normal ovarian tissue

Role of PET-CT in Radiotherapy Planning

The initial experience with FDG PET in radiation planning for uterine cancer has been promising, which should apply also to PET-CT.

The Role of PET-CT for Uterine and Cervical Cancers: Highlights and Recommendation

In Grade IA cervical cancer or tumor size <2 cm and Grade I endometrial carcinoma, there is a very low likelihood of extrauterine or extrapelvic disease. Pretreatment imaging including PET-CT is often not required [1].

The major usefulness of PET-CT is in detecting nodal and extrauterine disease, as well as for recurrence either locally or at distant sites in one examination. Important prognostic information can be conferred by the dual imaging.

In patients with invasive cervical cancer, the presence of full-thickness cervical involvement, parametrial invasion, lymphatic invasion, and positive resection margin infer a high probability of failed local control [28], and it is desirable to acquire a baseline and regular follow up PET-CT to deliver optimal therapy. The baseline study can also serve as RT planning. More vigilant surveillance should be carried out in patients with the following poor prognosticators: those who had been treated with radiation and are currently symptomatic with high SCC-Ag.

In patients with endometrial carcinoma, the following infer a high pretest likelihood of metastatic disease and recurrence rate: the presence of high grade or aggressive cell types such as clear cell, papillary serous or sarcomatous, positive endocervical curettage, myometrial invasion, abnormal liver function test, or raised CA-125 level [1]. PET-CT is an indispensable and accurate staging tool in establishing presence of extra-pelvic disease. This information is essential in deciding surgical from nonsurgical treatment and whether adjuvant therapy is required. It can also serve as a baseline study for monitoring therapy response and or RT planning.

PET-CT can be incorporated into the vigilant follow-up protocol to detect recurrence, especially when the above mentioned factors are present in patients with uterine cancer. For cervical cancer, PET-CT should be performed within the first 2 years and for corpus cancer the first 3 years from diagnosis. The first post treatment imaging investigation had been proposed at 3 months.

In case of equivocal PET-CT lesion (borderline FDG uptake with <1 cm functional size or prominent FDG uptake <1 cm anatomical size), either FNA or follow up CT or

PET-CT in 3 months is recommended. Small new pulmonary nodules may be below the detection threshold of FDG PET, and require follow up CT 3 months later [26].

References

1. Boles SM, Hricak H, Rubin P. Carcinoma of the cervix and endometrium. In: Bragg D, Rubin P, Hricak H (eds.). Oncologic Imaging, 2nd edn. Philadelphia: WB Saunders, 2002, pp. 523–548.
2. Herbst AL, Cole P, Colton T. Age-incidence and risk of diethylstilbestrol-related clear cell Adenocarcinoma of the vagina and cervix. Am J Obstet Gynecol 1977;128:43–50.
3. Giesinger KR, Stanley MW, Raab SS, Silverman JF, Abati A. Modern Cytopathology. Philadelphia: Churchill Livingstone, 2003.
4. Wright T, Ferenczy A, Kurman RJ. In: Kurman RJ (eds.). Carcinoma and other of the cervix Blaustein's Pathology of the Female Genital Tract, 5th edn. New York: Springer-Verlag, 2002, p. 346.
5. Umesaki N, Tanaka T, Miyama M, et al. Positron emission tomography with 18F-fluorodeoxyglucose of uterine sarcoma: a comparison with magnetic resonance imaging and power doppler imaging. Gynecol Oncol 2001;80:372–377.
6. Narayan K, Mckenzie AF, Hicks RJ, Fisher R, Bernshaw D, Bau S. Relation between FIGO stage, primary tumor volume and presence of lymph node metastases in cervical cancer patients referred for radiotherapy. Int J Gynecol Cancer 2003;13:657–663.
7. Richter E, Feyerabend T, Bondorf W (eds.). Normal Lymph Node Topography: CT Atlas. New York: Springer, 2004.
8. Aizer-Dannon A, Bar-Am A, Ron IG, Flusser G, Even-Sapir E. Fused functional-anatomic images of metastatic cancer of cervix obtained by a combined gamma camera and an X-ray tube hybrid system with an illustrative case and review of the 18F-Fluorodeoxyglucose literature. Gynecol Oncol 2003;90: 453–457.
9. Singh AK, Grigsby PW, Dehdashti F, Herzog TJ, Siegal BA. FDG-PET lymph node staging and survival of patients with FIGO stage IIIb cervical carcinoma. Int J Radiat Oncol Biol Phys 2003;56(2):489–493.
10. Miller TR, Pinkus E, Dehdashti F, Grigsby PW. Improved prognostic value of 18F-FDG PET using a simple visual analysis of tumor characteristics in patients with cervical cancer. J Nucl Med 2003;44:192–197.
11. Belhocine T. An appraisal of 18F-FDG PET imaging in post-therapy surveillance of uterine cancers: clinical evidence and a research proposal. Int J Gynecol Cancer 2003;13:228–233.
12. Grigsby PW, Singh AK, Siegel BA, Dehdashti F, Rader J, Zoberi I. Lymph node control in cervical cancer. Int J Radiat Oncol Biol Phys 2004;59(3):706–712.
13. Cosin JA, Fowler JM, Chen MD, et al. Pretreatment surgical staging of patients with cervical carcinoma: the case for lymph node debulking. Cancer 1998;82:2241–2248.
14. Goff BA, Muntz HG, Paley PJ, et al. Impact of surgical staging in women with locally advanced cervical cancer. Gynecol Oncol 1999;74:436–442.
15. Loft A, Berthelsen AK, Roed H, et al. The diagnostic value of PET/CT scanning in patients with cervical cancer: a prospective study. Gynecol Oncol 2007;106:29–34.
16. Sala E, Wakely S, Senior E, Lomas D. MRI of malignant neoplasms of the uterine corpus and cervix. Am J Roentgenol 2007;188: 1577–1587.
17. Miller TR, Grigsby PW. Measurement of tumor volume by PET to evaluate prognosis in patients with advanced cervical cancer treated by radiation therapy. Int J Radiat Oncol Biol Phys 2002;53: 353–359.
18. DiSaia P, Rich W. Advanced and recurrent carcinoma of cervix. In: Coppleson M (ed.). Gynecologic Oncology. London: Churchill Livingstone, 1981, pp. 517–527.
19. Yen T-C, Ng K-K, Ma S-Y, Chou H, et al. Value of dual-phase 2-fluoro-2-deoxy-D-glucose positron emission tomography in cervical cancer. J Clin Oncol 2003;21:3651–3658.
20. Bipat S, Glas AS, Van der Velden J, Zwinderman AH, Bossuyt PMM, Stoker J. Computed tomography and magnetic resonance imaging in staging of uterine cervical carcinoma: a systemic review. Gynecol Oncol 2003;91:59–66.
21. Walsh JW. Computed tomography of gynecologic neoplasms. Radiol Clin North Am 1992;30:817–830.
22. Sugawara Y, Eisbruch A, Kosuda S, Recker BE, Kison PV, Wahl RL. Evaluation of FDG PET in patients with cervical cancer. J Nucl Med 1999;40:1125–1131.
23. Yeh L-S, Hung Y-C, Shen Y-Y, Kao C-H, Lin C-C, Lee C-C. Detecting para-aortic lymph nodal metastasis by positron emission tomography of 18F-flurodeoxyglucose in advanced cervical cancer with negative magnetic resonance imaging findings. Oncology Reports 2002;9:1289–1292.
24. Reinhardt MJ, Ehritt-Braun C, Vogelgesang D, Ihling C, Hogerle S, Mix M, Moser E, Krause TM. Metastatic lymph nodes in patients with cervical cancer: detection with MR imaging and FDG PET. Radiology 2001;218(3):776–782.
25. Rose PG, Adler LP, Rodriguez M, Faulhaber PF, Abdul-Karim FW, Miraldi F. Positron emission tomography for evaluating para-aortic nodal metastasis in locally advanced cervical cancer before surgical staging: a surgicopathologic study. J Clin Oncol 1999;17:41–45.
26. Sun S, Chen T, Yen R, et al. Value of whole body 18-F-fluoro-2-deoxyglucose positron emission tomography in the evaluation of recurrent cervical cancer. Anticancer Res 2002;21:2957–2962.
27. Wong TZ, Jones EL, Coleman RE. Positron Emission Tomography with 2-deoxy-2-[18F] fluoro-D-glucose for evaluating local and distant disease in patients with cervical cancer. Mol Imaging Biol 2004;6:55–62.
28. Sironi S, Buda A, Picchio M, et al. Lymph node metastasis in patients with clinical early-stage cervical cancer: detection with integrated FDG PET/CT. Radiology 2006;238:272–279.
29. Subhas N, Patel PV, Pannau HK, Jacene HA, Fishman EK, Wahl RL. Imaging of pelvic malignancies with in-line FDG PET-CT: case examples and common pitfalls of FDG PET. Radiographics 2005;25:1031–1043.
30. Grisaru D, Almog B, Levine C, et al. The diagnostic accuracy of ^{18}F-Fluorodexoyglucose PET/CT in patients with gynecological malignancies. Gynecol Oncol 2004;94:680–684.
31. Yildirim Y, Sehirali S, Avci ME, et al. Integrated PET/CT for the evaluation of para-aortic nodal metastasis in locally advanced cervical cancer patients with negative conventional CT findings. Gynecol Oncol 2008;108:154–159.
32. Park J, Seo S, Kang S, et al. The comparison of accuracy between PET and PET/CT for detecting lymph node metastasis in cervical cancer: prospective surgicopathologic study. Abstract. JCO 2007 ASCO Annu Meet Proc Pt I 2007; 25(18S):5587.
33. Ryu S-Y, Kim M-H, Choi S-C, Choi C-W, Lee K-H. Detection of early recurrence with 18F-FDG PET in patients with cervical cancer. J Nucl Med 2003;44:347–352.
34. Ma S, See L, Lai C, et al. Delayed 18F-FDG PET for detection of para-aortic lymph node metastases in cervical cancer patients. J Nucl Med 2003;44:1775–1783.
35. Lin WC, Hung YC, Yeh LS, Kao CH, Yen RF, Shen YY. Usefulness of 18F-fluorodeoxyglucose positron emission tomography to detect para-aortic lymph nodal metastasis in advanced cervical cancer with negative computed tomography findings. Gynecol Oncol 2003;89:73–76.

36. Yen T-C, See L-C, Chang T-C, et al. Defining the priority of using 18F -FDG PET for recurrent cervical cancer. J Nucl Med 2004;45: 1632–1639.
37. Chung HH, Jo H, Kang WJ, et al. Clinical impact of integrated PET/CT on the management of suspected cervical cancer recurrence. Gynecol Oncol 2007;104:529–534.
38. Havrilesky LJ, Wong TZ, Secord AA, Berchuck A, Clarke-Pearson DL, Jones EL. The role of PET scanning in the detection of recurrent cervical cancer. Gynecol Oncol 2003;90:186–190.
39. Yau YY, Chan WS, Tam YM, et al. Is there a significant difference in the standardized uptake value measurement in 2D or 3D PET/CT [abstract]. J Nucl Med 2004;45(suppl):30P.
40. Belhocine T, Thille A, Fridman V, et al. Contribution of whole body 18FDG PET imaging in the management of cervical cancer. Gynecol Oncol 2002;87:90–97.
41. Grigsby PW, Siegel BA, Dehdashti F, Mutch DG. Posttherapy surveillance monitoring of cervical cancer by FDG-PET. Int J Radiation Oncology Biol Phys 2003;55:907–913.
42. Grigsby PW, Siegel BA, Dehdashti F, Rader J, Zoberi I. Posttherapy [18F]Fluorodeoxyglucose positron emission tomography in carcinoma of the cervix: response and outcome. J Clin Oncol 2004;22: 2167–2171.
43. Malyapa RS, Mutic S, Low DA, et al. Physiologic FDG-PET three-dimensional brachytherapy treatment planning for cervical cancer. Int J Radiation Oncology Biol Phys 2002;54:1140–1146.
44. Henrickson MR, Longacre TA, Kempson RL. The uterine corpus. In: Sternberg SS, Antonioli DA, Carter K, Mills SE, Oberman HA (eds.). Diagnostic Surgical Pathology, 3rd edn. Philadelphia: Lippincott Williams & Wilkins, 1999:2203–2305.
45. Park J, Kim EN, Kim DY, et al. Comparison of the validity of magnetic resonance imaging and positron emission tomography/computed tomography in the preoperative evaluation of patients with uterine corpus cancer. Gynaecol Oncol 2008; 108(3):486–492 [Abstract].
46. Torabi M, Aquino SL, Harisinghani MG. Current concepts in lymph node imaging. J Nucl Med 2004;45:1509–1518.

Chapter 27
PET-CT of Testicular Malignancies

Mark Tann and Paul Shreve

Testicular cancer (seminoma and non seminomatous germ cell tumor [NSGCT]) is a relatively rare malignancy comprising 1% of cancer diagnoses. However, it is the most frequent of tumors encountered in young males and the incidence is increasing. Compared to the relatively poor prognosis for other soft tissue tumors, testicular cancer shows great response to treatment at all stages of disease, including initial limited or advanced stages and even at relapse [1].

Due to differences in treatment and management, testicular disease is divided into two major subgroups based on histology: seminoma and non-seminomatous germ cell tumors. Approximately half of testicular tumors will be pure seminoma. The non-seminomatous germ cell type may contain two or more cell types, which can include seminoma, but also include choriocarcinoma, embryonal cell carcinoma, or yolk sac tumor. Seminomas are radiosensitive and spread by localized tissue invasion and fairly predictable lymphatic drainage patterns. NSGCT on the other hand are radioresistant, and in addition to spread along lymphatic drainage routes, can metastasize by hematogenous routes.

Management of patients with testicular cancer thus differs between pure seminoma histology and mixed histology of NSGCT. For the purposes of clinical staging, the primary site will usually be in the testes; however, in some rare cases the tumor may originate from the mediastinum or retroperitoneum. In part because there is relatively effective treatment even for metastatic testicular cancer, classification of patients regarding different treatment regimens depends on clinical stage and other criteria of prognosis such as histology, including fraction of embryonal cell and presence of vascular invasion at the primary site and rising serum tumor markers [2, 3]. There are a number of staging systems in use in addition to conventional TNM staging (Table 27.1), including staging criteria specifically for seminoma (Table 27.2) and for NSGCT (Table 27.3).

Due to the limited accuracy of anatomic size criteria for lymph node metastases, a retroperitoneal lymph node dissection (RPLND) is often performed for initial staging [4]. An additional criteria used at initial staging is decline of serum tumor markers following orchiectomy. After the initial surgery, if the tumor markers have not declined at the expected rate, this is indicative of metastatic disease, even in the absence of surgical or imaging evidence of metastases. Useful tumor markers include human chorionic gonadotropin (secreted by 20% of seminomas) and alfa-fetoprotein secreted by the embryonal cell variant.

Management of Nonmetastatic Testicular Cancer (Stage I)

For NSGCT testicular cancer with no evidence of metastatic spread, careful observation including clinical and imaging surveillance and serum tumor marker monitoring is followed at some centers and prophylactic chemotherapy withheld [2]. Since 20–30% of patients with nonenlarged retroperitoneal lymph nodes on initial diagnosis are found to have metastases on RPLND, however some centers withhold chemotherapy only if the RPLND is negative. The presence of vascular invasion at the primary site is an additional reason for prophylactic chemotherapy at some centers. Generally, cisplatin-based chemotherapy is initiated when there is evidence of relapse, such as rising serum tumor markers or development of imaging evidence of lymphadenopathy or visceral or pulmonary metastases.

For pure seminoma testicular cancer with no evidence of metastatic spread, radiotherapy of the retroperitoneal lymph node chains may be performed even without evidence of lymphadenopathy or abnormal serum human serum gonadotropin, due to the exquisite radiosensitivity of seminoma [2]. As with NSGCT, chemotherapy may be included, particularly

M. Tann (✉)
Department of Radiology and Imaging Sciences, Indiana University School of Medicine, 550 University Boulevard, Room 0663, Indianapolis, IN, 46202-5253, USA
e-mail: matann@iupui.edu

P. Shreve and D.W. Townsend (eds.), *Clinical PET-CT in Radiology: Integrated Imaging in Oncology*,
DOI 10.1007/978-0-387-48902-5_27, © Springer Science+Business Media, LLC 2011

Table 27.1 AJCC TNM and anatomic stage and prognostic groups for testicular tumor (Used with the permission of the American Joint Committee on Cancer (AJCC), Chicago, IL. The original source for this material is the *AJCC Cancer Staging Manual*, 7th edn (2010) published by Springer Science and Business Media LLC. www.springer.com)

Definitions OF TNM

Primary Tumor (T)[a]

The extent of primary tumor is usually classified after radical orchiectomy, and for this reason, a *pathologic* stage is assigned.

pTX	Primary tumor cannot be assessed.
pT0	No evidence of primary tumor (e.g., histologic scar in testis)
pTis	Intratubular germ cell neoplasia (carcinoma in situ)
pT1	Tumor limited to the testis and epididymis without vascular/lymphatic invasion; tumor may invade into the tunica albuginea but not the tunica vaginalis.
pT2	Tumor limited to the testis and epididymis with vascular/lymphatic invasion, or tumor extending through the tunica albuginea with involvement of the tunica vaginalis
pT3	Tumor invades the spermatic cord with or without vascular/lymphatic invasion.
pT4	Tumor invades the scrotum with or without vascular/lymphatic invasion.

Regional lymph nodes (N)

Clinical

NX	Regional lymph nodes cannot be assessed.
N0	No regional lymph node metastasis
N1	Metastasis with a lymph node mass 2 cm or less in greatest dimension; or multiple lymph nodes, none more than 2 cm in greatest dimension
N2	Metastasis with a lymph node mass more than 2 cm but not more than 5 cm in greatest dimension; or multiple lymph nodes, any one mass greater than 2 cm but not more than 5 cm in greatest dimension
N3	Metastasis with a lymph node mass more than 5 cm in greatest dimension

Pathologic (pN)

pNX	Regional lymph nodes cannot be assessed
pN0	No regional lymph node metastasis
pN1	Metastasis with a lymph node mass 2 cm or less in greatest dimension and less than or equal to 5 nodes positive, none more than 2 cm in greatest dimension
pN2	Metastasis with a lymph node mass more than 2 cm but not more than 5 cm in greatest dimension; or more than 5 nodes positive, none more than 5 cm; or evidence of extranodal extension of tumor
pN3	Metastasis with a lymph node mass more than 5 cm in greatest dimension

Distant metastasis (M)

M0	No distant metastasis
M1	Distant metastasis
M1a	Nonregional nodal or pulmonary metastasis
M1b	Distant metastasis other than to non-regional lymph nodes and lung

Anatomic stage • Prognostic groups

Group	T	N	M	S (Serum tumor markers)
Stage 0	pTis	N0	M0	S0
Stage I	pT1–4	N0	M0	SX
Stage IA	pT1	N0	M0	S0
Stage IB	pT2	N0	M0	S0
pT3	N0	M0	S0	
pT4	N0	M0	S0	
Stage IS	Any pT/Tx	N0	M0	S1–3 (measured post orchiectomy)
Stage II	Any pT/Tx	N1–3	M0	SX
Stage IIA	Any pT/Tx	N1	M0	S0
	Any pT/Tx	N1	M0	S1
Stage IIB	Any pT/Tx	N2	M0	S0
	Any pT/Tx	N2	M0	S1
Stage IIC	Any pT/Tx	N3	M0	S0
	Any pT/Tx	N3	M0	S1
Stage III	Any pT/Tx	Any N	M1	SX
Stage IIIA	Any pT/Tx	Any N	M1a	S0
Any pT/Tx	Any N	M1a	S1	

(continued)

Table 27.1 (continued)

Stage IIIB	Any pT/Tx	N1–3	M0	S2
Any pT/Tx	Any N	M1a	S2	
Stage IIIC	Any pT/Tx	N1–3	M0	S3
Any pT/Tx	Any N	M1a	S3	
Any pT/Tx	Any N	M1b	Any S	

[a]Except for pTis and pT4, extent of primary tumor is classified by radical orchiectomy. TX may be used for other categories in the absence of radical orchiectomy

Table 27.2 Staging of seminoma

Royal Marsden Hospital	M.D. Anderson Cancer Center	Memorial Sloan-Kettering Cancer Center	American Joint Committee on Cancer	Boden-Gibb Commission on Cancer
I: confined to testis	I: confined to testis	A: confined to testis	I: confined to testis	A: confined to testis
IIa: RPLN <2 cm	IIa: RPLN <5 cm		IIN1: microscopic disease in RPLN	B: RPLN involved
IIb: RPLN = 2 cm or more and <5 cm	IIb: RPLN = 5 cm or more and = 10 cm or less	B1: RPLN <5 cm	IIN2: 5 LNs or less involved, all <2 cm	
IIc: RPLN = 5 cm or more and <10 cm	IIc: RPLN >10 cm	B2: RPLN = 5 cm or more and <10 cm	IIN3: >5 LNs involved or LN >2 cm	
IId: RPLN = 10 cm or more		B3: RPLN = 10 cm or more	IIN4: unresectable LN	
III: LN above diaphragm involved	III: LN above diaphragm or visceral organs involved	C: LN above diaphragm or visceral organs involved		C: LN above diaphragm or visceral organs involved
IV: extranodal disease				

RPLN retroperitoneal lymph node, *LN* lymph node

Table 27.3 Staging of nonseminomatous germ-cell tumors

	Stage		
Description	MSKCC	WR	TNM
Confined to testis	A	I	N0
Microscopic nodal involvement only, 5 or less nodes involved, and all nodes <2 cm	B1	IIA	N1 or N2A
Grossly positive nodes, or 6 or more nodes involved	B2	IIB	N2B
Bulky retroperitoneal involvement, unresectable	B3	IIC	N3
Metastases above the diaphragm or spread to solid visceral organs	C	III	M1

MSKCC Memorial Sloan-Kettering Cancer Center, *WR* walter reed, *TNM* tumor-nodes-metastasis staging system

when findings at initial diagnosis suggest an elevated likelihood of relapse, including initial tumor size and tumor involvement of the rete testis. As with NSGCT, cisplatin-based chemotherapy is initiated when there is evidence of relapse.

The relapse rates for Stage I NSGCT and pure seminoma testicular cancers is roughly 15% for NSGCT and 20–30% for seminoma [1], but due to the success of cisplatin-based chemotherapy regimens, the overall cure rate for patients with initial Stage I classification approaches 100%.

Management of Metastatic Testicular Cancer (Stages II and III)

With the introduction of cisplatin-based BEP (Bleomycin, etoposide, and cisplatin) regimens, the cure rate for metastatic disease has increased greatly from 25% to 80% [3]. At present there is an emphasis on trying to improve on this successful protocol by dividing those with metastatic disease into two groups based on prognostic factors defined by the International Germ-Cell Cancer Collaborative Group (Table 27.4). Those with poor prognostic factors are more likely to relapse and die of their disease and therefore warrant an aggressive therapy. Those with good prognostic indicators have a higher likelihood for response to minimal treatment, with a low likelihood of relapse, and therefore can be offered a less toxic regimen. Hence a Stage II seminoma with low tumor burden may be treated with radiation therapy alone, while Stage II seminoma with bulky adenopathy would include cisplatin-based chemotherapy. Additional prognostic information can be gained from observing the rate of decline in serum concentrations of HCG and α-fetoprotein after initiation of chemotherapy. Differentiation between a satisfactory or unsatisfactory decrease in serum markers during the first two cycles of chemotherapy provides predictive information for eventual outcome that is independent of the prognostic grouping shown in Table 27.4. Staging

Table 27.4 The International Germ-Cell Cancer Collaborative Group prognostic grouping for seminoma and nonseminomatous germ-cell tumors (From [5]. With permission from Oxford University Press)

Parameter seminoma	Good	Intermediate	Poor
Alpha-fetoprotein	Normal	Normal	
HCG	Any	Any	
Lactate dehydrogenase	Any	Any	
Primary	Any	Any	
Other	No nonlung secondary tumors	Nonlung visceral secondary tumors	
Percent of patients	90%	10%	
5-year survival	86%	72%	
Nonseminomatous germ cell tumor			
Alpha-fetoprotein	<1,000	1,000–10,000	>10,000
HCG	<5,000	5,000–50,000	>50,000
Lactate dehydrogenase	<1 • 5 × ULN	1 • 5–10 × ULN	>10 × ULN
Primary	Testis/retroperitoneum	Testis/retroperitoneum	Mediastinal
Other	No nonlung	No nonlung secondary tumors	Nonlung secondary tumors
Percent patients	56%	28%	16%
5-year survival	92%	80%	48%

HCG human chorionic gonadotrophin

based on imaging findings is thus one of a handful of criteria used in determining the therapy plan in patients deemed to have disease spread beyond the testis at time of initial diagnosis.

After chemotherapy for metastatic NSGCT, residual lymph node masses may remain in the retroperitoneum, mediastinum, or supraclavicular nodal basins and there may be residual pulmonary masses. Based on anatomic imaging criteria, it cannot be determined whether such residual masses are purely necrotic tissue, contain residual viable tumor, or are transformed teratoma. Residual masses, if isolated, may be resected, especially if there are persistently elevated serum tumor markers, to advance the likelihood of cure by removing residual viable tumor and teratoma, which has a significant possibility of later relapsing into malignant germ cell neoplasm. For pure seminoma, the rate of residual tumor mass post therapy is four times lower than seen than with NSGCT, but there is a similar desire to remove isolated resectable masses as the prognosis is poor for patients with residual tumor masses and persistently elevated tumor markers.

Role of PET-CT in Initial Diagnosis of Testicular Cancer

There is no recognized role for FDG PET or CT in the initial diagnosis of testicular cancer. There is moderate physiologic FDG uptake by the normal testis [6]. Asymmetric testicular FDG uptake on PET imaging should be further evaluated, just as a testicular solid mass is incidentally seen on CT.

Staging of Testicular Cancer with PET-CT

Despite the multiple staging systems used for testicular cancers (see Tables 27.1, 27.2, and 27.3), for practical purposes, the most important distinction in initial staging of testicular cancer is between clinical Stage I (no metastases) and clinical Stage II or III (presence of metastases). Identification of true Stage I disease would allow the use of less toxic therapeutic regimens in this group. Approximately 25% of those initially classified as stage 1 by CT alone have more advanced disease at RPLND, with as many as 50% under staged and 25% over staged [4]. Hence current management often includes a diagnostic RPNLD or prophylactic retroperitoneal lymph node basin radiation, or more aggressive chemotherapy to account for the risk that the stage I assumption is often wrong.

Testicular cancer spreads by two routes, the more common pathway following lymphatic drainage (Fig. 27.1), and the second route being hematogenous spread, especially with NSGCT. The pattern of lymphatic spread of testicular cancer follows the lymphatic drainage pathways of the testes. Primary tumors of the left testicle can be expected to spread first to the left paraaortic and ipsilateral preaortic lymph nodes. Primary tumors of the right testicle can be expected to spread first to the ipsilateral precaval and preaortic and the aortocaval lymph nodes. Right side testicular cancer lymph node spread commonly "crosses over" to the left pre- and paraaortic nodal chains, while left side testicular cancer rarely involves aortocaval or precaval nodal chains. The common sentinel lymph node for left testicular cancer is left paraaortic at the level of the left renal hilum, while for right testicular cancer, the common sentinel node is aortocaval below the level of the right renal artery. Following these sentinel nodal basins, lymphatic spread continues to the retrocrural nodes, then above the diaphragm via the thoracic duct to the posterior mediastinum and left supraclavicular nodal basin. Lymphatic spread of testicular cancer can occur in "retrograde fashion" to the common iliac, external iliac, or inguinal nodal basins if there is bulky disease. Hematogenous spread most commonly involves pulmonary metastases, although abdominal organs and the brain can also be involved.

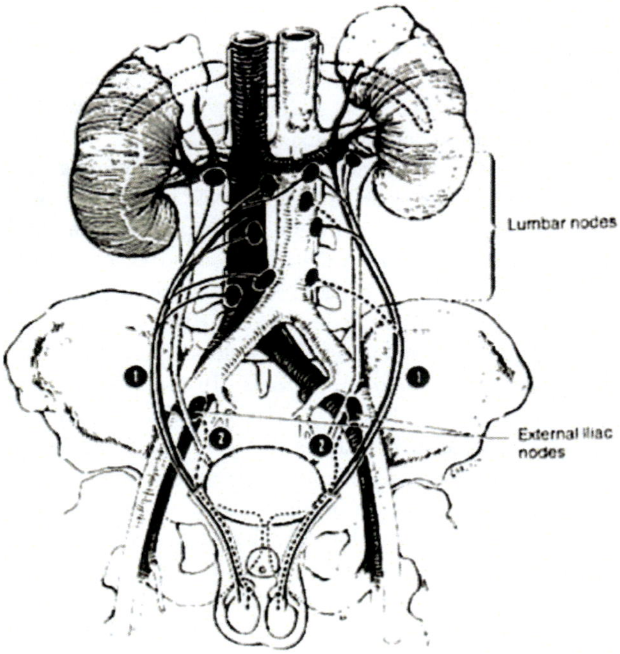

Fig. 27.1 Lymphatic drainage pathways of the testes (From [7]. With permission)

The role of CT in staging testicular cancer is well established, and CT has been the dominant modality used for all stages of imaging evaluation. The limitations of CT for the diagnosis of lymph node metastases are well known, and just as with other malignancies, adding the criteria of abnormal glucose metabolism improves the overall diagnostic accuracy. At present only a few studies evaluating the value of FDG-PET imaging for improved initial staging have been performed; however, the results have been promising but mixed, ranging from an accuracy of approximately 90% to no significant improvement over CT for detection of retroperitoneal lymph node metastases [6, 8–10]. These studies were performed with conventional PET scanners without the benefit of registered and aligned CT. The specific contribution of PET-CT to initial staging of testicular cancer has not been documented, but the potential for better accuracy, as has been shown in many different tumors, remains untapped. The results of the recent trial from the UK (TE22) on this subject are still pending.

In our experience FDG PET, and in particular PET-CT, with it's inherent advantages of whole-body scanning and combined modality imaging, has been useful for the detection and evaluation of above-diaphragm metastases and organ metastases (Fig. 27.2). With the general acceptance of

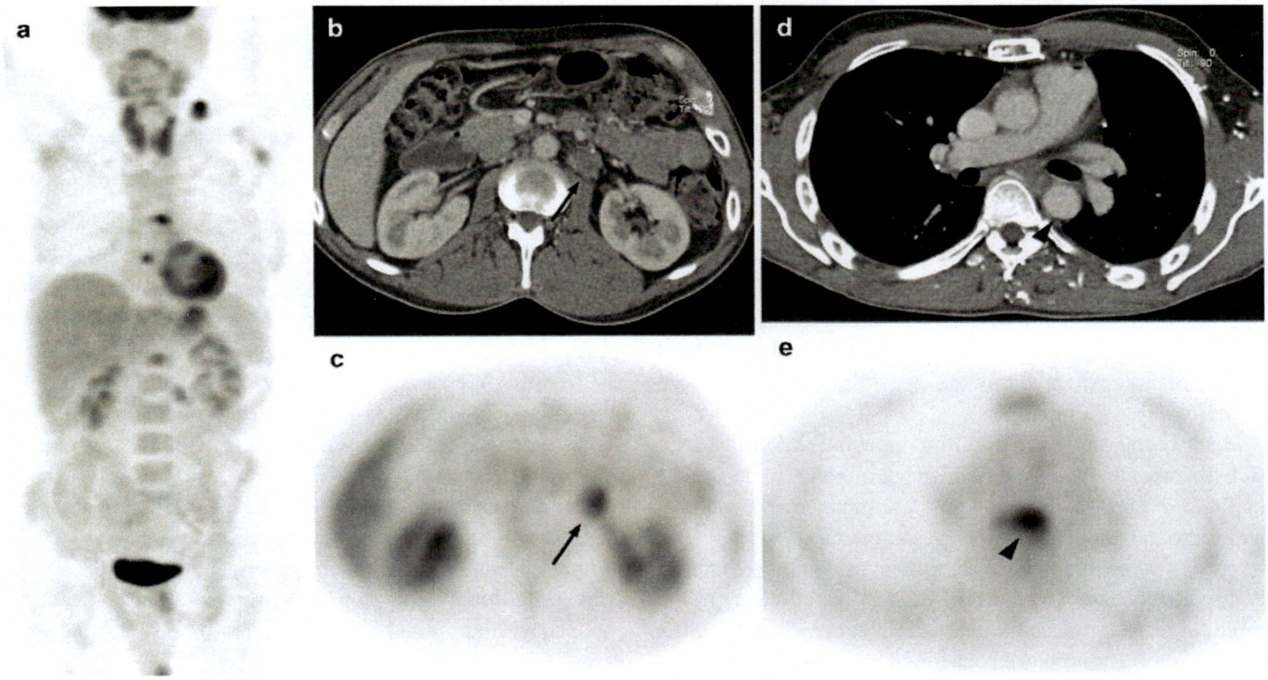

Fig. 27.2 Recurrent metastatic NSGCT. Anterior FDG PET MIP image (**a**) shows focal abnormal FDG tracer uptake at the left supraclavicular fossa, in the mediastinum and left mid abdomen. Transaxial CT (**b**) and FDG PET (**c**) image show the left mid-abdominal focus of abnormal tracer corresponds to a 2 cm left paraaortic lymph node with moderately abnormal FDG tracer uptake (*arrow*), and the mediastinal focus of abnormal tracer corresponds to a 1 cm left paraesophageal lymph node (*arrowhead*) with moderately intense abnormal FDG tracer uptake (**d, e**)

using oral and IV CT contrast, additional diagnostic power has been added to the PET-CT scan with fully optimized diagnostic CT. This enables the elimination of the need to perform two separate exams for the patient. Apart from providing attenuation and localization functions, the CT component of the PET-CT scanner also provides the same function as a stand-alone CT scanner, i.e., identification and evaluation of abnormal findings, which perhaps the PET could not, or abnormalities the FDG PET images identify but do not fully characterize. For example, the identification and serial evaluation of small lung nodules is very important in patients with NSGCT testicular cancer; lungs are the major site of hematogenous metastases. Small (<8 mm) pulmonary metastases may not be detected on the FDG PET images, but are readily demonstrated on CT. Lymph node necrosis as seen on CT is more specific for metastasis in lymph nodes, and extranodal extension of tumor as seen on CT is an important finding with negative prognostic implications.

Restaging of Testicular Cancer with PET-CT

Restaging testicular cancer includes restaging after therapy where residual tumor mass has management implications peculiar to testicular cancer, and restaging patients with rising tumor markers.

About 25% of seminoma patients will present with advanced disease, and after chemotherapy roughly 60% of this group will have residual masses on morphologic cross-sectional imaging [11]. There are many different approaches for managing these residual masses, with resection of masses larger than 3 cm and surveillance for smaller lesions being one of the more common options, relying on serial CT scan measurements [12, 13]. Unfortunately, these approaches result in a large fraction of patients being over- or undertreated. In this setting PET-CT can be most useful (Fig. 27.3). FDG-PET has been shown to reliably predict viability in residual tumor masses, with greater accuracy than the size criteria of 3 cm alone [14, 15]. A combined criteria of both the size and FDG avidity may even more correctly guide therapy.

For residual masses in NSGCT the contribution of FDG-PET to accurate diagnosis has also been shown to be greater than that of conventional imaging and tumor markers alone, but less so than in the case of pure seminoma [8, 16, 17]. The main reason for this is based on the occasional presence of teratomatous elements as part of the mixed cellularity of the initial tumor. After successful chemotherapy, while the other cell lines of the tumor have been killed, the low metabolic rate teratomatous elements may survive. Hence, while elevated glucose metabolism can be used to differentiate residual viable malignant neoplasm from fibrosis, necrosis, and elements of mature teratoma in a residual mass, the elements of mature teratoma cannot be reliably differentiated from fibrosis or necrosis based on morphologic criteria of CT or glucose metabolism demonstrated on FDG PET.

Analysis of SUV values for improved differentiation between viable tumor, scar, and teratoma has been tried, with a threshold value of 5 and above highly suggestive of tumor; however, there was still an overlap between the values of scar and teratoma [18]. It is because mature teratomatous elements can later dedifferentiate into a malignant germ cell neoplasm that it is desirable, when feasible, to remove residual masses with teratomatous elements. To further complicate matters, however, false positive elevation of glucose metabolism can occur in residual NSGCT masses due to the occasional presence of inflammatory necrosis in a nonviable tumor mass (Fig. 27.4). In our experience, the mediastinal residual lesions have shown more false positive PET results than in the retroperitoneum (Fig. 27.5). However, the precise etiology for this observation is not clear.

For patients without residual masses, assessment of residual viable neoplasm is also important as surgical resection of solitary or limited tumor sites may be performed. One third of patients with NSGCT will have residual viable tumor in retroperitoneal lymph nodes after initial chemotherapy [19]. Elevated tumor markers can be used to identify patients with residual disease or relapse, but the extent of recurrent disease and precise location of residual neoplasm is required to guide further treatment. Based on our experience and that of others [17, 20], PET, and in particular PET-CT, can outperform CT alone for the identification of residual or recurrent tumor deposits. The registered and aligned images generated by PET-CT permits localization of very small deposits of recurrent neoplasm such as nonenlarged lymph nodes (Fig. 27.6). If the PET-CT scan is negative in the setting of elevated serum markers, some limited studies and our own experience have shown that a recommendation to perform a repeat scan in 1–3 months time allowing the recurrent tumor time to reach sufficient size as to be detectable on FDG PET is useful (Fig. 27.7).

Overall in the setting of restaging, FDG PET was shown by Hain and coworkers to effect patient management in 57% of 55 treated patients presenting with residual masses or elevated serum markers [17]. Becherer and coworkers also showed improved accuracy by FDG PET versus CT alone in the detection of residual or recurrent disease [20]. To date, no comparable studies have been performed with PET-CT, but the expectations are higher, and it appears that at least in patients with abnormal serum markers or residual masses, PET-CT would be the preferred imaging study.

Important pitfalls in PET-CT of testicular cancer include residual masses in the setting of NSGCT tumors, which as

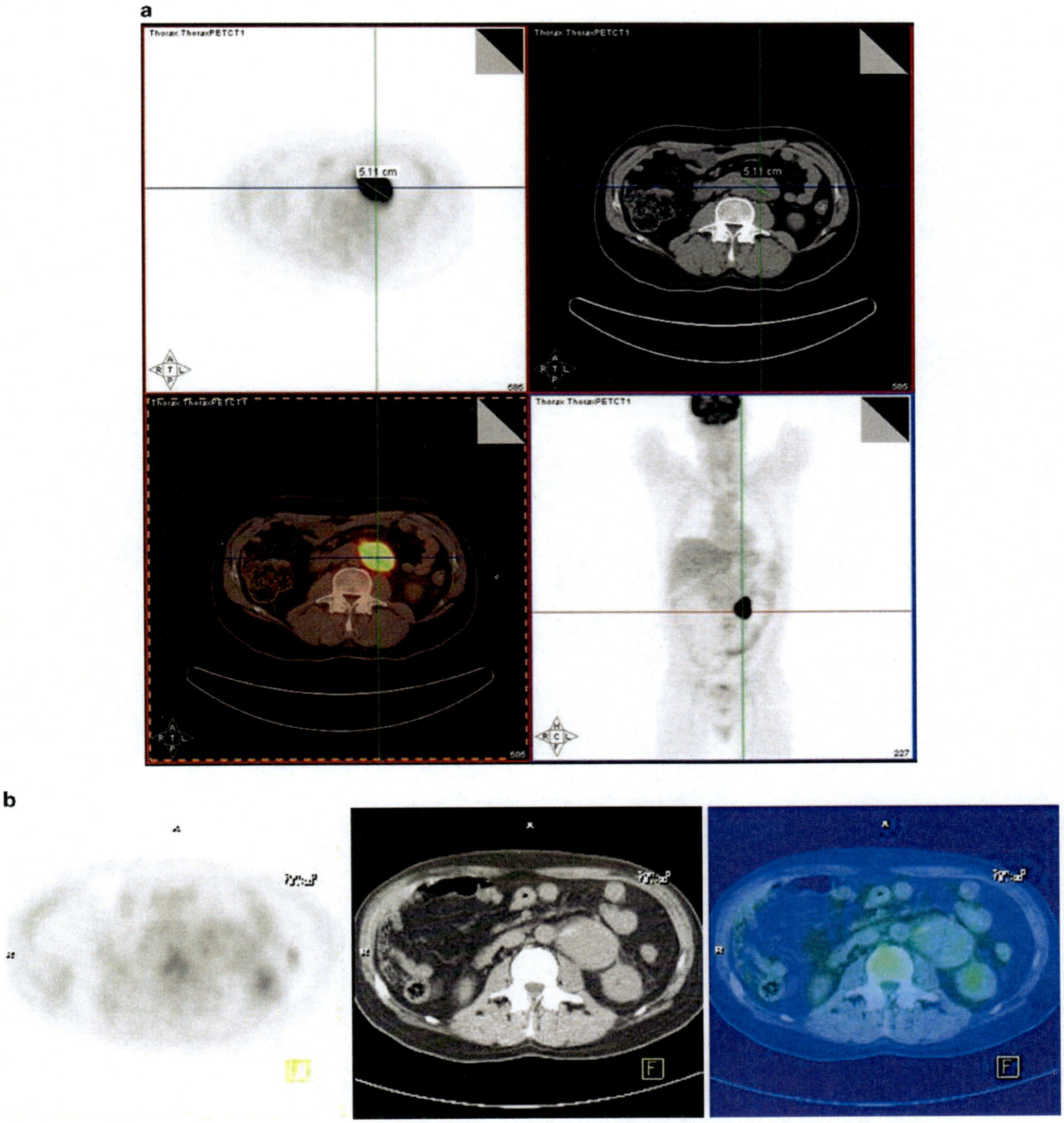

Fig. 27.3 Retroperitoneal masses. On the transaxial FDG PET, CT, FDG PET-CT fusion image, and whole torso coronal FDG PET (**a**) a left paraaortic mass is seen to be associated with intense abnormal FDG tracer uptake corresponding to a residual viable seminoma metastasis. In a different patient transaxial FDG PET, CT and FDG PET-CT fusion images (**b**) show a left paraaortic mass associated with FDG tracer activity no greater than soft tissue background corresponding to scar tissue

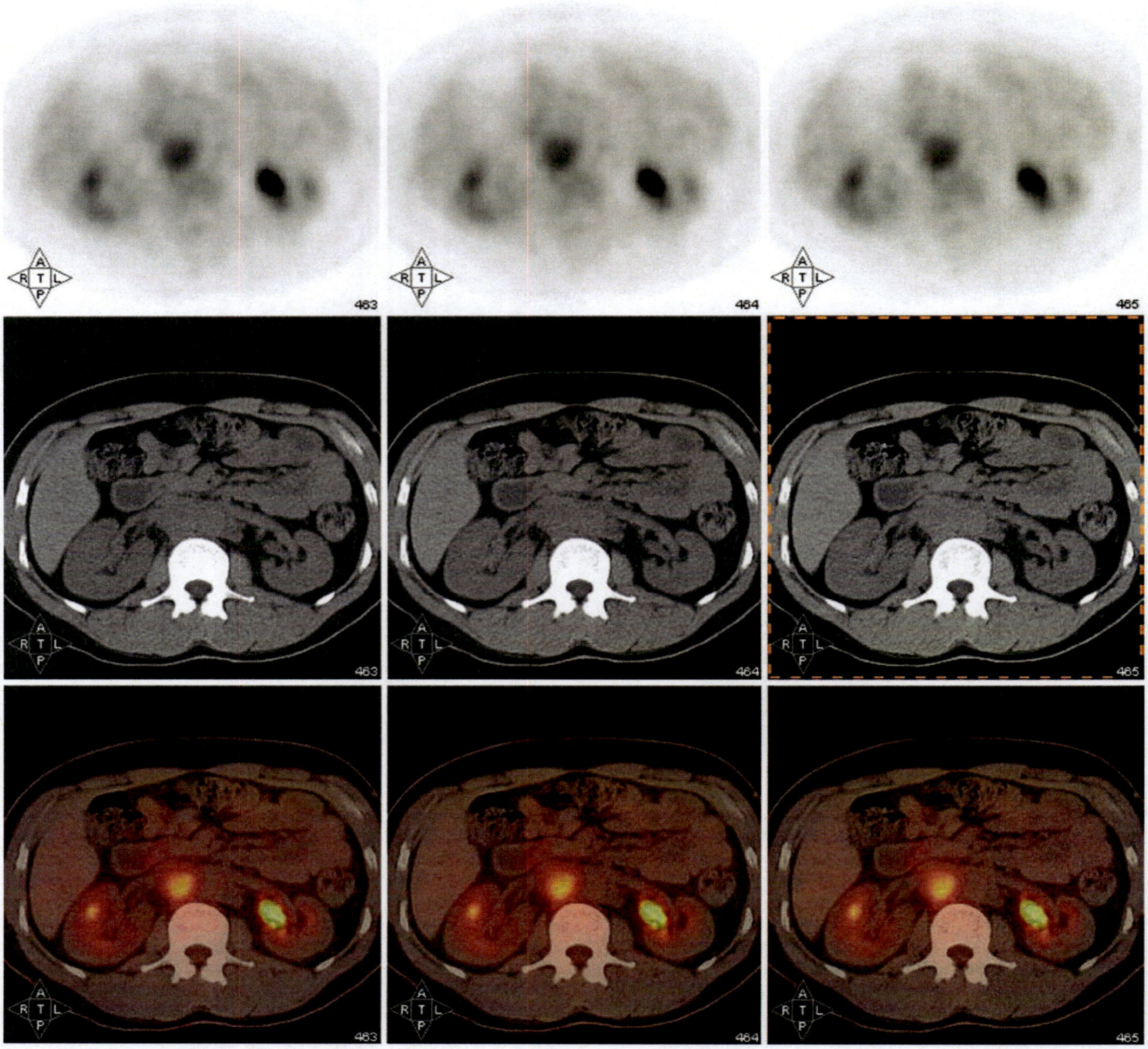

Fig. 27.4 False positive retroperitoneal node due to necrosis. Patient with rising serum markers and residual retroperitoneal lymphadenopathy following treatment. Sequential transaxial CT, FDG PET, and FDG PET-CT fusion images reveal moderately abnormal FDG tracer activity in a retrocaval lymph node mass, which on resection proved to contain only inflammatory necrotic tissue and no neoplasm

noted above, may contain teratomatous elements yet demonstrate no abnormal FDG tracer uptake. Also as noted above, when restaging a patient with NSGCT, residual masses can exhibit increased glucose metabolism due to inflammatory necrosis, and the necrotic feature may not be evident on morphologic imaging. Due to the possibility of suppression FDG tracer uptake in viable germ cell neoplasm during or shortly after chemotherapy, posttherapy restaging PET-CT should be performed a minimum of 2 weeks after therapy, with an optimal 4–12 week hiatus.

In reporting PET-CT exam for testicular cancer, the original histological diagnosis and treatment history is especially important. For instance, if there were known teratomatous elements and the indication was followup of a residual mass, then perhaps more diagnostic weight might be placed comparing the serial size of the residual

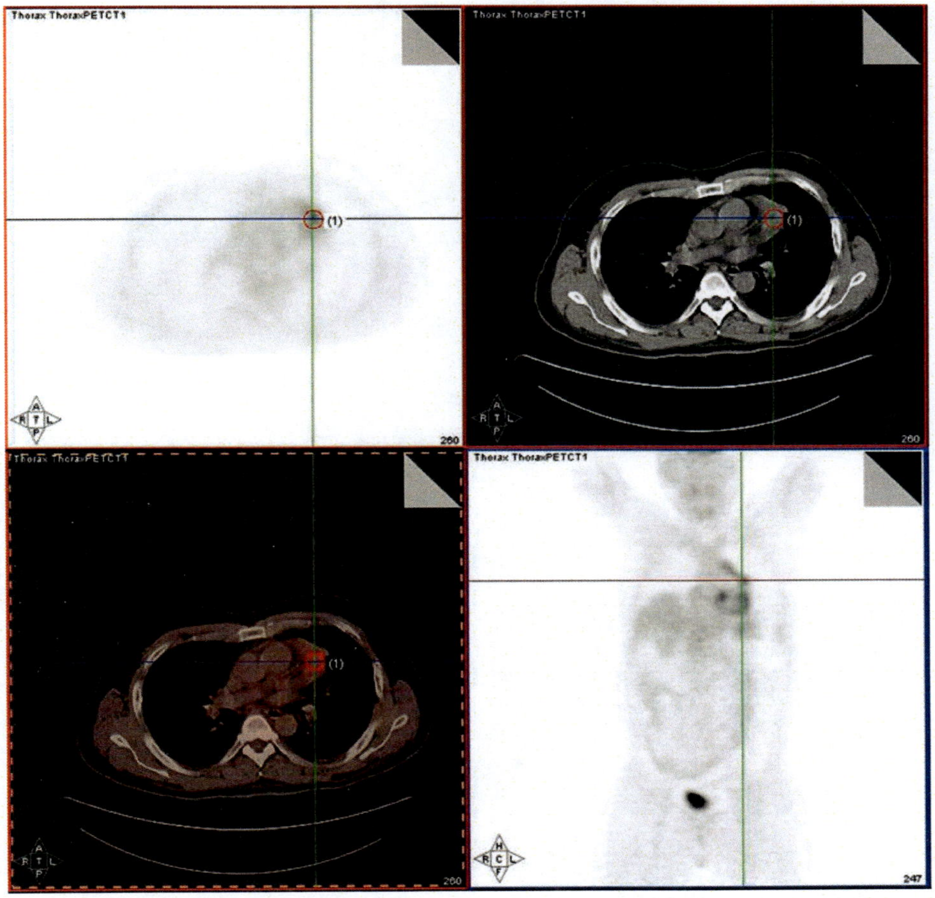

Fig. 27.5 False positive mediastinal mass. PET-CT performed 4 months post chemotherapy for residual mediastinal mass. Transaxial FDG PET, CT, and FDG PET-CT fusion images and whole torso FDG PET coronal image demonstrates moderately abnormal FDG tracer activity in the left mediastinum corresponding to a left prevascular space soft tissue mass. On resection only xanthogranulomatous inflammatory changes were found

mass or enhancement pattern on the CT component of the PET-CT, since the absence of abnormal glucose metabolism does not exclude the presence of teratomatous elements. In any case, if it is known there were teratomatous elements in the original histopathologic diagnosis, a caveat in the report concerning the likelihood of a false negative result and the importance of serial CT follow up should be included. In the case of positive and rising serum tumor markers, it is important to recommend the appropriate interval prior to the follow up PET-CT scan (1–3 months). As noted above, knowledge of the time elapsed since the last therapy and the scan is crucial for optimal patient scheduling; often the follow up scan is performed too early and this may lead to false negative FDG PET results. As with other cancers, FDG PET can neither reliably differentiate between a malignant neoplasm and a reactive enlarged inflammatory node nor between a small node involved by tumor and a non-enlarged benign node, and morphologic changes (chiefly size) on serial CT should always be included in the report.

Therapy Monitoring of Testicular Cancer with PET-CT

The application of FDG-PET for therapy monitoring of testicular cancer has only been minimally evaluated. Therapy monitoring using changes in glucose metabolism would be most helpful clinically in early prediction of treatment response for high-dose salvage chemotherapy. This group consists of patients who have relapsed with other regimens and are now being offered high dose chemotherapy with autologous bone marrow transplant/stem cell support. This

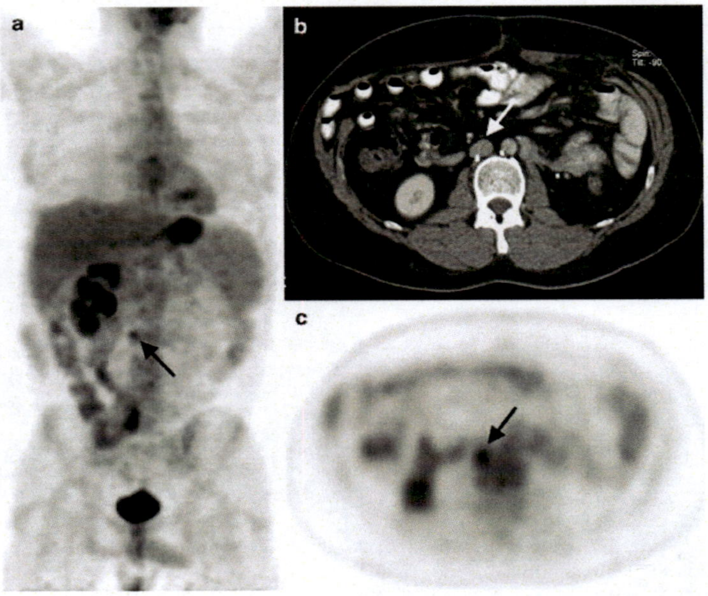

Fig. 27.6 Isolated recurrent metastasis. Mixed, primarily embryonal cell, testicular cancer diagnosed 9 years prior with prior treated recurrences. PET-CT performed for rising serum marker (alpha-fetoprotein). Anterior FDG PET MIP image (**a**) shows only a single small focus of abnormal FDG tracer activity in the mid abdomen projecting at the right margin of the spine (*arrow*). Transaxial CT and FDG PET images (**b**, **c**) reveal the small focus of intense abnormal FDG tracer activity corresponds to 4 mm soft tissue adjacent to a surgical clip (from the original retroperitoneal lymph node dissection), reflecting a retrocaval recurrent lymph node metastasis (*arrowhead*)

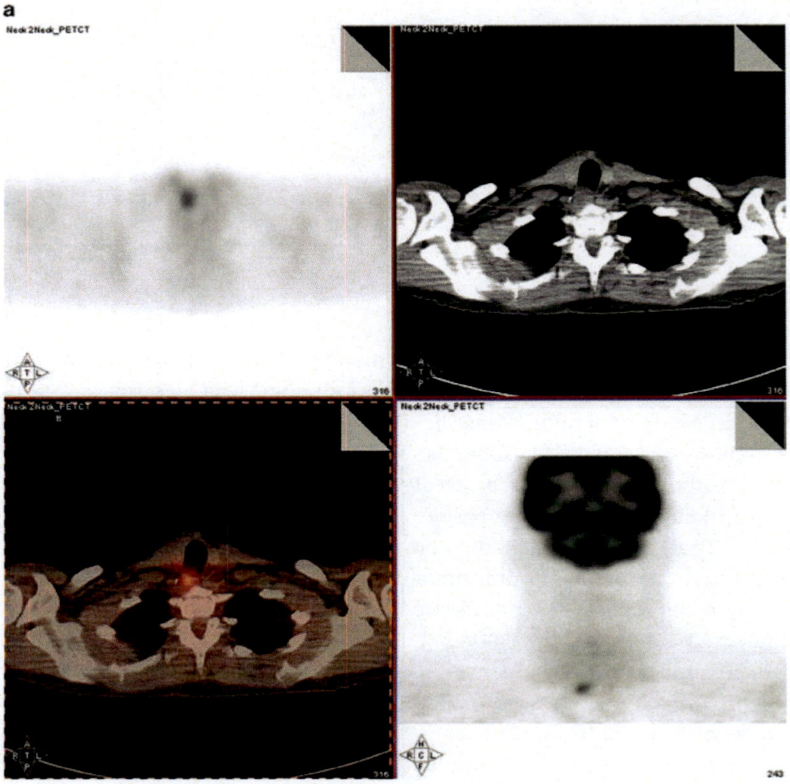

Fig. 27.7 Restaging for rising serum markers. Subtle high paratracheal FDG tracer uptake, shown on (*clockwise*) transaxial FDG PET, CT, FDG PET-CT fusion and coronal FDG PET images (**a**). Surgical exploration found no corresponding neoplasm. Repeat PET-CT scan performed 2 months later revealed two foci of moderately intense abnormal FDG tracer uptake corresponding to high paratracheal lymph nodes shown on transaxial FDG PET, CT, FDG PET and PET-CT fusion images (**b**), which on surgical exploration were positive for neoplasm

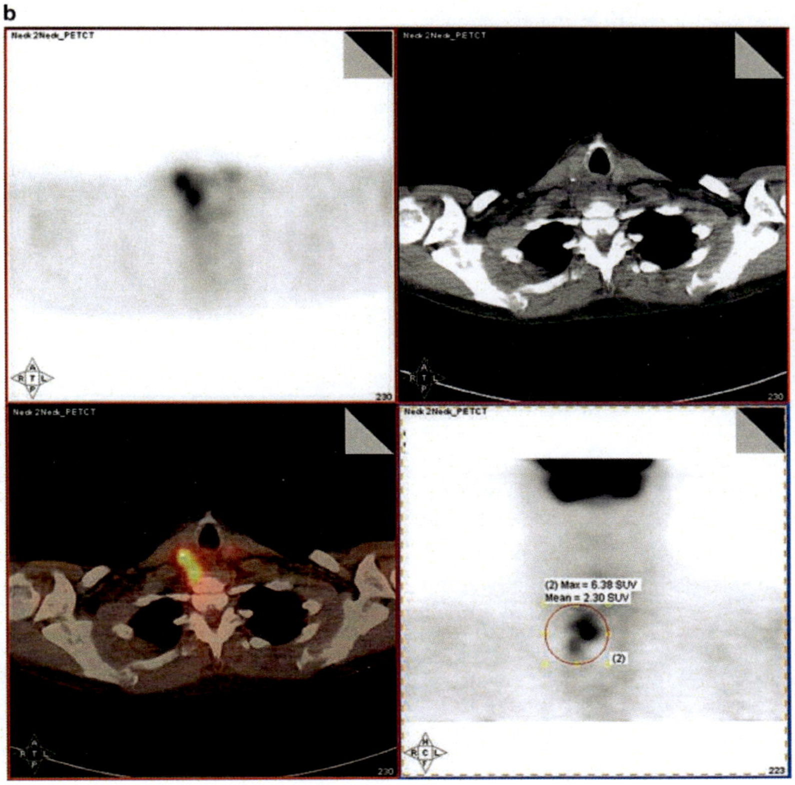

Fig. 27.7 (continued)

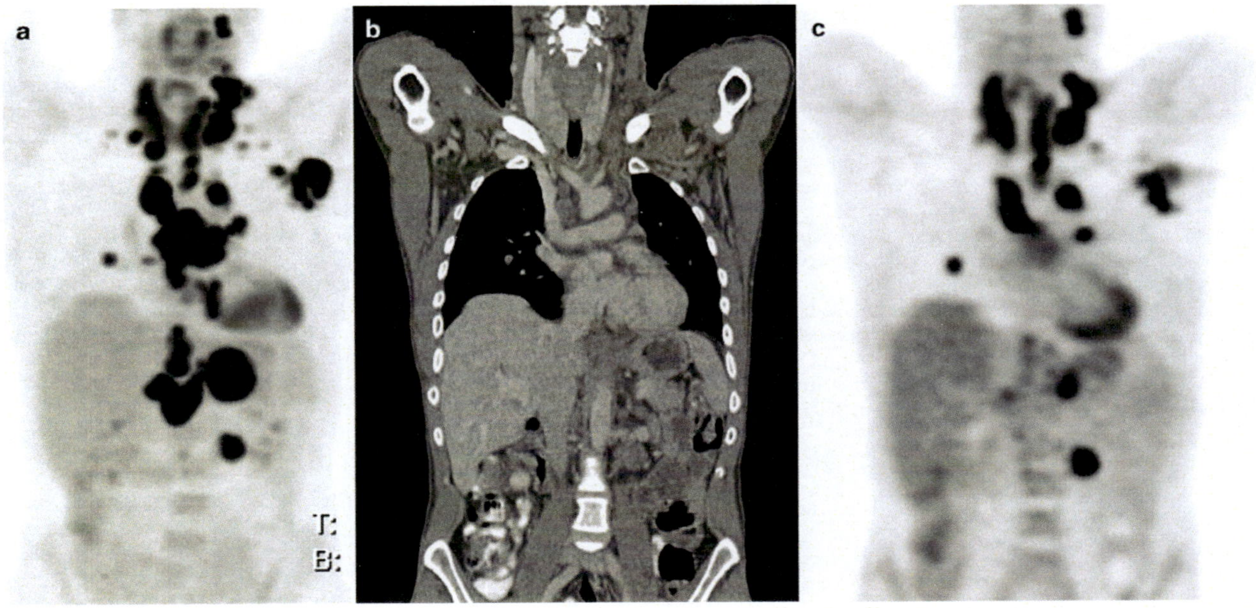

Fig. 27.8 NSGCT, poorly differentiated testicular cancer, following 3 cycles of chemotherapy. Anterior FDG PET MIP image (**a**) demonstrates extensive intense abnormal FDG tracer uptake at multiple sites including retroperitoneal, mediastinal, supraclavicular, lower cervical, and left axillary lymphadenopathy, as well as a small pulmonary and large left hepatic lobe metastasis. Coronal CT and FDG PET images (**b**, **c**) demonstrate the extensive retroperitoneal, mediastinal, cervical, and left axillary FDG avid lymphadenopathy and the isolated pulmonary metastasis. The persistent intense abnormal glucose metabolism in the metastatic lesions predicts a poor prognosis

therapy is suggested to have only a ~15% benefit and is expensive and toxic. Therefore it would be useful to be able to better predict during the induction phase those who would benefit from the therapy (Fig. 27.8). In one study FDG PET alone was shown to have a good level of accuracy in predicting responders compared to tumor marker decline and conventional imaging [21].

Radiation Therapy Planning for Testicular Cancer with PET-CT

As of yet, FDG PET or PET-CT scanning is not formally included into the initial staging of testicular cancers, and in particular Seminoma's. Therefore the possible improvement in radiation therapy planning based on PET-CT data has not been evaluated. Given the likelihood that the addition of FDG PET detection of metastases to nonenlarged lymph nodes may influence the extent of the treatment field; however, PET-CT may ultimately play a role in radiation therapy planning for testicular cancer.

References

1. Mead GM. Testes. In: Price P and Sikora K (eds.). Treatment of Cancer, 3rd edn. London: Chapman Hall, 1995, pp. 627–645.
2. Jones RH, Vasey PA. Part 1: Testicular cancer – management of early disease. Lancet Oncol 2003;4:730–737.
3. Einhorn LH, Williams SD, Troner M, et al. The role of maintenance therapy in disseminated testicular cancer. NEJM 1981;305:727–731.
4. Donohue JP, Thornhill JA, Foster RS, et al. Primary retroperitoneal lymph dissection in clinical stage A nonseminomatous germ cell testis cancer: a review of the Indiana University experience (196–1989). Br J Urol 1993;71:326–335.
5. Hartmann JT, Nicohls CR, Droz JP, et al. Prognostic variables for response and outcome in patients with extragonadal germ-cell tumors. Ann Oncol 2002;13(7):1017–1028.
6. Lassen U, Daugaard G, Eigtved A, et al. Whole-body FDG-PET in patients with stage 1 non-seminomatous germ cell tumours. Eur J Nucl Med 2003;30:396–402.
7. Richter E, Feyerabend T, Bondorf W (eds.). Normal Lymph Node Topography: CT Atlas. New York: Springer, 2004.
8. Albers P, Bender H, Yilmaz H, Schoeneich G, Biersack HJ, Mueller SC. Positron emission tomography in the clinical staging of patients with Stage 1 and II testicular germ cell tumors. Urology 1999;53:808–811.
9. Hain SF, O'Doherty MJ, Timothy AR, et al. Fluorodeoxyglucose PET in the initial staging of germ cell tumours, Eur J Nucl Med 2002;27:590–594.
10. Spermon JR, D Geus-Oei LF, Kiemeney LALM, et al. The role of ^{18}Fluoro-2-Deoxyglucose positron emission tomography in initial staging and re-staging after chemotherapy for testicular germ cell tumours, BJU Int 2002;89:549–556.
11. Pue HS, Heelen R, Mazumdar M, et al. Management of residual mass in advanced seminoma: results and recommendations from the Memorial Sloan-Kettering Cancer Center. J Clin Oncol 1996;14:454–460.
12. Schultz SM, Einhorn LH, Concer DJ, et al. Management of post chemotherapy residual mass in patients with advanced seminoma: Indiana University experience. J Clin Oncol 1989;7:1497–1503.
13. Steyerberg EW, Keizer HJ, Sleijfer DT, et al. Retroperitoneal metastases in testicular cancer: role of CT measurements of residual masses in decision making for resection after chemotherapy. Radiology 2000;215:437–444.
14. De Santis M, Bokemeyer C, Becherer A, et al. Predictive impact of 2-18fluoro-2-deoxy-D-glucose positron emission tomography for residual post chemotherapy masses in patients with bulky seminoma. J Clin Oncol 2001;19:3740–3744.
15. De Santis M, Becherer A, Bokemeyer C. 2-18fluoro-deoxy-D-glucose positron emission tomography is a reliable predictor for viable tumor in postchemotherapy seminoma: an update of the prospective multicenter SEMPET trail. J Clin Oncol 2004;22:1034–1039.
16. Cremerius U, Wildberger JE, Borchers H, Zimny M, Jakse G, Bunther RW, Buell U. Does positron emission tomography using 18-fluoro-2-deoxyglucose improve clinical staging of testicular cancer?- Results of a study of 50 patients. Urology 1999;54:900–904.
17. Hain SF, O'Doherty JM, Timothy AR, Leslie MD, Harper PG, Huddart RA. Fluorodeoxyglucose positron emission tomography in the evaluation of germ cell tumours at relapse. Br J Cancer 2000;83:863–869.
18. Sugarwara Y, Zasadny KR, Grossman HB, et al. Germ cell tumor: differentiation of viable tumor, mature teratoma, and necrotic tissue with FDG PET and kinetic modeling. Radiology 1999;211:249–256.
19. Oldenburg J, Alfsen C, Lien HH, Aass N, Waehre H, Fossa SD. Postchemotherapy retroperitoneal surgery remains necessary in patients with nonseminomatous testicular cancer and minimal residual tumor masses. J Clin Oncol 2003;21:3310–3317.
20. Becherer A, De Santis M, Karanikas G, et al. FDG PET is superior to CT in the prediction of viable tumour in post-chemotherapy seminoma residuals. Eur J Radiol 2005;54(2):284–288.
21. Bokemeyer C, Kollmannsberger C, Oechsle K, et al. Early prediction of treatment response to high-dose salvage chemotherapy in patients with relapsed germ cell tumors using [18F]FDG PET. Br J Cancer 2002;86:506–511.

Chapter 28
PET-CT in Pediatric Malignancies

Joseph J. Junewick and Paul Shreve

Virtually every imaging strategy for children has been adapted from adults and PET-CT is no different. Many of the pediatric applications of PET-CT have been inferred from the success of FDG PET and PET-CT in adults. Other than the overlap with certain adult malignancies, there have been very few PET clinical trials in pediatric oncology. Consequently, integration of PET-CT into pediatric oncology imaging algorithms has been slow, but continues to advance.

The slow adoption of PET-CT into pediatric oncology imaging algorithms is due to several factors: (1) Dedicated in-house PET-CT scanners are not widely available at pediatric centers. (2) While costs have decreased and some examinations are increasingly covered by insurance, adding an additional expensive imaging procedure to existing imaging algorithms is seem by payers as adding to overall costs. (3) Due to the relative rarity of many pediatric tumors, much of the experience with PET and PET-CT has been anecdotal. (4) Management of the developmental and psychosocial needs of children in the scanner requires special skills of the technologists and nurses and modification of imaging procedure and technical parameters. (5) As with the introduction of other new imaging techniques in pediatrics, it takes time before the imaging technique is incorporated in the patient care protocols, safety margins are assured, and protocols are adapted for children.

The potential of PET-CT to direct management in pediatric oncology is enormous [1–4]. PET-CT provides greater diagnostic information than conventional imaging for non-CNS malignancies [2, 4]. Initial experience suggests that PET is useful to assess residual post-therapeutic masses regardless of the type of neoplasm [3, 5]. Unfortunately, pediatric PET-CT lacks the same degree of validation as adult PET-CT. As a result, this chapter varies somewhat from others in this text. The emphasis will be placed on developing an understanding of various pediatric malignancies; to the extent possible, the influence of PET-CT on the diagnosis, staging/restaging, treatment planning, and treatment response will be discussed.

Lymphoma

Lymphoma (Hodgkin's disease and non-Hodgkin's lymphoma) is a neoplastic proliferation of immune cells and represents the third most common pediatric malignancy. While lymphoma is not just a pediatric disease, there are unique features of the disease in the pediatric population, presumably because of the age-related differences in the immune system and unique considerations related to treatment.

Hodgkin's Disease

Hodgkin's disease has a bimodal incidence with one age peak in adolescence and young adulthood and the other in late adulthood. Hodgkin's disease is rare in children less than 5 years of age. Under the age of 10 years, males are more commonly affected, whereas in adolescence males and females are equally affected. Patients most often present with painless cervical or supraclavicular adenopathy. The mediastinum is involved at diagnosis in nearly two thirds of patients. There are several subtypes of Hodgkin's disease with the nodular sclerosing histologic subtype being the most common, followed by mixed cellularity, lymphocyte predominance, and others. Histology predicts sites of involvement, stage, comorbid conditions, and clinical course.

Hodgkin's disease usually spreads in a contiguous lymphatic pattern (Fig. 28.1). Extranodal dissemination (typically stage IV) occurs as a result of direct extension or hematogenous spread, with the lung, liver, bones and bone marrow being the most common sites. Staging for Hodgkin's

J.J. Junewick (✉)
Department of Radiology, Spectrum Health Hospitals, Helen de Vos Children's Hospital, Grand Rapids, MI, USA
and
Michigan State University College of Human Medicine, Grand Rapids, MI, USA
e-mail: jjunewick@advancedrad.com

P. Shreve and D.W. Townsend (eds.), *Clinical PET-CT in Radiology: Integrated Imaging in Oncology*,
DOI 10.1007/978-0-387-48902-5_28, © Springer Science+Business Media, LLC 2011

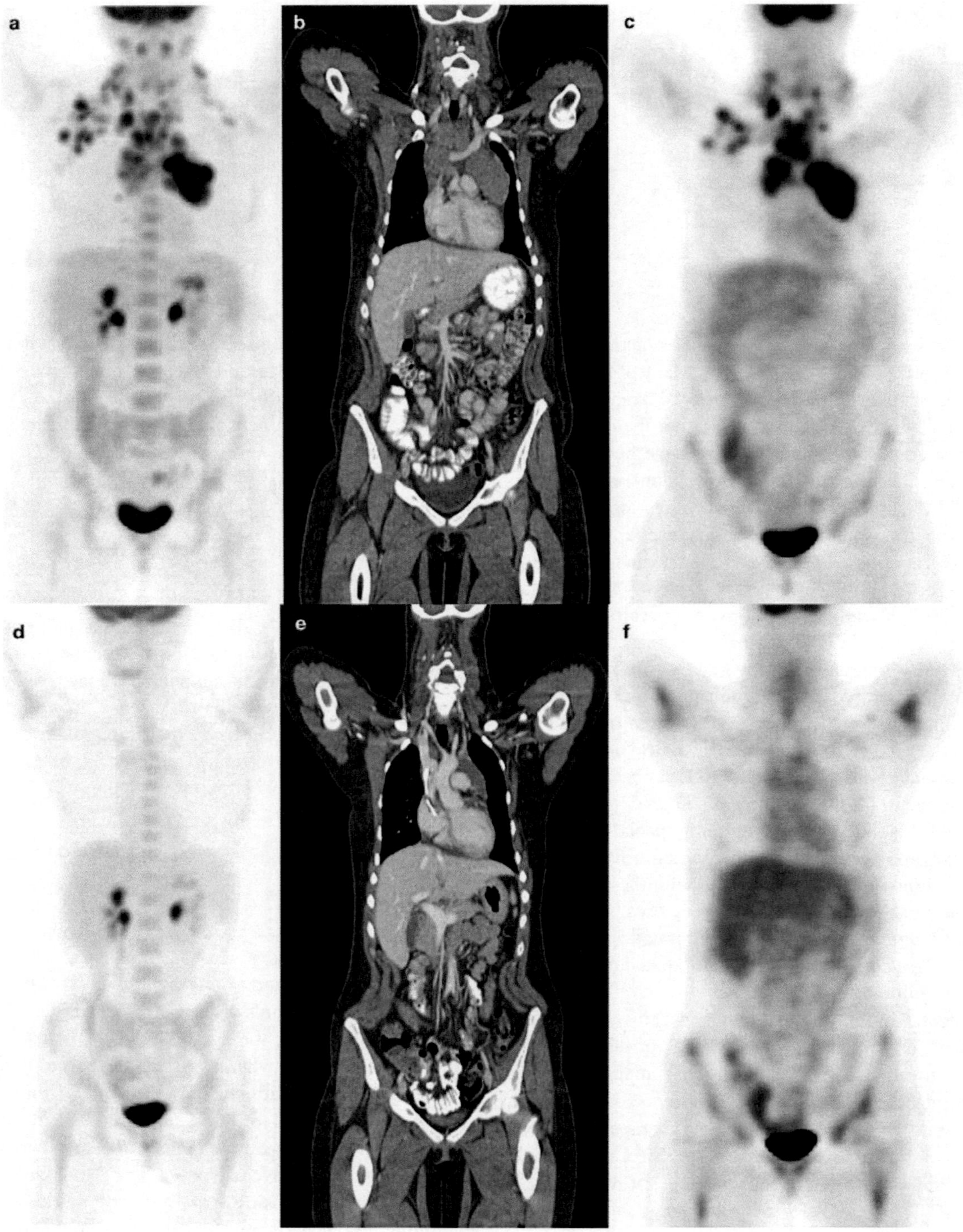

Fig. 28.1 Classic Hodgkin's lymphoma at presentation and following completion of chemotherapy. Anterior maximum intensity projection image (*MIP*) intensely FDG avid bulky lymphadenopathy in the mediastinum with additional FDG avid lymph nodes in the supraclavicular and right deep axially nodal basins (**a**). Coronal CT (**b**) and FDG PET (**c**) image reconstructions demonstrate the bulky lymphadenopathy. On the posttherapy anterior MIP image there is no abnormal FDG activity in the thorax or neck (**d**). Coronal CT (**e**) shows residual soft tissue in the left mediastinum AP window and right mediastinum between the superior vena cava and right brachiocephalic artery, which is completely without FDG tracer uptake on the PET image (**f**), consistent with residual scar tissue

disease is based on clinical and imaging evaluations. Clinical parameters include physical examination, sedimentation rate, liver function tests, and bone marrow aspiration and biopsy. Bone marrow aspiration and biopsy are performed in patients with stage III or IV disease or in patients exhibiting "B" symptoms (fever, night sweats, or weight loss). Imaging evaluation includes chest radiography, CT and/or MR examinations, Gallium-67 or FDG PET scan, and occasionally whole body bone scan. CT and MR examinations predominantly determine anatomic extent of disease based on enlarged lymph nodes and evidence of visceral infiltration. FDG PET is now the preferred modality to assess metabolic activity although Gallium-67 scanning currently remains an acceptable alternative. Chest radiography remains an important method to assess for the presence of bulky disease (mediastinal mass >33% of the transverse diameter of the chest at the level of the diaphragm), although this can also be achieved by CT. Bone scan may be necessary if there is bone pain or an elevated alkaline phosphatase level. The Ann Arbor classification is most commonly used for staging on Hodgkin's disease (Table 28.1).

Treatment strategies for Hodgkin's disease are determined based on risk. Low-risk disease represents stage I or IIA with no bulky lymphadenopathy or B symptoms. High-risk disease is stage III and IV with B symptoms, and intermediate-risk disease is composed of all other stages. Most pediatric patients with Hodgkin's disease receive combined chemotherapy as initial treatment. Chemotherapy is tailored based on risk stratification to minimize known long-term side effects, which include diminished fertility, leukemia, pulmonary fibrosis, and cardiovascular damage. Radiation therapy (treatment volume and radiation dose) is usually protocol-specific. If radiation therapy is utilized in the treatment protocol it is usually low-dose-involved field radiation therapy, because growth disturbance, breast vulnerability, and cardiovascular complications are associated with standard dose radiation therapy. High-dose chemotherapy with autologous or allogenic bone marrow transplantation may be used for refractory disease. The goal of treatment is complete response; any other outcome is considered a failure.

Table 28.1 Hodgkin's disease staging (Ann Arbor system)

Stage	Definition
I	Involvement of a single lymph node group or localized involvement of an extralymphatic organ
II	Involvement of more than one lymph node group or localized involvement of an extralymphatic organ on the same side of the diaphragm
III	Involvement of more than one lymph node group on both sides of the diaphragm with or without localized involvement of an extralymphatic organ
IV	Diffuse involvement of one or more extralymphatic organs with or without lymph node involvement

Fever, night sweats, and weight loss indicate "B" symptoms; lack of these symptoms represents "A" symptoms

Lymph node group refers to anatomically defined lymph node clusters or lymphatic organs (thymus or spleen). Subdiaphragmatic involvement or bulky disease (mass larger than 10 cm or greater than one third the diameter of the chest) has negative prognostic implications. Direct extension of adjacent adenopathy to an organ is not considered extranodal organ involvement

Non-Hodgkin's Lymphoma

Pediatric non-Hodgkin's lymphoma is usually high grade and of the small noncleaved cell type (Burkitt's lymphoma), lymphoblastic lymphoma, or large cell lymphoma. Multiple sites of involvement are common in Burkitt's lymphoma. An abdominal mass (Fig. 28.2) is the most common presentation followed by a jaw mass (endemic Burkitt's). Bone marrow, central nervous system, lymph node, pleura, and paraspinous involvement occur less frequently. A mediastinal mass is the most common presentation in patients with lymphoblastic lymphoma. If there are other sites of involvement, they tend to be supradiaphragmatic. Large cell lymphomas may involve the mediastinum but otherwise have similar distribution to Burkitt's lymphomas.

Tumor burden at diagnosis, central nervous system involvement, and bone marrow involvement are the major prognostic indicators. Tumor burden may be at least partially quantifiable by evaluating tumor breakdown products such as LDH, uric acid, lactic acid, and others. The St. Jude staging system is the most often used and parallels the Ann Arbor system for Hodgkin's disease with the following distinctions: (1) A primary gastrointestinal tumor with or without mesenteric adenopathy is Stage II. (2) Extensive intraabdominal or paraspinal primary disease is Stage III. (3) Bone marrow or CNS involvement is Stage IV. The Children's Oncology Group segregates between limited and extensive disease, corresponding respectively to Stage I/II and Stage III/IV of the St. Jude system. The St. Jude Staging system is summarized in Table 28.2.

Children with non-Hodgkin's lymphoma tend to have advanced stage disease and a high incidence of bone marrow and central nervous system involvement. Despite this, more than 70% will survive beyond 5 years. Patients with single abdominal organ or isolated bone disease have a survival rate of about 90%; whereas patients with extensive intrathoracic, bone marrow, or abdominal disease or central nervous system disease have a lower survival rate. Accurate initial staging is probably the most important factor in determining the optimal therapy and consequently patient outcome. Systemic chemotherapy regimens differ depending upon the specific type of non-Hodgkin's lymphoma. Intrathecal chemotherapy and neuroaxis irradiation are administered to prevent and treat central nervous system disease.

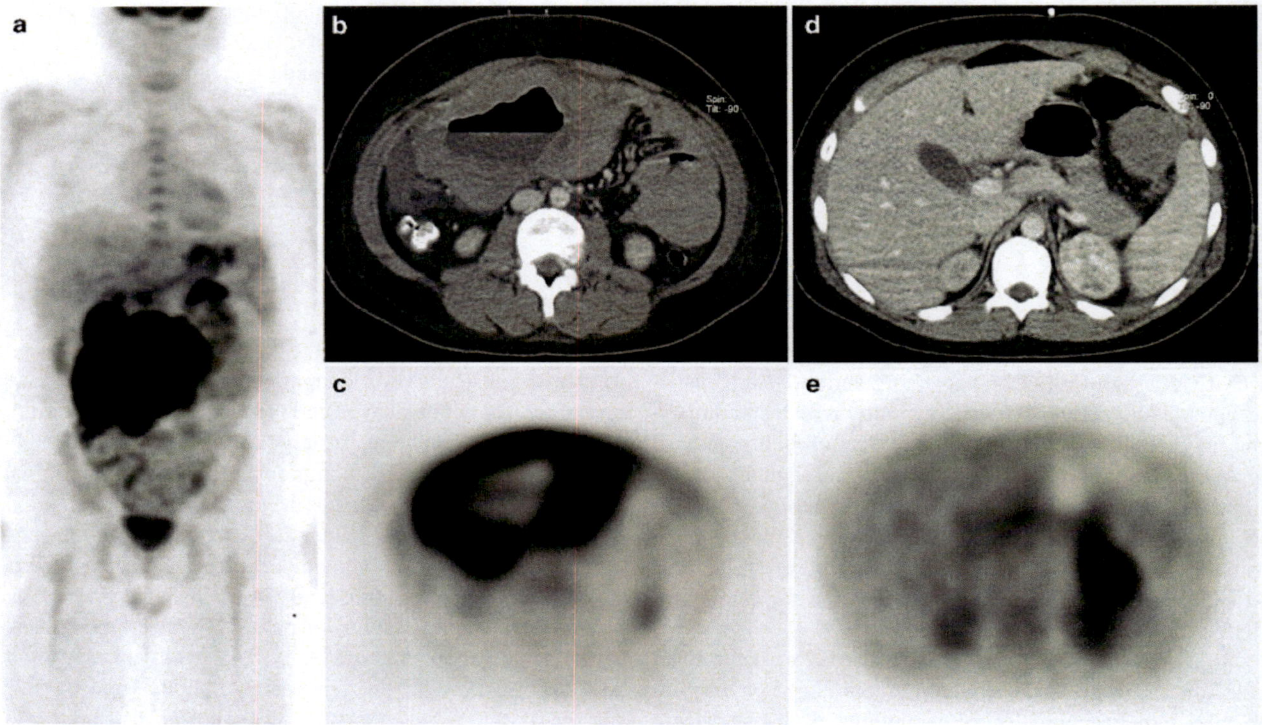

Fig. 28.2 Burkitt's lymphoma presenting as abdominal mass. Whole body anterior FDG PET MIP image (**a**) shows a large highly FDG avid mass in the mid abdomen with separate foci of abnormal FDG uptake in the left upper abdomen. Transaxial CT (**b**) and FDG PET (**c**) images show a large mass in the mid abdomen with central necrosis that is intensely FDG avid. A separate FDG avid mass (CT **d**, FDG PET **e**) involves the pancreatic tail

Table 28.2 Non-Hodgkin lymphoma staging (modified St. Jude)

Stage	Description
I	A single tumor or lymph node group (not involving the mediastinum or abdomen)
II	Either a single tumor with regional nodal involvement, two or more nodal groups on the same side of the diaphragm, or a primary gastrointestinal tumor (with or without regional nodal involvement) which is completely resected
III	Either involvement of nodal groups on both sides of the diaphragm, any primary intrathoracic tumor, extensive intraabdominal disease, paraspinal disease, or epidural disease
IV	Bone marrow involvement or central nervous system involvement

PET-CT increasingly plays an integral role in the initial staging of lymphomas. The combined anatomic and metabolic assessment of disease significantly improves the accuracy of staging, especially in non-Hodgkin's lymphomas where tumor distribution is less predictable [6, 7]. Response to therapy has strong prognostic importance in pediatric lymphomas and dictates duration of chemotherapy. Lymphomas usually respond well to treatment and dramatically decrease in size. Residual mass in lymphoma, however, is very common, especially with nodular sclerosing type Hodgkin's disease, and PET-CT allows differentiation of viable from sterilized residual neoplasm (see Fig. 28.1). Knowledge of viable residual tumor allows early modification of the treatment regimen before relapse is becomes evident on the basis of increasing size of a residual mass [6–10]. Radiation therapy is now being meticulously tailored based on initial bulk disease and/or areas of residual metabolic activity of disease depicted on PET-CT to decrease in treatment volume and patient exposure. Residual FDG tracer avidity after completion of treatment (Fig. 28.3) has a high predictive value for relapse of lymphoma and a negative PET-CT strongly correlates with absent disease [6, 10].

Rhabdomyosarcoma

Rhabdomyosarcoma is the most common soft tissue sarcoma in childhood. Its clinical, biologic and pathologic characteristics vary considerably. Rhabdomyosarcoma is almost exclusively a pediatric malignancy; the adult counterpart is malignant fibrous histiocytoma. Occurrence is bimodal, with are two age peaks: 2–6 years (usually head and neck and genitourinary tract sites) and 15–19 years (usually extremity, trunk, and paratesticular sites).

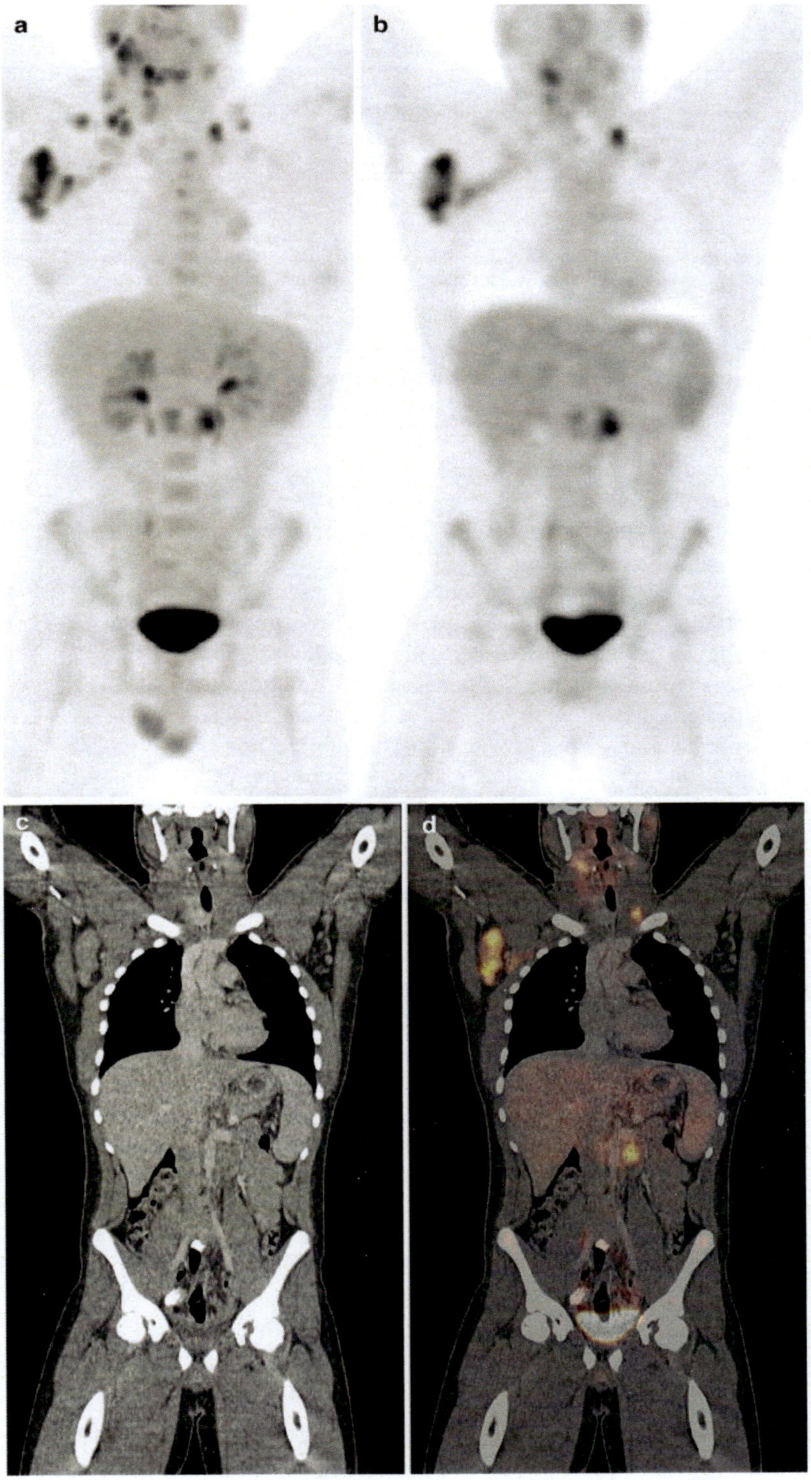

Fig. 28.3 Residual viable disease after treatment of non-Hodgkin's lymphoma. Whole torso anterior FDG PET MIP image (**a**) shows multiple foci of nodal lymphoma above and below diaphragm. The posttreatment coronal FDG PET (**b**), CT (**c**), and PET-CT fusion image (**d**) demonstrate residual right axillary lymphadenopathy remains FDG avid as well as FDG uptake in a nonenlarged left supraclavicular node and a left paraaortic node

Rhabdomyosarcoma derives from primitive mesenchymal cells which demonstrate muscle differentiation on histologic, immunochemical, or electron microscopic evaluation. There are four histologic types in decreasing order of frequency: embryonal, alveolar, undifferentiated, and botryoidal. Each of these types may predict the location and prognosis. The embryonal type predominantly involves the head and neck and the genitourinary tract and has an intermediate prognosis.

Table 28.3 Pretreatment rhabdomyosarcoma staging

Stage	Sites	Tumor (T)	Size	Nodes (N)	Metastasis (M)
I	Orbit, head and neck(excluding parameningeal), GU (non bladder, nonprostate)	T1 or T2	a or b	N0, N1, or Nx	M0
II	Bladder/prostate, extremity, cranial, parameningeal	T1 or T2	a	N0 or Nx	M0
III	Bladder/prostate, extremity, cranial, parameningeal	T1 or T2	a	N1	M0
			b	N0, N1, Nx	
IV	All	T1 or T2	a or b	N0 or N1	M1

T1 is confined to site of origin. T2 extends beyond site of origin and/or is fixed to adjacent tissues. Size less than or equal to 5 cm is "a" and greater than 5 cm is "b." N0 indicates region lymph nodes are not involved, whereas N1 indicates neoplastic involvement and Nx indicates unknown clinical status

The undifferentiated and alveolar types tend to affect the extremities and have a poor prognosis. The botryoid type usually involves the urinary bladder, vagina, middle ear, or nasopharynx and has a good prognosis.

The head and neck region account for about 28% rhabdomyosarcomas, whereas the extremities account for 24%, the genitourinary tract accounts for 18%, the trunk accounts for 11%, and the orbit accounts for 7%. These tumors grow rapidly and invade adjacent structures and disseminate by lymphatic or hematogenous pathways. Rhabdomyosarcomas, especially of the extremity, trunk and paratesticular locations, present most often as a painless mass. Additionally, orbital lesions present with proptosis and ophthalmoplegia; bladder lesions may present with urinary tract infection or hematuria; uterine and cervical lesions may present with menorrhagia or metrorrhagia; and, vaginal lesions may present with protruding mass or serosanguinous discharge.

Rhabdomyosarcoma most commonly spreads to regional lymph nodes. Paratesticular rhabdomyosarcomas often metastasize to regional lymph nodes, while orbital lesions rarely have nodal metastases, given few lymphatic channels in this region. Less commonly, there is distant spread to the lung, bone, and bone marrow. Treatment failures can either manifest as local or regional recurrence or metastatic disease.

Rhabdomyosarcoma is a curable disease with more than 70% survival at 5 years after the diagnosis. Relapses are uncommon after 5 years although more often with stage III, stage IV disease, or large primary tumors; relapse survival is best with initial low stage and low risk disease. Operative management is the initial treatment of choice, although surgery may be limited by the location and extent of tumor and the desire to preserve function. Hyperfractionated radiation or conventional fractionated radiation is employed for local control when surgery cannot ablate the mass or with infiltrative lesions. Chemotherapy (usually vincristine, dactinomycin, and cyclophosphamide or ifosfamide and etoposide) regimens are continually being refined. Recurrent disease is treated with combination chemotherapy; intensive chemotherapy followed by autologous bone marrow transplantation is also being investigated.

The Intergroup Rhabdomyosarcoma Study (IRS-IV) pretreatment clinical staging is based on TNM classification scheme (Table 28.3). Imaging studies and surgical findings determine the extent of disease. Further, treatment is prescribed by a postsurgical grouping classification (Table 28.4).

Table 28.4 Postsurgical rhabdomyosarcoma staging

Group	Definition
1	Localized disease, completely excised, no microscopic residual
	1A Confined to site of origin, completely resected
	1B Infiltrating beyond site of origin, completely resected
2	Total gross resection
	2A Microscopic residual disease
	2B Regional lymph node involvement; no microscopic residual
	2C Microscopic residual and regional lymph node involvement
3	Incomplete resection or biopsy with gross residual
4	Distant metastasis

Rhabdomyosarcoma and other soft tissue sarcomas have been shown to be FDG avid, and PET-CT is a useful adjunct for initial diagnosis and staging as well as in the detection of recurrent disease [11–14]. On initial staging PET-CT examination, evaluation of size and extension of the primary tumor and the presence of local lymph node spread and metastatic sites is important [11]. On restaging PET-CT examinations, locoregional recurrence is most common; however, pulmonary, osseous, and bone marrow metastatic disease need to be excluded (see Fig. 28.4). PET-CT has been successful in assessing the efficacy of neoadjuvant chemotherapy, with reduction in avidity of greater that 50% in soft tissue sarcomas associated with increased time to recurrence and improved overall survival [14].

Neuroblastoma

Neuroblastoma is the most common extracranial solid neoplasm in childhood. Considered one of the "small round blue cell" tumors, it arises from primitive pluripotent sympathetic cells in neural crests. The three classic histopathologic forms in order of increasing maturation and differentiation (and hence decreasing malignancy) are: neuroblastoma, ganglioneuroblastoma, and ganglioneuroma.

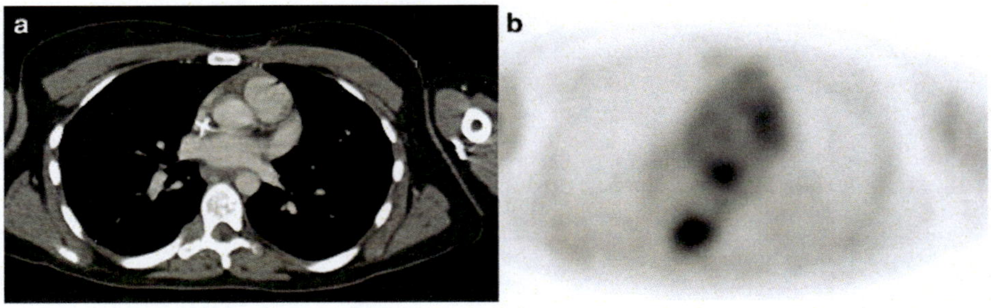

Fig. 28.4 Recurrent rhabdomyosarcoma. Transaxial CT (**a**) and FDG PET (**b**) demonstrate a FDG avid subcarinal lymph node and abnormal FDG avid soft tissue at the right costovertebral junction extending into the spinal canal

Neuroblastoma has an incidence of 10.5 cases per million per year. The average age at diagnosis is 22 months, with 36% occurring before 1 year of age, 79% occurring before 4 years of age, and 97% occurring before 10 years of age. The etiology of neuroblastoma is unknown, but numerous environmental exposures and germinal mutation have been implicated. Neuroblastoma occasionally undergoes spontaneous differentiation and maturation to more benign forms such as ganglioneuroma.

Neuroblastoma can arise anywhere along the sympathetic chain. The abdomen (fairly evenly divided between the adrenal gland and the remainder of the abdominal sympathetic chain) is by far the most common location, accounting for two thirds of cases. The paraspinal (thoracic more than cervical), pelvic, and other regions account for the remainder, in decreasing order. Regional lymph node metastasis occurs in 35% of apparently localized tumors. Lymph node metastasis outside of the body cavity of origin represents disseminated disease. Hematogenous metastases are most common to bone marrow, bone, liver, and skin and infrequently to lung and brain. The incidence of metastatic disease increases with age at diagnosis; disseminated disease occurs in 25% under the age of 1 year and 68% over the age of 1 year.

Pathology and staging are essential to determine therapy and risk group. Numerous staging systems have been employed. While all provided similar prognostic information, the International Neuroblastoma Staging System (Table 28.5) was developed to give uniformity for clinical trials around the world.

Surgery plays an important role in management of neuroblastoma. It establishes the diagnosis, obtains tissue for biologic studies, aids in staging, and attempts excision when possible. Many times a second operation is performed after chemotherapy to assess treatment response and reattempt excision. Chemotherapy is the predominant means of treatment. The goal is to take advantage of drug synergies, targeting noncell cycle and cell cycle-dependent phases. Induction therapy with alkylating agents, platinum compounds, topoisomerase II inhibitors, and vincristine is followed by myeloablative therapy with a combination of alkylators, etoposide and carboplatin. Subsequently, local irradiation to the primary site is added in an effort to prevent local recurrence.

Table 28.5 Neuroblastoma staging

Stage	Definition
1	Tumor confined to organ/region of origin
	Complete gross excision and/or microscopic residual disease
	Microscopically negative lymph nodes not attached to primary tumor
2A	Unilateral tumor with incomplete gross excision
	Microscopically negative lymph nodes not attached to primary tumor
2B	Unilateral tumor with complete or incomplete excision
	Positive ipsilateral lymph nodes
	Microscopically negative contralateral lymph nodes
3	Midline with or without regional lymph node involvement
	Unilateral tumor with contralateral lymph node involvement
	Midline tumor with bilateral lymph node involvement
4	Dissemination to distant lymph nodes and organs
4S	Localized primary tumor (Stage 1 or 2)
	Dissemination limited to skin, bone marrow and/or liver

Anatomic (CT) and metabolic (MIBG) evaluation have been important in the diagnosis and staging of neuroblastoma [15, 16]. Two to three trips to the department (1 for injection and 1–2 for imaging), multiple sedations, iodine drops, and scheduling issues make MIBG scanning inconvenient. Since FDG uptake is directly proportional to tumor burden and cell proliferation, FDG PET as part of PET-CT may substitute for MIBG imaging. It follows then that neuroblastoma patients may benefit from the synergy of PET-CT in initial staging and follow up.

FDG PET imaging has advantages in spatial resolution and in detecting hepatic disease compared to MIBG [17]. FDG also detects more osseous involvement of neuroblastoma than conventional bone scanning. However, FDG PET does not image marrow disease well, and further hematopoietic stimulation used in many chemotherapy regimens can obscure neuroblastoma involvement of bone marrow. Calvarial lesions can be obscured by adjacent brain activity on conventional stand-alone PET, and physiologic activity and inflammation can result in false-positive findings. These deficiencies are largely overcome by concurrent CT. It has been suggested that 18F-FDG PET-CT can be used in conjunction with bone marrow aspiration/biopsy to monitor for recurrent disease after resection of the primary tumor if there is no known skull involvement [17, 19].

Osteosarcoma and Ewing Sarcoma

Osteosarcoma

Osteosarcoma is the most common non-lymphoproliferative malignancy in adolescence. Osteosarcoma derives from bone-forming mesenchymal cells and can differentiate toward fibrous tissue, cartilage, or bone. The presence of osteoid is necessary for the pathologic diagnosis of osteosarcoma. Most cases occur between the ages of 5 and 25 years, with the peak centered at the time of the adolescent growth spurt. Speculation that this tumor is related to disordered bone growth is supported by the occurrence in (1) rapidly growing bones, (2) girls earlier than boys, and (3) tall children. The majority of patients presents with pain over the affected area.

Generally speaking, osteosarcoma can be categorized as localized or metastatic. Metastatic disease is actually present in most patients at the time of diagnosis although it is usually occult. The usual route of metastases for osteosarcoma is hematogenous; lymphatic spread is usually to regional nodes but uncommon and carries a poor prognosis. Staging of osteosarcoma is based upon the TNM stage as well as the histologic grade (Table 28.6).

Osteosarcoma is managed by a combination of surgery and chemotherapy. Pre- and postoperative multidrug chemotherapy is necessary for local control of tumor and treatment of micrometastatic disease. Preoperative chemotherapy also provides prognostic information, since chemotherapy-induced tumor necrosis is correlated with survival. Location of the disease is very important, since complete surgical excision is necessary for long-term disease control. Limb-sparing resections, as an alternative to amputation, are less morbid, but are associated with slightly higher recurrence rates. Chemotherapy is continued in the postoperative period. Osteosarcomas are relatively radioresistant and radiotherapy is reserved for inoperable tumors or tumors which cannot be totally resected.

Initial experience with FDG PET found generally high FDG uptake by osteosarcoma [20], and detection of recurrences by FDG PET compared favorably with conventional modalities [21]. FDG PET alone was at lease as accurate as a combination of conventional bone scan, MRI, and chest CT in evaluating intraosseous skip lesions (more than two discontinuous lesions in the same bone) and multifocal osseous disease (more than one bone involvement), regional lymph node involvement, and generalized metastatic disease [22]. Pulmonary metastases however, are most sensitively detected on CT due to resolution limitations of FDG PET. Hence the combination of PET and CT provides obvious advantages in a single imaging examination (Fig. 28.5).

Osteosarcomas demonstrate varied histology within the lesion and grade is assigned based on the least differentiated portion. Initial experience suggests tumor grade of sarcoma can be directly related to the level of FDG avidity [23]. Therefore, PET-CT directed biopsy potentially could improve initial staging information by directing the biopsy to the site of least differentiated tumor.

FDG PET has been shown to be useful in assessing and predicting response to therapy [24]. Tumor response to presurgical adjuvant chemotherapy is the most important prognostic indicator in osteosarcoma. Tumor necrosis is highly correlated with disease-free survival. Until now, tumor necrosis could only be evaluated after surgical resection and examination of the surgical specimen, or by site directed MRI [25]. PET-CT may provide assessment of post chemotherapy tumor necrosis by direct metabolic assessment of the necrosis rate by visually comparing avidity or by calculating tumor to nontumor ratios on pretreatment and posttreatment imaging, allowing for modification of neoadjuvant therapy regimens prior to surgery.

MR imaging of the local site for recurrent disease, CT imaging of the lungs for metastatic disease, and bone scan for surveillance of metastatic and recurrent disease will likely remain in the imaging armamentarium for the monitoring of osteosarcoma. While there is no clear indication to routinely employ PET-CT in the evaluation of osteosarcoma, it will play an important role in complex cases. For example, local recurrence is very difficult to assess in patients who have undergone limb-sparing procedures, given the inherent artifacts on MR imaging and bone scanning. Occasionally, osteolysis at the amputation site or sclerotic foci (reparative bone or cement) adjacent to prostheses can be problematic on followup radiographic examinations, and PET-CT imaging may be particularly helpful in differentiating these posttreatment changes from recurrent disease.

Table 28.6 AJCC osteosarcoma staging (Used with the permission of the American Joint Committee on Cancer (AJCC), Chicago, IL. The original source for this material is the *AJCC Cancer Staging Manual*, 7th edn. (2010) published by Springer Science and Business Media LLC. www.springer.com)

Anatomic stage • Prognostic groups					
Stage IA	T1	N0	M0	G1, 2	Low grade, GX
Stage IB	T2	N0	M0	G1, 2	Low grade, GX
	T3	N0	M0	G1, 2	Low grade, GX
Stage IIA	T1	N0	M0	G3, 4	High grade
Stage IIB	T2	N0	M0	G3, 4	High grade
Stage III	T3	N0	M0	G3, 4	
Stage IVA	Any T	N0	M1a	Any G	
Stage IVB	Any T	N1	Any M	Any G	
	Any T	Any N	M1b	Any G	

The American Joint Commission on Cancer defines T1 as tumor less than or equal to 8cm, T2 as greater than 8cm, and T3 as skip lesions of bone; N0 as no regional lymph node spread and N1 as regional lymph node spread; M0 as no distant metastasis, M1a metastasis to lung only and M1b metastasis to other site; G1 or G2 as low grade, and G3 or G4 as high grade

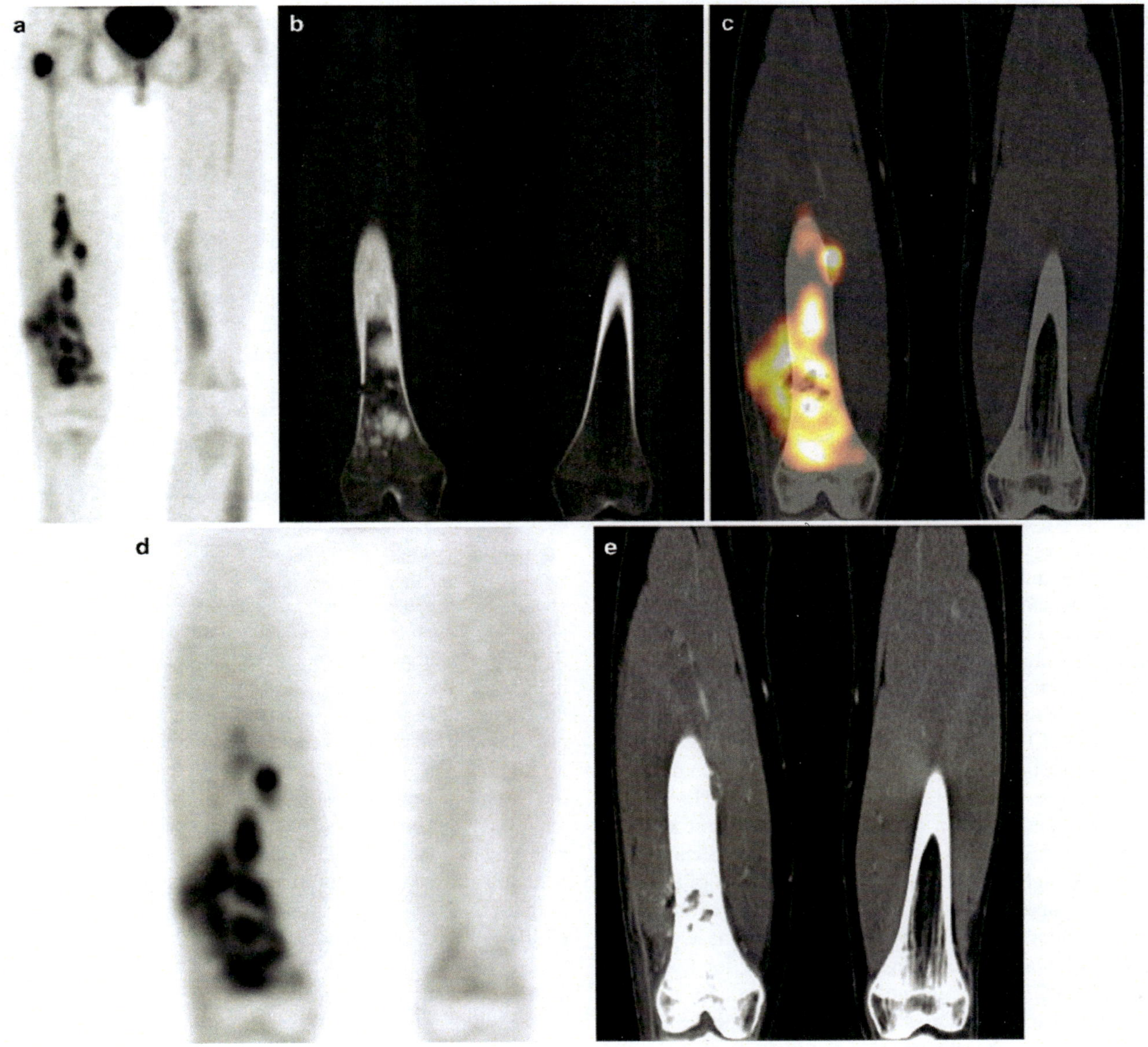

Fig. 28.5 Osteosarcoma of the right lower extremity. Anterior FDG PET MIP image (**a**) shows multiple foci of abnormal FDG tracer activity in the mid and distal right thigh; some located in the expected location of the femur, others in the adjacent soft tissue. An intense focus at the right intertrochanteric region (*arrow*) represents a skip lesion. Coronal CT bone window images (**b**) and FDG PET-CT fusion (**c**) images show multiple FDG avid osteoblastic lesions in the femoral diaphysis as well as FDG tracer uptake well lateral of the femoral cortex. Coronal CT soft tissue window images (**d**) and FDG PET (**e**) show subtle abnormal soft tissue contrast enhancement in the adjacent musculature which is FDG avid (*arrows*) reflecting extensive soft tissue involvement

Ewing Sarcoma

Ewing sarcoma represents a spectrum of small round cell tumors including Ewing sarcoma of bone, extraosseous Ewing sarcoma, and peripheral primitive neuroectodermal tumors. Patients often present in the second decade of life with pain, swelling, and/or fever. Ewing sarcoma is more common in males and rare in those of African descent. Distribution of Ewing sarcoma of bone is nearly equally distributed between the axial and appendicular skeleton. Peripheral primitive neuroectodermal tumor and extraosseous Ewing sarcoma tend to occur in the spine, pelvis, and chest regions.

Metastatic disease most commonly occurs by the hematogenous route with lung, bone, and bone, marrow being the most common sites. Hepatic metastasis is unusual and lymphatic spread is rare. Like osteosarcoma, micrometastatic disease is present in most patients at the time of diagnosis.

Approximately one-quarter of patients will have detectable metastatic disease at presentation.

Currently, no accepted staging system for Ewing sarcoma exists [25]. Disease is defined as localized when, by imaging or clinical means, it has not extended beyond the primary site or regional lymph nodes. Further, localized disease is divided into groups based on complete excision (Group I), microscopic residual disease (Group II), and gross residual disease (Group III). Similar to rhabdomyosarcoma, treatment protocols are often stratified based on the presence or absence of metastatic disease (Group IV) and on size, location and extent of the primary lesion. Extraosseous Ewing sarcoma is grouped similar to rhabdomyosarcoma, based on the presence of residual disease after resection.

Intensive combination chemotherapy is the mainstay of treatment. It is effective in reducing the volume of the primary tumor and treatment of metastatic disease. Local control is ideally achieved with surgical resection and/or radiation therapy. The overall survival is nearly 70% at 5 years with an event-free survival of 50% at 10 years. Major prognostic factors at the time of diagnosis include tumor site (resectablity), tumor volume, and the presence of metastases at the time of diagnosis. Younger children have better event free survival than older children and adults. However, response to preoperative chemotherapy is the most important variable.

PET-CT may be helpful in both initial assessment and for restaging of Ewing sarcoma. Although studies are currently lacking, PET-CT likely will more accurately determine the extent of disease at initial staging by defining the local extent of tumor and detection of unsuspected metastatic deposits. FDG PET has shown advantages in detecting recurrent disease [26] and offers the additional information of the metabolic response on preoperative chemotherapy and restaging examinations [24]. Like osteosarcoma, response to initial chemotherapy is a key prognostic indicator for Ewing sarcoma [26, 27]. It is also not uncommon to have anatomic distortions at the primary site related to treatment, and residual mass following therapy, and hence PET-CT will likely play a role in the differentiation of post-treatment changes from recurrent Ewing sarcoma (Fig. 28.6).

Other Tumors and Tumor-like Conditions

Hepatic Malignancies

Hepatoblastoma

Hepatoblastoma is the most common primary hepatic neoplasm in childhood. Patients usually present with abdominal mass; less commonly with anorexia, weight loss, anemia, hemihypertrophy, or isosexual precocity. There is a higher incidence of hepatoblastoma in patients with Beckwith-Wiedemann syndrome and familial polyposis. The median age of onset is 1 year, with most cases occurring before 5 years. Hepatoblastoma occurs more frequently in males.

The malignant component is comprised of either fetal or embryonal epithelial cells, but can also demonstrate a malignant mesenchymal component. Pure fetal histology is associated with a better prognosis. Hepatoblastoma typically presents as a large, homogeneous, unifocal, well-circumscribed hepatic mass. Serum alpha-fetoprotein is elevated in about 80% of patients, although patients with low or normal alpha-fetoprotein levels are associated with a poor prognosis. Serum alpha-fetoprotein is none-the-less a useful serum tumor marker for hepatoblastoma, and is used to assess response to treatment and surveillance. A rise in serum alpha-fetoprotein often heralds recurrent or metastatic hepatoblastoma.

Approximately 40% of patients have advanced disease at the time of presentation. Regional spread of hepatoblastoma includes lymph node metastasis to the porta hepatis and invasion of the portal vein. Distant metastatic disease is most commonly to the lungs while osseous metastasis are unusual. Staging is based upon post-surgical extent of disease (Table 28.7).

Cure rate for hepatoblastoma approaches 90% although cure requires local and systemic control. Treatment requires local control with surgical resection and systemic control with chemotherapy. Chemotherapy can convert unresectable to resectable disease. Recurrent tumor or progression of tumor during treatment results in poor survival rates.

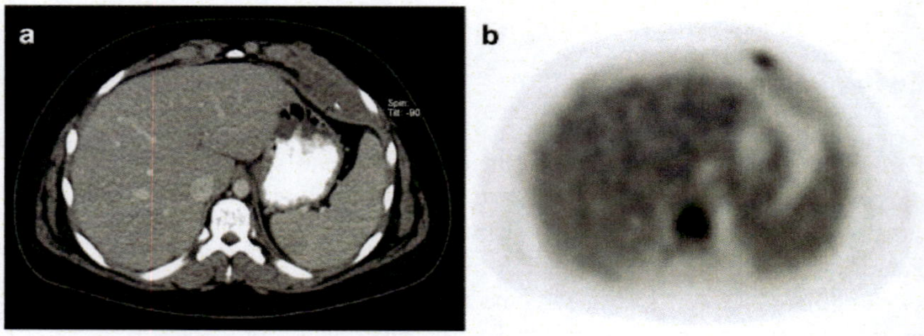

Fig. 28.6 Treated Ewing's sarcoma of the lower left chest wall. Transaxial CT (**a**) and FDG PET (**b**) images reveal residual soft tissue mass involving the ribs and intercostal musculature, which is found with any abnormal FDG tracer activity except a tiny focus at a nodule at the margin of the mass corresponding to residual viable Ewing's sarcoma

Table 28.7 Hepatoblastoma staging

Stage	Definition
1	Completely resected tumor; no clinical or radiographic metastatic disease.
2	Microscopic residual at margins of resection; no metastatic disease
3	Partial resected or unresected tumor confined to the liver or tumor spill into peritoneum at surgery or positive regional lymph nodes
4	Distant metastatic disease

To date, assessment of the utility of PET and PET-CT in the management of hepatoblastoma is limited. A few cases of recurrent hepatoblastoma diagnosed with FDG PET and PET-CT have been reported [29, 30]. PET-CT may have a role in followup of problem cases where chemotherapy and/or surgical alteration of local anatomy make differentiation of sterile or residual/recurrent disease difficult on CT alone or MRI. PET-CT, especially with 3D reconstructions, may be the preferred modality for detecting recurrence in such settings and for surgical planning. Also in the setting of hepatoblastoma that does not elaborate alpha-fetoprotein, PET-CT may be the preferred modality for monitoring recurrence.

Hepatocellular Carcinoma

Hepatocellular carcinoma in children is similar pathologically to adult disease. Pediatric disease often occurs in the absence of cirrhosis and demonstrates the fibrolamellar histology. Similar to hepatoblastoma, hepatocellular carcinoma is usually infiltrative or multicentric and is associated with elevated alpha fetoprotein levels. In contrast, hepatocellular carcinoma occurs in older children and is associated with underlying metabolic disease. Metastatic spread is to regional lymph nodes and lungs and rarely to bone.

Hepatocellular carcinoma is F18-FDG avid [31]. Normal hepatocytes have relatively high glucose-6 phosphatase activity; accumulation of FDG in hepatocellular carcinoma is variable related to the degree of activity of this enzyme. FDG PET has been shown to be helpful in the management of patients with metastatic liver disease and assessing lesions after radiofrequency ablation [31].

Langerhans' Cell Histiocytosis

Langerhans' cell histiocytosis refers to a spectrum of disease formerly unified by the term histiocytosis X and previously referred to in various clinical scenarios as eosinophilic granuloma, Hand-Schuller-Christian disease and Letterer-Siwe disease. Langerhans' cell histiocytosis is a disorder of immune regulation. The Langerhans' cell is a dendritic cell that occurs in epithelial surfaces. It is a bone marrow-derived antigen-processing cell involved in T-cell-mediated and non-immune antigen responses. Overproliferation of the Langerhans' cell and its accumulation in various organs results in the disease. Langerhans' cell histiocytosis may present as local or systemic disease and may affect virtually any organ system.

Manifestations of Langerhans' cell histiocytosis can be quite protean. The hallmark is the lytic bone lesion. Other clinical features include mild discomfort and irritability, diabetes insipidus, chronic otitis, fever, rash, pancytopenia, weight loss, hepatomegaly, and exophthalmos. Once the diagnosis is established histologically, radiographic bone survey, conventional total body bone scan, and CT of the chest and abdomen, and magnetic resonance imaging of the brain are performed to evaluate the extent of disease.

Langerhans' cell histiocytosis is categorized as (1) single system disease affecting a single site, (2) single system disease affecting multiple sites or (3) multisystem disease. Typically, however, disease is self-limited disease with single system involvement. Multiple system involvement is associated with poor outcome. Additional poor prognostic factors include age less than 2 years and organ dysfunction.

Treatment protocols vary based on the severity of disease. Single system disease (e.g., bone, lymph node, or skin) is usually treated locally with resection, when possible. Multisystem disease requires systemic therapy, usually initial therapy with vinblastine, etoposide, and prednisone and maintenance therapy with the same drugs and 6-mercaptopurine and methotrexate. Cyclosporin A therapy may be added in severe disease. Focused low dose radiation therapy may used in large or painful lesions, surgically inaccessible lesions, or to prevent permanent organ damage. Bone marrow transplantation may be employed in refractory cases.

Since Langerhans' cells rely on intracellular glucose metabolism for their energy, FDG imaging, is suitable with the neoplasm typically demonstrating FDG tracer uptake [32, 33]. At least in limited experience, FDG imaging appears to have greater specificity than scintigraphy and conventional radiography in determining osseous involvement. Lung, thymus, and liver involvement are more common manifestations of multisystem disease but multisystem disease is relatively uncommon with Langerhans' cell histiocytosis. Given the FDG avidity of this disease, however, PET-CT is likely to be the preferred single imaging examination, especially in suspected multisystem Langerhans' cell histiocytosis.

Inflammatory Pseudotumor

Inflammatory pseudotumor also known as atypical fibromyxoid tumor, pseudosarcomatous fibromyxoid tumor,

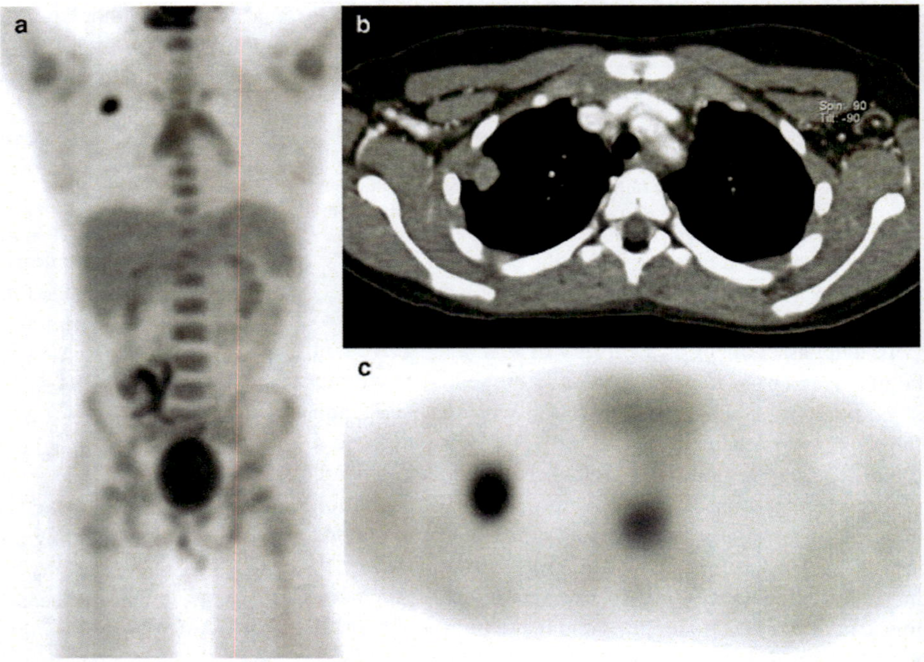

Fig. 28.7 Inflammatory pseudotumor. Whole torso anterior FDG PET MIP image (**a**) reveals intense abnormal focal FDG tracer activity in the right lateral lung. Physiologic FDG tracer activity is seen in thymus and bowel. Transaxial CT (**b**) and FDG PET (**c**) images demonstrate a 1.4 cm subpleural pulmonary nodule that shows contrast enhancement and intense FDG uptake. The intense FDG uptake is due to the inflammatory stroma composing the tumor

plasma cell granuloma, pseudosarcomatous myofibrotic proliferation, or postoperative spindle cell nodule is a rare soft tissue tumor found in children and young adults. It is characterized by spindle cell proliferation within an inflammatory stroma. Inflammatory pseudotumor has an intermediate or low malignant potential with risks of invasion and recurrence but not metastasis. Most lesions are related to a defect in the ALK gene, similar to anaplastic large cell lymphoma. Treatment is usually surgical however antiinflammatory medication has also been employed. The tumor is associated with intense FDG tracer uptake (Fig. 28.7), not unlike active granulomatous infection. Metastatic inflammatory pseudotumor has been reported to be diagnosed on PET-CT [34]. PET-CT is likely to be most useful in monitoring therapy or recurrence.

Renal Tumors

Wilms Tumor

Wilms tumor, clear cell sarcoma and rhabdoid tumor account for about 6% of pediatric neoplasms with Wilms tumor being by far the most common. While renal tumors do accumulate FDG, the utility of PET-CT in the evaluation of renal tumors is somewhat limited. Conventional anatomic imaging is usually adequate for diagnosis and staging. Renal excretion of FDG can impede visualization of small renal tumors and perinephric spread. Regardless, PET-CT may have a role in problem solving in the assessment of renal malignancies in children.

Wilms tumor (nephroblastoma) is derived from pluripotent metanephric blastema and is the most common renal neoplasm in children. It is strongly associated with aniridia, hemihypertrophy, and genital malformations and occurs in conjunction with neurofibromatosis, Beckwith-Wiedemann syndrome, Drash syndrome, and nephroblastomatosis. Peak incidence occurs between 2 and 3 years of age. Wilms tumors are often round and confined by an inflammatory pseudocapsule, although occasionally Wilms tumors are multicentric and/or bilateral [35]. Tumor penetration through the pseudocapsule into lymphatics, blood vessels, and renal sinus results in local spread. Lung and liver are the usual sites of metastasis, with other sites being very uncommon. Currently, experience is limited; however, PET-CT may be helpful in differentiating nephroblastomatosis from multicentric Wilms tumors and in the evaluation of recurrent and metastatic disease.

Clear Cell Sarcoma

Clear cell sarcoma of the kidney shares some features with Wilms tumor in terms of site of origin and age of onset, and is intensely FDG avid (Fig. 28.8). Clear cell sarcoma tends to much more readily permeate the perirenal lymphatic system, likely accounting for the high rate of local recurrence. Micrometastatic disease, similar to other sarcomas, may also contribute to distant metastasis to the brain, liver, lung and bone.

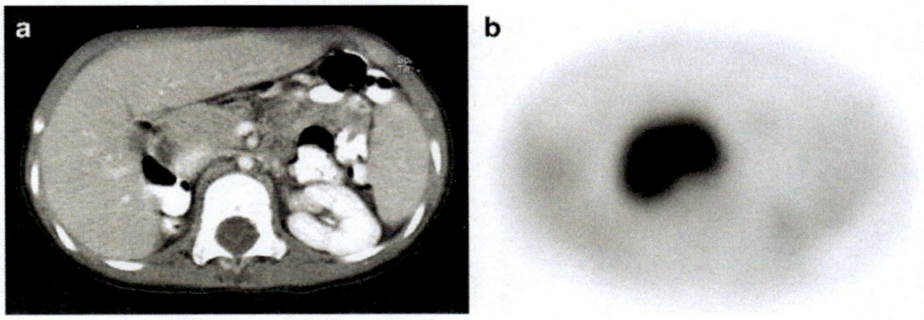

Fig. 28.8 Recurrent clear cell carcinoma of the kidney. Transaxial CT (**a**) and FDG PET (**b**) demonstrate a soft tissue mass in the retroperitoneum which is intensely FDG avid

Rhabdoid Tumor of Kidney

Rhabdoid tumor of the kidney is a highly malignant tumor. It occurs in infants and very young children. Primitive neuroectodermal tumors of the nervous system are associated with this tumor. Common sites of metastasis include regional lymph nodes and lung, and less commonly the liver, brain, and bone. Relapse and death are unfortunately common. The utility of FDG PET or PET-CT for management of this rare tumor has not yet been investigated; a single case report suggests that PET was useful in differentiating local recurrence from postsurgical change and in identifying occult distant metastases [36].

Imaging Pitfalls in PET-CT of Pediatric Malignancies

PET-CT Imaging pitfalls in the pediatric population can be divided into the CT portion of the study and those related the FDG portion of the examination. The CT-related pitfalls in the pediatric population are primarily those associated with imposed limitations in image contrast resolution and motion-related artifacts (physiologic as well unintentional patient movement). The FDG PET pitfalls are primarily those associated with physiologic and nonmalignant pathologic sources of FDG tracer uptake, and are relatively similar to those encountered in adult patients, with the exception of certain sources of physiologic tracer uptake such as the thymus gland and brown fat. Developmental variations on both CT and FDG PET images, such as growth plates and cellular marrow add complexity, and parallel the difficulties encountered with other imaging examinations in the pediatric population.

CT Dose and Image Contrast

Radiation dose is always an important consideration in radiology, but particularly so in pediatric imaging. Lowing the radiation dose on CT scanning by using reduced mA, kVp, as well as dose modulation features of contemporary scanners, is routine in pediatric imaging. Even in children with malignancies there is a desire to reasonably limit radiation exposure, as many of these patients will survive into adulthood, and can expect to undergo a large number of imaging studies involving ionizing radiation. These strategies, however, lower the signal to noise ratio on the CT images, and consequently the anatomy is more difficult resolve. This is further exacerbated by the overall paucity of fat in children relative to adults. Optimized use of oral and intravenous contrast material is thus particularly important to compensate for low inherent contrast and absence of fat planes in pediatric patients undergoing PET-CT [37].

Patient Movement During Scan Acquisition

Motion is the bane of pediatric imaging. Patient movement can interfere with the image acquisitions, PET, and CT image registration, and the CT-derived PET attenuation correction. Technologists and nurses familiar with children are often able to use distraction techniques and other methods to optimize the examination acquisition in CT, but for PET-CT the total acquisition time can be as much as 30 min, and hence in younger children sedation may be necessary, or at the least, anxiolysis. Older children, especially those who have already undergone imaging studies, often can understand the need for and comply with directions to remain still throughout the entire CT and PET image acquisitions. Physiologic motion secondary to respiration can be difficult to control in pediatric patients. Children often have difficulty cooperating for breath-hold techniques and this can lead to misregistration between CT and PET images. Unless it is certain that patients can comply, the CT imaging acquisition is usually performed during uniform quiet breathing. In some instances a separate breath-hold CT acquisition of the chest and upper abdomen may be obtained. With 16 or more channel multidetector CT, the respiratory-related artifacts in children with quiet breathing are usually minimal and acceptable for most applications.

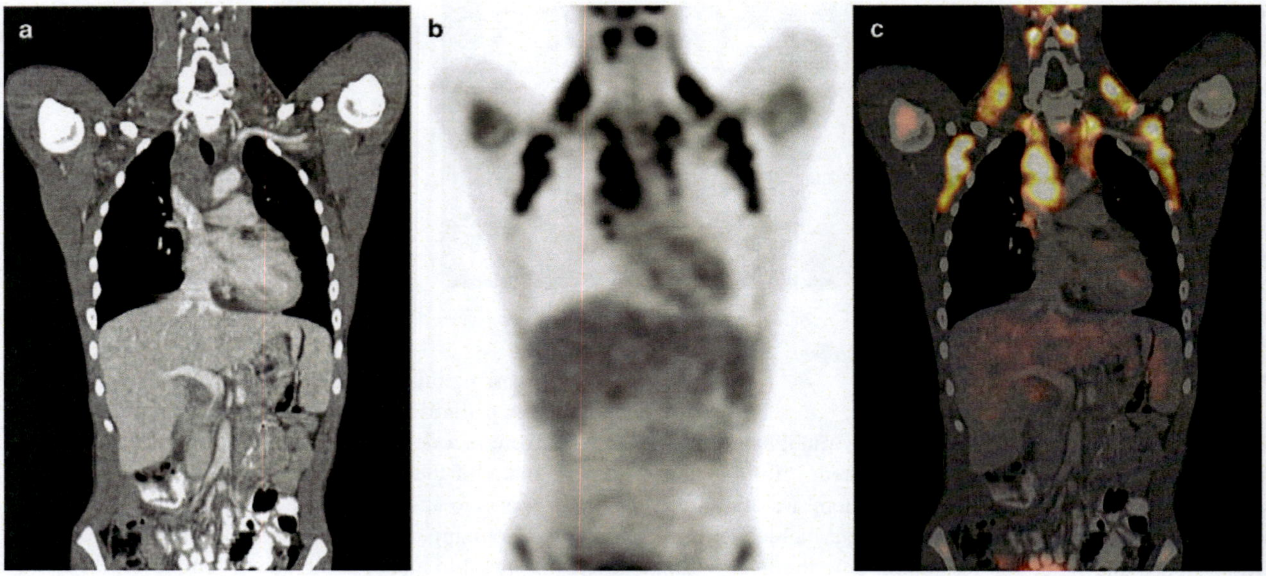

Fig. 28.9 Brown fat physiologic FDG uptake. Coronal CT (**a**), FDG PET (**b**), and FDG PET-CT fusion image (**c**) show intense FDG tracer uptake in brown fat at the neck base and in the axilla. Intense FDG uptake in the mediastinum however corresponds to lymphadenopathy in this patient being staged for lymphoma. In the present of brown fat physiologic FDG uptake there should be careful review of the CT images for the presence of lymph nodes or abnormal soft tissue in the regions of brown fat uptake

Brown Fat FDG Uptake in Children

Brown fat, a hypervascular form of fat tissue rich in mitochondria, is thought to function primarily in the regulation of body temperature. Brown fat comprises as much as 5% of the body mass in a neonate and then decreases with age. Adrenergic stimulation of brown fat leads to increased glycolytic activity and heat production, and the increased glycolytic activity results in marked FDG tracer uptake in the brown fat tissue. Intense brown fat FDG uptake is now a well recognized potential pitfall in FDG PET imaging of adult patients, and it can be especially problematic in FDG imaging of school age children and adolescents. Exposure to cold and anxiety in general are thought to be the major causes of elevated FDG uptake in brown fat on FDG PET imaging. Anxiolytics and beta blocking drugs can be used to reduce or eliminate brown fat FDG tracer uptake [38, 39].

Brown fat FDG tracer uptake is commonly seen at the base of the neck in the fat adjacent to the lateral edge of the trapezius muscle, the suboccipital regions, in the fat adjacent to the sternocleidomastoid muscles, near the cupola of the lungs, and the fat adjacent to the costovertebral junctions along the thoracic spine [40]. Brown fat FDG uptake can also be seen within the mediastinal fat and intraabdominal fat under the diaphragm. While brown fat FDG tracer uptake is usually easy to identify on PET-CT due to the registered and aligned images; in children the relative paucity of fat and potential misregistration of the PET and CT images due to patient movement can confound interpretation. More important, the presence of brown fat FDG tracer uptake does not exclude the presence of abnormal lymph nodes or masses (Fig. 28.9), and the FDG tracer activity in fat may obscure pathologic lymph nodes on the FDG PET images such as in the setting of lymphoma [41].

Thymus Gland Enlargement and FDG Uptake

The mutability of the thymus gland at different ages and during various states of disease and health adds complexity to both the PET and CT evaluation of the mediastinum in the pediatric population. Anatomic criteria for normal thymus are vague and there can be significant overlap of metabolic activity in normal thymus, inflammatory disease, thymic hyperplasia, and neoplasm. Consequently, anatomic and metabolic features of the thymus and some of its disease states deserve some discussion.

The thymus accounts for a large portion of the anterior mediastinum during infancy and usually extends from the brachiocephalic vessels toward the right cardiophrenic angle. Occasionally, thymus is seen extending into the neck, toward the left cardiophrenic angle, or even into the posterior mediastinum. The gland assumes a more quadrilateral shape and tends to occupy the superior mediastinum as the child approaches school age. The thymus assumes a more triangular shape in adolescents and young adults. Attenuation coefficients of the thymus as measured on CT decrease with age, likely related to normal fibrofatty involution; but in general, attenuation of the thymus gland should appear homogeneous on CT. During infancy, thymic margins may be undulating (“thymic wave”), although with increasing age, margins of the thymus are usually straight or gently curving. Lobulated or nodular margins are not normally seen. The superior-inferior dimension of the thymus increases, the medial-lateral dimension stays fairly constant, and the anterior-posterior dimension (thickness) decreases with age. The thickness is probably the best dimension to predict thymic disease; >2.42 cm in patients less than 10 years of age and >1.77 cm in patients older than 10 years of age can be considered enlarged [42].

Metabolic activity of the normal thymus gland can be variable [43, 44]. In general, the observed FDG tracer activity decreases with age, corresponding to normal involutional change of the thymus. The distribution of FDG tracer, however, should remain uniform throughout the gland. The level of tracer activity observed in the thymus gland deemed “normal physiologic” is largely based on studies with correlation to morphologic features on CT, lack of clinical symptoms, and absence of mediastinal disease on follow-up imaging.

The thymus usually undergoes involution during cytotoxic chemotherapy and then typically returns to normal after cessation of chemotherapy, or between courses of chemotherapy. Thymic hyperplasia is defined as a 50% increase in gland volume compared to baseline. Thymic hyperplasia occurs in approximately one fourth of patients undergoing chemotherapy. In these cases, the thymus maintains its usual shape and attenuation and FDG activity is uniformly and diffusely increased (Fig. 28.10).

Heterogeneous or focally increased activity usually indicates thymic disease. It can be difficult if not impossible to differentiate between neoplasm and inflammatory/infectious etiologies that involve the thymus and mediastinum. Granulomatous disease and incompletely treated neoplasm have considerable overlap; SUV greater than 4 has been suggested to reliably indicate neoplasm. Perhaps the best means of discrimination between normal and abnormal thymus is by combining anatomic and metabolic data, but it is still sometimes difficult to differentiate its various disease states.

Other Variants

Bone marrow is more FDG avid in children compared to adults on PET imaging. A greater cellular (red marrow) component likely accounts for this difference. Hematopoietic drug stimulation accentuates normal marrow activity in children just as the case with adults [45]. Other drugs, including interferon, have also been reported to induce increased bone marrow activity [46].

Dietary restriction is difficult in children and consequently cardiac activity is difficult to suppress. Regardless, cardiac activity is usually easy to differentiate from mediastinal malignancy with CT registration.

Focal FDG tracer uptake due to inflammation can be misinterpreted as a metastatic deposit. Inflammatory cells exhibit increased glycolytic activity and thus FDG avidity. FDG PET has been shown to be useful in evaluation of various inflammatory processes including chronic granulomatous disease of childhood, inflammatory bowel disease, and even occult infection. In general, the pediatric immune system is more reactive than in adults and it is not uncommon to see small lymph nodes in the neck, chest, abdomen, pelvis, and extremities (axillae, groins, and popliteal fossae) associated with elevated FDG tracer uptake as well due to normal physiologic inflammatory reaction.

There are numerous examples of infectious and inflammatory mimics of oncology. FDG tracer uptake in lymph nodes can be entirely indistinguishable from FDG tracer uptake due to neoplasm, especially when intense such as seen with granulomatous infection. Histoplasmosis, tuberculosis, and other granulomatous diseases in children often do not calcify, and consequently involved lymph nodes associated with intense FDG tracer uptake are easily mistaken for lymphoma and recurrent lymphoma (Fig. 28.11). Round pneumonia is a common pediatric malady and can present a diagnostic challenge in oncologic imaging; these pneumonias are mass-like and demonstrate increased activity at PET-CT imaging [47]. Meckel’s diverticulum, the most common congenital anomaly of the gastrointestinal tract, can also simulate neoplasia on metabolic imaging [48].

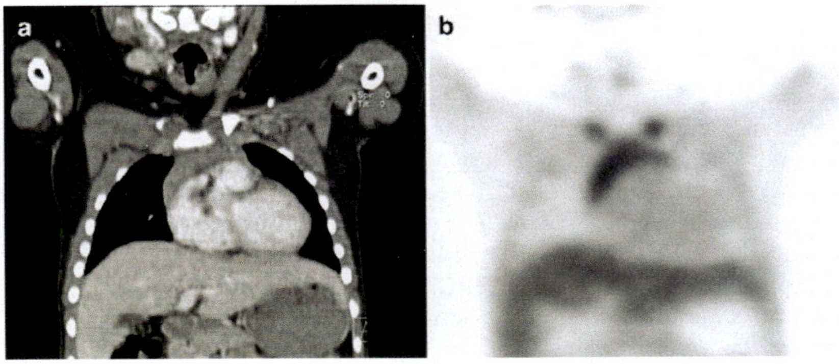

Fig. 28.10 Thymic hyperplasia following chemotherapy. Coronal CT (**a**) and FDG PET (**b**) shows a normal configuration and size (for the patient’s age) thymus gland which is moderately intensely FDG avid. The configuration and uniform appearance on the CT images confirms the FDG uptake on the PET image is due to thymus gland and not nodal or other soft tissue mass in the anterior mediastinum

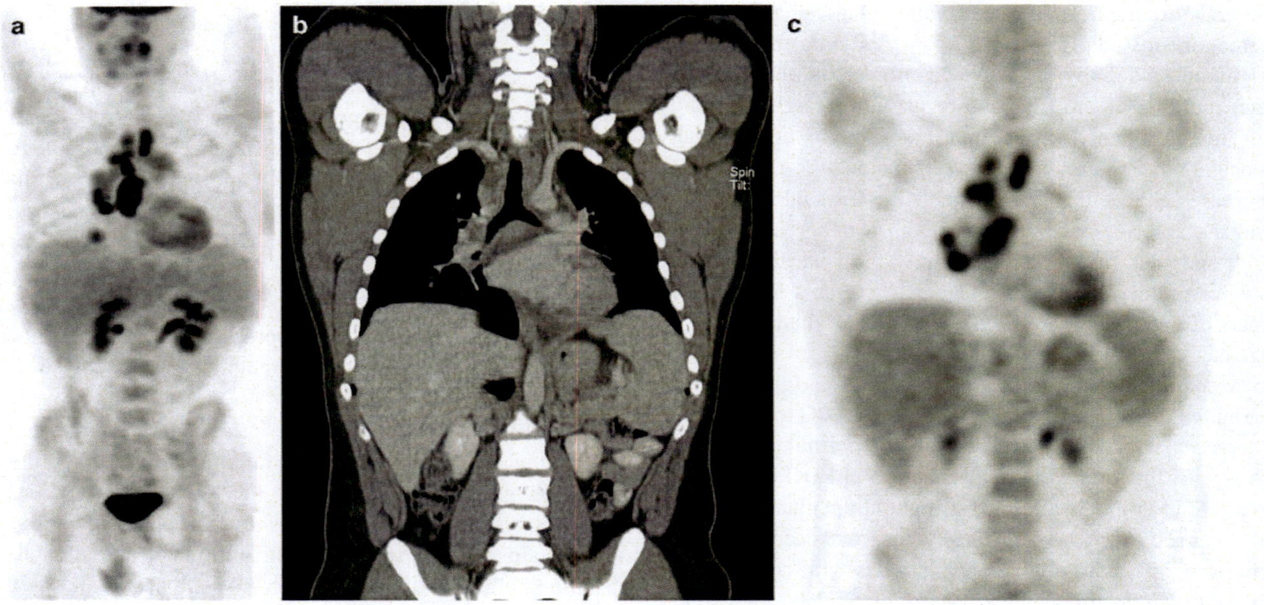

Fig. 28.11 Intensely positive lymph nodes on FDG PET due to histoplasmosis. (**a**) Anterior FDG PET MIP image demonstrates intense FDG tracer activity in the mediastinum of this 9 year old child. Coronal CT (**b**) and FDG PET (**c**) images show intense FDG uptake is in borderline enlarged noncalcified low paratracheal, subcarinal and right hilar lymph nodes subsequently shown to be entirely to active histoplasmosis infection

Various musculoskeletal pathologies can also cause abnormal FDG tracer uptake that may be mistaken for malignancy. Avascular necrosis, fractures, Scheuermann's disease and bone infarction in the reparative phase can be FDG avid. Myositis, muscle trauma, and muscle overuse can lead to focal or asymmetric uptake and simulate disease. Several pediatric PET-CT nuances such as variation of maturation of the ischiopubic synchondrosis [49] and nonossifying fibroma [50] have been recently described.

Another source of interpretive error is extravasation of radiopharmaceutical, which can occur more frequently in the pediatric population due to difficult venous access. Focal areas of increased activity may be seen at the injection site, in the lymphatic system and in skeletal muscle. Extravasation patterns are similar to those observed with other radiopharmaceuticals. Extravasation is usually easy to recognize since activity tends to be very intense and regionally related to the injection site.

Conclusion

The purpose of this chapter has been to provide a basic overview of pediatric oncology with insight into the important although nascent role of PET-CT in the diagnosis and management of childhood tumors. As time goes on, availability of pediatric PET-CT technology will increase, indications and opportunities for pediatric PET-CT will expand, and anecdotal observations will give way to statistically valid studies in children.

References

1. Hahn K, Pfluger T. Has PET become an important clinical tool in paediatric imaging? Eur J Nucl Med Mol Imaging 2004;31(5):615–621.
2. Connolly JH, Fahey FH, Shulkin BL. PET and PET/CT in pediatric oncology. Semin Nucl Med 2007;37(5):316–331.
3. Stauss J, Franzius C, Phluger T, Jurgens KV, Biassani L. Guidelines for 18F-FDG PET and PET/CT in pediatric oncology. Eur J Nucl Med Mol Imaging 2008;35(8):1581–1588.
4. Tatsumi M et al. 18F-FDG PET/CT in evaluating non-CNS pediatric malignancies. J Nucl Med 2007;48(12):1923–1931.
5. Pirro V et al. FDG PET and evaluation of post-therapeutic residual tumors in pediatric oncology: preliminary experience. J Pediatr Hematol Oncol 2008;30(5):343–346.
6. Rhodes MM et al. Utility of FDG Pet/CT in follow up of children treated for Hodkin's and non-Hodgkin's lymphoma. J Pediatr Hematol/Oncol 2006;28:300–306.
7. Cheng G, Servaes S, Alavi A, Zhuang H. FDG PET and PET/CT in the management of pediatric lymphoma patients. PET Clin 2008;3(1): 621-634.
8. Friedberg JW et al. FDG-PET is superior to Gallium scintigraphy and more sensitive in the follow-up of patients with de novo Hodgkin lymphoma comparison. Leuk Lymphoma 2004;45(1):85–92.
9. Juweid ME, Cheson BD. Role of positron emission tomography in lymphoma. J Clin Oncol 2005;23(21):4577–4580.
10. Terasawa T et al. 18F-FDG PET for Post-therapy assessment of Hodgkin's disease and aggressive non-Hodgkin's lymphoma: a systematic review. J Nucl Med 2008;49(1): 13–21.
11. Arush B et al. Assessing the use of FDG PET in the detection of regional and metastatic nodes in alveolar rhabdomyosarcoma of the extremities. J Pediatr Hematol/Oncol 2006;28:440–445.
12. Klem ML et al. PET for staging in rhabdomyosarcoma: an evaluation of PET as a adjunct to current staging tools. J Pediatr Hematol/Oncol 2007;29:9–14.
13. Tateishi U, Hosono A, Makimoto A, Nakamoto Y, Kaneta T. Comparative study of FDG PET/CT and conventional imaging

in the staging of rhabdomyosarcoma. Ann Nucl Med 2009;23(2): 155–161.
14. McCarville MB. PET and PET/CT in pediatric sarcomas. PET Clin 2008;3(4):563–575.
15. Iagaru A et al. F-18 FDG PET and PET/CT evaluation of response to chemotherapy in bone and soft tissue sarcomas. Clin Nucl Med 2008;33(1):8–13.
16. Kushner BH. Neuroblastoma: a disease requiring a multitude of imaging studies. J Nucl Med 2004;45:1172–1188.
17. Shulkin BL, et al. Neuroblastoma: positron emission tomography with 2-[fluorine-18]-fluoro-2-deoxy-D-glucose compared with metaiodobenzylguanidine scintigraphy. Radiology 1996;199:743–750.
18. Kushner BH et al. Extending positron emission tomography scan utility for high risk neuroblastoma: fluorine-18 fluoro-deoxyglucose positron emission tomography as sole imaging modality in follow-up of patients. J Clin Oncol 2001;19(14):3397–3405.
19. McDowell H, Losty P, Barnes N, Kokai G. Utility of FDG-PET/CT in the follow-up of neuroblastoma which became MIBG negative. Pediatr Blood Cancer 2009;52(4):552.
20. Brenner W, Bohuslavizki KH, Eary JF. PET imaging in osteosarcoma. J Nucl Med 2003;44(6):930–942.
21. Franzius C, Daldrup-Link HE, Wagner-Bohn A, et al. FDG-PET for the detection of recurrences from malignant primary bone tumors: comparison with conventional imaging. Ann Oncol 2002;13:157–160.
22. Volker T et al. Positron emission tomography for staging pediatric sarcoma patients: results of a prospective multicenter trial. J Clin Oncol 2007;25(34):5435–5411.
23. Aoki J, Wantanabe H, Shinozaki T, et al. FDG PET of primary benign and malignant bone tumors: standardized uptake values in 52 lesions. Radiology 2001;219:774–777.
24. Hawkins DS, Rajendran JG, Conrad EU, et al. Evaluation of chemotherapy response in pediatric bone sarcomas by (F-18)-fluorodeoxy-d-glucose positron emission tomography. Cancer 2002;94(12):3277–3284.
25. Dyke JP et al. Osteogenic and Ewing sarcomas: estimation of necrotic fraction during induction chemotherapy with dynamic contrast-enhanced MR imaging. Radiology 2003;228(1):271–278.
26. Raney RB et al. Ewing sarcoma of soft tissues in childhood: a report from the intergroup rhabdomyosarcoma study, 1972 to 1991. J Clin Oncol 1997;15(2):574–582.
27. Wunder JS et al. The histological response to chemotherapy as a predictor of the oncological outcome of operative treatment of Ewing sarcoma. J Bone Joint Surg Am 1998;80(7):1020–1033.
28. Hawkins DS et. al. [18F] Fluorodeoxyglucose positron emission tomography predicts outcome for Ewing sarcoma family of tumors. J Clin Oncol 2005;23:8828–8834.
29. Sironi S, Messa C, Cistaro A, et al. Recurrent Hepatoblastoma in orthotopic transplanted liver: detection with FDG positron emission tomography. AJR 2004;182:1214–1216.
30. Figarola MS et al. Recurrent hepatoblastoma with localization by PET-CT. Pediatr Radiol 2005;35:1254–1258.
31. Mody RJ, Pohlen JA, Malde S, Strouse PJ, Shulkin BL. FDG PET for the study of primary hepatic malignancies in children. Pediatr Blood Cancer 2006;47(1):51–55.
32. Binkovitz LA, Olshefski RS, Adler BH. Coincidence FDG-PET in the evaluation of Langerhans' cell histiocytosis: preliminary findings. Pediatr Radiol 2003;33(9):598–602.
33. Kaste SC, Rodriguez-Galindo C, McCarville ME, Shulkin BL. PET-CT in pediatric Langerhans cell histiocytosis. Pediatr Radiol 2007;37(7):615–622.
34. Kuo PH et al. Metastatic inflammatory myofibroblastic tumor imaged by PET-CT. Clin Nucl Med 2006;31(2):106–108.
35. Prasad SR et al. Neoplasms of the renal medulla: radiologic-pathologic correlation. Radiographics 2005;25:369–380.
36. Pirro V et al. 18F-Fluorodeoxyglucose positron emission tomography in the characterization of suspected rhabdoid renal tumor recurrence: a case report. J Pediatr Hematol Oncol 2007;29(1): 69–71.
37. Nadel HR, Shulkin B. Pediatric positron emission tomography-computed tomography protocol considerations. Semin Ultrasound, CT MRI 2008;29:271–278.
38. Gelfand MJ et al. Pre-medication to Block [^{18}F] FDG uptake in the brown adipose tissue of pediatric and adolescent patients. Pediatr Radiol 2005;35:984–990.
39. Shammas A, Lim R, Charron M. Pediatric FDG PET/CT physiologic uptake, normal variants, and benign conditions. Radiographics 2009;29(5):1467–1486.
40. Paidsetty S, Blodgett TM. Brown fat: atypical locations and appearance encountered in PET/CT. AJR (2009);193(2):359–366.
41. Kazama T et al. FDG PET in the evaluation of treatment for lymphoma: clinical usefulness and pitfalls. Radiographics 2005;25: 191–207.
42. Francis IR et al. The thymus: reexamination of the age-related changes in size and shape. AJR 1985;145:249–254.
43. Brink L et al. Increased metabolic activity in the thymus gland studied with ^{18}F-FDG PET: age dependency and frequency after chemotherapy. J Nucl Med 2001;42:591–595.
44. Ferdinand B, Gupta P, Kramer E. Spectrum of thymic uptake at 18F-FDG PET. Radiographics 2004;24:1611–1616.
45. Sugawara Y, Fischer SJ, Zasadny KR. Pre-clinical and clinical studies of bone marrow uptake of fluorine-18-fluorodeoxy-glucose with or without granulocyte colony-stimulating factor during chemotherapy. J Clin Oncol 1998;16:173–180.
46. Cone LA et al. PET positive generalized lymphadenopathy and splenomegaly following interferon – alpha 2b adjunctive therapy for melanoma. Clin Nucl Med 2007;32(10):793–796.
47. Shie P et al. Round pneumonia mimicking pulmonary malignancy on F-18 FDG PET/CT. Clin Nucl Med 2007;32(1):55–56.
48. Tennant SL, Ganatra R. Meckel's diverticulum – an incidental finding on PET/CT. Clin Nucl Med 2007;32(7):555–558.
49. Drubach LA et al. The ischipubic synchondrosis: changing appearance of PET/CT as a mimic of disease. Clin Nucl Med 2006;31(7): 414–417.
50. vonFalck C et al. Non-ossifying fibroma can mimic residual lymphoma in FDG PET: additional value of combined PET/CT. Clin Nucl Med 2007;32(8):640–642

Further Reading

1. Pizzo PA, Poplack DG. Principles and Practice of Pediatric Oncology, 5th edn. Philadelphia: Lippincott, 2005.

Chapter 29
PET-CT of Renal Cell Carcinoma

Todd M. Blodgett and Sanjay Paidisetty

Renal malignancy accounts for about 3–4% of all cancers, with approximately 54,000 new diagnoses and 13,000 deaths estimated in the USA in 2008 [1]. Renal cell carcinoma is the most common malignancy of the kidney, accounting for 85% of renal malignancies. Renal cell carcinoma most commonly occurs in the sixth through eighth decades of life, and there is a 1.6:1 male to female predominance. Risk factors for renal cell carcinoma include cigarette smoking, obesity, hypertension, a positive family history, acquired cystic kidney disease-associated end-stage renal disease, and the rare autosomal dominant Von Hippel-Lindau disease [2, 3]. Classic signs and symptoms of renal cell carcinoma leading to diagnosis include flank pain (40%), hematuria (50%), or palpable mass (35%), with only 10% presenting with the classic triad of all three. However, today nearly half of renal cell carcinoma is detected incidentally on ultrasound or CT scans ordered for other indications, with the majority of these patients being asymptomatic [4]. Overall, 30% of patients will present with metastatic disease, with lung, bone, lymph nodes, liver, and opposite kidney being the most common sites for metastases [5].

Renal cell carcinoma is primarily a surgically managed malignancy, offering little improvement in outcomes with additional chemotherapy or radiation. Unless there is more than isolated metastatic disease, the primary renal tumor is usually resected. Preoperative imaging is important, however, in determining surgical planning and approach. The size of the tumor and involvement of the perinephric tissues, ipsilateral adrenal gland, and extension beyond Gerota's fascia determine the need for simple versus radical nephrectomy. Partial nephrectomy and laparoscopic nephrectomies are increasingly offered to selected patients with smaller tumors confined to the kidney and adjacent perinephric fat. Local extension of renal cell carcinoma into the renal vein and inferior vena cava or the presence of regional lymph node metastases indicate the need for radical nephrectomy and more extensive lymph node dissection and vascular resection. Even when the primary renal mass has extended beyond Gerota's fascia, radial nephrectomy and debulking, often following tumor embolization to reduce potential blood loss, may be indicated if metastatic disease is not present. Although rare, spontaneous regression of renal cell carcinoma metastases can occur, sometimes in response to resection of the primary mass. In addition, in selected patients, isolated metastases such as a solitary pulmonary nodule will be resected. Otherwise, treatment of metastatic disease is palliative. Several cytokine-based therapy regimens such as interferon alpha have been extensively investigated for metastatic cases; however, partial or complete remission rates after therapy have been low with a median increase of 3–4 months in survival [5]. Other novel therapeutic approaches, such as tyrosine kinase inhibitors and vascular endothelial growth factor signaling targets, are in clinical trials.

Role of PET-CT for Initial Diagnosis of Renal Cell Carcinoma

PET-CT has a limited role in the diagnosis of renal cell carcinoma or the differential diagnosis of a renal mass. Typically, a combination of morphologic imaging modalities including ultrasound (US), CT, or MR, are used to characterize a renal mass. Solid masses on morphologic imaging are almost always considered malignant, whereas cystic masses are placed into categories originally described by Bosniak [6]. CT and US can usually readily differentiate a purely cystic (Bosniak category 1) from solid mass, with purely cystic masses requiring no further evaluation or follow-up imaging. Bosniak category 1 lesions all have the imaging criteria of imperceptible nonenhancing walls and measure near water attenuation (<20 HU). Cysts that contain proteinaceous material can be problematic, as they can have a solid appearance on CT (>20 HU), but there should be no enhancement of the lesion between the non-contrast and contrast enhanced series. Category II lesions are subdivided into minimally complicated cysts (category II), and those with more complexity

T.M. Blodgett (✉)
FRG Molecular Imaging, Foundation Radiology Group, 401 Liberty Avenue, Suite 2000, Pittsburgh, PA, 15222, USA
e-mail: toddblodgett@yahoo.com

P. Shreve and D.W. Townsend (eds.), *Clinical PET-CT in Radiology: Integrated Imaging in Oncology*,
DOI 10.1007/978-0-387-48902-5_29, © Springer Science+Business Media, LLC 2011

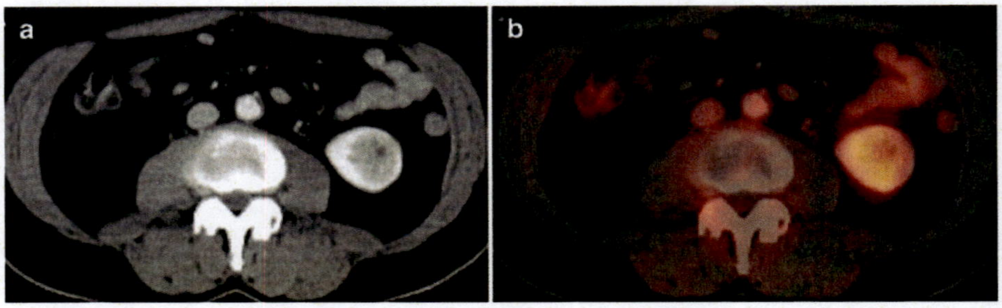

Fig. 29.1 Isometabolic primary renal cell carcinoma. Transaxial CT (**a**) shows a solid enhancing renal mass in the inferior pole left kidney, with only mild FDG activity, approximately equal to background renal parenchyma, seen on fused PET-CT (**b**)

(category IIF) or nonenhancing hyper-attenuation (40–90 HU). Unlike category II, category IIF lesions require further imaging evaluation or follow-up imaging at 3, 6, and 12 month intervals, to ensure stability or document interval lesion growth. For more complex or solid lesions (Bosniak categories 3 and 4) with irregular and thickened septa, multilocular appearance or irregular margination, it is often not possible to differentiate renal cell carcinoma from other solid renal masses. Therefore, these are almost always treated empirically as malignant lesions with surgical resection [7].

The primary differential diagnosis for a solid renal mass includes renal oncocytoma, hemorrhagic renal cyst, angiomyolipoma, transitional cell carcinoma, and lymphoma. Angiomyolipoma can be reliably distinguished from malignancy on CT or US. The presence fat attenuation (HU = −30 to −150) within a renal mass on CT or echotexture features of fat within the mass on US is a fairly specific sign for angiomyolipoma. Aside from angiomyolipomas, CT is generally unreliable in distinguishing other benign solid renal masses from renal cell carcinoma.

In limited published studies, FDG PET alone has not been shown to be useful for differentiating between renal cell carcinoma and other solid renal masses [8–11]. This primarily reflects the wide range of FDG tracer uptake in renal cell carcinoma, with well over a third of primary renal cell carcinoma exhibiting FDG tracer uptake equal to or less than the normal renal parenchyma 1–2 h following FDG tracer administration. For smaller intraparenchymal renal masses, urinary tracer in the intrarenal collecting system can further confound identification of FDG tracer uptake by the renal mass. Oncocytomas have been reported to exhibit FDG tracer uptake in the same range as renal cell carcinoma [11]. Although not reported in the literature, in our experience, angiomyolipomas do not take up FDG. The largest published study to date examining FDG PET for evaluating primary renal cell carcinoma showed an overall sensitivity of 60% compared to 92% for contrast enhanced CT [9].

While large or exophytic FDG avid renal masses are readily identified on PET-CT, this is largely a reflection of the morphologic abnormality. An intraparenchymal renal cell carcinoma, which does not exhibit FDG tracer uptake greater than the adjacent renal cortex, will be identified entirely based on the CT findings (Fig. 29.1). A solid mass identified on CT images, which is not unequivocally an angiomyolipoma, must be considered a renal cell carcinoma, even if it does not exhibit abnormal FDG tracer uptake. Uncommonly, the contrast enhanced CT findings will be subtle, while abnormal FDG tracer uptake of the RCC will be clearly depicted on the FDG PET images (Fig. 29.2).

In summary, based on the limited available data, it is possible the FDG PET images of PET-CT may be helpful in differentiating benign from malignant renal lesions in selected patients, possibly including complex cystic masses that fall into the Bosniak 3 and 4 categories prior to performing a nephrectomy. However, the current role of PET-CT for differentiating benign from malignant renal masses is complementary, rather than as a first line diagnostic tool.

Staging of Renal Cell Carcinoma with PET-CT

Renal cell carcinoma spreads by local extension beyond the renal capsule to perinephric tissue within Gerota's fascia, and the ipsilateral adrenal gland. Local extension beyond Gerota's fascia includes adjacent includes the liver, abdominal wall, and retroperitoneal space. Lymphatic spread is to renal hilar and retroperitoneal lymph nodes initially and subsequently to mediastinal lymph nodes. Hematogenous metastases are principally to lung, liver, bone and kidneys, although renal cell carcinoma is known to metastasize to brain, thyroid and soft tissues.

The staging of renal cell carcinomas is performed using the preferred TNM classification (Table 29.1), rather than the more outdated Robson criteria. The local extent of the primary tumor, as denoted by T stage, is especially important with renal cell carcinoma, as the T stage alone can determine stage I through IV. The T stage with renal cell carcinoma also strongly influences survival, with higher 5-year survival rates (71–97%) for patients who have disease confined to Gerota's fascia and not involving the renal vein or adrenal gland, than those with local involvement of the renal vein or adrenal

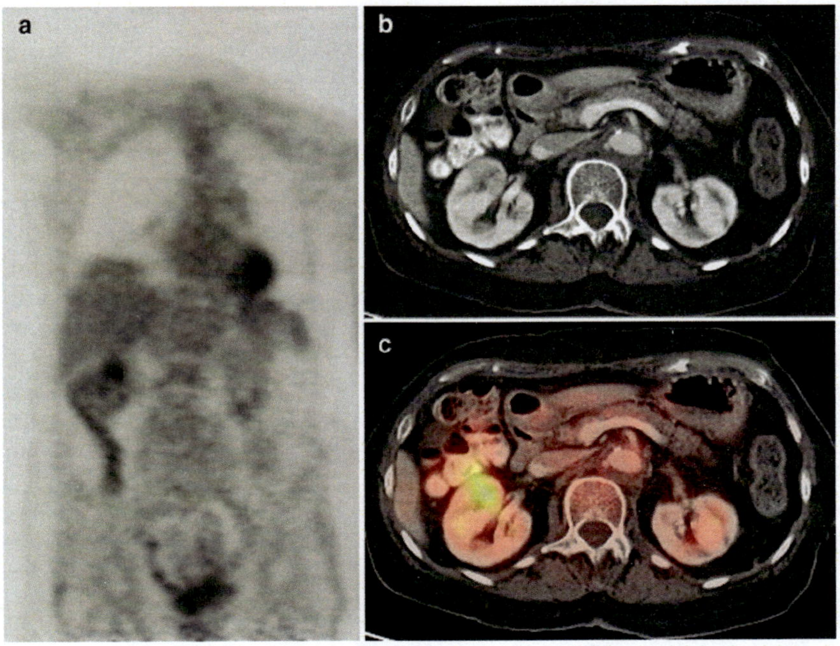

Fig. 29.2 Hypermetabolic primary renal cell carcinoma. Coronal FDG PET (**a**) shows asymmetrical FDG uptake in the right kidney above background parenchyma. Transaxial CT (**b**) shows only minimally different attenuation difference between the tumor and normal cortex. Axial FDG PET-CT fusion image (**c**) shows the increased FDG activity to correlate to the subtle mass

Table 29.1 Renal cell carcinoma definitions of TNM and anatomic stage and prognostic groups (Used with the permission of the American Joint Committee on Cancer (AJCC), Chicago, IL. The original source for this material is the *AJCC Cancer Staging Manual*, 7th edn (2010) published by Springer Science and Business Media LLC. www.springer.com)

Definitions of TNM	
Primary tumor (T)	
TX	Primary tumor cannot be assessed
T0	No evidence of primary tumor
T1	Tumor 7 cm or less in greatest dimension, limited to the kidney
T1a	Tumor 4 cm or less in greatest dimension, limited to the kidney
T1b	Tumor more than 4 cm but not more than 7 cm in greatest dimension limited to the kidney
T2	Tumor more than 7 cm in greatest dimension, limited to the kidney
T2a	Tumor more than 7 cm but less than or equal to 10 cm in greatest dimension, limited to the kidney
T2b	Tumor more than 10 cm, limited to the kidney
T3	Tumor extends into major veins or perinephric tissues but not into the ipsilateral adrenal gland and not beyond Gerota's fascia
T3a	Tumor grossly extends into the renal vein or its segmental (muscle containing) branches, or tumor invades perirenal and/or renal sinus fat but not beyond Gerota's fascia
T3b	Tumor grossly extends into the vena cava below the diaphragm
T3c	Tumor grossly extends into the vena cava above the diaphragm or invades the wall of the vena cava
T4	Tumor invades beyond Gerota's fascia (including contiguous extension into the ipsilateral adrenal gland)
Regional lymph nodes (N)	
NX	Regional lymph nodes cannot be assessed
N0	No regional lymph node metastasis
N1	Metastasis in regional lymph node(s)
Distant metastasis (M)	
M0	No distant metastasis
M1	Distant metastasis

Anatomic stage • Prognostic groups			
Stage I	T1	N0	M0
Stage II	T2	N0	M0
	T1 or T2	N1	M0
Stage III	T3	N0 or N1	M0
Stage IV	T4	Any N	M0
	Any T	Any N	M1

gland (37–53%), and those with extension of the primary tumor beyond Gerota's fascia (20%) [12]. While TNM stage strongly influences survival of patients diagnosed with renal cell carcinoma, histologic classification is important as, for example, spindle cell and anaplastic cell types carry a worse prognosis for a given clinical stage. Histologic classification including Fuhrman grade and general health of the patient also influence survival and are further taken into account in some integrated staging systems for renal cell carcinoma [13]. No significant correlation was found, however, between the degree of FDG uptake on PET as measured by standardized uptake values and histologic classification or Fuhrman grade of primary renal cell carcinoma in one study [11]. Five year survival of patients with distant metastatic disease is 0–20% depending in part on these other factors [14].

T Stage

T staging is determined by the size of the primary tumor and relationship with adjacent tissues and organs. T1 denotes tumors confined to the kidney and less than 7 cm in greatest dimension while T 2 denotes tumors greater than 7 cm greatest dimension but still confined to the kidney. In the newer 2002 TNM classification, the T1 category for staging of patients is subdivided into T1a, those less than 4 cm and T1b, those 4–7 cm. This new T1 subdivision reflects the differential recurrence and survival rates between the two categories, as well as the current practice of treating T1a (those having primary peripheral exophytic tumors less than 4 cm) with partial, rather than full, nephrectomies. Furthermore, the new classification is supported by an independent validation study, which demonstrated superior predictive ability compared to the older TNM classification [12]. However, the size cutoff between T1 and T2 is still debated [15].

T3 denotes any size tumor that extends beyond the renal capsule and directly invades the perinephric tissues or the adrenal gland (T3a), or extends into the major veins (T3a and T3b), but otherwise has not extended beyond Gerota's fascia. The subdivisions of T3 denote the extent of tumor spread into the venous system, with T3b limited to venous structures below the diaphragm, while T3c has tumor extension in the venous structures above the diaphragm. Although patients with venous spread of tumor above the diaphragm are still considered surgical candidates, a thoracotomy is typically required in addition to a laparotomy to remove all viable intravascular tumor. Patients with T3 tumors undergo radical nephrectomy unless precluded by metastatic disease or the condition of the patient.

T4 denotes a tumor of any size that has breached Gerota's fascia, with or without adjacent organ involvement. The prognosis for T4 stage primary renal cell carcinoma, even in the absence of nodal or distant metastatic disease, is poor. T4 tumors are classified as Stage IV, even in the absence of nodal or distant metastases. In selected patients, radical nephrectomy may be performed, but generally stage IV disease is considered incurable.

T staging of renal cell carcinoma with PET-CT is almost entirely determined by the findings on the CT images (Fig. 29.3). While the extent of the margins of FDG avid tumor is sometimes delineated by FDG PET images, with renal cell carcinoma the size of the tumor within the kidney will be best depicted for measurement on contrast enhanced CT images. Direct involvement of the adrenal gland will be largely a CT diagnosis. Similarly, the extension of tumor or presence of tumor thrombus in the renal vein and vena cava is sensitively depicted on the CT images when appropriate contrast enhanced technique is used. FDG tracer uptake in venous tumor or tumor thrombus is typically modest or absent, and thus is only of limited utility. Extension beyond Gerota's fascia into adjacent organs such as the liver, abdominal and

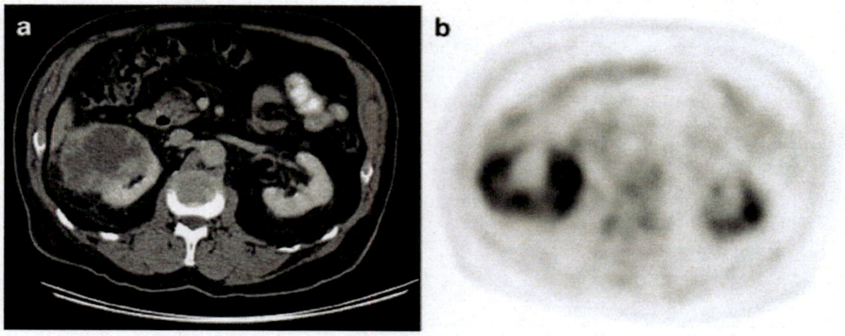

Fig. 29.3 T-Stage of RCC. Transaxial contrast enhanced CT (**a**) shows a right renal mass greater than 7 cm in maximum dimension which extend beyond the renal parenchyma into the perirenal fat but not through Gerota's fascia for a T3 T-stage. The corresponding FDG PET image (**b**) shows the renal cell carcinoma having greater uptake than renal parenchyma but less than urinary tracer seen just medial to the mass. Focal FDG tracer in the left kidney is urinary tracer

paraspinous musculature is also largely diagnosed on the CT images, although in some instances the true extent of the neoplasm will be grossly delineated by the FDG PET findings.

Patients undergoing PET-CT for newly diagnosed renal cell carcinoma will often already have an imaging evaluation of the primary renal mass, usually a CT or ultrasound. The T stage may be adequately diagnosed on these studies, although it is not uncommon, as noted above, that a renal mass was incidentally found on an imaging study, such as a CT, performed for another indication. Such CT scans may not have been properly optimized for evaluation of renal cell carcinoma, including phases of contrast for the renal mass and adequacy of renal vein and vena cava contrast opacification. Additional valuable staging information may be obtained from the properly performed PET-CT exam. In addition, renal cell carcinoma can be an incidental finding on PET-CT exams performed for evaluation of a different cancer.

N Staging

N staging for renal cell carcinoma involves detecting abnormal regional lymph nodes, with the most commonly involved nodes at the time of diagnosis being renal hilar, paracaval, paraaortic, aortocaval, and other retroperitoneal lymph nodes. Nodal laterality does not affect the N classification. N staging is divided into only three categories, N0 (no regional nodal metastases), N1 (metastases to a single regional lymph node), and N2 (metastases in more than one regional lymph node). While the presence of lymph node metastases does result in Stage III (N1) and Stage IV (N2), and portends a poor prognosis, the presence of lymph node metastases does not preclude surgical management. Radical nephrectomy with retroperitoneal lymph node dissection may be performed, as a small minority of cases with regional lymph node metastases can be cured with surgery.

CT criteria for abnormal lymph nodes considered suspicious for metastatic involvement include size >1 cm in the short axis and/or necrosis. These criteria are nonspecific, however, as nonenlarged lymph nodes can be replaced by metastatic neoplasm and benign processes can result in enlarged lymph nodes. Central necrosis is more specific finding for metastatic involvement on CT images that occasionally occurs with renal cell carcinoma, although usually the lymph node is substantially enlarged when central necrosis occurs due to a RCC metastasis. As with other cancers, FDG PET images can identify lymph node metastases of renal cell carcinoma in non-enlarged lymph nodes, improving the accuracy of N staging over CT alone (Fig. 29.4). Renal cell carcinoma, including metastases, can be associated with only modest, or no appreciable FDG tracer uptake at all. The absence of abnormal FDG tracer uptake in a borderline enlarged or enlarged lymph node on the FDG PET images does not have the same negative predictive value for renal cell carcinoma as typically encountered with FDG PET of other commonly imaged cancers. Hence enlarged, contrast-enhancing or necrotic regional lymph nodes should be considered

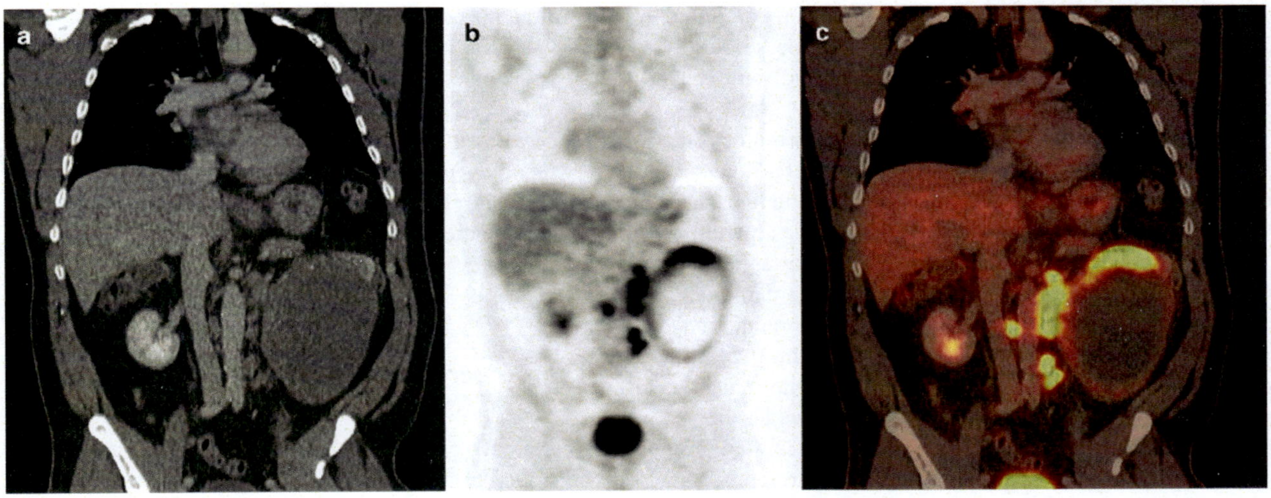

Fig 29.4 Primary renal cell carcinoma with retroperitoneal lymph node metastases. Coronal contrast enhanced CT (**a**) show a large left renal mass occupying much of the left kidney and borderline enlarged left paraaortic and aortocaval nodes. Coronal FDG PET (**b**) and FDG PET-CT fusion image (**c**) demonstrates intense FDG tracer uptake in the retroperitoneal lymph nodes and varying intensity of FDG tracer uptake along the rim of the renal mass. Central necrosis manifest in absent FDG tracer activity and decreased attenuation is common in large renal cell carcinoma masses

suspicious even when not abnormal on the FDG PET images, especially when the primary renal mass is not itself highly FDG avid.

M Staging

Distant metastases of renal cell carcinoma most commonly are to the lung, liver, and skeleton and mediastinal lymph nodes, but can occur in other organs including the ipsilateral or contralateral adrenal glands, contralateral kidney, brain, thyroid gland, and soft tissues including muscle. As with other cancers, PET-CT is particularly useful in evaluating the whole body for distant metastatic disease. FDG PET alone has been reported to have a sensitivity ranging from 63% to 77% and a specificity ranging from 75% to 100% [9, 16, 17]. In general, FDG PET lacked sensitivity due to the fraction of renal cell carcinoma metastases that were associated with limited or absent FDG tracer uptake. The presence of an abnormality on FDG PET, however, is reported to have a high positive predictive value, although true positive lesions were anatomically abnormal by size criteria in one study [17, 18]. While one study found FDG PET to be more sensitive for detection of the typical lytic osseous metastases of renal cell carcinoma than bone scan alone, FDG PET alone was less sensitive than combined CT and bone scan [9, 19]. Studies evaluating the effect of FDG PET alone on the management of patients with renal cell carcinoma have reported changes in overall management in 13–35% of patients [9, 10]. Studies systemically evaluating the performance of integrated PET-CT on the staging of renal cell carcinoma are not yet available; however, the contribution of the CT to overall diagnostic performance of PET-CT of renal cell carcinoma likely will be important, compensating for the sensitivity limitations secondary to the low FDG avidity of some renal cell carcinomas (Fig. 29.5).

The chief pitfall in PET-CT of renal cell carcinoma is the relatively low or absent FGD uptake encountered in a substantial portion (well over a third) of primary and metastatic renal cell carcinoma. Hence the false negative fraction of lymph node and distant organ and osseous metastases on the FDG PET images can be significant, requiring particularly careful attention to CT technique and interpretation. As noted above, enlarged regional lymph nodes must be considered suspicious even in the absence of abnormal FDG tracer uptake on the PET images, especially when the primary renal cell carcinoma is known to be of limited FDG avidity. Pulmonary metastases of renal cell carcinoma may be equivocal or negative on the FDG PET images, and hence the usual approach to pulmonary nodules should not be applied regarding negative predictive value of an FDG PET negative nodule. Osseous metastases of renal cell carcinoma are often purely lytic and hence very careful review of properly displayed CT images is necessary. Also, since T stage is of central importance in operative planning, CT technique should be optimized for T stage evaluation in those patients that have not been adequately staged on prior imaging studies.

On unenhanced CT images, renal cell carcinomas can be hyperdense, isodense, or hypodense to normal renal tissue, with heterogeneous areas due to variable amounts of hemorrhage and necrosis. Some renal cell carcinomas may not be visible at all on noncontrast CT images, except for the presence of calcification (10%) or cystic areas (2–5%). On contrast-enhanced CT, renal cell carcinoma becomes readily apparent in most cases, and can have several different appearances, but typically a primary renal cell carcinoma is a solid cortically based mass with variable contrast enhancement. CT evaluation of a renal mass, in general, and renal cell carcinoma in particular, is best performed without and with intravenous contrast material optimally depicting both calcifications and the soft tissue features of the mass. Also, hyperdense cysts can be differentiated from other potentially malignant renal masses by the lack of contrast enhancement. Renal cell carcinoma tends to be hypervascular, showing arterial phase enhancement on multiphase CT imaging, although they tend to be most conspicuous on the nephrographic phase (later) than on the arterial or corticomedullary phases of the CT imaging.

Minimizing urinary tracer activity in the upper urinary tract can improve the FDG PET images of the kidneys and reduce potential false positive FDG PET findings due to focal urinary tracer accumulation within the kidneys. Intravenous hydration and loop diuretics can reduce, although not always completely eliminate, urinary FDG tracer activity in the intrarenal collecting system.

It is also important to evaluate the ipsilateral adrenal gland, as the current practice is to spare the gland at radical nephrectomy. Although both PET and CT portions of a PET-CT will offer information, interpreting physicians should report even small abnormalities involving the ipsilateral adrenal on CT, such as displacement or enlargement, as this is an indication of adrenalectomy as part of the surgical exploration.

Restaging Renal Cell Carcinoma with PET-CT

The routine use of PET-CT in the posttreatment period has not been well established. Limited data regarding restaging renal cell carcinoma on FDG PET alone are similar to results for staging, with high positive predictive values but sensitivity limited by the low FDG avidity of some renal cell carcinoma [18, 20].

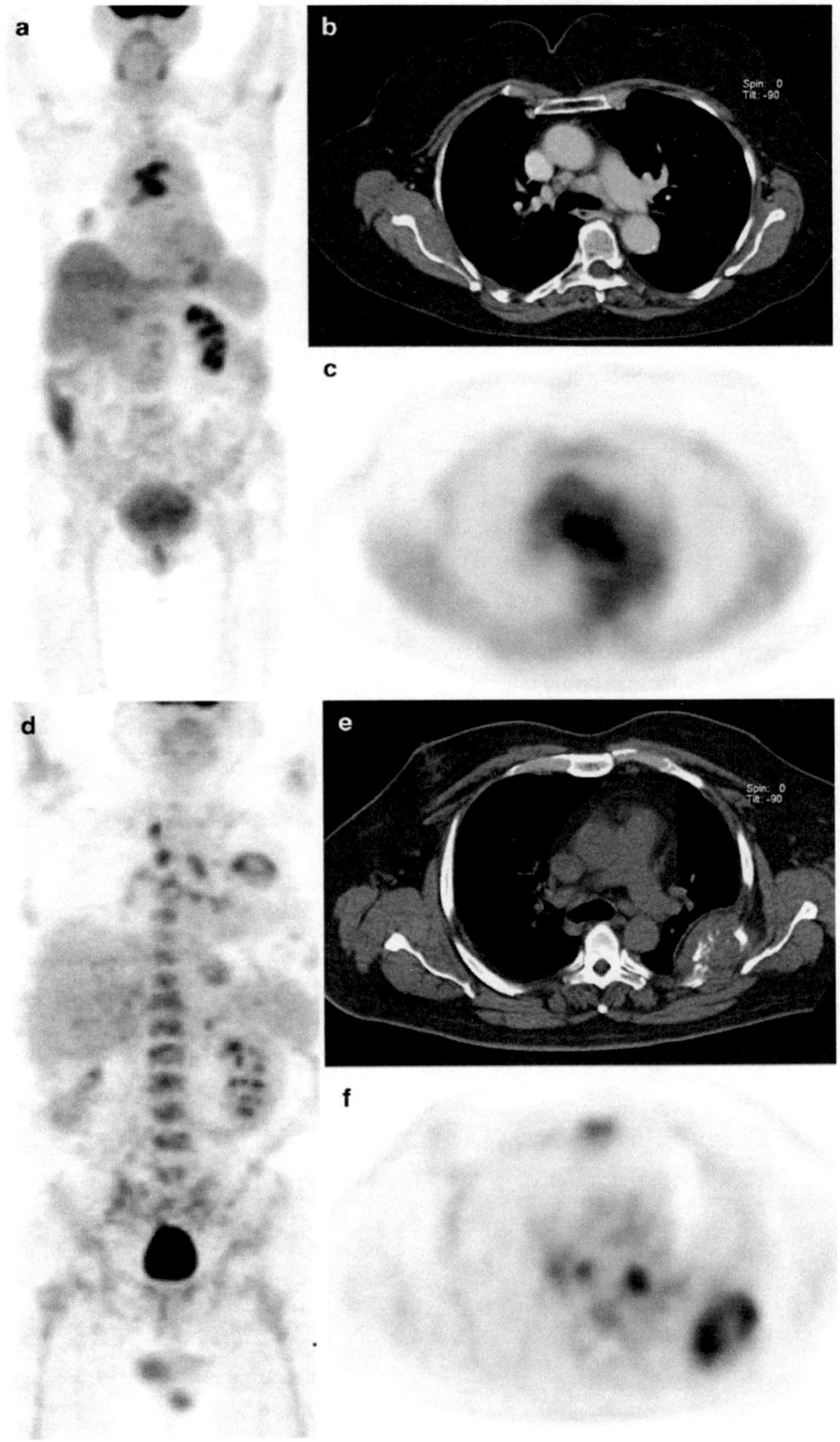

Fig. 29.5 Metastatic renal cell carcinoma. (**a**) Anterior FDG PET maximum intensity projection (*MIP*) image in patient 2 years post right nephrectomy for renal cell carcinoma demonstrates intense abnormal FDG tracer uptake in the lower mediastinum. Transaxial CT (**b**) and FDG PET (**c**) reveal borderline enlarged enhanced precarinal lymph nodes associated with intense abnormal FDG tracer uptake. In another patient the anterior FDG PET MIP image (**d**) shows small foci of FDG tracer uptake in the mediastinum and an ovoid area of modest FDG tracer activity in the left chest wall. Transaxial CT (**e**) and FDG PET (**f**) images show the modest abnormal FDG tracer activity in the left chest wall focal FDG tracer activity corresponds to a large expansile and destructive rib metastasis. FDG tracer uptake by metastatic renal cell carcinoma is widely variable and can be minimal or intense

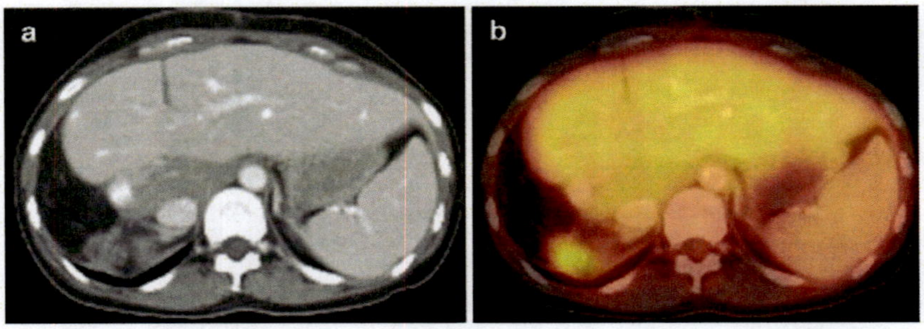

Fig. 29.6 Local recurrence of renal cell carcinoma. Transaxial CT (**a**) shows ill defined soft tissue in the superior right nephrectomy bed in a patient 5 years after right nephrectomy for renal cell carcinoma. Corresponding FDG PET-CT fusion image (**b**) demonstrates definite abnormal FDG tracer uptake in the soft tissue confirming recurrent neoplasm rather than scar tissue

There are certainly potential applications in which PET-CT will be very useful, such as is in differentiating residual/recurrent tumor form scar in the nephrectomy bed (Fig. 29.6). Both scar and tumor at the nephrectomy bed often appear similar on CT, making less appealing as a single modality for evaluating patients following a nephrectomy. The detection of unsuspected metastases is important in patients with renal cell carcinoma as there is some benefit to survival when isolated or limited metastases are resected. Pulmonary metastases are a frequent finding for which resection may be considered, but the presence of other sites of metastases as well as local recurrence must be excluded before such resection, and PET-CT may be the preferred modality for the restaging of such patients.

As with staging, the principal pitfall of restaging renal cell carcinoma with PET-CT is the modest to absent FDG avidity of some renal cell carcinoma, and this appears to be true for recurrent disease on restaging. Small pulmonary metastases are more sensitively detected on CT than FDG PET in general, and particularly with renal cell carcinoma, which may exhibit limited or absent FDG tracer uptake. A new pulmonary nodule in a patient with renal cell carcinoma or a history of renal cell carcinoma must be considered highly suspicious for a metastasis, even if it is not associated with abnormal FDG tracer uptake.

Renal Cell Carcinoma Therapy Monitoring and Planning with PET-CT

As renal cell carcinoma is largely managed surgically, it is unclear what role PET-CT will play in terms of evaluating response to systemic therapies. It is possible that as more useful chemotherapy and radiation therapy regimens are implemented, that PET-CT could help determine responders from nonresponders. However, there are no large studies to date evaluating PET-CT for this purpose.

Conclusion

There is a paucity of studies looking at the role of combined PET-CT in the evaluation of primary renal masses, staging and restaging of patients with renal cell carcinomas. However, given the preliminary evidence from the individual modalities, possible roles of PET-CT would include staging and restaging of selected patients with renal cell.

References

1. Jemal A, Siegel R, Ward E, et al. Cancer statistics, 2008. CA Cancer J Clin 2008;58:71–96.
2. Lipworth L, Tarone RE, McLaughlin JK. The epidemiology of renal cell carcinoma. J Urol 2006;176:2353–2358.
3. Rini BI, Rathmell WK, Godley P. Renal cell carcinoma. Curr Opin Oncol 2008;20:300–306.
4. Smith SJ, Bosniak MA, Megibow AJ, Hulnick DH, Horii SC, Raghavendra BN. Renal cell carcinoma: earlier discovery and increased detection. Radiology 1989;170:699–703.
5. Janzen NK, Kim HL, Figlin RA, Belldegrun AS. Surveillance after radical or partial nephrectomy for localized renal cell carcinoma and management of recurrent disease. Urol Clin North Am 2003;30:843–852.
6. Bosniak MA. The current radiological approach to renal cysts. Radiology 1986;158:1–10.
7. Wolf JS, Jr. Evaluation and management of solid and cystic renal masses. J Urol 1998;159:1120–1133.
8. Goldberg MA, Mayo-Smith WW, Papanicolaou N, Fischman AJ, Lee MJ. FDG PET characterization of renal masses: preliminary experience. Clin Radiol 1997;52:510–515.
9. Kang DE, White RL, Jr., Zuger JH, Sasser HC, Teigland CM. Clinical use of fluorodeoxyglucose F 18 positron emission tomography for detection of renal cell carcinoma. J Urol 2004;171:1806–1809.
10. S, Thomas GW, Berlangieri SU, et al. Clinical role of F-18 fluorodeoxyglucose positron emission tomography for detection and management of renal cell carcinoma. J Urol 2001;166:825–830.
11. Shreve PD, Miyauchi T, Wahl RL. Characterization of primary renal cell carcinoma by FDG PET. Radiology 1998;209P:94.
12. I, Blute ML, Leibovich BC, Cheville JC, Lohse CM, Zincke H. Independent validation of the 2002 American Joint Committee on

cancer primary tumor classification for renal cell carcinoma using a large, single institution cohort. J Urol 2005;173:1889–1892.
13. Fuhrman SA, Lasky LC, Limas C. Prognostic significance of morphologic parameters in renal cell carcinoma. Am J Surg Pathol 1982;6:655–663.
14. Mekhail TM, Abou-Jawde RM, Boumerhi G, et al. Validation and extension of the Memorial Sloan-Kettering prognostic factors model for survival in patients with previously untreated metastatic renal cell carcinoma. J Clin Oncol 2005;23:832–841.
15. Shuch B, La Rochelle JC, Pantuck AJ, Belldegrun AS. The staging of renal cell carcinoma. Curr Opin Urol 2008;18:455–461.
16. Aide N, Cappele O, Bottet P, et al. Efficiency of [(18)F]FDG PET in characterising renal cancer and detecting distant metastases: a comparison with CT. Eur J Nucl Med Mol Imaging 2003;30:1236–1245.
17. Majhail NS, Urbain JL, Albani JM, et al. F-18 fluorodeoxyglucose positron emission tomography in the evaluation of distant metastases from renal cell carcinoma. J Clin Oncol 2003;21:3995–4000.
18. Jadvar H, Kherbache HM, Pinski JK, Conti PS. Diagnostic role of [F-18]-FDG positron emission tomography in restaging renal cell carcinoma. Clin Nephrol 2003;60:395–400.
19. Seto E, Segall GM, Terris MK. Positron emission tomography detection of osseous metastases of renal cell carcinoma not identified on bone scan. Urology 2000;55:286.
20. Safaei A, Figlin R, Hoh CK, et al. The usefulness of F-18 deoxyglucose whole-body positron emission tomography (PET) for restaging of renal cell cancer. Clin Nephrol 2002;57:56–62.

Further Reading

1. Cohen HT, McGovern FJ. Renal-cell carcinoma. NEJM 2005;353:2477–2490.
2. Federle MP, Chen, J.J. Renal cell carcinoma. In: Federle MP (ed.). Diagnostic Imaging: Abdomen. Salt Lake City: Amirsys, 2004:III-3–96.
3. Hain SF, Maisey MN. Positron emission tomography for urological tumours. BJU Int 2003;92(2):159–164.
4. Shreve P. PET imaging in urologic tumors. In: Valk PE Bailey DL, Townsend DW, Maisey MN (eds.). Positron Emission Tomography: Basic Science and Clinical Practice Part IV: Oncology. London: Springer, 2003:637–644.
5. Shvarts O, Han KR, Seltzer M, Pantuck AJ, Belldegrun AS. Positron emission tomography in urologic oncology. Cancer Control 2002;9(4):335–342.

Chapter 30
PET-CT in Soft Tissue Malignancies

Edwin L. Palmer, James A. Scott, and Thomas F. DeLaney

Tumors of soft tissue arise from mesenchymal elements of muscle, connective tissues, adipose tissue, blood vessels, and peripheral nerves. Soft tissue neoplasms therefore comprise a very diverse group of tumors. Benign soft tissue tumors such as lipomas, fibromas, and desmoids are usually incidental findings noted by the patient. Fortunately, malignant soft tissue tumors are very rare, occurring only about one hundredth as frequently as benign soft tissue neoplasms. When considered together, all types of soft tissue sarcomas comprise less than 1% of newly diagnosed cancers in adults, although they represent a higher fraction of pediatric malignancies. Soft tissue sarcomas are two to three times as common as the even more rare primary bone sarcomas. It is currently believed that most soft tissue sarcomas originate from primitive mesenchymal cells that differentiate into a specific tumor type as they undergo malignant degeneration. The prognosis in soft tissue sarcomas is guarded, with eventual mortality from the tumor in about one half of patients with aggressive sarcomas [1].

Skin cancers originating from epithelioid elements are clinically and pathologically distinct from those soft tissue tumors of mesenchymal origin. Common skin cancers such as basal cell and squamous carcinomas tend to invade locally and to have a natural history distinct from sarcomas. Treatment of these involves local excision, and there is no established role for PET-CT in these tumors.

In this chapter, we deal primarily with the numerous types of soft tissue sarcomas. Because these tumors are so rare, clinical experience with the entire group of sarcomas is very limited in comparison to more common malignancies such as lung or breast cancer. Trying to understand the specific appearance and natural history of each histologic tumor type is even more challenging. To complicate matters further, the behavior of specific tumor types that arise in different body regions, such as retroperitoneum or extremity, may differ significantly. There is often insufficient clinical experience with individual tumor types to permit an in-depth understanding of their differences.

Fortunately, a number of generalizations about all soft tissue sarcomas can be made, allowing reasonable understanding about both the clinical approach and imaging appearances of these tumors. The more common sarcoma types are listed in Table 30.1. These include both mesoderm-derived sarcomas and ectodermal malignant neural tumors that are embryologically divergent from, but tending to behave similarly to, sarcomas.

Soft issue sarcomas occur primarily in older adults, with most cases diagnosed in patients over age 50. These tumors are very rare in children, and the vast majority of tumors in the pediatric age group are embryonal rhabdomyosarcomas. In both adults and children, most tumors are noted incidentally, typically when the patient identifies a soft tissue mass. The mass is usually asymptomatic, although lesions can be painful depending on location and involvement of adjacent nerves or bone. Superficial masses may be detected very early, while deep tumors, such as those in the retroperitoneum, are often not identified until they have grown quite large and have compressed or invaded abdominal or pelvic organs. Most tumor histologies follow a general distribution, although some tumor types have specific anatomic predilections. For example, epithelioid sarcoma is very commonly found in the forearm or finger. Leiomyosarcoma and liposarcoma have a particular predilection for the retroperitoneum, accounting for most of the tumors detected in this region.

Definitive treatment of sarcomas consists of complete surgical resection of the tumor, if possible. Sarcomas often infiltrate adjacent tissue extensively, so wide local resection is necessary. Adjunctive radiation therapy significantly reduces local recurrence rate in comparison to surgery alone, and is therefore standard practice. Radiotherapy is particularly important in extremity sarcomas, in which limb sparing surgical resection is desirable. Careful resection of the entire tumor, with adequate disease-free margins is essential, requiring considerable experience and expertise by the oncologic surgeon.

E.L. Palmer (✉)
Division of Nuclear Medicine and Molecular Imaging & PET-CT, Massachusetts General Hospital, 32 Fruit Street, Boston, MA, USA, 02114
e-mail: epalmer@partners.org

P. Shreve and D.W. Townsend (eds.), *Clinical PET-CT in Radiology: Integrated Imaging in Oncology*, DOI 10.1007/978-0-387-48902-5_30, © Springer Science+Business Media, LLC 2011

Table 30.1 Common soft tissue sarcomas (Used with the permission of the American Joint Committee on Cancer (AJCC), Chicago, IL. The original source for this material is the *AJCC Cancer Staging Manual*, 7th edn. (2010) published by Springer Science and Business Media LLC. www.springer.com)

Malignant fibrous histiocytoma
Liposarcoma
Leiomyosarcoma
Synovial sarcoma
Malignant peripheral nerve sheath tumors
Rhabdomyosarcoma
Fibrosarcoma
Extraosseous Ewing's sarcoma
Angiosarcoma
Extraosseous osteosarcoma
Epithelioid sarcoma
Clear cell sarcoma
Alveolar soft part sarcoma
Malignant hemangiopericytoma
Gastrointestinal stromal tumor

Randomized clinical trials have demonstrated a clear improvement in local tumor control with the addition of adjuvant radiation therapy to conservative surgery in the management of extremity and truncal soft tissue sarcomas. Adjuvant radiation therapy can be given by external beam radiation or brachytherapy, or a combination thereof. External beam radiation can be given either preoperatively or postoperatively. There are potential advantages to both preoperative and postoperative administration of radiation. Preoperative radiation therapy might be expected to reduce tumor burden prior to resection, theoretically allowing more conservative surgical therapy. Radiation fields can be limited to the tumor and adjacent tissues at risk for microscopic infiltration, a volume that is considerably smaller than that which must be treated following surgery, where the entire surgical bed, incision, and drain site tracts are included in the initial target volume irradiated to 50 Gy. Preoperative radiation therapy allows lower administered doses (50 Gy pre-op vs 60–66 Gy postop). Postoperative radiotherapy, however, allows histologic examination of the tumor specimen, especially the margins, aiding in further treatment planning. It is also associated with fewer acute wound complications.

There is one randomized, controlled trial comparing preoperative versus postoperative radiotherapy in patients with potentially curable extremity soft-tissue sarcoma [2]. In this Canadian trial, a significantly higher percentage of preoperatively treated patients had acute wound complications (35% versus 17%). Other factors associated with wound complications were the volume of resected tissue and lower limb tumor location. There were no differences in local control between the patients in the two arms of the study, with over 90% local control. The regional and distant failure rates as well as the progression-free and overall survival rates were also no different between the two arms of the study. Over time, however, as a consequence of the higher doses and larger fields, the postoperative radiation therapy patients have developed more late subcutaneous fibrosis [3].

There is thus a difference in the morbidity profile between preoperative and postoperative radiotherapy, with a higher rate of generally reversible acute wound healing complications in the patients receiving preoperative treatment, in comparison to a higher rate of generally irreversible late complications, including grade 3–4 fibrosis, in those patients receiving postoperative radiation therapy. Because very few acute wound-healing complications occurred in either group when the tumor was in the upper extremity, pre-operative radiation therapy is favored for these patients. Some centers also continue to favor preoperative radiation for the majority of lower extremity patients, because acute wound complications generally do go on to heal with appropriate wound care, whereas the late treatment effects are usually irreversible.

Compared to external beam radiation therapy, brachytherapy minimizes the radiation dose to surrounding normal tissues, maximizes the radiation dose delivered to the tumor, and shortens treatment times. There have been no randomized comparisons of the relative efficacy or morbidity of external beam radiation therapy compared with brachytherapy. In the usual brachytherapy schedule, treatment is completed within 6 days and requires only one hospitalization. Afterloading catheters are placed in a target area of the tumor operative bed defined by the surgeon, and spaced at 1 cm intervals to cover the entire area of risk.

Intraoperative radiotherapy with electron beam or orthovoltage is delivered to the tumor or tumor bed at the time of surgery. It can be particularly useful to boost the dose to retroperitoneal, paraspinal and spinal, and pelvic sarcomas [4, 5]. At the time of surgery, radiation-sensitive normal tissues not involved by the tumor can be moved outside of the intraoperative radiation field, thus allowing higher doses to be delivered to the tumor while sparing adjacent normal tissues.

Role of PET-CT in the Initial Diagnosis of Soft Tissue Tumors

Although there is significant experience in PET evaluation of sarcomas, our understanding is very limited in comparison to more common tumors such as lung cancer or lymphoma. Most published series are small, and often have significant methodologic deficiencies. In addition, we have at present very incomplete knowledge of the differences between the PET appearances of various histologic types of tumors. For all of these reasons, our current understanding should be seen as a preliminary approach that will evolve over time.

Once a soft tissue mass has been detected, a biopsy is usually required to determine whether it is benign or malignant,

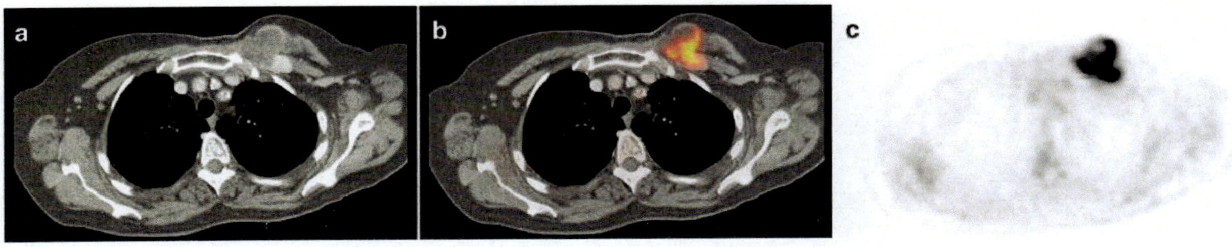

Fig. 30.1 A 56-year-old woman who is 14 years status post left modified radical mastectomy and radiation therapy for breast cancer, followed 8 years ago by chest wall recurrence, treated with surgical resection and additional radiation therapy. The patient recently noted growth of an upper chest wall mass, shown on PET images (**a**), CT (**b**), and CT-PET (**c**). Biopsy showed fibrosarcoma, grade 1/3

and if malignant, to establish the histologic diagnosis and tumor grade. Although some have advocated the use of PET imaging in the initial diagnosis of soft tissue sarcomas, no definitive role has yet been established. In selected patients, PET might be useful in guiding biopsy, as discussed below.

Extensive experience has shown that most malignant soft tissue tumors are FDG avid [6, 7]. As a general rule, most high-grade and many intermediate grade tumors are intensely FDG positive, and the intensity of FDG uptake, as determined by several techniques, correlates well with tumor grade [8, 9]. Benign soft tissue tumors generally do not show FDG uptake greater than adjacent normal muscle, and are usually not visible on PET images as separate identifiable structures. Figures 30.1, 30.2, and 30.3 show typical examples of newly diagnosed sarcomas that are FDG avid.

Despite these differences, it is not possible to confidently differentiate benign from malignant soft tissue tumors using PET imaging for several reasons. Many low-grade tumors have FDG uptake that is little or no greater than adjacent normal soft tissue structures or than benign tumors. Therefore, it is not always possible to differentiate *low-grade* sarcomas from benign tumors with pet imaging [7, 10]. To further complicate matters, some benign tumors may show intense FDG avidity. For example, benign schwannomas and desmoids may show FDG uptake comparable to that seen in many high-grade sarcomas [6]. This mirrors the experience with primary bone tumors, where many histologically benign but clinically aggressive tumors such as giant cell tumors may show intense uptake similar to high-grade sarcomas. Avid FDG uptake, however, does not necessarily imply that a benign lesion is biologically aggressive. In bone, even non-aggressive conditions, such as fibrous dysplasia and Paget's disease may show very intense uptake. In soft tissue, sarcoidosis and infectious or noninfectious inflammatory processes may show uptake as intense as any sarcoma.

Semiquantitative evaluation of sarcoma FDG uptake using SUV has been advocated to reproducibly evaluate the known general correlation between FDG uptake and tumor grade. For example, one study showed that median SUV was 1.3 in low-grade, 2.7 in intermediate grade, and 4.5 in high-grade sarcomas [9]. These findings mirror similar results with primary bone sarcomas. Because FDG uptake often varies greatly from one part of the tumor to another, the maximum SUV value within the tumor is typically used. Low uptake areas, such as zones of necrosis, might artifactually reduce the SUV calculation were the average value used.

Existing evidence suggests that the use of quantitative parameters such as SUV or metabolic rates does not significantly improve upon visual assessment of FDG uptake for the purposes of differentiating sarcomas from benign tumors [7]. Although the average or median SUV values differ even between low-grade sarcomas and benign tumors, these data are true only for large *populations* of patients. In an *individual* patient, it is not possible to distinguish benign from malignant, or to attribute a tumor grade, based upon the SUV. There is significant overlap between the ranges of SUV shown in benign, low-grade, and higher-grade tumors, and an individual patient's SUV does not allow assignment of the tumor to a pathologic group. With this important understanding in mind, it is generally true that most intermediate and high-grade malignancies show an SUV of ≥ 2 [7]. It is possible that FDG evaluation of tumor metabolic activity may someday add to our clinical understanding of tumor grade and tumor biology, but there is at present insufficient evidence to support that role. It has been suggested that the intensity of FDG uptake is an independent predictor of poor prognosis [11].

At the present time, our understanding of the variability in FDG uptake between the different histologic types of sarcomas is insufficient to make definitive statements. Some studies have shown differences between the median FDG uptakes of varying histologic types, but the differences have been small, and the individual variation in tumor uptake is great.

Some investigators have suggested that more complicated metabolic evaluation of the tumor obtained by using dynamic acquisition PET imaging may be superior to SUV alone. Even these parameters, however, have not been able to confidently differentiate all benign from malignant soft tissue lesions.

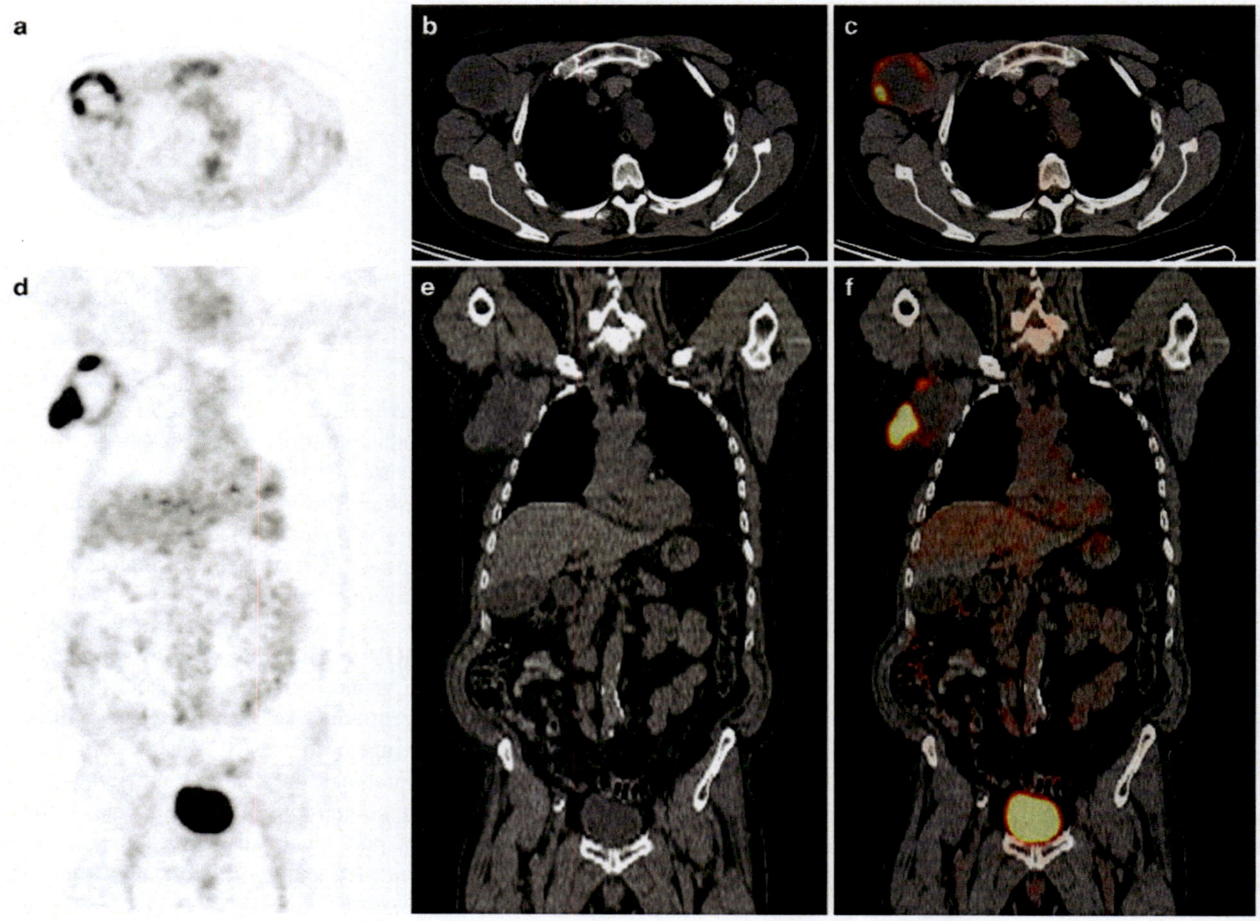

Fig. 30.2 A 72-year-old man with new diagnosis of right axillary mass shown on axial (**a–c**) and coronal (**d–f**) PET-CT images. Biopsy showed grade 2–3/3 malignant peripheral nerve sheath tumor. Note that PET images show intense uptake in the periphery of the tumor, but little uptake in the central regions, corresponding to lower attenuation on CT, and likely necrosis. At resection, most of the central tumor was non-viable

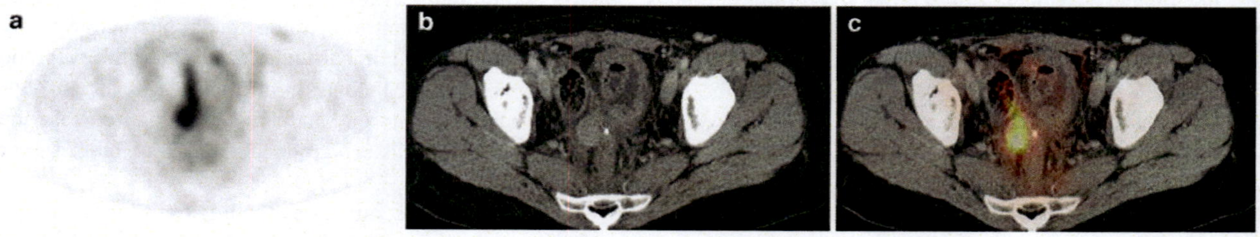

Fig. 30.3 A 45-year-old woman previously operated on for right lower quadrant mass initially thought to be an abscess. Review of outside pathology slides demonstrated a high-grade (3/3) leiomyosarcoma, incompletely resected. PET scan (**a**) shows intense, linear uptake in the pelvis. CT (**b**) shows an abnormal soft tissue density, close to a surgical clip, located posterior and superior to the bladder, and corresponding well to the PET uptake as shown on PET-CT fusion image (**c**). At surgery, residual leiomyosarcoma was found adherent to the sigmoid colon

Although PET imaging does not play a routine role in the initial diagnosis of soft tissue sarcoma, its use has been advocated to direct biopsy in selected patients, by identifying those regions of the tumor that show high metabolic activity. This might, in tumors with substantial necrosis, avoid biopsy of a necrotic zone and yield a better pathologic specimen. In this application, PET-CT provides a substantial advantage over conventional stand-alone PET imaging by allowing confident correlation of intense tumor uptake with easily identifiable regional anatomy shown on CT to plan a CT guided

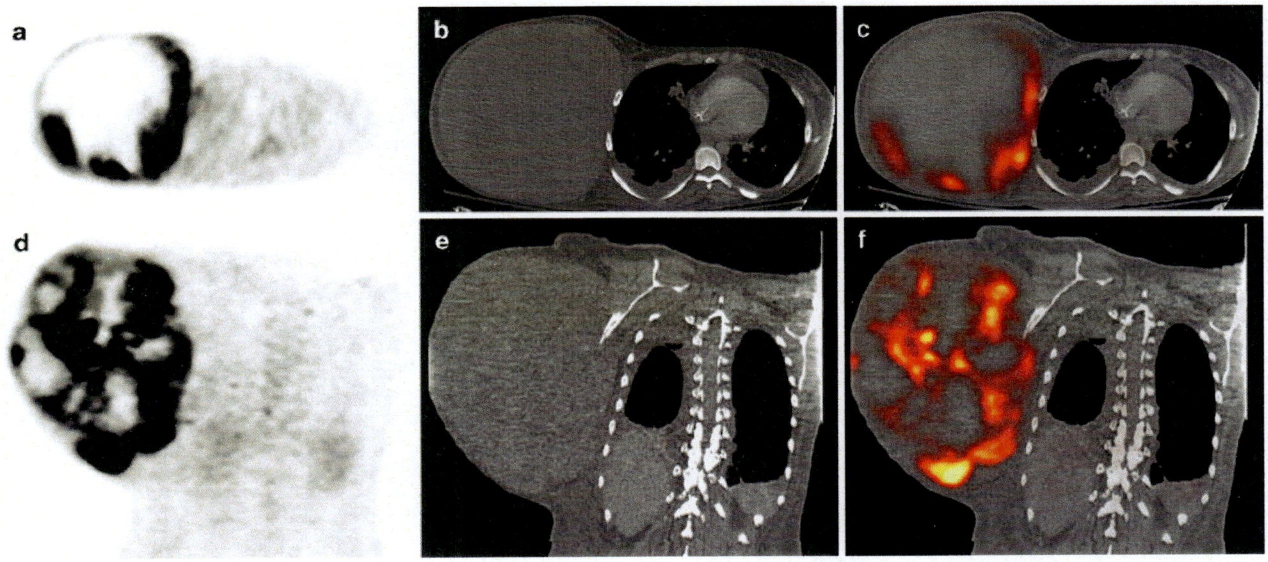

Fig. 30.4 A 32-year-old woman with neurofibrosis-1, and rapidly expanding right axillary mass. Axial PET, CT, and PET-CT images (**a–c**) show a massive soft tissue mass with very intense peripheral tracer uptake, but little metabolic activity centrally. Coronal images (**d–f**) show that activity is very heterogeneous. Biopsy showed high-grade (2–3/3) malignant peripheral nerve sheath tumor

biopsy. Although showing great promise, this use of PET has not been clearly validated at this time.

An example of another clinical setting in which PET might play a role in guiding biopsy is in patients with neurofibromatosis type 1 (von Recklinghausen's disease). These individuals often have innumerable cutaneous and subcutaneous benign tumors. If a patient develops pain, the rare possibility of malignant degeneration to neurofibrosarcoma or malignant schwannoma needs to be considered. If there are numerous masses, it may be impossible to determine by clinical evaluation or MRI what lesions might be of concern. In this setting, relatively increased FDG uptake in a single lesion is a suspicious finding, and can direct biopsy (Fig. 30.4). In this setting, increased FDG uptake does not necessarily indicate malignancy. It may simply allow a rational approach to biopsy.

Soft Tissue Sarcoma Staging

Sarcomas tend to grow locally, and spread by direct extension into adjacent tissue. Complete evaluation of tumor staging requires knowledge of the size of the primary tumor, and the presence of locoregional nodal disease and hematogenous metastases.

Although several soft tissue sarcoma staging systems exist, one of the most commonly used systems is that of the American Joint Committee on Cancer (AJCC). The AJCC staging system is summarized in Table 30.2. Clinical staging of soft tissue sarcomas uses the TNM status that is familiar from other, more common tumors. In addition, however, pathologic assessment of the tumor grade is an essential element of staging. This reflects the primary importance of histologic grade as a determinant of biologic behavior and clinical outcome. Several histologic grading systems exist, incorporating evaluation of such factors as histologic type, mitotic activity, degree of differentiation, atypia, cellularity, pleomorphism, and necrosis. The goal of all of these systems is to differentiate low-grade from high-grade tumors. Some physicians use a simple binary system in which tumors are classified as either "low" or "high" grade. The most commonly used system employs three grades. In this system, Grade 1 is considered a low-grade tumor, while Grades 2 and 3 are considered high-grade tumors. To further complicate matter, some physicians utilize a four level system, in which Grades 1 and 2 are considered "low grade," and Grades 3 and 4 are considered "high grade."

Tumor size, as measured by either clinical or radiologic assessment, is classified as ≤5 cm or >5 cm. This distinction reflects the fact that tumors larger than this dimension have a worse prognosis, with a higher incidence of nodal and hematogenous metastasis, and greater ultimate mortality. The 5 cm size used in the TNM staging has an arbitrary element, however. As a general rule, there is also proportionality between tumor size greater than 5 cm and poor clinical outcome, so tumors that are 10 cm in diameter likely carry a worse prognosis than those that are 5 cm, despite being assigned the same "T" score.

In addition to simply measuring tumor size, accurate staging requires knowledge of the depth of tumor involvement.

Table 30.2 AJCC staging system for soft tissue sarcoma

Definition of TNM				
Primary tumor (T)				
TX		Primary tumor cannot be assessed		
T0		No evidence of primary tumor		
T1		Tumor 5 cm or less in greatest dimension[a]		
	T1a	Superficial tumor		
	T1b	Deep tumor		
T2		Tumor more than 5 cm in greatest dimension[a]		
	T2a	Superficial tumor		
	T2b	Deep tumor		
Regional lymph nodes (N)				
NX		Regional lymph nodes cannot be assessed		
N0		No regional lymph node metastasis		
N1[b]		Regional lymph node metastasis		
Distant metastasis (M)				
M0		No distant metastasis		
M1		Distant metastasis		
Anatomic stage • Prognostic groups[c]				
Stage IA	T1a	N0	M0	G1, GX
	T1b	N0	M0	G1, GX
Stage IB	T2a	N0	M0	G1, GX
	T2b	N0	M0	G1, GX
Stage IIA	T1a	N0	M0	G2
	T1b	N0	M0	G2
Stage IIB	T2a	N0	M0	G2
Stage III	T2b	N0	M0	G3
	T2b	N1	M0	G3, GX
	Any T	N1	M0	Any G
Stage IV	Any T	Any N	M1	Any G

[a] Superficial tumor is located exclusively above the superficial fascia without invasion of the fascia; deep tumor is located either exclusively beneath the superficial fascia, superficial to the fascia with invasion of or through the fascia, or both superficial yet beneath the fascia

[b] Presence of positive nodes (N1) in M0 tumors is considered Stage III

[c] Various systems for histologic grading of sarcomas exist, in which tumors are assigned to "high" or "low," or, more commonly, to Grade 1–3 or Grade 1–4. The appropriate stage is listed here for each approach

A distinction is made between truncal or extremity tumors that lie superficial to the muscular fascia and those that lie deep to or that penetrate the fascia. Deep involvement carries a less favorable prognosis than does a superficial location. All tumors of retroperitoneum, pelvis, mediastinum, and visceral organs are considered to have deep involvement.

Regional lymph node metastasis carries great implication in sarcoma staging, with a significance comparable to the presence of distant metastasis. The presence of either regional lymph node involvement or hematogenous distant metastasis renders the tumor grade IV, regardless of the histologic grade.

In addition to standard staging evaluation parameters of tumor grade, size, and spread, there are numerous molecular and cytogenetic factors that appear likely to influence the biologic behavior of sarcomas. Our current understanding of these if very incomplete, and these factors are therefore not included in the staging system.

Role of PET-CT in Tumor Staging

PET-CT imaging shows great promise in the initial evaluation of sarcomas, although its definitive role has not yet been established. Conventional imaging of soft tissue tumors entails the use of MRI with gadolinium contrast, which provides definition superior to that available from CT. MR imaging is typically limited to evaluation of the primary tumor, with CT used to evaluate the chest, and if necessary the abdomen. When PET-CT is employed, the whole body is imaged, providing assessment of distant metastases as well as the extent of local tumor. Most sarcomas are well shown by PET, and the extent of tumor involvement can be easily identified. In this application, PET-CT offers particular advantages over conventional stand-alone PET imaging, as there are few anatomic landmarks in the soft tissues for orientation on PET images alone. Comparative data on the value of PET and MRI for local tumor extent is limited.

To understand the value of PET in assessing lymph node and hematogenous metastasis, it is important to be aware of the patterns of sarcoma spread. In most soft tissue sarcomas, spread to regional lymph nodes is rare, occurring in only 6% of patients overall [12]. Nodal metastasis is especially uncommon in low-grade tumors and in those tumors less than 5 cm in diameter. Thus, the likelihood of finding regionally involved lymph nodes is quite small. Among the various histologic types of sarcomas, nodal disease is most common in epithelioid sarcoma, rhabdomyosarcoma, synovial sarcoma, and vascular sarcomas [12].

At the time of initial staging, it is also uncommon to detect distant metastases, which are present in less than 10% of tumors [13]. Metastases rarely occur in low-grade tumors. In general, the incidence of distant metastasis in intermediate and high-grade lesions is greater in large tumors. Among most histologic tumor types, lung metastases are by far the most common location for hematogenous spread. This is particularly true when dealing with tumors of the extremity or head and neck. Retroperitoneal tumors may alternatively spread to liver, a pattern of metastasis uncommon in extremity sarcomas. Liposarcoma appears to differ from most other tumor types, with a particular predilection to metastasize to soft tissue locations. In one series, solitary extra pulmonary metastasis occurred in 59% of patients [14].

Conventional sarcoma staging uses chest CT to search for pulmonary metastases. Although chest CT has a low yield at the time of initial diagnosis, if negative, it provides an important baseline evaluation. Most lung metastases are small at presentation, and can be very challenging to diagnose without a baseline CT for comparison. Even in the small percentage of patients in whom lung metastases are present at initial staging, PET imaging of the chest is rarely diagnostic. The small nodules typically present, often in the range of 2 or 3 mm, are well below the limits of PET resolution.

Some patients with sarcoma may receive neoadjuvant therapy prior to tumor resection. In these patients, imaging reevaluation is usually undertaken before definitive surgical resection. PET imaging can provide an assessment of the residual metabolic activity in the primary tumor, as well as reevaluation of sites of nodal or hematogenous metastasis. There is very limited data regarding the usefulness of PET in comparison to standing imaging modalities in this application.

Restaging with PET-CT

Those sarcomas that recur usually do so in the first several years following initial diagnosis and treatment. For that reason, frequent imaging reevaluation of the patient is usually undertaken, both to search for local recurrence and for distant metastasis (Figs. 30.5 and 30.6). PET imaging can assist in both of these evaluations, although there is very little data about the relative utility of PET in comparison to MRI and CT for the evaluation of metastatic disease. The limited information that exists suggests that PET is roughly comparable to conventional imaging [7].

When evaluating the location of primary tumor, it is important to realize that recent radiation therapy or surgery can cause intense uptake indistinguishable from residual tumor. The precise time frame for the resolution of postsurgical or radiation changes is difficult to determine, but inflammatory uptake may persist for months, gradually declining in intensity. PET-CT imaging provides a substantial advantage in comparison to standard PET imaging by providing correlation of high FDG uptake regions with the CT appearance, sometimes allowing an inference about the likelihood of residual tumor versus inflammation.

Following treatment, it may be difficult to differentiate residual tumor from posttreatment inflammatory changes by either MRI or CT. In some cases, PET can be very useful in this instance. Most posttreatment change is associated with low-level FDG uptake, corresponding to minor inflammation. In this setting, the presence of identifiable residual tumor is unlikely. A more challenging situation arises when

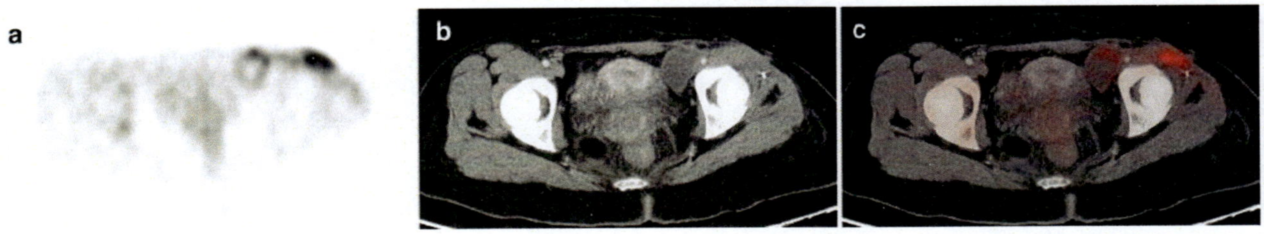

Fig. 30.5 A 20-year-old woman status post resection of synovial cell sarcoma in the proximal left thigh, now with left groin mass. PET images show moderate, peripheral uptake in the groin (**a**), corresponding to a soft tissue mass with central low attenuation just medial to the acetabulum on CT and PET-CT images (**b–c**). Surgical resection of an iliac lymph node showed synovial sarcoma, grade 2/3. PET images also show more intense uptake in the anterior thigh, corresponding to the region of prior surgery. There was no soft tissue mass in this region, consistent with uptake in residual postoperative changes. This highlights the occasional difficulty in differentiating residual or recurrent tumor from posttreatment changes by PET imaging alone

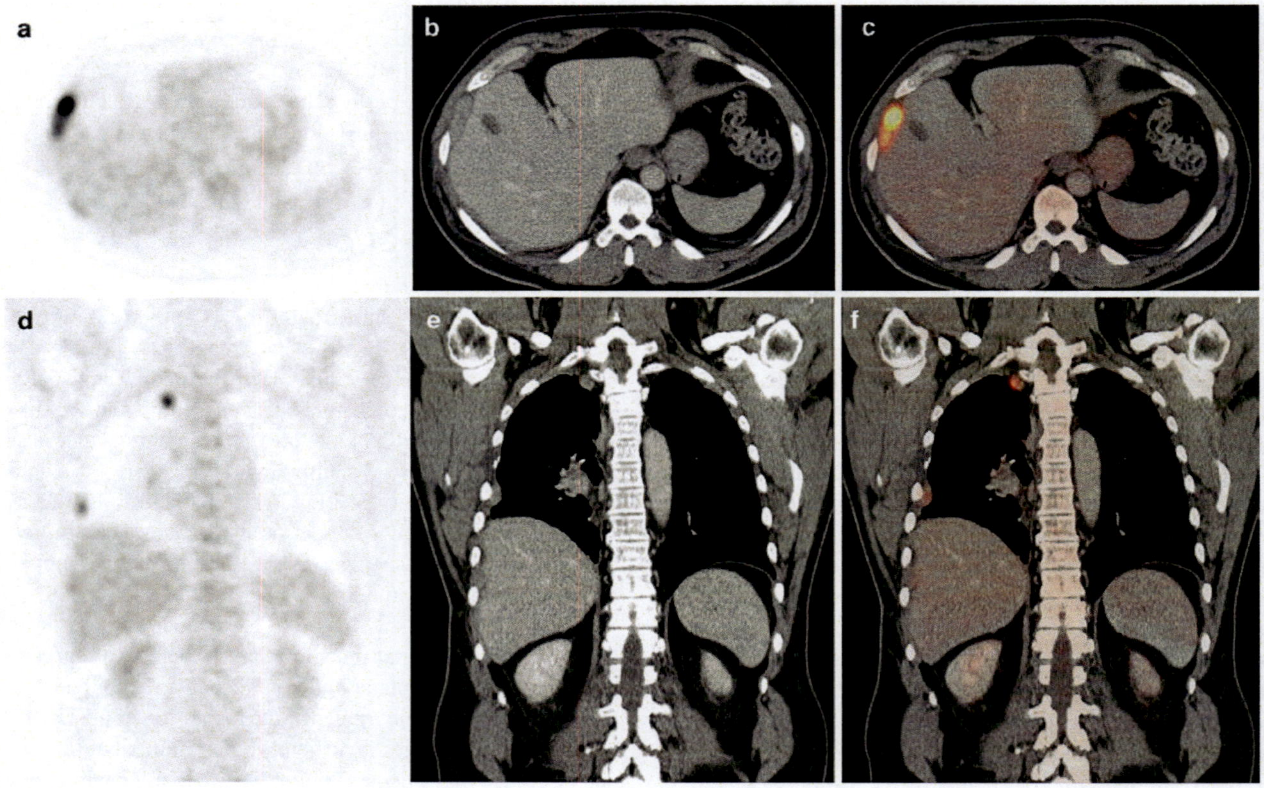

Fig. 30.6 A 65-year-old man who had resection of synovial cell sarcoma of the right arm 14 years earlier, with subsequent metastatic right lung nodules resected 7 years earlier. Surveillance CT scans show new pleural nodules. Axial and coronal PET images (**a, d**) show intense peripheral chest uptake. Axial and coronal CT (**b** and **e**) and PET-CT fusion images (**c, f**) show correlation with the pleural nodules, consistent with metastatic disease

the PET scan shows intense tracer accumulation. Here, the distinction between residual tumor and inflammatory changes is not always possible. Short interval followup or PET-directed biopsy may be needed to resolve the question.

The ultimate cause of death in patients with recurrent sarcoma is metastatic disease. Metastatic disease that develops after treatment almost always involves the lungs. Although pulmonary metastases initially present as tiny nodules, they may enlarge greatly with time, reaching a size that is easily shown by PET imaging. The combination of FDG avidity and progressive enlargement in comparison to baseline chest CT allows a confident diagnosis of malignancy. In patients who have failed systemic chemotherapy, resection of pulmonary metastases may be contemplated if the number of lung lesions is limited. In this setting, evaluation with PET can be very helpful to evaluate the full extent of disease before resection is undertaken.

Recurrent disease that manifests in a location other than the primary site or lung is rare, presenting in only about 14% of patients with recurrence [15]. These less-frequent sties of recurrence include bone, liver, and subcutaneous tissues. Retroperitoneal tumors have a greater incidence of local recurrence or liver metastases than do sarcomas originating from the extremities.

Therapy Monitoring with PET-CT

There is very limited data available about the response of sarcomas to treatment with either chemotherapy or radiation therapy. In some cases, it has not been possible to differentiate complete from partial response. There is presently no defined use for PET imaging to monitor treatment response.

Pitfalls and Pearls

- Soft tissue sarcoma recurrence tends to be predictable with regard to location. If the PET-CT scan shows unexpected uptake, carefully evaluate the CT images for a possible cause of confusion. Bear in mind, for example, that bone metastases are rare, so rib uptake may simply represent a fracture. Except for primary abdominal tumors, intraabdominal metastases are rare, so evaluate the images carefully before diagnosing abnormal retroperitoneal or pelvis lymph nodes; the uptake may represent confusing physiologic bowel or urinary activity, or rarely a second malignancy.

- When evaluating a region of prior surgery, carefully correlate the location of abnormal uptake with the finding on contrast enhanced MRI. Most sarcomas are treated with adjuvant radiation therapy, which can result in mildly increased FDG uptake for weeks to months after treatment. Low level uptake probably reflects post-treatment change, but the distinction from residual tumor with minimal metabolic activity may not be possible.
- At either initial diagnosis or follow-up examination, even very intense FDG uptake may not represent malignancy. In published series, false positive PET scans often resulted from infectious or inflammatory changes that mimicked tumor. PET-CT provides an advantage over conventional PET imaging because the precise location of tissue hypermetabolism can be shown on CT, and is thus easily correlated with MRI findings for anatomic clues about the likely nature of uptake. In some cases, definitive evaluation is not possible, and careful follow up scans or biopsy is needed for diagnosis.

References

1. Cormier JN, Pollock RE. Soft tissue sarcomas. CA Cancer J Clin 2004;54:94–109.
2. O'Sullivan B, Davis AM, Turcotte R, et al. Preoperative versus postoperative radiotherapy in soft-tissue sarcoma of the limbs: a randomized trial. Lancet 2002;359:2235–2241.
3. O'Sullivan B, Davis AM, Turcotte R, et al. Five-year results of a randomized phase III trial of pre-operative vs. post-operative radiotherapy in extremity soft tissue sarcoma. Proc Am Soc Clin Oncol 2004;23:815.
4. Gieschen HL, Spiro IJ, Suit HD, et al. Long-term results of intraoperative electron beam radiotherapy for primary and recurrent retroperitoneal soft tissue sarcoma. Int J Radiat Oncol Biol Phys 2001;50(1):127–131.
5. Hoekstra HJ, Sindelar WF, Szabo BG, Kinsella TJ. Hemipelvectomy and intraoperative radiotherapy for bone and soft tissue sarcomas of the pelvic girdle. Radiother Oncol 1995;37(2):160–163.
6. Aoki J, Watanabe H, Shinozaki T, et al. FDG-PET for preoperative differential diagnosis between benign and malignant soft tissue masses. Skeletal Radiol 2003;32:133–138.
7. Ioannidis JPA, Lau J. ^{18}F-FDG PET for the diagnosis and grading of soft-tissue sarcoma: a meta-analysis. J Nucl Med 2003;44:717–724.
8. Eary JF, Conrad EU, Bruckner JB, et al. Quantitative [F-18] fluorodeoxyglucose positron emission tomography in pretreatment and grading of sarcoma. Clin Cancer Res 1998;4:1215–1220.
9. Schwarzbach MHM, Dimitrakopoulou-Strauss A, et al. Clinical value of [18-F] fluorodeoxyglucose positron emission tomography imaging in soft tissue sarcomas. Ann Surg 2000;231:380–386.
10. Bastiaannet E, Groen H, Jager PL, et al. The value of FDG-PET in the detection, grading and response to therapy of soft tissue and bone sarcomas; a systematic review and meta-analysis. Cancer Treat Rev 2004;30:83–101.
11. Eary JF, O'Sullivan F, Powitan Y, et al. Sarcoma tumor FDG uptake measured by PET and patient outcome: a retrospective analysis. Eur J Nucl Med 2002;29:1149–1154.
12. Mazeron JJ, Suit HD. Lymph nodes as sites of metastases from sarcomas of soft tissue. Cancer 1987;60:1800–1808.
13. Rydholm A, Berg NO, Gullberg B, et al. Epidemiology of soft-tissue sarcoma in the locomotor system. A retrospective population-based study of the inter-relationships between clinical and morphologic variables. Acta Pathol Microbiol Immunol Scand [A] 1984;92:363–374.
14. Cheng EY, Springfield DS, Mankin HJ. Frequent incidence of extrapulmonary sites of initial metastasis in patients with liposarcoma. Cancer 1995;75:1120–1127.
15. Potter DA, Glenn J, Kinsella T, et al. Patterns of recurrence in patients with high-grade soft-tissue sarcomas. J Clin Oncol 1985;3:353–366.

Chapter 31
PET-CT of Pancreatic Cancer

Todd M. Blodgett, Sanjay Paidisetty, and Paul Shreve

Pancreatic cancer is the fourth leading cause of death in the USA, with an estimated 37,680 new cases diagnosed in 2008, accounting for 25% of all deaths due to digestive tract malignancies [1]. The mean age at diagnosis is 55 years and pancreatic cancer is rare in patients under 40. Historically, men have been affected more often than women, although the rate for women is now approaching that of men.

There are no definitive causes of pancreatic cancer; however, associations have been made with smoking, diabetes mellitus, obesity, and chronic pancreatitis, as well as several hereditary syndromes such as hereditary pancreatitis and Gardner's syndrome. Increased incidence of pancreatic adenocarcinoma has also been reported in chemists and metal industry workers.

The vast majority (90%) of pancreatic cancers are adenocarcinomas of ductal origin. Carcinomas of acinar cell origin, sarcomas, malignant lymphomas, and malignant islet cell tumors comprise the remainder of cancers originating in the pancreas. The pancreatic head is the most common location (70%), with approximately 20% of tumors arising in the body, 5% in the tail, and 15% involving more than one section.

Most patients are asymptomatic until late in the course of disease, accounting for its dismal overall 5-year survival of less than 10% [2]. The most common presenting symptoms depend on the tumor location, with those in the head of the pancreas presenting with obstructive jaundice, pain, and weight loss, while those in the body and tail typically present later with problems associated with metastatic disease or local invasion of adjacent organs. Over the last 30 years, survival rates for patients with carcinomas of the pancreatic head have improved, mostly due to the success with surgical resection techniques.

Patients with adenocarcinoma of pancreas often have elevated tumor markers (CA 19-9) at diagnosis, which has been used for predicting prognosis and relapse in patients with known or suspected disease. However, CA 19-9 is not specific for pancreatic carcinoma. Other laboratory tests often reveal elevated bilirubin, with other obstructive liver function values being elevated in patients with biliary obstruction. At presentation, approximately 65% of patients will have advanced local or metastatic disease, 20% will have localized disease with spread to regional lymph nodes, and only 15% will have disease localized to the pancreas.

The uncommon islet cell tumors of the pancreas can present similar to adenocarcinoma of the pancreas due to mass effect if the islet cell tumor is a nonsecreting neoplasm. Those islet cell tumors that secrete peptide hormones (insulinoma, glucagonoma, gastrinoma, VIPoma) will present with clinical consequences of the excess hormone production.

Treatment of pancreatic cancer for those with limited disease at the head of the pancreas is surgical resection with a pancreaticoduodenectomy (Whipple procedure). Resectable cancer in the tail or body of the pancreas is treated with a distal pancreatectomy. Secreting islet cell tumors are likewise resected as the primary treatment. Even so, the 5-year survival rate for localized adenocarcinoma of the pancreas is at best about 20% [3–5]. Chemotherapy after resection of pancreatic adenocarcinoma may increase survival; however, adjunctive chemoradiation therapy appears to offer no advantage [6]. For the majority of patients, pancreatic cancer will be diagnosed when it is unresectable, and a combination of chemoradiation with palliative surgical bypass or endoscopic stenting of common bile duct obstruction is the mainstay of treatment. For these patients, overall 5-year survival is less than 5%.

Evaluation of a patient with known or suspected pancreatic carcinoma thus centers on whether the tumor is a malignant neoplasm and whether it is resectable. The presence of metastatic spread beyond local lymph nodes or involvement of local major vascular structures precludes resection. Histologic confirmation of the primary tumor or of a metastatic lesion is usually obtained by CT or ultrasound-guided percutaneous needle biopsy, endoscopic ultrasound guided needle biopsy, or endoscopic retrograde cholangiopancreatographic brushings before treatment. Patients with a pancreatic mass that appears resectable based on imaging findings,

T.M. Blodgett (✉)
FRG Molecular Imaging, Foundation Radiology Group, 401 Liberty Avenue, Suite 2000, Pittsburgh, PA 15222, USA
e-mail: toddblodgett@yahoo.com

P. Shreve and D.W. Townsend (eds.), *Clinical PET-CT in Radiology: Integrated Imaging in Oncology*,
DOI 10.1007/978-0-387-48902-5_31, © Springer Science+Business Media, LLC 2011

however, may undergo definitive surgery even without preoperative histologic diagnosis of malignancy. Pancreatic head masses are treated by pancreaticoduodenectomy (Whipple procedure) and tail masses by direct resection of the tail of the pancreas. Careful exploration at the time of attempted resection is performed to confirm there is no vascular involvement and search for undetected metastatic disease. In 10–15% of patients, small liver metastases or peritoneal metastases will be discovered at the time of exploration. Extensive lymph node sampling (at least 15 nodes) also is performed at attempted resection to accurately determine the status of lymph node metastases. Patients determined to be unresectable at the time of exploration with obstructive jaundice may undergo a palliative biliary bypass procedure.

Diagnosis of Pancreatic Carcinoma with PET-CT

Primary pancreatic carcinoma, at the time of diagnosis, varies in size, typically ranging from 2 to 8 cm. Carcinomas originating in the head of the pancreas tend to be smaller than those in the body or tail of the pancreas at diagnosis. The typical appearance of pancreatic cancer on non-contrast-enhanced CT is an isodense mass. Without intravenous contrast enhancement, it is often not possible to see small- to moderate-sized tumors. Hemorrhage and calcification are rare findings. Common associated imaging findings include variable amounts of pancreatic and/or common bile duct dilatation and obstruction (the double duct sign) and distal pancreatic atrophy.

The mainstay diagnostic test for differentiating and evaluating pancreatic masses has been contrast-enhanced helical CT. Typically the CT scan is performed with thin collimation (3 mm or less) and rapid bolus injection of intravenous contrast material in at least two phases of contrast enhancement (arterial and portal venous phases). In addition, negative or water-based oral contrast is usually employed to fill and define the adjacent duodenum. The most common findings on contrast-enhanced CT of pancreatic carcinoma are a heterogeneous, poorly enhancing (and thus relatively lower attenuation) mass associated with lymphadenopathy or other findings of metastatic disease, such as liver metastases. Properly performed contemporary contrast-enhanced multiphase helical CT can detect primary pancreatic cancers as small as 1–2 cm, and determine whether the pancreatic cancer is resectable with high accuracy [7, 8]. The high positive predictive value of CT in determining resectability (over 95%) is largely due to the detection of metastases and depiction of direct involvement of adjacent major vessels by the cancer. Sensitivities of FDG PET alone in identifying pancreatic adenocarcinoma have been reported to range between 85% and 96% [9–13]. SUV uptake has been shown to be beneficial, as statistically significant differences between malignant and benign lesions have been demonstrated by some studies; however, definitive cutoff values have not been determined [12, 14]. Although it remains controversial as to whether CT alone is superior to FDG PET alone in regards to sensitivities in the diagnosis of primary pancreatic cancer, the inability of FDG PET alone to provide exact anatomic localization precludes the modality from being the test of choice [15–19]. Four recent studies examining the use of PET-CT demonstrated high sensitivities (89–100%), high positive predictive values (89–92%) but a wide range in specificity (69–88%), and negative predictive values (64–100%) in identifying primary cancer [9, 14, 20, 21]. The wide range in the statistical measures can be explained by the different protocols utilized for the CT portion of the exam (noncontrast, biphase, and triple phase contrast enhancement). A recent prospective study found no significant differences in diagnostic capability were found between PET-CT and US, EUS, and ERCP in identifying malignancy in individuals with solid pancreatic masses ≥1cm [14].

Differential diagnosis of a pancreatic mass includes distinguishing a pancreatic adenocarcinoma from the pseudomass of chronic pancreatitis, cystic primary neoplasms of the pancreas, islet cell tumors, metastasis to the pancreas (melanoma, renal cell carcinoma), and primary pancreatic lymphoma. Long-term prognosis of cystic pancreatic neoplasms, pancreatic lymphoma, and islet cell tumors is significantly better than that of adenocarcinoma of the pancreas. Islet cell carcinomas are generally easy to differentiate from adenocarcinoma by the presence of hypervascularity (enhancement on arterial phase of contrast enhanced CT imaging), but this requires careful attention to the CT protocol, as small islet cell tumors may not be seen on other phases of contrast enhanced CT.

Most problematic is the differentiation between the pseudomass of chronic pancreatitis and primary pancreatic adenocarcinoma. Chronic pancreatitis can form a mass-like lesion, indistinguishable on anatomical imaging from pancreatic adenocarcinoma. Tumor markers are usually not helpful in distinguishing between these two, as they may be elevated in both. FDG PET has been shown to be superior to contrast-enhanced CT alone in several studies for differentiating the benign mass of chronic pancreatitis from malignant pancreatic masses, with the overall sensitivity, specificity, and accuracy ranging from 85% to 100%, 67–99%, and 85–95%, respectively, compared to sensitivity of 65–79% and specificity of 44–62% for CT [15, 22–26]. A recent study examining FDG uptake patterns found autoimmune pancreatitis to be characterized by heterogenous accumulation, which was statistically significantly different than the pattern seen in pancreatic cancer characterized by nodular shape and solitary localization. Furthermore, uptake to hilar lymph

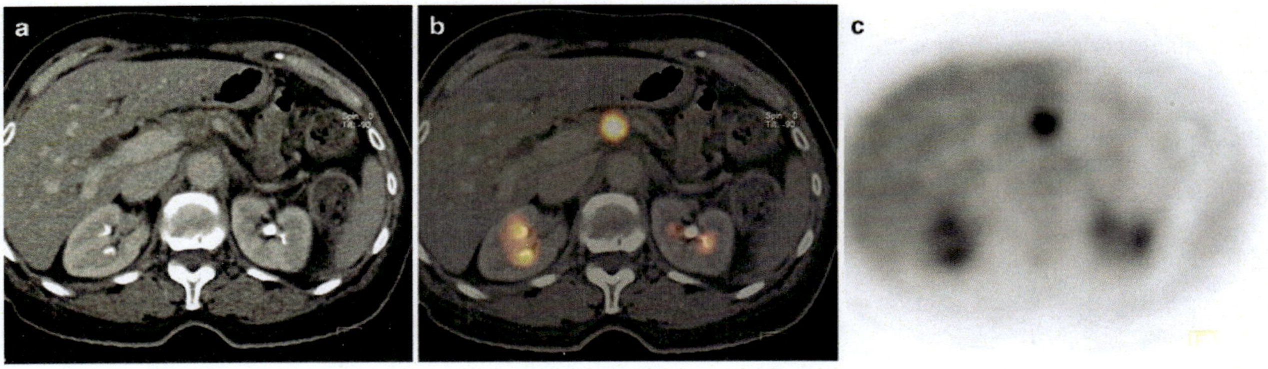

Fig. 31.1 Small primary adenocarcinoma of the pancreas. (**a**) Transaxial contrast-enhanced CT at portal venous phase demonstrates subtle low attenuation in the head of the pancreas with associated moderate dilatation of the pancreatic duct. (**b, c**) Transaxial FDG PET and PET-CT fusion images reveal intense abnormal FDG tracer uptake at the site, reflecting the 1.8 cm primary tumor

node was seen significantly more frequently in autoimmune pancreatitis than in pancreatic cancer [27]. It should be noted that FDG uptake in the setting of distinguishing pancreatitis from malignancy can be influenced by other nondisease factors. In patients with insulin requiring diabetes, the level of FDG tracer uptake in a primary pancreatic malignancy has been found in some series to be decreased, reducing sensitivity. Furthermore, false positives also were reported due to focal mass forming acute pancreatitis and acute-on-chronic pancreatitis [28].

A small pancreatic malignancy can be difficult to delineate on CT, especially in younger patients, as the pancreas is of a more uniform density. Focal FDG tracer uptake can pinpoint a site of subtle abnormality depicted on CT (Fig. 31.1), corresponding to a small primary neoplasm. This is especially useful in the setting of patients with a normal appearing pancreas on initial anatomic imaging, but with secondary signs of a pancreatic mass such as unexplained common bile duct or pancreatic duct dilatation. Also, in a series of patients with metastatic disease of unknown primary, PET-CT identified an unsuspected pancreatic primary cancer in 6 of the 24 patients in which the primary was identified, out of a total of 68 patients [29]. Whether PET-CT can improve detection of small islet cell tumors in patients with the clinical syndrome of a secreting islet cell tumor has not yet been fully evaluated due to the rarity of this condition.

Cystic pancreatic neoplasms, while uncommon, present a particular diagnostic challenge, as there are both benign and malignant as well as borderline malignant cystic neoplasms of the pancreas, and their appearance on anatomic imaging can overlap with inflammatory cystic masses. Serous cystadenomas represent roughly a third of cystic neoplasms of the pancreas and are almost always benign. They are typically identified on CT by uniform distributed tiny cysts in a honeycomb pattern. Mucinous cystic neoplasms (including intraductal papillary mucinous neoplasms) are characterized by large cysts of fluid or near fluid attenuation associated with thin enhancing septa. These cystic pancreatic masses can be benign, low-grade malignant, or malignant. On anatomic imaging, it is generally not possible to reliably determine the presence of malignancy in these masses. On CT, cystic tumor size has been significantly correlated with likelihood of malignancy; however, a similar relationship was not made in regard to the presence of septa and thickness of septa [30]. There is limited experience reported with the use of FDG PET in identifying malignant cystic pancreatic neoplasms and studies comparing FDG PET to CT or MR have not demonstrated consistent results in firmly identifying one modality superior to the other [30–33]. The FDG tracer uptake in cystic pancreatic neoplasms is, however, generally modest, and completely overlaps the FDG tracer uptake that can occur in inflammatory cystic masses. Thus, it remains debatable if FDG PET alone can be routinely used to determine the presence of malignancy. A recent study demonstrated PET-CT (CT and PET studies performed separately but both images used together to evaluate cystic neoplasms) to have significantly higher sensitivity compared to CT alone and higher sensitivity and specificity compared to PET alone [30].

Staging of Pancreatic Carcinoma with PET-CT

Because only a small percentage of patients undergo surgical resection, a single TNM classification is used for both clinical and pathologic staging (Table 31.1). Patients who undergo surgical resection have a median survival of less roughly 18 months and a 5-year survival rate of, at best, 20–25%. Poor prognostic indicators for those found to be resectable include the size of the primary pancreatic mass, regional lymph node involvement, and poorly differentiated histology of the tumor. Patients with unresectable pancreatic cancer have a very poor prognosis, with a typical survival of 3–6 months from the time of diagnosis. It has been supported

Table 31.1 Pancreatic carcinoma TNM and stage grouping (Used with the permission of the American Joint Committee on Cancer (AJCC), Chicago, IL. The original source for this material is the *AJCC Cancer Staging Manual*, 7th edn (2010) published by Springer Science and Business Media LLC. www.springer.com)

Definitions of TNM			
Primary tumor (T)			
TX	Primary tumor cannot be assessed		
T0	No evidence of primary tumor		
Tis	Carcinoma in situ[a]		
T1	Tumor limited to the pancreas, 2 cm or less in greatest dimension		
T2	Tumor limited to the pancreas, more than 2 cm in greatest dimension		
T3	Tumor extends beyond the pancreas but without involvement of the celiac axis or the superior mesenteric artery		
T4	Tumor involves the celiac axis or the superior mesenteric artery (unresectable primary tumor)		
Regional lymph nodes (N)			
NX	Regional lymph nodes cannot be assessed		
N0	No regional lymph node metastasis		
N1	Regional lymph node metastasis		
Distant metastasis (M)			
M0	No distant metastasis		
M1	Distant metastasis		
Anatomic stage • Prognostic groups			
Stage 0	Tis	N0	M0
Stage IA	T1	N0	M0
Stage IB	T2	N0	M0
Stage IIA	T3	N0	M0
Stage IIB	T1	N1	M0
	T2	N1	M0
	T3	N1	M0
Stage III	T4	Any N	M0
Stage IV	Any T	Any N	M1

[a]This also includes the "PanInIII" classification

by several recent studies that higher SUV uptake values (≥4.0) of malignancy in FDG PET can be correlated with shorter survival and can also serve as an independent prognostic factor and help select patients for surgical therapy [19, 26, 34–38].

Pancreatic cancer spreads by local extension quite readily, as there is no true capsule surrounding the pancreas. Tumors of the pancreatic head, in addition to obstructing the common bile and pancreatic ducts, will extend beyond the pancreas proper into the retropancreatic fat to involve the mesenteric artery, celiac axis, and celiac nerve plexus. Additional typical local invasion of a pancreas head tumor includes the adjacent duodenum, portal and mesenteric vasculature, and transverse colon or gastric antrum. Tumors originating in the body or tail of the pancreas will extend into the adjacent splenic vein, spleen, stomach, left adrenal gland or colon.

The pancreas is vested with a rich lymphatic network, allowing lymphatic spread to parapancreatic lymph nodes, and then outward along the celiac axis and mesenteric artery nodal chains, along hepatic artery lymphatics to porta hepatis lymph nodes, as well as to gastrohepatic ligament and splenic hilar lymph nodes, and paraaortic and paracaval lymph nodes at the level of the renal veins, depending on the location of the primary tumor. Distant lymphatic spread of tumors in the body and tail of the pancreas include pleura and lung.

Because the pancreas blood flow drains into the portal venous system, hepatic metastases are nearly always the first manifestation of hematogenous spread of pancreatic cancer. Pancreatic cancer also has a proclivity for peritoneal metastases. Lung metastases tend to occur later, and less commonly adrenal, renal, and bone and thoracic lymph nodes, particularly in the setting of recurrence.

T Stage

Potentially resectable patients are those with T1, T2, or T3 tumors. T4 tumors are too locally advanced, involving major vessels or adjacent organs to be resected. T1 tumors are limited to the pancreas and 2 cm or less in size in greatest dimension, while T2 tumors are larger than 2 cm but remain limited to the pancreas. T3 tumors extend beyond the pancreas, or involve the bile duct or duodenum, but do not involve the adjacent major vessels, or other adjacent organs. When the primary tumor involves the celiac axis, superior mesenteric artery (SMA), hepatic artery, or portal vein, or the stomach, spleen or colon, the tumor is considered T4 stage and is not resectable.

Typically patients with uncinate or head lesions are candidates for resection, as those that involve the body or tail almost always are advanced at the time of diagnosis. Tumors in the body and tail of the pancreas discovered incidentally on imaging examinations, however, may still be confined to the pancreas, and particularly those less than 2 cm, potential candidates for primary resection.

T staging of pancreatic cancer on PET-CT imaging is nearly entirely based on the CT images. FDG PET has little role in determining T stage, due to the lack of anatomic detail and the inability to resolve the relationship of FDG activity with small pertinent structures. Usually, when proper contrast enhanced CT technique is used, the size of the primary pancreatic tumor can be delineated. Extension beyond the pancreas and into adjacent organs is also based almost entirely on the CT images. In some instances the extent of abnormal FDG tracer activity on the FDG PET images can be of value in assessing the full extent of the neoplasm. Of particular importance is soft tissue encasement of the celiac axis or SMA, involvement of the proximal hepatic artery, and extension into the portal vein or involvement of the proximal superior mesenteric vein. Obvious encasement of the origin of the celiac axis or SMA is readily diagnosed on the CT images, although full delineation of the FDG avid neoplasm as depicted on the PET images is helpful (Fig. 31.2). When the extent of soft tissue involving the vessels is limited, the abnormal glucose metabolism associated with this minimal soft tissue may not be resolved on the FDG PET images, and the diagnosis of vessel involvement is based on the CT findings. The vessels should be surrounded by a fat plane on the CT images, and any soft tissue thickening or absent fat plane depicted on CT must be considered suspicious. When there is any question of possible involvement of the celiac axis or SMA based on suspicious PET-CT findings or proximity of the primary mass to these vessels, endoscopic ultrasound provides the most sensitive evaluation [39]. Tumor involvement of the adjacent major vessels precludes resection because these vessels cannot removed en bloc and then repaired. Encasement of the celiac axis or SMA always precludes resection, as generally does encasement of invasion of the portal vein or portal confluence. Limited tumor involvement of the superior mesenteric vein, portal vein, or splenic vein, on the other hand, are relative contraindications to surgery, as patch repairs can be fashioned depending on the extent and location of the involvement.

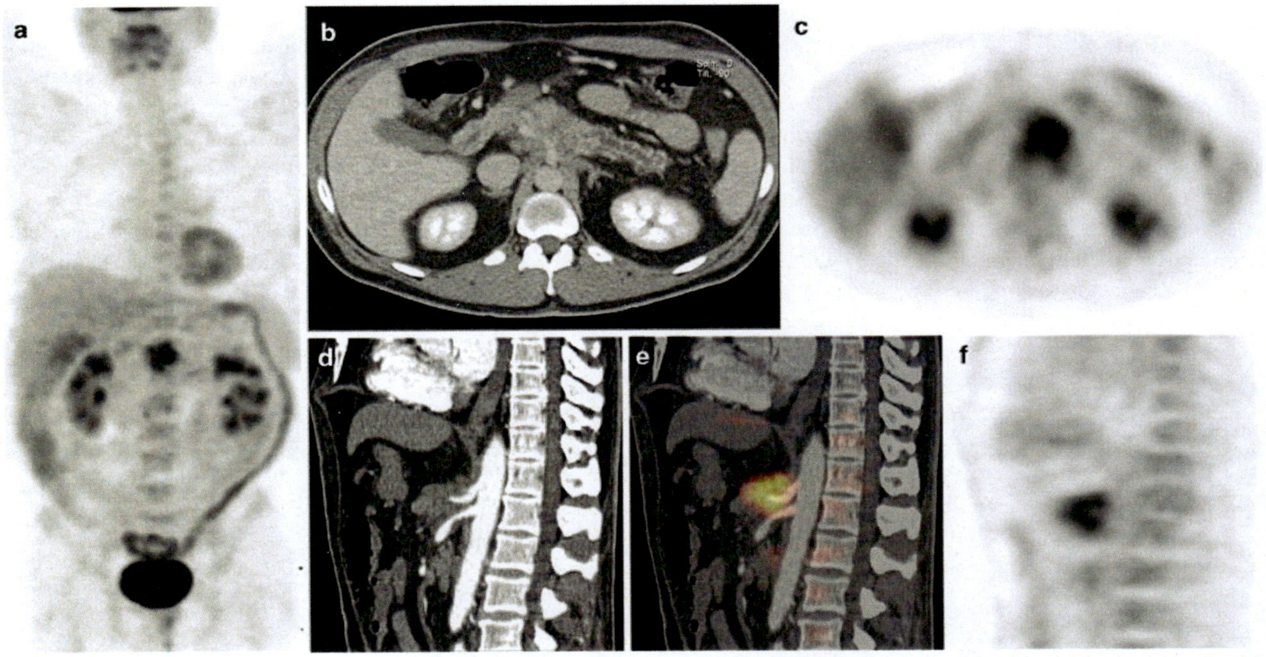

Fig. 31.2 Unresectable pancreatic cancer. (**a**) Anterior FDG PET MIP image reveals intense focal FDG tracer uptake in the upper mid abdomen corresponding to a primary pancreatic cancer, without evidence of additional regional or distant metastatic disease. (**b**, **c**) Transaxial contrast enhanced CT at the portal venous phase reveals a pancreatic head fullness with associated pancreatic duct dilatation and the transaxial FDG PET image reveals intense abnormal FDG tracer uptake in the region of pancreatic fullness corresponding to the primary pancreatic neoplasm. (**d–f**) Sagittal contrast-enhanced CT in the late arterial phase demonstrates bulky soft tissue encasement of the celiac axis with soft tissue extending to the proximal superior mesenteric artery which is associated with abnormal FDG tracer uptake seen on the sagittal FDG PET and PET-CT fusion images

N Stage

At the time of presentation, 40% of patients will have locoregional lymph node metastases. Due to the rich lymphatic network of the pancreas, pancreatic carcinoma readily spreads to peripancreatic lymph nodes and on to the regional nodal basins including paraceliac axis and SMA, portocaval, porta hepatis, gastrohepatic ligament, splenic hilum, and lesser curvature of the stomach regions.

N staging of patients with pancreatic adenocarcinoma is limited to N0 (no detectable metastatic lymph nodes) and N1 (presence of malignant lymph node involvement). The CT criteria for lymph node involvement, as with other cancers, are based on size. Generally, lymph nodes are considered abnormally enlarged if they exceed 1 cm in short axis diameter. Size criteria are relatively nonspecific, as benign lymph nodes can be enlarged and a subcentimeter lymph node can be filled with neoplasm. Central necrosis within a lymph node depicted on CT is considered a more specific sign of metastatic involvement, but this is almost always only seen in enlarged lymph nodes. While nodal enlargement in lymph nodes in regional nodal basins is relatively easy to identify on properly performed CT images, parapancreatic lymph nodes, especially lymph nodes directly abutting the pancreas itself, can be difficult to delineate on CT images alone.

As with other cancers, the FDG PET images of PET-CT facilitate identification of lymph node metastases, especially to non-enlarged and borderline enlarged lymph nodes (Fig. 31.3). Aligned and registered FDG PET and CT images have been shown to further improve identification of involved lymph nodes in patients with pancreatic cancer [40]. This in part reflects the difficulty in identifying lymph nodes closely associated with the pancreas itself and the difficulty in identifying lymph nodes generally in patients with little intraabdominal fat, a not uncommon condition in patients with pancreatic cancer. It should be noted, however, that the presence of lymph node metastases does not in itself render a patient unresectable. Lymph nodes that would be removed at the time of resection such as parapancreatic lymph nodes, do not preclude resection if involved, even though under the staging criteria such involvement renders the N stage N1, and hence Stage IIB.

PET-CT cannot detect microscopic metastatic involvement of lymph nodes, and it is not uncommon for a patient with a PET-CT examination negative for lymph node metastases to have multiple lymph nodes positive for metastatic disease on histopathologic examination at the time of resection. EUS, especially with the combined capability for directed biopsy, has been shown to have the highest accuracy for determination of N stage in patients with cancer, especially in patients with primary tumors involving the head and uncinate process of the pancreas. A recent study demonstrated superior ability for the combination of EUS, staging CT, and PET-CT compared to each alone in identifying local regional disease; however, the percentage of patients identified was still low (53%) [9]. Thus, there are no imaging techniques that have the ability to identify nodal metastasis with acceptable sensitivity.

M Stage

Pancreatic adenocarcinoma metastasizes most frequently to the liver, peritoneal cavity and lungs, pleura, and intrathoracic lymph nodes. At diagnosis, 50% of patients have liver metastases and 35% have peritoneal metastases (Fig. 31.4). Unlike N staging, FDG PET has been shown to be superior to other imaging modalities for determining the presence of metastatic disease, detecting distant metastatic involvement in 33% of patients in which the lesions were not detected on CT [20]. By identifying distant metastases, one study found

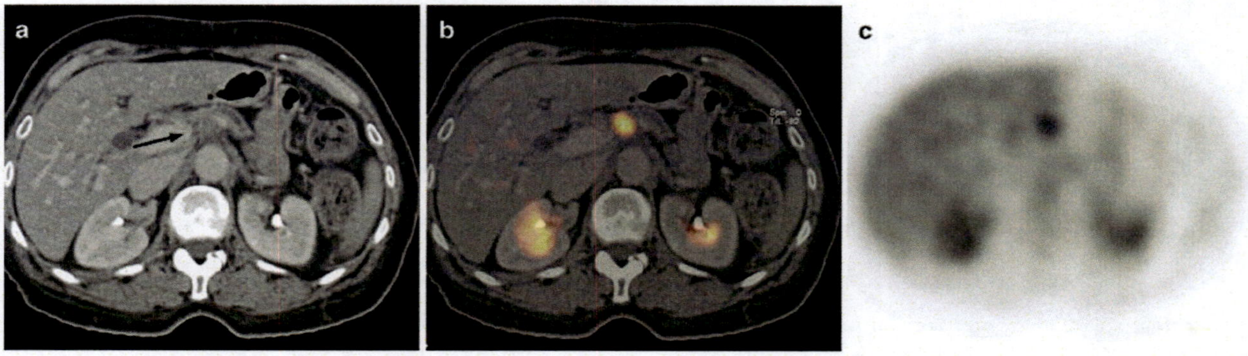

Fig. 31.3 Metastasis to a celiac axis lymph node. (**a**) Transaxial contrast enhanced CT demonstrates ill defined soft tissue adjacent to the celiac axis (*arrow*), which is associated with an isolated intense focal abnormal FDG tracer uptake on the FDG PET and PET-CT fusion images (**b, c**). Identification of abnormal lymph nodes on CT alone becomes more difficult as intraabdominal fat is reduced

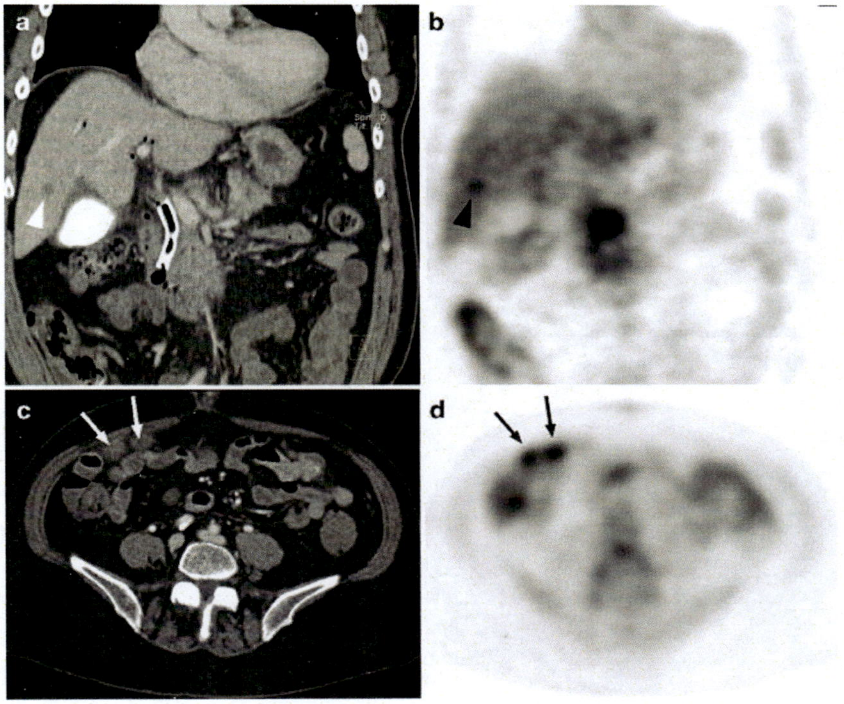

Fig. 31.4 Distant metastases. Liver metastases (**a, b**) Coronal CT and FDG PET images demonstrate the primary pancreatic head adenocarcinoma adjacent to the common bile duct stent and a small hepatic metastasis in the right hepatic lobe (*arrowhead*). (**c, d**) Peritoneal metastases: Transaxial CT and FDG PET images reveal two ill-defined 1 cm nodules associated with moderately abnormal FDG tracer uptake in the intraperitoneal fat at the level of the pelvic inlet (*arrows*)

that the use of FDG PET led to a change in management in 16% of patients, which had a significant impact on patient selection for surgery and consequently led to a significant cost savings [41]. In another study, clinical stage was changed in 12% of patients due to FDG PET findings, although in some instances liver and lung metastases were detected on CT that were not resolved on FDG PET [42]. The FDG PET sensitivity reported for detecting hepatic metastatic lesions by less than 1 cm was reported to be 43% compared to a sensitivity of 97% for lesions greater than 1 cm [43]. These latter two studies emphasize the potential for the complimentary role of PET with CT. A recent study found the use of PET-CT in combination with staging CT (use of coregistered image and CT image concurrently) to have a higher sensitivity in identifying metastatic lesions compared to PET-CT or staging CT alone and changed management in 11% of patients [9]. Another recent study found contrast-enhanced PET-CT to have high sensitivity and specificity and significantly superior to PET alone and a trend of being superior to unenhanced PET-CT in identifying liver, lung, and bone metastases, peritoneal carcinomatosis, and arterial infiltration for the preoperative assessment of resectability [44].

R Stage

Although not part of the TNM staging algorithm, the extent of resection margin positive for tumor revealed on histopathologic examination of the surgical specimen has significant prognostic implications for the patient. A resection of the primary mass with negative surgical margins is designated R0, positive microscopic margins is R1, and gross positive margins is categorized R2. Patients with grossly positive tumor margins (R2) have no survival advantage to those that do not undergo resection and receive chemotherapy alone. Conversely, those with negative surgical margins (R0) and no lymph node involvement on histopathologic examination have a 5 year survival of 20–25%.

Restaging Pancreatic Carcinoma with PET-CT

In the setting of restaging pancreatic cancer, local recurrence at the site of resection and regional lymph node involvement, as well as distant metastases, are important findings. The PET-CT can be particularly useful in diagnosing local recurrence, where

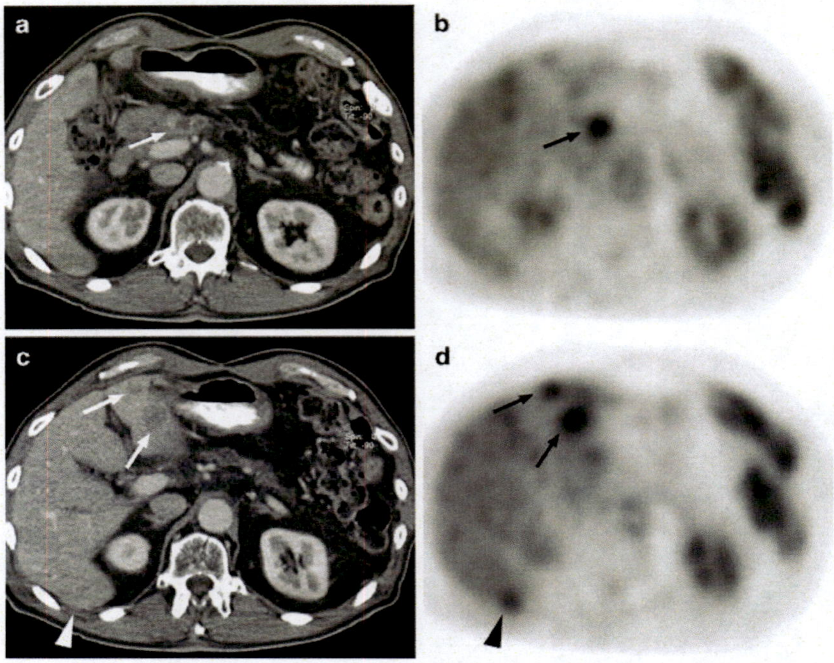

Fig. 31.5 Recurrent adenocarcinoma of the pancreas. (**a, b**) Transaxial CT and FDG PET images reveal a small area of decreased attenuation in the pancreatic body that is intensely FDG avid (*arrow*), corresponding to recurrent pancreatic cancer at the resection margin. (**c, d**) Additional transaxial CT and FDG PET images demonstrate two metastases in the lateral segment of the left hepatic lobe (*arrows*) and a 6 mm metastasis in the posterior right hepatic lobe (*arrowhead*)

post operative changes can confound both CT and FDG PET interpretation when registered and aligned CT and FDG PET images are not available (Fig. 31.5). In addition, since peritoneal metastases are an important pattern of metastases for pancreatic cancer, the complimentary nature of both PET and CT imaging should facilitate the detection of peritoneal spread. Lung metastases are also an important site of metastatic spread for pancreatic cancer, and here CT would be the most sensitive modality. Pleural involvement and thoracic lymph node involvement would be most sensitively detected on the FDG PET images. FDG PET had been shown to be useful in identifying recurrent disease in patients with rising CA 19-9 tumor markers, particularly when CT is negative or equivocal [42]. In a recent study of 23 patients with recurrent pancreatic cancer comparing FDG PET with contrast CT or MR, the FDG PET images were most accurate in detecting intra-abdominal recurrence, although the sensitivity of FDG PET for hepatic metastases was only 42% compared to 92% for CT/MR [45].

Pitfalls and Issues of Reporting in PET-CT Imaging of Pancreatic Carcinoma

As noted to above, there are independent and complimentary advantages of FDG PET and CT in the imaging of pancreatic cancer. For example, small pulmonary metastases will be most sensitively detected on the CT images, while nonenlarged lymph node metastases will be detected on the FDG PET images. Both in the setting of initial staging and in restaging of pancreatic cancer, proper CT technique including thin section collimation and rapid bolus of intravenous contrast material are important to take full advantage of PET-CT. Multiphase CT technique is especially important for determining the status of vasculature involvement. Islet cell pancreatic neoplasms are hypervascular and difficult to detect as primary lesions or hepatic metastases on portal venous phase CT images, and are best seen on late arterial phase CT (Fig. 31.6).

Pancreatic carcinoma is not, on average, as FDG avid as other cancers commonly imaged by FDG PET, and this in part contributes to a lower sensitivity for hepatic metastases on the FDG PET images than would be expected. Hence, optimized CT technique for detecting hepatic metastases should be employed when performing PET-CT in the setting of pancreatic cancer. Peritoneal metastases are an important pattern of distant metastases (M1 disease). The FDG PET images will facilitate identification of the larger formed peritoneal implants (generally >8 mm), but smaller peritoneal implants may only be detected on the CT images. Hence optimal CT technique in terms of contrast enhancement, collimation, breath hold, and beam current should be employed while scanning the abdomen and pelvis in patients at initial diagnosis and restaging of pancreatic cancer. Ascites is a

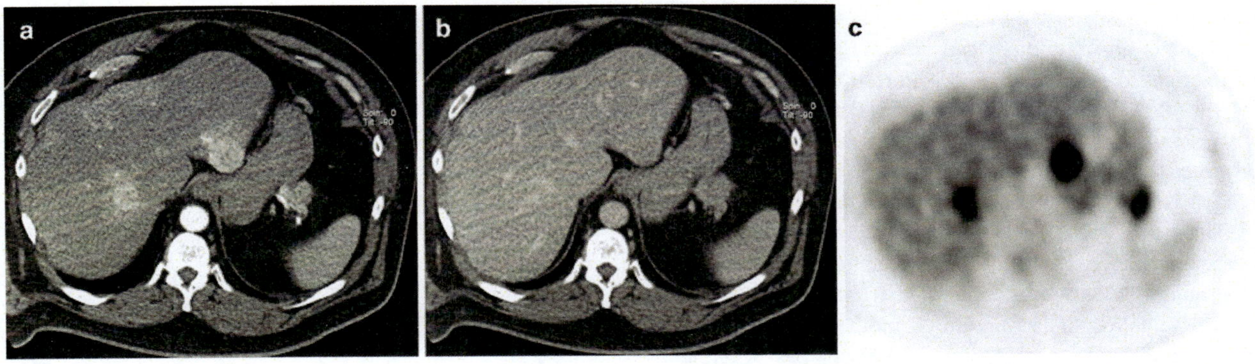

Fig. 31.6 Islet cell pancreatic cancer with liver metastases. Transaxial CT in late arterial phase (**a**) and portal venous phase (**b**) of contrast enhancement and FDG PET images (**c**) reveal a 12-mm enhancing mass in the tail of the pancreas that is intensely FDG avid. Two large hepatic metastases are demonstrated on the FDG PET images and seen as hypervascular masses on the arterial phase CT images, but are isointense on the portal venous phase CT images

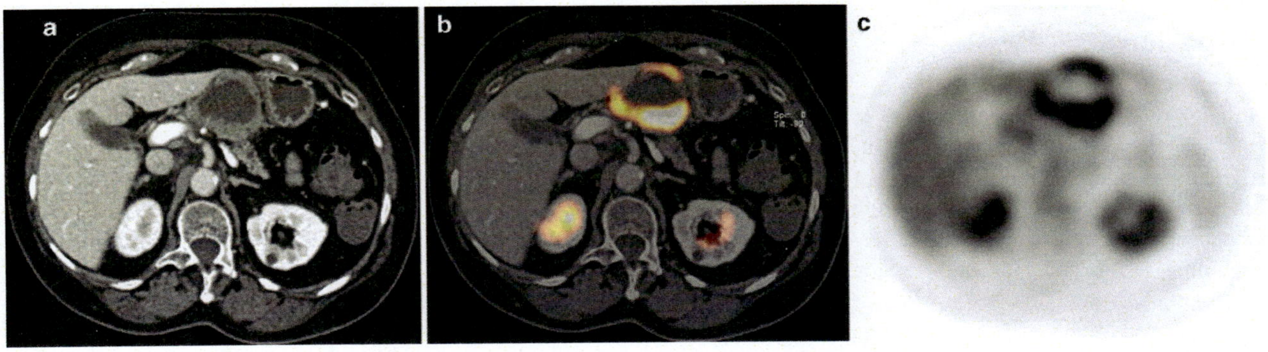

Fig. 31.7 Cystic pancreatic mass. Transaxial CT (**a**) and FDG PET (**b**) and PET-CT fusion (**c**) images reveal a large cystic mass in the pancreas that is associated with abnormal FDG tracer uptake at portions of the thicken rim. The imaging findings of an inflammatory cystic mass or malignant cystic pancreatic neoplasm can be indistinguishable

potentially important finding on the CT images as this may reflect presence of occult peritoneal metastases.

A thorough description of the relationship of the mass to adjacent vascular structures and organs should be included in the PET-CT report. The extent of abutment vs. encasement of vessels with soft tissue, and presence of any venous thrombosis should be described, as different degrees and extent of venous tumor involvement can render a patient non-resectable. The location of all enlarged or FDG avid lymph nodes should be noted as metastatic involvement of lymph nodes which would be resected as part of the contemplated procedure would not preclude resection. The absence or presence, and the degree of, biliary ductal and pancreatic ductal dilatation should be noted. FDG tracer uptake can occur in an obstructed biliary tract or in the setting of cholangitis, and should not be mistaken for hepatic metastases or a pancreatic head tumor.

On restaging PET-CT examinations, it is also important to recognize that there is increased FDG tracer uptake associated with pancreatitis, and focal acute mass forming pancreatitis can potentially yield false positive findings for a pancreatic neoplasm on the FDG PET images. In addition, phlegmatous masses can be very FDG avid, even after clinical and laboratory signs of pancreatitis have resolved [46]. As noted above, cystic masses in the pancreas can be difficult to correctly classify, as benign vs. malignant, in part due to the overlap of abnormal FDG uptake due to neoplasm versus inflammation (Fig. 31.7). Hence, careful attention must be made to any morphologic features of pancreatic inflammatory disease depicted on the CT images of a PET-CT examination when evaluating a cystic pancreatic mass, as well as corroborative clinical history, and clinical and laboratory findings relevant to present or past pancreatic inflammatory disease.

Role of PET-CT in Post Treatment Monitoring

There have been no large studies to date evaluating the potential utility of FDG PET or PET-CT to predict or assess response to chemotherapy and/or radiation. Two studies using small cohorts (n = 10,15) have supported the use of FDG PET in evaluating the effectiveness of chemoradiotherapy [26, 38].

It has also been supported by several studies that SUV uptake values of the primary tumor can be correlated to predicting effectiveness for chemotherapy in unresectable cases; however, specific value ranges have not been defined [19, 26, 34–38]. A small study has suggested that a negative FDG PET study after chemoradiation in a patient who had a positive pretherapy scan may be a good prognostic indicator [35]. In general, since no effective therapy currently exists for treating unresectable pancreatic cancer, and the anticipated survival of unresectable patients is measured in months, there is little practical value in monitoring the chemotherapy or chemoradiation therapy of adenocarcinoma of the pancreas. Treatment regimens utilizing preoperative adjunctive chemotherapy or chemoradiation therapy, on the other hand, if developed, would be potential settings for PET-CT therapy monitoring.

Conclusion

Although there are currently a paucity of studies comparing the efficacy of PET-CT with CT and FDG PET alone, results from current studies are promising and PET-CT is likely to play a significant role in the evaluation and management of patients with pancreatic carcinoma. Its major benefit is in combining the benefits of both anatomic and functional imaging into a single imaging session.

References

1. Jemal A, Siegel R, Ward E, et al. Cancer statistics, 2008. CA Cancer J Clin 2008;58:71–96.
2. Rosewicz S, Wiedenmann B. Pancreatic carcinoma. Lancet 1997;349:485–489.
3. Li D, Xie K, Wolff R, Abbruzzese JL. Pancreatic cancer. Lancet 2004;363:1049–1057.
4. Pakzad F, Groves AM, Ell PJ. The role of positron emission tomography in the management of pancreatic cancer. Semin Nucl Med 2006;36:248–256.
5. Yeo CJ, Cameron JL, Lillemoe KD, et al. Pancreaticoduodenectomy for cancer of the head of the pancreas. 201 patients. Ann Surg 1995;221:721–731; discussion 31–33.
6. Neoptolemos JP, Stocken DD, Friess H, et al. A randomized trial of chemoradiotherapy and chemotherapy after resection of pancreatic cancer. NEJM 2004;350:1200–1210.
7. Diehl SJ, Lehmann KJ, Sadick M, Lachmann R, Georgi M. Pancreatic cancer: value of dual-phase helical CT in assessing resectability. Radiology 1998;206:373–378.
8. Lu DS, Reber HA, Krasny RM, Kadell BM, Sayre J. Local staging of pancreatic cancer: criteria for unresectability of major vessels as revealed by pancreatic-phase, thin-section helical CT. AJR Am J Roentgenol 1997;168:1439–1443.
9. Farma JM, Santillan AA, Melis M, et al. PET-CT fusion scan enhances CT staging in patients with pancreatic neoplasms. Ann Surg Oncol 2008;15:2465–2471.
10. Imdahl A, Nitzsche E, Krautmann F, et al. Evaluation of positron emission tomography with 2-[18F]fluoro-2-deoxy-D-glucose for the differentiation of chronic pancreatitis and pancreatic cancer. Br J Surg 1999;86:194–199.
11. Keogan MT, Tyler D, Clark L, et al. Diagnosis of pancreatic carcinoma: role of FDG PET. AJR Am J Roentgenol 1998;171: 1565–1570.
12. Zimny M, Bares R, Fass J, et al. Fluorine-18 fluorodeoxyglucose positron emission tomography in the differential diagnosis of pancreatic carcinoma: a report of 106 cases. Eur J Nucl Med 1997;24: 678–682.
13. Zimny M, Buell U. 18FDG-positron emission tomography in pancreatic cancer. Ann Oncol 1999;10(Suppl 4):28–32.
14. Schick V, Franzius C, Beyna T, et al. Diagnostic impact of (18) F-FDG PET-CT evaluating solid pancreatic lesions versus endosonography, endoscopic retrograde cholangio-pancreatography with intraductal ultrasonography and abdominal ultrasound. Eur J Nucl Med Mol Imaging 2008;35(10):1775–1785.
15. Inokuma T, Tamaki N, Torizuka T, et al. Evaluation of pancreatic tumors with positron emission tomography and F-18 fluorodeoxyglucose: comparison with CT and US. Radiology 1995;195:345–352.
16. Koyama K, Okamura T, Kawabe J, et al. Diagnostic usefulness of FDG PET for pancreatic mass lesions. Ann Nucl Med 2001;15: 217–224.
17. Lytras D, Connor S, Bosonnet L, et al. Positron emission tomography does not add to computed tomography for the diagnosis and staging of pancreatic cancer. Dig Surg 2005;22:55–61; discussion 62.
18. Sendler A, Avril N, Helmberger H, et al. Preoperative evaluation of pancreatic masses with positron emission tomography using 18F-fluorodeoxyglucose: diagnostic limitations. World J Surg 2000; 24:1121–1129.
19. WakabayashiH,NishiyamaY,OtaniT,etal.Roleof18F-fluorodeoxyglucose positron emission tomography imaging in surgery for pancreatic cancer. World J Gastroenterol 2008;14:64–69.
20. Heinrich S, Goerres GW, Schafer M, et al. Positron emission tomography/computed tomography influences on the management of resectable pancreatic cancer and its cost-effectiveness. Ann Surg 2005;242:235–243.
21. Saif MW, Cornfeld D, Modarresifar H, Ojha B. 18F-FDG positron emission tomography CT (FDG PET-CT) in the management of pancreatic cancer: initial experience in 12 patients. J Gastrointest Liver Dis 2008;17:173–178.
22. Bares R, Klever P, Hauptmann S, et al. F-18 fluorodeoxyglucose PET in vivo evaluation of pancreatic glucose metabolism for detection of pancreatic cancer. Radiology 1994;192:79–86.
23. Ho CL, Dehdashti F, Griffeth LK, Buse PE, Balfe DM, Siegel BA. FDG-PET evaluation of indeterminate pancreatic masses. J Comput Assist Tomogr 1996;20:363–369.
24. Mertz HR, Sechopoulos P, Delbeke D, Leach SD. EUS, PET, and CT scanning for evaluation of pancreatic adenocarcinoma. Gastrointest Endosc 2000;52:367–371.
25. Stollfuss JC, Glatting G, Friess H, Kocher F, Berger HG, Reske SN. 2-(fluorine-18)-fluoro-2-deoxy-D-glucose PET in detection of pancreatic cancer: value of quantitative image interpretation. Radiology 1995;195:339–344.
26. Bang S, Chung HW, Park SW, et al. The clinical usefulness of 18-fluorodeoxyglucose positron emission tomography in the differential diagnosis, staging, and response evaluation after concurrent chemoradiotherapy for pancreatic cancer. J Clin Gastroenterol 2006;40:923–929.
27. Ozaki Y, Oguchi K, Hamano H, et al. Differentiation of autoimmune pancreatitis from suspected pancreatic cancer by fluorine-18 fluorodeoxyglucose positron emission tomography. J Gastroenterol 2008;43:144–151.

28. van Kouwen MC, Jansen JB, van Goor H, de Castro S, Oyen WJ, Drenth JP. FDG-PET is able to detect pancreatic carcinoma in chronic pancreatitis. Eur J Nucl Med Mol Imaging 2005;32:399–404.
29. Pelosi E, Pennone M, Deandreis D, Douroukas A, Mancini M, Bisi G. Role of whole body positron emission tomography/computed tomography scan with 18F-fluorodeoxyglucose in patients with biopsy proven tumor metastases from unknown primary site. Q J Nucl Med Mol Imaging 2006;50:15–22.
30. Tann M, Sandrasegaran K, Jennings SG, Skandarajah A, McHenry L, Schmidt CM. Positron-emission tomography and computed tomography of cystic pancreatic masses. Clin Radiol 2007;62: 745–751.
31. Sperti C, Pasquali C, Decet G, Chierichetti F, Liessi G, Pedrazzoli S. F-18-fluorodeoxyglucose positron emission tomography in differentiating malignant from benign pancreatic cysts: a prospective study. J Gastrointest Surg 2005;9:22–28; discussion 68–69.
32. Mansour JC, Schwartz L, Pandit-Taskar N, et al. The utility of F-18 fluorodeoxyglucose whole body PET imaging for determining malignancy in cystic lesions of the pancreas. J Gastrointest Surg 2006;10:1354–1360.
33. Sperti C, Bissoli S, Pasquali C, et al. 18-fluorodeoxyglucose positron emission tomography enhances computed tomography diagnosis of malignant intraductal papillary mucinous neoplasms of the pancreas. Ann Surg 2007;246:932–937; discussion 937–939.
34. Maemura K, Takao S, Shinchi H, et al. Role of positron emission tomography in decisions on treatment strategies for pancreatic cancer. J Hepatobiliary Pancreat Surg 2006;13:435–441.
35. Maisey NR, Webb A, Flux GD, et al. FDG-PET in the prediction of survival of patients with cancer of the pancreas: a pilot study. Br J Cancer 2000;83:287–293.
36. Nakata B, Nishimura S, Ishikawa T, et al. Prognostic predictive value of 18F-fluorodeoxyglucose positron emission tomography for patients with pancreatic cancer. Int J Oncol 2001;19:53–58.
37. Sperti C, Pasquali C, Chierichetti F, Ferronato A, Decet G, Pedrazzoli S. 18-Fluorodeoxyglucose positron emission tomography in predicting survival of patients with pancreatic carcinoma. J Gastrointest Surg 2003;7:953–959; discussion 959–960.
38. Yoshioka M, Sato T, Furuya T, et al. Role of positron emission tomography with 2-deoxy-2-[18F]fluoro-D-glucose in evaluating the effects of arterial infusion chemotherapy and radiotherapy on pancreatic cancer. J Gastroenterol 2004;39:50–55.
39. Gress FG, Hawes RH, Savides TJ, et al. Role of EUS in the preoperative staging of pancreatic cancer: a large single-center experience. Gastrointest Endosc 1999;50:786–791.
40. Lemke AJ, Niehues SM, Hosten N, et al. Retrospective digital image fusion of multidetector CT and 18F-FDG PET: clinical value in pancreatic lesions – a prospective study with 104 patients. J Nucl Med 2004;45:1279–1286.
41. Nishiyama Y, Yamamoto Y, Yokoe K, et al. Contribution of whole body FDG-PET to the detection of distant metastasis in pancreatic cancer. Ann Nucl Med 2005;19:491–497.
42. Franke C, Klapdor R, Meyerhoff K, Schauman M. 18-FDG positron emission tomography of the pancreas: diagnostic benefit in the follow-up of pancreatic carcinoma. Anticancer Res 1999;19:2437–2442.
43. Frohlich A, Diederichs CG, Staib L, Vogel J, Beger HG, Reske SN. Detection of liver metastases from pancreatic cancer using FDG PET. J Nucl Med 1999;40:250–255.
44. Strobel K, Heinrich S, Bhure U, et al. Contrast-enhanced 18F-FDG PET-CT: 1-stop-shop imaging for assessing the resectability of pancreatic cancer. J Nucl Med 2008;49(9):1408–1413.
45. Ruf J, Lopez Hanninen E, Oettle H, et al. Detection of recurrent pancreatic cancer: comparison of FDG-PET with CT/MRI. Pancreatology 2005;5:266–272.
46. Shreve PD. Focal fluorine-18 fluorodeoxyglucose accumulation in inflammatory pancreatic disease. Eur J Nucl Med 1998;25:259–264.

Further Reading

1. Federle MP, Anne, V.S. Pancreatic ductal carcinoma. In: Federle MP (ed.). Diagnostic Imaging: Abdomen. Salt Lake City: Amirsys, 2004:II-3–50.
2. Kalra MK, Maher MM, Mueller PR, Saini S. State-of-the-art imaging of pancreatic neoplasm. Br J Radiol 2003;76:857–865.
3. Kim YH, Saini S, Sahani D, Hahn PF, Mueller PR, Auh YH. Imaging diagnosis of cystic pancreatic lesions: pseudocyst versus nonpseudocyst. RadioGraphics 2005;25:671–685.
4. Sahani DV, Kadavigere R, Saokar, A, Castillo CF, Brugge WR, Hahn PF. Cystic pancreatic lesions: a simple imaging-based classification system for guiding management. RadioGraphics 2005;25: 1471–1485.

Chapter 32
PET-CT of Bone Metastases

James A. Scott and Edwin L. Palmer

From the seventeenth century perspective of Randle Holme, the skeleton of man was the "emblem of mortality." A physician of today might wryly concur, perhaps adding some functions less well known to Mr. Holme. The human skeleton does, in fact, serve several nonemblematic functions. As a primary calcium storage site, it facilitates calcium homeostasis and provides the necessary calcium for physiologic processes in a balance controlled by a closely regulated hormonal system. It provides scaffolding for the muscular activity associated with locomotive functions, houses the bone marrow, and protects the central nervous system. Bone is continually being remodeled to store or free calcium and to optimize its structure in response to changes in mechanical loading. All of these tasks are disrupted by metastatic disease.

Bone is subdivided into cortical and cancellous regions. The former constitutes the dense bone that surrounds a central honeycomb of thin interweaving plates that compose cancellous bone, within which resides the bone marrow. In the adult, about four fifths of the total bone mass is cortical, and this remodels at about one tenth the rate of cancellous bone. The normal adult turns over 10% of their total bone mass per year. This normal bone remodeling is a coordinated process in which the bone resorptive, or osteoclastic function, lasts about 2–4 weeks, followed by a brief transition phase, after which bone formation takes place over the ensuing 4 months.

Metastatic disease derails much of this useful activity [1–3]. The process of bone resorption, intrinsically faster than that of bone formation, favors osteolytic metastases. Most bone metastases spread by the hematogenous route. Particularly important in this regard is Batson's paravertebral plexus, where the absence of valves permits retrograde tumor dissemination, and also metastasis to the proximal long bones through anastomotic veins. Bone metastases prefer regions with high blood flow, such as the red marrow, their progression stimulated by growth factors released and activated during bone resorption. However, metastasis to specific areas of the skeleton is not determined simply by the geography of blood flow with respect to the primary tumor site. Direct invasion of bone by adjacent tumor and invasion from adjacent lymph nodes, particularly in the spine, also causes bone metastasis. Unlike hematogenous dissemination, these forms are usually associated with a soft tissue mass.

The process of metastasis involves a sequence of steps that determine the final point of lodgement of the tumor cells in bone. Initially tumor cells must detach from the primary tumor site and enter tumor capillaries to reach the general circulation. This initial step involves the attachment to, and proteolytic disruption of the basement membrane, followed by migration of the tumor cells through this membrane into the blood stream. After vascular dissemination to bone, the tumor cells adhere to marrow endothelial cells before passing through fenestrations in this layer to reach the bone marrow. Research suggests that the tumor then releases factors that stimulate osteoclasts while ensuing resorptive processes release factors that further promote the growth of the metastases. In this manner, the normally tightly controlled interaction of osteoblasts and osteoclasts is disrupted, leading to uncontrolled osteolysis. Interestingly, the therapeutic application of bisphosphonates not only inhibits osteoclastic resorption, but also exerts pro-apoptotic and anti-proliferative effects on tumor cells. These latter effects of bisphosphonates, unexpected and potentially important clinically, are the target of extensive research.

Bone metastasis is a critical issue in cancer patients, as more than 2 out of 3 patients who die from cancer have bone metastases. Complications of bone metastasis include pain, spinal cord compression, pathologic fracture, and hypercalcemia, the latter being the most rapidly fatal complication. Most common in breast, prostate, and renal cancers, bone metastases occur with lower but still sizeable frequencies in other tumor types. In breast carcinoma, bone is the most frequent site of recurrence following resection of the primary tumor and is associated with a median life expectancy of less than 2 years. Treatment of bone metastases is largely palliative, consisting of radiation, pain medication, and the

J.A. Scott (✉)
Department of Radiology, Massachusetts General Hospital, 55 Fruit St, Boston, MA, 02114, USA
e-mail: scott@helix.mgh.harvard.edu

P. Shreve and D.W. Townsend (eds.), *Clinical PET-CT in Radiology: Integrated Imaging in Oncology*, DOI 10.1007/978-0-387-48902-5_32, © Springer Science+Business Media, LLC 2011

use of antiresorptive agents of the diphosphonate class. The presence of bone metastasis is also critical to the clinical management of tumors. In lung cancer, for instance, the high cost of surgery together with its associated morbidity and the limited life expectancy in the presence of bone metastasis requires an accurate staging process to limit needless iatrogenic morbidity.

The traditional workup for bone metastasis relies upon the radionuclide bone scan employing technetium labeled diphosphonates. The advent of positron-labeled radiopharmaceuticals, however, portends a change in this tradition. Although this evolution is still in its early stages, we can expect significant changes in how bone metastases are identified and monitored during treatment.

Radiographic Evaluation

Traditional

Bone metastases have traditionally been separated into osteoblastic and osteolytic types based upon the relative proportion of bone formation and destruction. In both types of metastasis it is the osteoblasts and osteoclasts rather than the actual tumor cells (excepting in the case of bone forming tumors) that cause the bone formation or destruction associated with the metastatic deposit. Despite this binary terminology, metastases show a continuum of appearances on radiographs, ranging from the pure osteolytic lesions of multiple myeloma to the dense sclerotic lesions of prostate cancer metastases. With the prototypic exception of myeloma, most osteolytic lesions tend to produce a reactive response in normal adjacent bone. Classic osteolytic tumor types include thyroid, lung, and renal, while tumor types associated with varying degrees of sclerosis include prostate, breast, various endocrine tumors, and carcinoid.

Radiologic techniques get mixed reviews in the evaluation of metastatic disease involving bone [4, 5]. Plain film radiographs require that approximately half the bone mineral content be lost before an osteolytic lesion in the vertebra becomes visible on a standard radiograph of the spine. This accounts for a sensitivity of 50% or less, depending upon tumor type, for detection of bone metastases using the standard radiograph. The conventional radiograph is also poorly suited to monitor treatment because of the slow rate of change in radiographic density during therapy and the inherent difficulties in even relative quantification of the image appearance. CT performs better than the plain film, with sensitivities ranging from 70% to 100% in detecting bone metastases. CT shows early tumor deposits within the bone marrow by an increase in attenuation values due to replacement of marrow fat by tumor cells. Intrinsically limited by the relatively small area imaged and by the observational subtlety of findings limited to the marrow, CT is more remediably hampered by the underutilization of bone windows by most radiologists. Compared with CT, MRI offers superior imaging of the bone marrow and marrow-based abnormalities and poorer depiction of the bone cortex. Metastases appear as areas of diminished signal intensity on T1-weighted images (owing to the high content of fat in bone marrow) and as foci of increased signal on T2-weighted images because of their high water content. The adjunctive use of gadolinium additionally permits differentiation of viable tumor tissue from necrotic tissue. Reported sensitivities of MRI for osseous metastatic disease are in the 80–90% range, superior to bone scanning, particularly for detecting metastases in the spine. MRI has been most often used as a focused examination rather than as a general skeletal screening tool, although its application to the appendicular skeleton may widen with the advent of faster pulse sequences.

The radionuclide bone scan has been the traditional workhorse for the diagnosis of bone metastasis. It displays the entire skeleton in an easy-to-interpret format with generally high sensitivity for metastases. The labeled diphosphonates used in bone scanning accumulate at sites of osteoblastic activity and thus reflect the intensity of this process throughout the skeleton. As normal physiology requires osteoblastic activity, the mere presence of increased tracer uptake is not necessarily pathologic. Uptake can also be prominent in benign lesions and is not always present in malignant abnormalities. Thus the specificity of the bone scan is reduced by the fact that common arthritic changes, trauma, infection, and benign tumors can have an appearance similar to metastases. For example, the bone scan effectively identifies osteoblastic tumors, such as prostate carcinoma metastases, but may fail to distinguish these from intense degenerative uptake often seen in the spine and pelvis, the usual sites of initial tumor dissemination. Although the location or pattern of this uptake may help to distinguish benign from malignant abnormalities, this method is hardly infallible.

False positive scans can also be observed in the setting of serial studies showing the "flare" phenomenon. This term describes a pattern of increasing tracer uptake in known lesions, with the occasional appearance of new foci, resulting from a reparative osteoblastic response of preexisting metastases to treatment. Usually seen during the early stage of treatment, this pattern is easily confused with the progression of disease and usually requires clinical correlation to assist in the distinction.

With the exception of bone-forming tumors such as osteosarcoma, it is reactive bone rather than the metastatic tissue that takes up the radiotracer. This is why purely osteolytic tumors (myeloma) and very rapidly growing metastases (renal, thyroid) that show little reactive bone formation may show a falsely normal appearance or present as subtle "cold lesions." Thus, despite the many successes of the bone scan, its failures in aggressive osteolytic lesions, marrow-based tumors, subcentimeter lesions, and in foci located in poorly resolved areas such as the anterior spine, have led many oncologists to look for alternatives.

PET

The clinical advent of positron imaging makes possible the labeling of a number of agents that may be suitable for bone imaging. The primary agents for this application are ^{18}F fluoride and ^{18}F fluorodeoxyglucose (FDG). Both of these tracers permit tomographic imaging of the whole body at a higher image resolution than can be achieved with standard ^{99m}Tc-MDP bone scanning or SPECT. Of the two agents, ^{18}F fluoride is the more similar to the standard single photon bone agents in clinical use, imaging the osteoblastic response to tumor tissue. ^{18}F FDG, on the other hand, measures tumor metabolic activity itself. These differing tracer characteristics create differing clinical applications for the two agents.

^{18}F Fluoride and ^{18}F FDG – Mechanisms

^{18}F fluoride was first reported in 1962 and, now, a generation later, is making its unfeigned clinical debut. Fluoride has a mechanism of uptake similar to single-photon bone agents whereby it exchanges with hydroxyl groups in the hydroxyapatite crystals to form fluoroapatite. Fluoride produces higher bone to soft tissue contrast at 1 h after injection than does MDP and, by virtue of positron imaging technology, has better resolution than do conventional single photon bone scans. The inherent tomographic nature of ^{18}F fluoride images is a potential advantage in imaging the spine, a difficult site to evaluate with planar scans. Fluoride also permits quantitative assessment of uptake, potentially useful in evaluating bone metastases, assessing healing in bone grafts, and monitoring antiresorptive therapy in focal bone disorders such as Paget's disease.

Fluoride PET has been compared to both standard bone scanning as well as SPECT to determine their relative efficacy in identifying bone metastases [6]. In a testimonial to the adage that "you get what you pay for," planar single photon imaging is both the least sensitive and the least expensive method. SPECT was intermediate in both performance and expense while ^{18}F PET was the high-ticket diagnostic winner (Fig. 32.1).

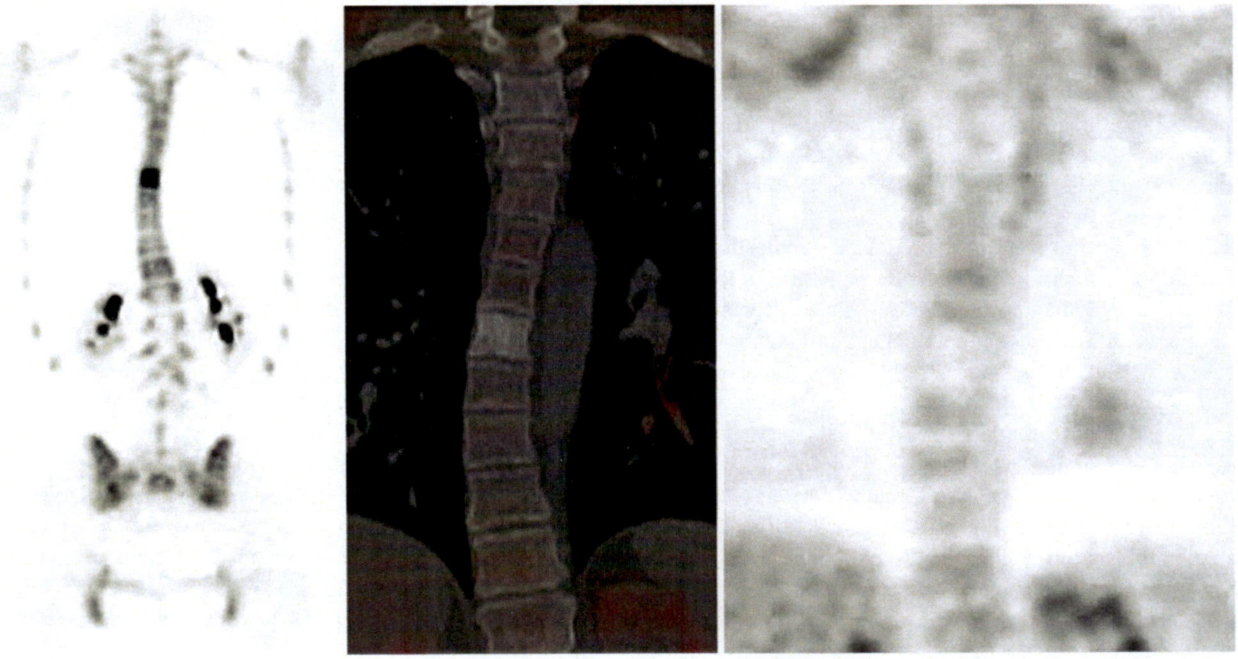

Fig. 32.1 27 year old woman breast cancer after chemotherapeutic treatment of T7 metastasis. Fluoride ion PET (*left*) shows markedly increased uptake at the T7 vertebral body. CT scan (*middle*) shows sclerosis at T7 while FDG PET (*right*) shows a photopenic area indicating the absence of metabolic activity in the non-viable metastatic deposit

^{18}F labeled deoxyglucose (FDG) localizes in tissues by a different mechanism than does ^{18}F fluoride. The uptake of FDG is proportional to the metabolic rate for glucose rather than the level of osteoblastic activity. The two agents can be expected to show differing image appearances depending upon the relative metabolic and osteoblastic characteristics of the lesion in question. This difference becomes important in clinical practice. For example, FDG does not appear as sensitive as either MDP or fluoride in the detection of the osseous metastatic lesions in prostate cancer. Conversely, FDG is more sensitive than is ^{18}F fluoride for the detection of marrow-based abnormalities.

^{18}F Fluoride and ^{18}F FDG – Applications

We will discuss FDG imaging of bone in three respects: its use in studying cortical versus intramedullary metastases, its ability to differentiate malignant versus benign processes, and its role in monitoring the treatment of bone metastases. The additional anatomic information provided by PET-CT will be considered in the context of these two agents as they compare with stand-alone PET and with other imaging methods.

Location of the Metastasis Within Bone

Most authors have found that FDG better detects metastasis in soft tissue than in bone. This difference partially results from variations in target to background activity between bone and soft tissue. Areas of higher background metabolic activity, such as active bone marrow, require higher tumor metabolic rates to achieve the requisite diagnostic contrast. Within bone, sclerotic metastases usually have a lower level of FDG uptake than do lytic lesions. This difference results from several factors, including the less cellular nature of blastic metastases, an intrinsically lower glycolytic rate in blastic lesions, and the outstripping of blood supply in aggressive lytic lesions that creates relative tissue hypoxia and thus increased FDG uptake.

The relative utility of fluoride ion or MDP (the two are similar pharmacologically) and FDG will differ depending on the location of the metastasis within bone and the discordance between tumor metabolic activity and the local reactive osteoblastic response to the tumor. It is important to note that the local osteoblastic response does not correlate well with the degree of malignancy either before or after treatment. A significant shortcoming of traditional bone scanning agents in following the treatment of bone metastases is the persistence of tracer uptake after the local tumor has been eradicated. Since ongoing bone remodeling takes place both in response to continued bone destruction by the tumor and as a reparative response to successful treatment, the interpretation of such uptake during the course of treatment may be difficult. This distinction is most difficult in the short-term, when the scan has the most potential to usefully call attention to a failing treatment. Given the shorter time course of changes in tumor viability compared to those of accompanying reactive osseous changes, one would predict that FDG would more rapidly evaluate treatment response in metastases, at least in those with higher glycolytic rates. Metastases known to be metabolically inactive may be better studied with MDP or fluoride than with FDG (although serial scans will likely be required).

With this framework in mind, let's look at the data regarding imaging of bone metastases from various tumor types. Lymphoma is prototypic of tumors primarily involving the bone marrow. Single photon imaging has proven unreliable in evaluating lymphomatous bone disease because of the relative lack of osteoblastic response to marrow-based lesions. FDG, on the other hand, reflects the metabolic activity of the tumor itself rather than that of reactive osteoblasts, and appears superior to standard bone scanning [7], particularly in more aggressive types of lymphoma (Fig. 32.2). FDG is not invariably useful, however, as low grade lymphomas may show uptakes that are indistinguishable from normal. It is likely that MRI will remain the procedure of choice in imaging known low-grade lymphomas. Higher-grade lesions should prove suitable for FDG imaging, both for initial staging and treatment follow-up.

Daldrup-Link et al., reporting in children, showed that FDG PET had a higher sensitivity for metastatic disease to bone marrow than did either whole body MRI or standard bone scanning [8]. This study included a wide variety of tumor types with a spectrum of metabolic activity, underscoring the impressiveness of the results. Again, one might expect less impressive results in low-grade tumors.

A potential difficulty in interpreting post-treatment FDG images of marrow metastases is the occurrence of benign myeloid hyperplasia (Fig. 32.3). This hyperplastic response appears as diffusely increased marrow activity and can mimic the appearance of lymphomatous involvement. Although correlation with the clinical setting will usually help to distinguish between these two possibilities, differentiation based upon image findings alone can be difficult or impossible. Of some assistance is the pattern of abnormal uptake. If the uptake is diffuse and homogeneous, the process is most likely reactive. On the other hand, focal involvement strongly suggests tumor. Although the intensity of FDG uptake is often lower with marrow hyperplasia than with lymphomatous involvement, this distinction is not reliable in clinical practice, particularly if the original tumor was low grade.

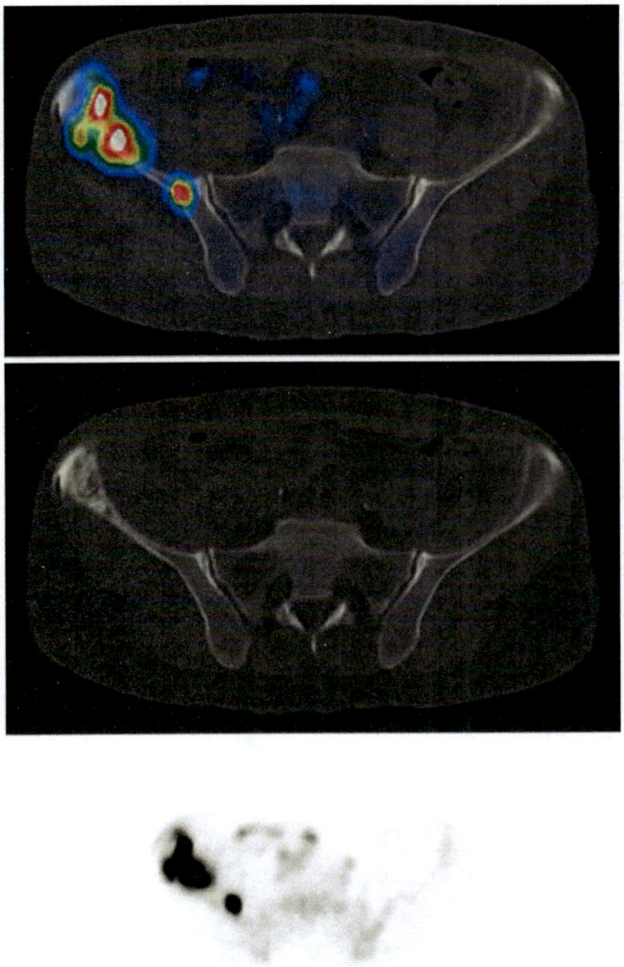

Fig. 32.2 PET-CT overlay (*top*), CT (*middle*), and FDG-PET (*bottom*) images in a 59 year old male with lymphoma involving bone. Note the mixed lytic and sclerotic abnormalities on CT. The smaller focus near the sacroiliac joint is more evident on the FDG images than it is on the bone-windowed CT

Several authors have examined the use of FDG PET in the identification of bone metastases from solid tumors. Most work has been performed with regard to the more common tumors metastasizing to bone, particularly breast, lung, and prostate.

The sensitivity of FDG-PET is equal or superior to the bone scan in identifying metastases from breast cancer (see Fig. 32.1). Differing results reported between studies likely result from patient selection. If the study population consists of patients with lesions in areas where the bone scan is insensitive (for example, bone marrow or anterior vertebral bodies), the tomographic FDG study will show relatively higher sensitivity. FDG has clearly better specificity than does the bone scan [9], particularly in the setting of PET-CT, but even stand-alone PET shows this superiority. The improvement in specificity results from the inability of the standard bone scan to distinguish benign abnormalities (such as arthritic change) from tumor foci, and its inability to distinguish persistent viable tumor foci from ongoing reparative osteoblastic activity.

In non-small cell lung cancer (NSCLC), the bone scan shows similar or slightly better sensitivity than FDG imaging [10] (Fig. 32.4). The difference between the relative sensitivity of FDG and of MDP in breast cancer and NSCLC results from proportionately higher cortical involvement with NSCLC metastasis. For the same reasons that hold for breast cancer metastases, the bone scan has a significantly lower specificity than does FDG imaging in NSCLC. Certainly PET-CT is best able to demonstrate the anatomic cause of increased uptake. Although the advent of FDG imaging has led some oncologists to entirely abandon the bone scan in NSCLC, this is probably ill-advised [11]. Many bone metastases are asymptomatic at presentation. A solitary asymptomatic metastasis in an extremity might not be included on PET images, resulting in potentially unnecessary surgery. Unless the whole body, including the extremities, is imaged in the FDG study, this should not be regarded as a replacement for the standard bone scan in the staging process.

Tumors such as renal cell and thyroid carcinoma may be difficult to detect on the standard bone scan. These tumor types are often associated with little osteoblastic reaction, leading either to a falsely negative scan or to "cold areas" that can be relatively difficult to identify. A relatively recent study by Schirrmeister and colleagues found that more than half of bone metastases from thyroid primaries showed little or no activity on ^{18}F fluoride scans and all appeared lytic on CT [12]. The combination of bone scanning and ^{131}I-whole body scanning, however, identified all of the metastatic lesions. With renal [13] and thyroid primaries, FDG shows clearly improved sensitivity compared to bone scanning, as it images the tumor itself rather than the minimal associated osteoblastic reaction. As with NSCLC, although PET identifies more metastases on a lesion-by-lesion basis, the entire skeleton, including the extremities, must be imaged on the FDG study to provide a better clinical result than that obtained with the standard bone scan.

The role of PET in prostate carcinoma has not yet been determined. Despite initial discouraging results in the evaluation of prostate bone metastases [14], FDG has some theoretical advantages over traditional imaging methods. Although prostate metastases are primarily osteoblastic, FDG can identify an early bone marrow phase of disease that precedes visibility on standard bone scan or ^{18}F fluoride images. Furthermore, FDG might be able to identify a positive response to the treatment before changes become apparent on the standard bone scan. The bone scan may require

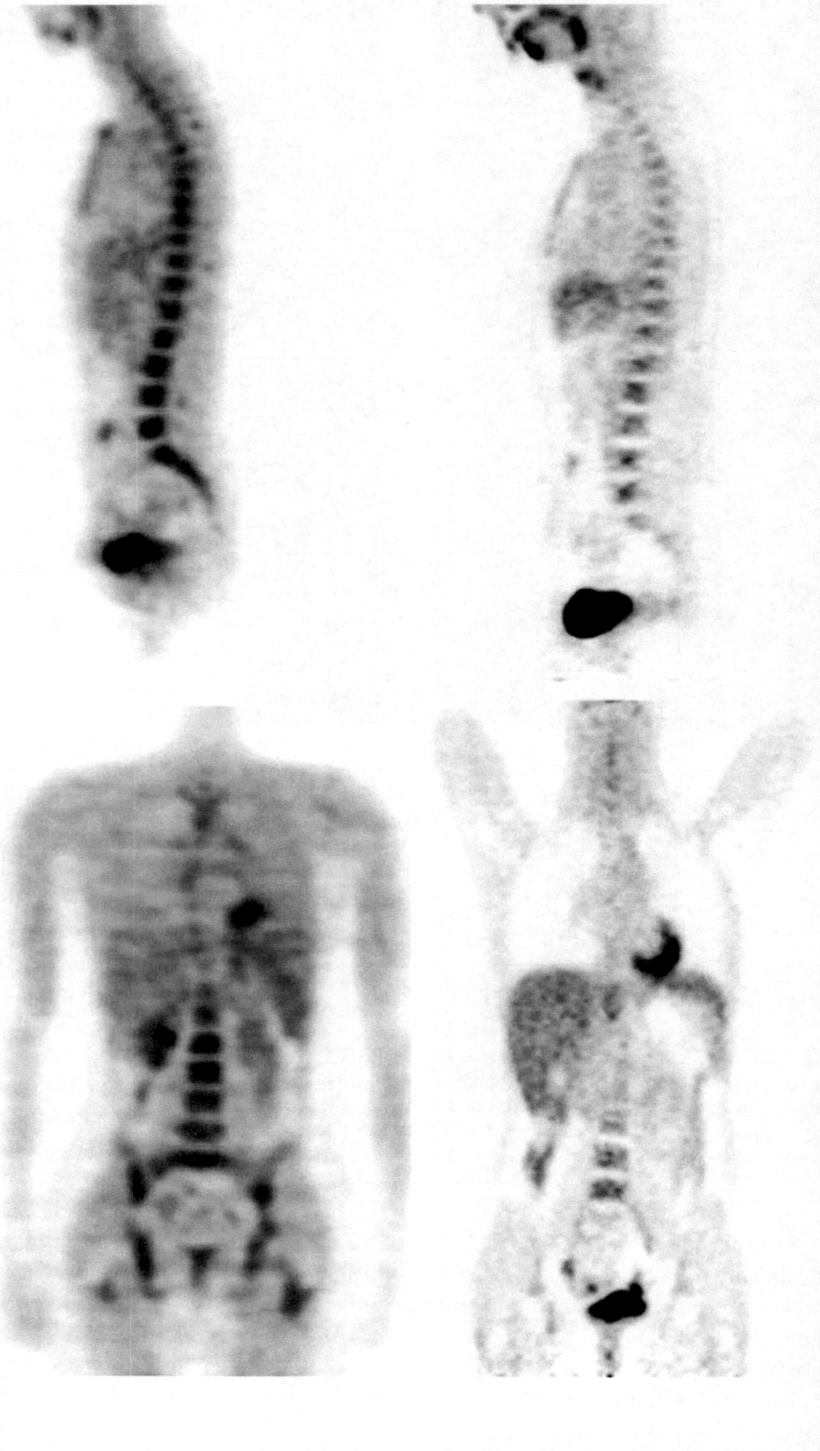

Fig. 32.3 A 39 year old woman with breast carcinoma shows diffusely increased bone marrow uptake on FDG-PET after treatment including marrow-stimulating factors (*left two images*) with a return to a normal appearance on a scan obtained 8 months later (*right two images*)

several months, and sometimes over 2 years, for complete resolution of abnormal findings after successful treatment. It is likely that FDG would be less susceptible to false positives related to the "flare" phenomena, in which pseudo-progression of disease results from a reparative osteoblastic response to successful treatment. On the other hand, FDG is less sensitive than are standard diphosphonates or ^{18}F fluoride in detecting osteoblastic metastases, despite a higher specificity [13]. Critically important to scan interpretation is the observation that commonly used anti-hormonal therapies, although limiting disease progression, usually do not actually kill the viable tumor cells at metastatic foci. These treatments appear

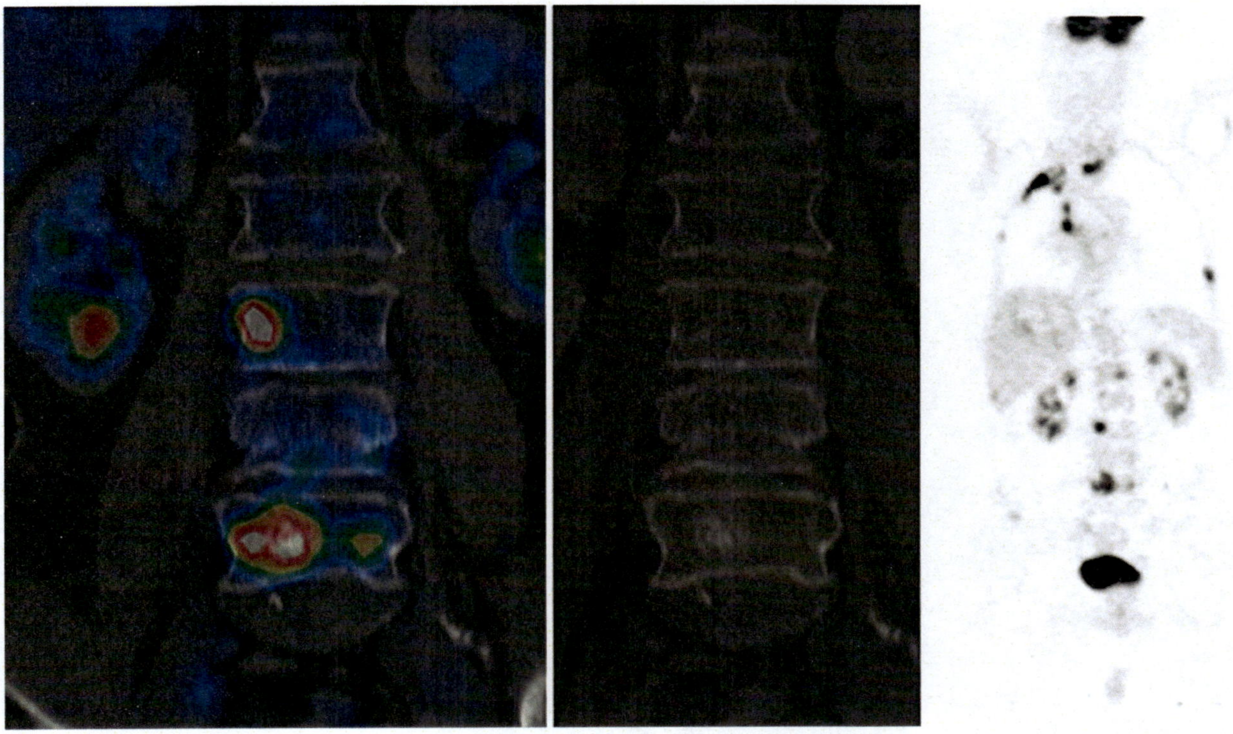

Fig. 32.4 PET-CT overlay (left), CT (*middle*) and FDG-PET (*right*) images in a 72 year old male with NSCLC. FDG abnormalities are evident in the ribs bilaterally as well as in multiple cervical, thoracic, and lumbar vertebral bodies. Mixed lytic and sclerotic foci are evident in the L3 and L5 vertebrae, showing intensely increased uptake on the FDG images

to cause cell cycle arrest rather than apoptosis. Thus absent FDG uptake at metastatic sites during hormonal therapy is consistent with quiescent but still viable tumor and it is most correct to conclude that FDG can distinguish active osseous metastatic foci from quiescent disease [15]. Given these uncertainties together with the lack of reliable outcome measurements in metastatic prostate carcinoma, the ultimate clinical role of FDG remains in question.

FDG is superior to normal radiographs in the evaluation of plasmacytoma/multiple myeloma, showing greater extent of disease than standard radiographs in over 60% of patients [16]. This results from a better ability of FDG to detect smaller metastatic foci, particularly in the setting of osteoporosis. The bone scan is insensitive in detecting myelomatous deposits, which show a notable absence of osteoblastic activity. The fluoride scan faces a similar limitation.

Differentiation of Benign and Malignant Bone Processes on PET-CT Imaging

Both benign and malignant processes can cause either diffuse or focal abnormalities of FDG uptake. The clinical history and the CT component of the PET-CT study assist in this distinction. Diffuse osseous abnormalities are of most concern in malignant processes that involve the bone marrow, such as lymphoma, for which this appearance is typical. These must be distinguished from benign abnormalities with a similar appearance. Colony stimulating factors (CSFs), including hematopoietic growth factors, granulocyte-macrophage colony stimulating factors and erythropoietin can all cause diffusely increased FDG uptake that mimics diffuse tumor infiltration of the marrow (see Fig. 32.3). Delaying FDG imaging by a week or more after CSF therapy helps to minimize this potentially confusing appearance. A similar situation may occur after radiation treatment. Rodent experiments suggest that a transient rise of FDG activity follows soon after radiation treatment, with an ensuing reduction of uptake to below baseline levels [17]. Although this transient increase in marrow uptake should conform to the radiation port, correlation with the presence and timing of radiation treatment helps to identify the iatrogenic origin of the finding (Fig. 32.5).

Focal areas of increased FDG uptake can be diagnostically challenging in the spine and sacrum, where osteoporotic compression fractures can mimic or coexist with pathologic fractures of the vertebrae. The standard bone scan

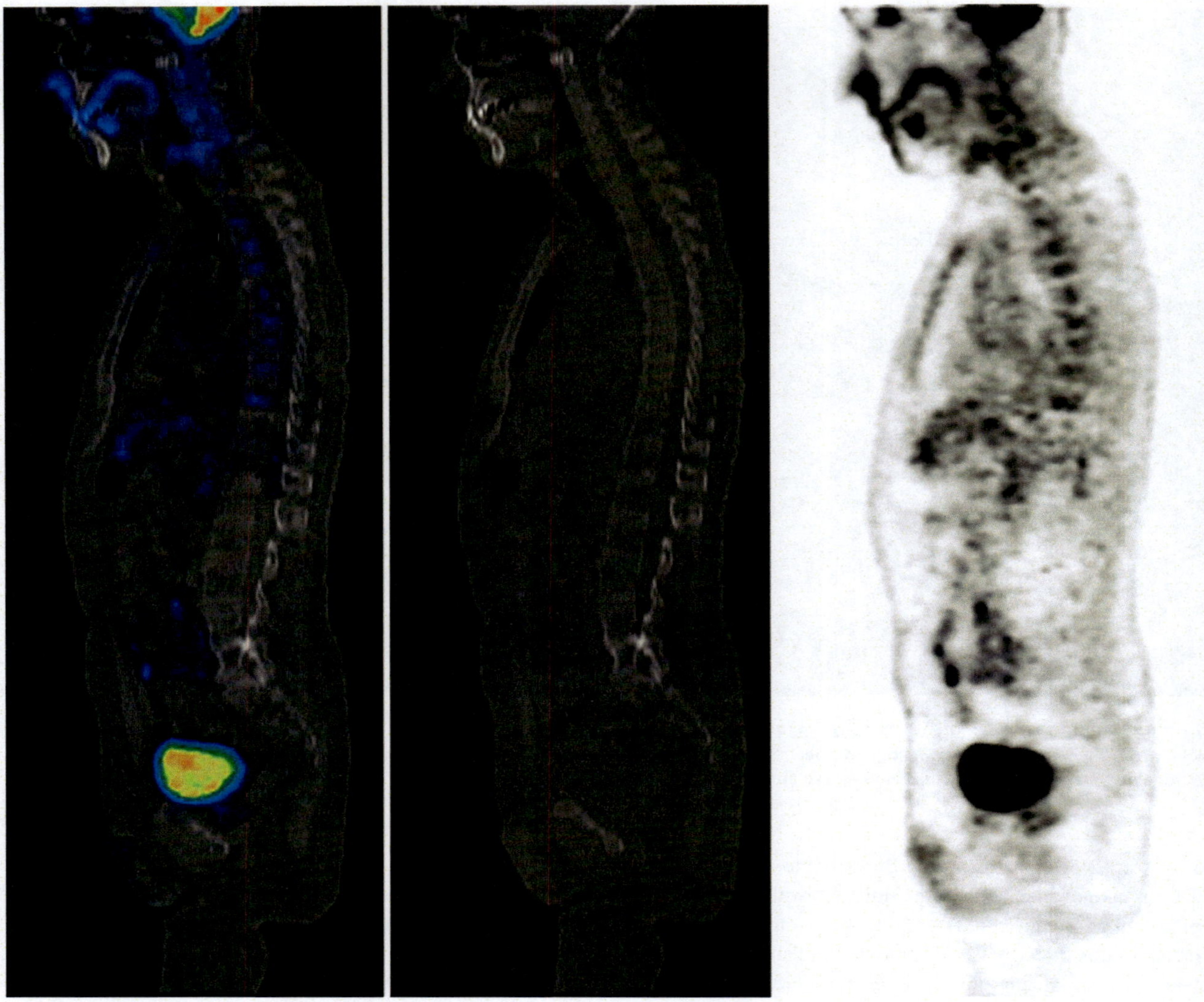

Fig. 32.5 PET-CT images in a 51 year old male with lymphoma show diminished FDG uptake in the lower thoracic and lumbar spine at the site of radiation treatment

has shown little success in making this distinction without the addition of inferential support from foci outside the spine to suggest a metastatic origin. It appears that acute vertebral fractures resulting from osteoporosis show less FDG uptake than do those resulting from malignant or inflammatory processes [18]. Certainly relative FDG uptake may be a useful indicator. Yet despite relative differences in the quantified mean FDG uptake between benign and malignant processes, the variability in each group is too great to permit clinical reliance on quantified SUV values. Substantial overlap between individual members of two statistically distinct populations inevitably limits real-life clinical application to individuals.

Fractures in areas outside the spine can also produce focally increased uptake similar to that usually associated with tumor. FDG abnormalities can precede CT findings, further confounding distinction (Fig. 32.6). As in the spine, benign fractures generally show less FDG uptake than do pathologic fractures [19]. Even so, benign fractures can show increased uptake soon after injury owing to the acute inflammatory reaction, later returning to a normal or near normal appearance several weeks after the acute event [20]. The meaning of increased FDG accumulation in a fracture should be probably be viewed in the context of when the fracture was sustained relative to the imaging procedure. While all fractures will likely show increased FDG accumulation

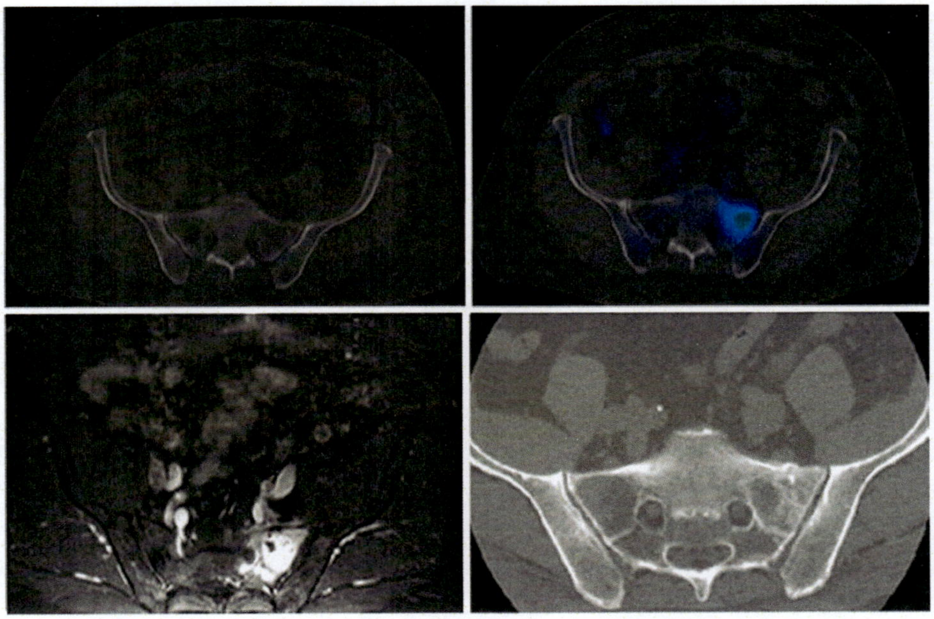

Fig. 32.6 A 64 year old male with sarcoma of the paranasal sinus and insufficiency fracture of the left sacrum. Initial PET-CT (*top left*) shows a normal CT appearance of the sacrum with increased FDG uptake in the left sacrum (*top right*). An MRI performed 1 month later (*bottom left*) shows marrow edema in the left sacrum and a repeat CT performed 3 months after the initial scan (*bottom right*) now shows the insufficiency fracture in the left sacrum

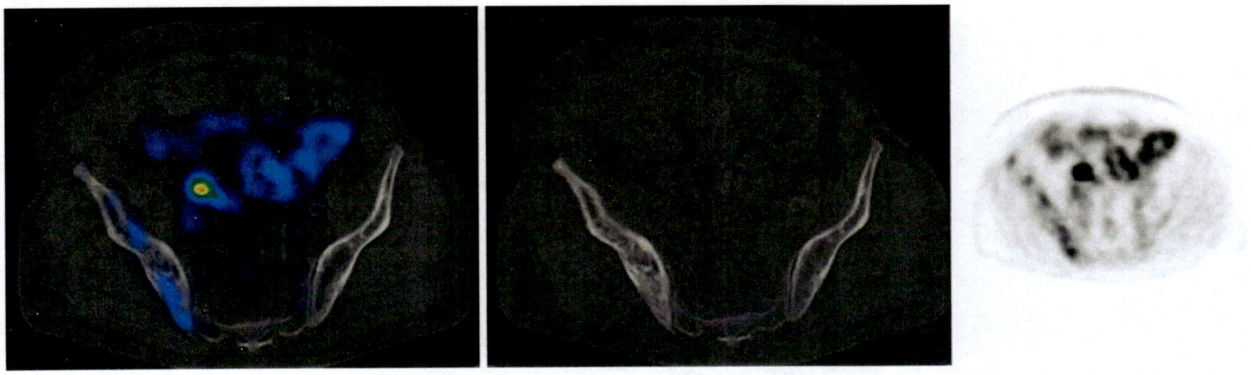

Fig. 32.7 A 73 year old male with melanoma and known Paget's disease involving the right iliac crest. Bone scans and plain films had shown Paget's disease in this area 7 years prior to the PET-CT. This case of Paget's disease is associated with increased FDG uptake

soon after injury, uptake should persist longer in pathologic fractures both because of local metabolic tumor activity and a prolonged healing response. Unfortunately, it is most often in the early stages after injury when diagnosis is needed and it is in this early stage that the imaging distinction is most difficult.

Benign tumors may also show increased uptake simulating malignancy [21]. Paget's disease, although often negative on FDG images, can show increased uptake (Fig. 32.7). Given the metabolic spectrum inhabited by Paget's disease, it isn't surprising that its appearance can vary on FDG studies. Similarly, sarcoidosis involving bone (Fig. 32.8), enchondromas, the pseudofractures of osteomalacia, chondroblastomas, Langerhans cell histiocytosis, and bone infarcts have all been reported to show increased FDG accumulation. There are likely many others. Many of these benign processes show an intensity of uptake indistinguishable from malignant tumors. Even common degenerative changes (because of an associated inflammatory component) can show increased FDG uptake. In view of their frequency, the location of degenerative changes is a fortunate indicator as to their identity (Figs. 32.9, 32.10, and 32.11). Given the poor discriminatory power of lesion intensity, the anatomic information supplied by PET-CT is of significant value in comparison to stand-alone PET imaging.

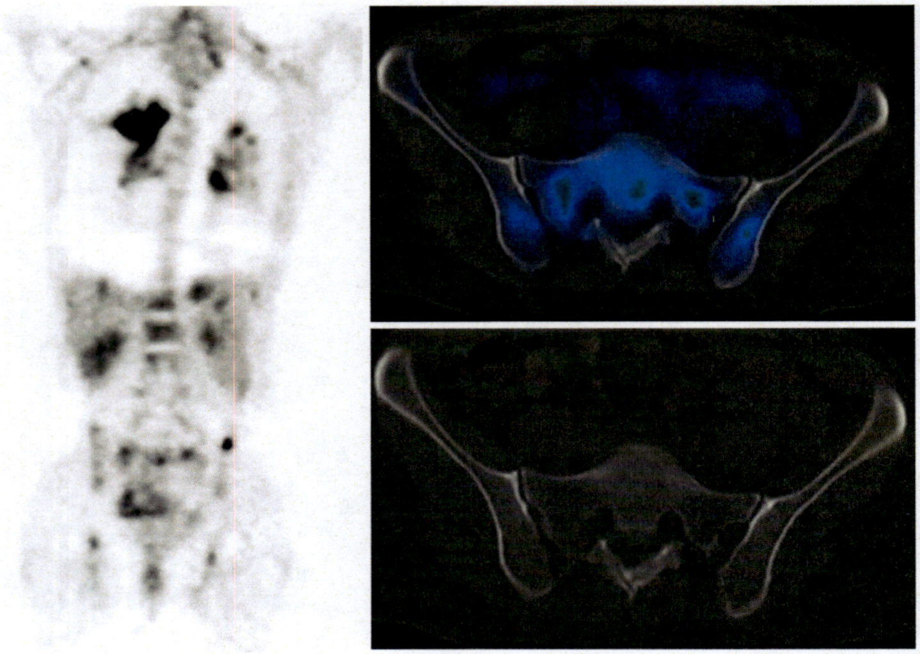

Fig. 32.8 PET-CT scan in a 42 year old woman with sarcoidosis. Abnormal FDG uptake in both iliac wings, sacrum, spine, and bilateral femurs is consistent with known sarcoidosis. Note the relatively unremarkable CT appearance in the areas of the pelvic FDG abnormalities. Other findings in the chest are also related to sarcoidosis

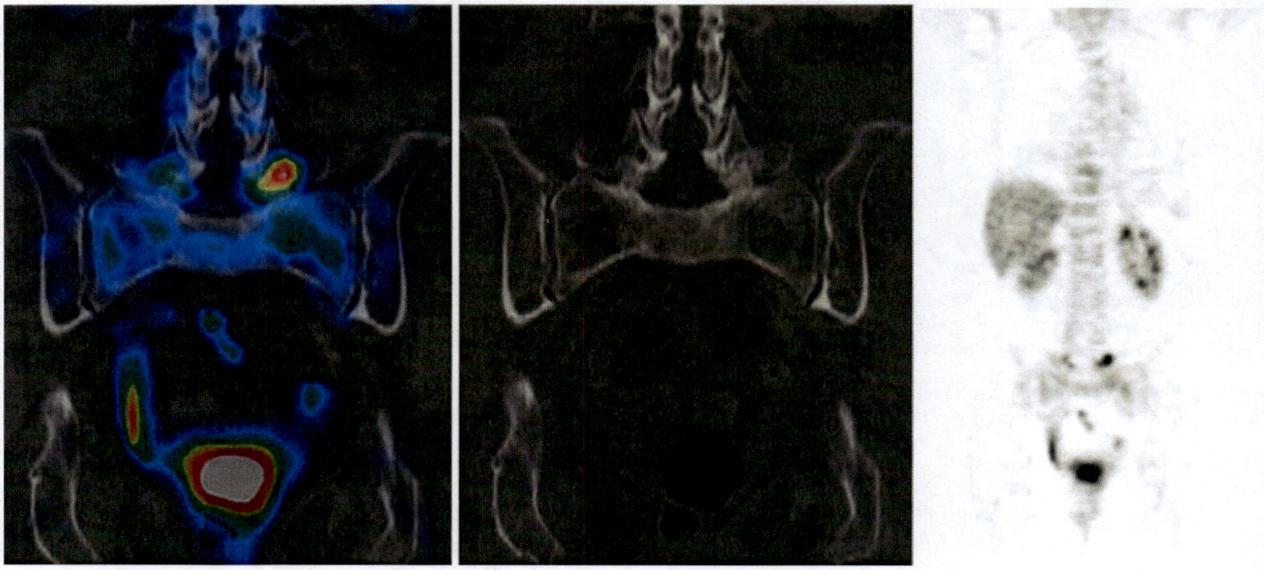

Fig. 32.9 PET-CT in a 65 year old woman with colon carcinoma showing increased FDG activity at (*left* greater than *right*) facet joints of L5 with corresponding osteoarthritic changes on CT. MRI confirmed the absence of metastatic disease

Monitoring Therapy and Quantification

Stafford and colleagues examined the potential of serial FDG PET studies in monitoring the response of bone metastases to therapy in cases of breast carcinoma [22]. The authors found a correlation between the maximum SUV value of the most prominent focus with blood tumor markers, conventional images and subjective symptom changes. This correlation suggests a potential role for FDG in monitoring the therapeutic response of bone metastases. The authors caution, however, that imaging too soon after the institution of therapy could lead to a false positive increase in FDG uptake related to a short-lived metabolic flare response.

The use of SUV in monitoring the response to treatment in bone metastases (and for determining whether individual foci are malignant or benign) is fraught with potential problems [23, 24]. A number of quantitative methods and parameters

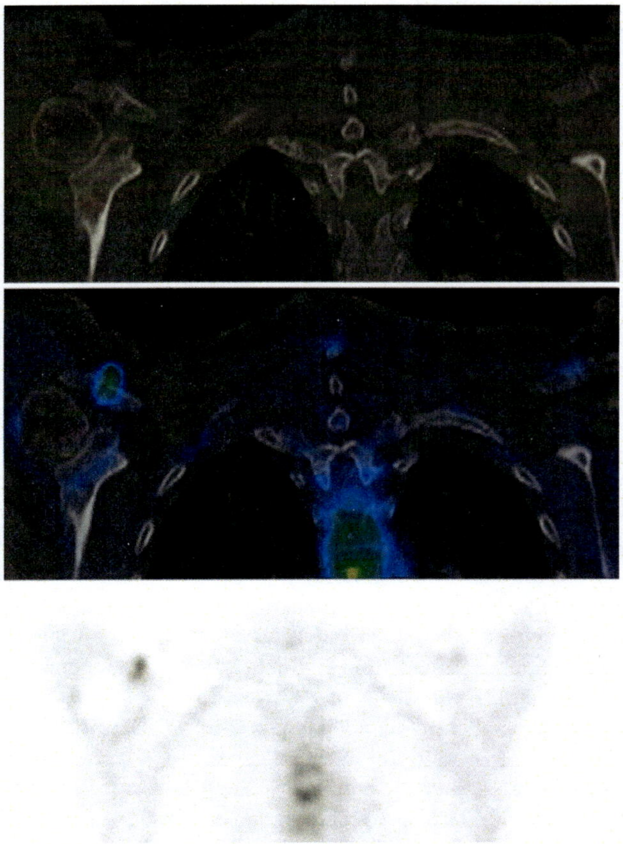

Fig. 32.10 PET-CT images in a 46 year old female with ovarian carcinoma and degenerative change at the right acromioclavicular joint associated with locally increased FDG uptake

have been proposed in this regard. In varying degrees, all these methods trade accuracy for simplicity. Detailed kinetic analysis to determine the tissue deoxyglucose metabolic rate (MRDGlc) is the "gold standard" and provides the most accurate quantitative data. Its calculation requires invasive and cumbersome procedures, placing an often unjustifiable burden on both the patient and physician. Less unwieldy but reasonably accurate approximations to the MRDGlc, such as the Simplified Kinetic Analysis, employ population-based approximations such that a single timed blood sample and a 15 min static image suffice to approximate the MRDGlc [25]. At the extreme "simple" end of this spectrum is the SUV, a beguilingly uncomplicated parameter that can be derived from a single image without the need for blood sampling. Although the SUV correlates with the MRDGlc, it oversimplifies complex physiologic issues, fails to account for temporal changes in the amount of tracer available to the tumor, and unjustifiably assumes that all of the FDG in a given voxel is metabolically important. Poorly standardized times between injection and imaging (difficult in a busy clinical department), imaging too early after injection, and not accounting for differences in blood glucose activity render the SUV insensitive to important changes in the MRDGlc. Enforcing a standardized image acquisition time 3 or more hours after injection (to achieve the mathematically required plateau of tracer blood concentration) solves some of these problems, but such measures may not accord with practical scheduling demands. Until these issues are clearly addressed and standardized, it is best to avoid clinical reliance upon unpredictably inaccurate parameters such as the SUV.

Fig. 32.11 PET-CT images in a 61 year old man with rectal carcinoma. The FDG images show uptake at sites of osteoarthritic change on CT. The bone lesions were not metastatic

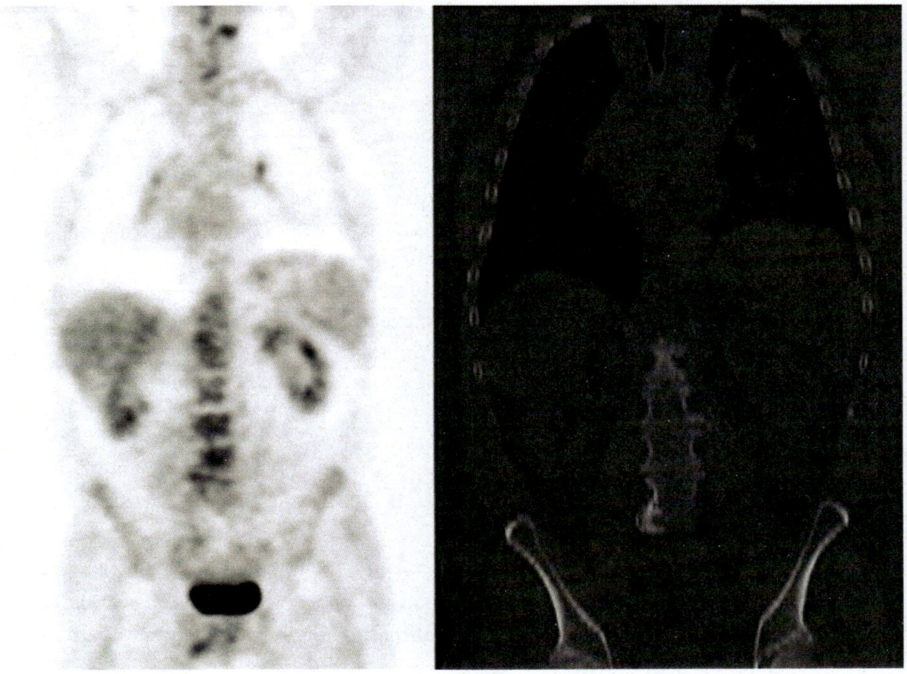

Formal Kinetic Analysis

The physiology of tracer metabolism in bone suggests a potential value for detailed kinetic analysis [26, 27]. Regional clearance of fluoride ion from plasma to bone mineral, Ki, is more than three times higher in regions of bone metastasis than it is in areas of normal bone. This fact might enable kinetic analysis to help differentiate benign from malignant osseous processes. Such analysis requires a dynamic PET study, obtained continuously during the initial 60 min after tracer injection, to define FDG kinetic parameters. This detailed analysis revealed differences in the SUV and in individual kinetic parameters between benign and malignant groups, but again, overlap between the two groups would limit clinical application. After employing additional discriminant analysis of different kinetic parameters (including the fractal dimension of the lesion), the authors were able to achieve a sensitivity of 76% and a specificity of 97%. This work illustrates the potential value of multifactorial analysis to improve upon the ability of any single factor alone to distinguish benign from malignant processes. Such detailed applications are procedurally intensive but worthy of investigation.

Integration of CT Findings

We have noted that correlative CT images improve the diagnostic specificity of the PET scan. Certainly the coexistence of a lytic or sclerotic bone lesion in association with an abnormal area of FDG uptake signals the likelihood of tumor. And as we have seen, a CT abnormality (usually sclerotic) associated with absent or minimal FDG uptake may indicate a low-grade malignancy or a benign process.

The changing appearance of the PET-CT scan during treatment often transmits useful information. A reduction in FDG uptake generally signals a favorable response to therapy. This may be accompanied by increasing sclerosis on the CT images, usually progressing from the periphery of the lesion inward. Occasionally such increasing sclerosis can make a metastasis more visually apparent, falsely suggesting disease progression on the CT images. Similarly the appearance of necrosis in metastatic lesions may incorrectly suggest interval progression. Fortunately FDG uptake will decline in the suspect areas in both of these cases.

PET-CT Compared with Other Imaging Methods

PET appears to be an excellent method to detect skeletal metastatic disease. The additional anatomic information provided by CT increases the specificity of the radionuclide image. How does PET-CT compare to a stand-alone PET scan?

A comparison between fluoride PET and hybrid ^{18}F fluoride PET-CT in diagnosing bone metastases found the hybrid study to be, not surprisingly, superior [28]. The hybrid study had a higher specificity of 97%, as compared to 72% for the PET study alone, as well as better sensitivity than stand-alone PET. Improved sensitivity results from the detection of metastases associated with limited osteoblastic activity. Although the sensitivity and specificity figures should not be overly trusted, being population dependent and lacking a universal and satisfactory gold standard, the superiority of PET-CT to stand-alone PET in terms of specificity seems well established.

Another study by the same group compared PET-CT to stand-alone PET in the evaluation of malignant involvement of the spine, this time using FDG [29]. This study showed superior sensitivity of PET and PET-CT compared to CT alone (98% for PET and PET-CT vs 74% for CT alone). There was no difference in sensitivity between PET and PET-CT. Specificity was significantly improved by PET-CT when compared to either PET or to CT alone. The improvement in specificity largely resulted from the correlation of degenerative changes on CT with areas of increased FDG uptake and by identifying suspected vertebral uptake as muscular artifact.

While CT is useful for attenuation correction and for providing detailed anatomic correlation, some authors have taken the approach of using a second radionuclide agent for anatomic correlation. Hoegerle and colleagues employed ^{18}F-FDG and ^{18}F-fluoride ion at a 3:1 activity radio and imaged 90 min after tracer injection [30]. The incorporation of the lower dose fluoride study permitted superior localization of FDG abnormalities when compared to FDG used alone. The combined method was most useful in distinguishing bone from nonbone localization when soft tissue lesions were located adjacent to the spine and in determining the anatomic level of a soft tissue abnormality, using the skeleton as a reference structure. This method would likely prove less satisfactory than FDG imaging alone were the clinical concern assessment of tumor viability (as FDG and fluoride uptake cannot be distinguished from one another). The FDG-fluoride scan clearly lacks the anatomic resolution of PET-CT, although it shows promise as a screening tool on stand-alone PET studies.

Conclusions

PET-CT is a step forward in the imaging evaluation of osseous metastatic disease. PET imaging alone improves the depiction of bone marrow using ^{18}F-FDG and of bone cortex using ^{18}F-fluoride, as compared with traditional imaging methods, particularly the standard bone scan. The addition of registered CT information on the PET-CT study improves specificity by correlating specific anatomic structures with fluoride or FDG accumulation, and thus establishing a more precise diagnosis. Many benign tracer accumulations, such as those related to osteoarthritic changes and muscle artifact, are readily identifiable on correlative CT images.

It is likely that the primary tracer used for PET-CT studies in the near future will be FDG. We can anticipate that ^{18}F fluoride, given its superiority to standard single photon imaging, will show increasing application, both in stand-alone and PET-CT applications. We can also look forward to the wider application of clinically practical, standardized methods of quantifying FDG uptake in bone metastases, probably using one of the simplifications of the multicompartmental analysis scheme. As these applications evolve, we might bear in mind Thomas Kuhn, "What a man sees depends both upon what he looks at and also upon what his previous visual-conceptual experience has taught him to see."

References

1. Kakonen S-M, Mundy GR. Mechanisms of osteolytic bone metastases in breast carcinoma. Cancer 2003;97:834–839.
2. Roodman GD. Mechanisms of disease: mechanisms of bone metastasis. N Engl J Med 2004;50:1655–1664.
3. Rodan GA. The development and function of the skeleton and bone metastases. Cancer 2003;97:726–732.
4. Hamaoka T, Madewell JE, Podoloff DA, Hortobagyi GN, Uemo NT. Bone imaging in metastatic breast cancer. J Clin Oncol 2004;22:2942–2953.
5. Rybak LD, Rosenthal DI. Radiological imaging for the diagnosis of bone metastases. Q J Nucl Med 2001;45:53–64.
6. Arslandemir HM, Konig HH, Buck AK, Nussle K, Glatting G, Gabelmann A, Hetzel J, Hombach V, Schirrmeister H. F-18 NaF PET for detection of bone metastases in lung cancer: accuracy, cost effectiveness and impact on patient management. J Bone Miner Res 2003;18:2206–2014.
7. Moog F, Kotzerke J, Reske SN. FDG-PET can replace bone scintigraphy in the staging of malignant lymphoma. J Nucl Med 1999;40: 1407–1413.
8. Daldrup-Link HE, Franzius C, Link TM, Laukamp D, Sciuk J, Jürgens H, Schober O, Rummeny EJ. Whole-body MR imaging for detection of bone metastases in children and young adults. Am J Roentgenol 2001;177:229–236.
9. Ohta M, Tokuda Y, Suzuki Y, Kubota M, Makuuchi H, Tajima T, Nasu S, Suzuki Y, Yasuda S, Shohtsu A. Whole body PET for the evaluation of bony metastases in patients with breast cancer: comparison with 99mTc-bone scintigraphy. Nucl Med Commun 2001;22:875–879.
10. Gayed I, Vu T, Johnson M, Macapinlac H, Podoloff D. Comparison of bone and 2-deoxy-2-[18F]fluoro-D-glucose positron emission tomography in the evaluation of bony metastases in lung cancer. Mol Imaging Biol 2003;5:26–31.
11. Schirrmeister H, Arslandemir C, Glatting G, Mayer-Steinacker R, Bommer M, Dreinhofer K, Buck A, Hetzel M. Omission of bone scanning according to staging guidelines leads to futile therapy in non-small cell lung cancer. Eur J Nucl Med Mol Imaging 2004;31: 964–968.
12. Schirrmesiter H, Buck A, Guhlmann A, Reske SN. Anatomical distribution and sclerotic activity of bone metastases from thyroid carcinoma associated with F-18 sodium fluoride positron emission computed tomography. Thyroid 2001;11:677–683.
13. Wu HC, Yen RF, Shen YY, Kao CH, Lin CC, Lee CC. Comparing whole body 18F-2-deoxyglucose positron emission tomography and technetium 99 m methylene diphosphonate bone scan to detect bone metastases in patients with renal cell carcinomas: a preliminary report. J Cancer Res Clin Oncol 2002;128:503–506.
14. Shreve PD, Grossman HB, Gross MD, Wahl RL. Metastatic prostate cancer: initial findings of PET with 2-deoxy-2-[F-18] fluoro-D-glucose. Radiology 1996;199:751–755.
15. Morris MJ, AkhurstT, Osman I, Nunez R, Macapinlac H, Siedlecki K, Verbel D, Schwartz L, Larson SM, Scher HI. Fluorinated deoxyglucose positron emission tomography imaging in progressive metastatic prostate cancer. Urology 2002;59:913–918.
16. Schirrmeister H, Bommer M, Buck AK, Muller S, Messer P, Bunjes D, Dohner H, Bergmann L, Reske SN. Initial results in the assessment of multiple myeloma using 18F-FDG PET. Eur J Nucl Med Mol Imaging 2002; 29:361–366.
17. Higashi T, Fisher SJ, Brown RS, Nakada K,, Walter GL, Wahl RL. Evaluation of the early effect of local radiation on normal rodent bone marrow metabolism using FDG: preclinical PET studies. J Nucl Med 2000;41:2026–2035.
18. Schmitz A, Risse JH, Textor J, Zander D, Biersack HJ, Schmitt O, Palmedo H. FDG-PET findings of vertebral compression fractures in osteoporosis: preliminary results. Osteoporos Int 2002;13:755–761.
19. Kato K, Aoki J, Endo K. Utility of FDG-PET in differential diagnosis of benign and malignant fractures in acute to subacute phase. Ann Nucl Med 2003;17:41–46.
20. Shon IH, Fogelman I. F-18 FDG positron emission tomography and benign fractures. Clin Nucl Med 2003;28:171–175.
21. Aoki J, Watanabe H, Shinozaki T, Takagishi K, Ishijima H, Oya N, Sato N, Inoue T, Endo K. FDG PET of primary benign and malignant bone tumors: standardized uptake value in 52 lesions. Radiology 2001;219:774–777.
22. Stafford SE, Gralow JR, Schubert EK, Rinn KJ, Dunnwald LK, Livingston RB, Manakoff DA. Use of serial FDG PET to measure the response of bone-dominant breast cancer to therapy. Acad Radiol 2002;9:913–921.
23. Thie JA. Understanding the standardized uptake value, its methods, and implications for usage. J Nucl Med 2004;45:1431–1434.
24. Keyes JW Jr. SUV: standard uptake or silly useless value? J Nucl Med 1995;36:1836–1839.
25. Hunter GJ, Hamberg LM, Alpert NM, Choi NC, Fischman AJ. Simplified measurement of deoxyglucose utilization rate. J Nucl Med 1996;37:950–955.
26. Dimitrakopoulou-Strauss A, Strauss LG, Heichel T, Wu H, Burger C, Bernd L, Ewerbeck V. The role of quantitative (18) F-FDG PET studies for the differentiation of malignant and benign bone lesions. J Nucl Med 2002;43:510–518.
27. Cook GJ, Blake GM, Marsden PK, Cronin B, Fogelman I. Quantification of skeletal kinetic indices in Paget's disease using dynamic 18F-fluoride positron emission tomography. J Bone Miner Res 2002;17:854–859.
28. Even-Sapir E, Metser U, Flusser G, Zuriel L, Kollender Y, Lerman H, Lievshitz G, Ron I, Mishani E. Assessment of malignant skeletal disease: initial experience with 18F-fluoride PET-CT and comparison between 18F-fluoride PET and 18F-fluoride PET-CT. J Nucl Med 2004;45:272–278.
29. Metser U, Lerman H, Blank A Lkievshitz G, Bokstein F, Evan-Sapir E. Malignant involvement of the spine: Assessment by ^{18}F-FDG PET-CT. J Nucl Med 2004;45:279–284.
30. Hoegerle S, Juengling F, Otte A, Altehoefer C, Moser EA, Nitzsche EU. Combined FDG and [F-18] fluoride whole body PET: a feasible two-in-one approach to cancer imaging. Radiology 1998;209: 253–258.

Index

P. Shreve and D.W. Townsend (eds.), *Clinical PET-CT in Radiology: Integrated Imaging in Oncology*, DOI 10.1007/978-0-387-48902-5, © Springer Science+Business Media, LLC 2011

F

G

H

I

K

L

M

N

O

P